Veterinary Biostatistics

SECOND EDITION

Veterinary Biostatistics

SECOND EDITION

PV Sreenivasaiah
PhD, FNAVS
Former Professor and Head
Department of Livestock Production Management
Rajiv Gandhi Institute of Veterinary Education and Research
Puducherry 605 009

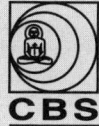

CBS

CBS Publishers & Distributors Pvt Ltd

New Delhi • Bengaluru • Chennai • Kochi • Kolkata • Mumbai
Hyderabad • Nagpur • Patna • Pune • Vijayawada

Veterinary Biostatistics
Second Edition

ISBN: 978-93-86217-70-7

Copyright © Author

Second Edition: 2017
First Edition: 2007

Published by Satish Kumar Jain and produced by Varun Jain for
CBS Publishers & Distributors Pvt Ltd
4819/XI Prahlad Street, 24 Ansari Road, Daryaganj, New Delhi 110 002, India.
Ph: 23289259, 23266861, 23266867   Website: www.cbspd.com
Fax: 011-23243014   e-mail: delhi@cbspd.com; cbspubs@airtelmail.in.
Corporate Office: 204 FIE, Industrial Area, Patparganj, Delhi 110 092
Ph: 4934 4934   Fax: 4934 4935   e-mail: publishing@cbspd.com; publicity@cbspd.com

Branches

- **Bengaluru:** Seema House 2975, 17th Cross, K.R. Road,
  Banasankari 2nd Stage, Bengaluru 560 070, Karnataka
  Ph: +91-80-26771678/79   Fax: +91-80-26771680   e-mail: bangalore@cbspd.com
- **Chennai:** 7, Subbaraya Street, Shenoy Nagar, Chennai 600 030, Tamil Nadu
  Ph: +91-44-26680620, 26681266   Fax: +91-44-42032115   e-mail: chennai@cbspd.com
- **Kochi:** Ashana House, No. 39/1904, AM Thomas Road, Valanjambalam,
  Ernakulam 682 016, Kochi, Kerala
  Ph: +91-484-4059061-65   Fax: +91-484-4059065   e-mail: kochi@cbspd.com
- **Kolkata:** 6/B, Ground Floor, Rameswar Shaw Road, Kolkata-700 014, West Bengal
  Ph: +91-33-22891126, 22891127, 22891128   e-mail: kolkata@cbspd.com
- **Mumbai:** 83-C, Dr E Moses Road, Worli, Mumbai-400018, Maharashtra
  Ph: +91-22-24902340/41   Fax: +91-22-24902342   e-mail: mumbai@cbspd.com

Representatives

- **Hyderabad** 0-9885175004   • **Nagpur**   0-9021734563   • **Patna**   0-9334159340
- **Pune**   0-9623451994   • **Vijayawada** 0-9000660880

Printed at: Rashtriya Printers, Dilshad Garden, Delhi, India

Preface to the Second Edition

It is indeed a pleasure to note that the first edition of *Veterinary Biostatistics* has received overwhelming response by the readers, which has prompted publication of the second edition.

This edition also aims to help researchers understand the very basis of the analytical procedure, decide "when" and "how" to apply statistical tools while processing animal science data, and to overcome difficulties in interpreting the results obtained in relation to the aim of the experiment. Ultimately, it is necessary that an animal science worker should not only be able to understand the statistical treatment but also "feel" the data and the results.

As in the first edition, technical terms are used with no explanation(s) assuming that an animal scientist does not need them. Proofs for formulae are not discussed primarily because it is not mandatory that an animal scientist should know them but not due to their nonavailability; many books dedicated to mathematical statistics elaborately deal with those details. All steps in calculations are shown only in those cases where the calculations are likely to be complicated for an animal scientist, otherwise final results are given. Exercises are not included mainly to reduce the bulk of the book and also because, for each of the tests, an example is discussed with calculations.

Many of the readers did feel that if statistical applications which mandate the use of computers are also included, it would definitely add a new dimension to the book. This was particularly true with those dealing with animal breeding, marketing of products, extension workers and the like. All opinions have been well received.

It is true that computer application has become a part and parcel of statistical analyses even for those which were earlier carried out by scientific calculators. Further, each of the computer software comes with its own tutorial and complete description of the product. Therefore, procedure for the use of computer software has not been included in this book.

Notwithstanding the above, it is mandatory that concepts of such analyses need to be provided so that the research workers can select a suitable method of analysis. In addition, it is equally important to outline interpretation of the results given by the computer. Basis of test statistics and its significance are extremely important in arriving at logical conclusions.

In view of the above, a chapter entitled "Multivariate Analysis" is added providing primarily the underlying concepts and interpretation of the computer output. Actual method of statistical analysis is not detailed because of many reasons. Firstly, such an analysis involves mathematical techniques which require knowledge of matrix algebra, differentiation, etc. Secondly, such calculations are not possible manually, even by use of scientific calculator and hence, even if such details are not included, the reader will be able not only to plan and conduct investigation but also to comprehend and derive valid conclusions from the research data.

All said and done, it is noteworthy that the 'joy' of analyzing the data manually and interpreting the results thereafter is unique and it need not be 'bartered' for the 'convenience' offered by a computer; except in case of multivariate analysis. It is hoped, most readers would subscribe to this view. Only those statistical tables which are frequently used are given as appendices; others can be accessed in many publications; this is to facilitate location of the tables by the users.

My special thanks are due to my mother (for having opened my "babe" eyes into the field of basic mathematics); guardian Dr SK Susheela Bai, who has been and continues to be my guiding force; teachers of mathematics during my primary and secondary schooling, Mr Krishnaswamy, Mr Guruswamy and Mr Gurusiddappa; teachers during my BVSc program at UAS, Bangalore; Mr Rajender Singh and Mr Singhal during MVSc at IVRI, Izatnagar; and Dr Nageshwara Rao and Dr Eshwar Reddy during PhD at APAU, Hyderabad, who gave me insight into the vast ocean of statistics.

I thank one and all at Rajiv Gandhi Institute of Veterinary Education and Research, Puducherry, who are directly or indirectly helpful in this endeavour; especially to Mr R Ganesan, Associate Professor (Statistics), Department of Animal Genetics and Breeding.

I am thankful to my parents-in-law, brothers-in-law, brothers, sister, wife and children, who, as always, stood by me while preparing this book. My special thanks are due to Mr Satish Kumar Jain and his team of CBS Publishers & Distributors Pvt Ltd for bringing out this edition in an elegant manner.

PV Sreenivasaiah

Preface to the First Edition

It is still ringing in my ears that Dr PV Rao, one of my beloved teachers and Professor and Head (since Retd), Department of Poultry Science, APAU, Hyderabad, when I showed him the First Edition of "Scientific Poultry Production" told "... You are supposed to be good at statistics; but details on Poultry Genetics and Breeding are not included, why?" I couldn't give a reply satisfactory to either of us. In any case, I did make up for that lapse in the second and third editions. More importantly, the conversation seeded a dream in me; why not attempt a book on Statistics for Animal Scientists? That was way back during 1987.

After near two decades of incubation, during publication of third edition of Scientific Poultry Production, I informally put across my dream to the Publisher of Poultry book, Mr Suneel Gomber. He virtually took me by surprise by telling spontaneously that "... For many years now we have no statistics book exclusively for Veterinarians and please give me your book ...". I could not believe what was heard for once. He was so magnanimous, firm on the decision and went on imploring me on the issue every time we spoke, that I had to force him get some of the chapters, at preliminary stage, reviewed by qualified statistician(s) before I venture into such a project. Mr Gomber confirmed that he will publish the book and the reviewer(s), at best, can only suggest modifications; I need not have to wait for review. I can't thank him enough for the enormous confidence he has in me and so willingly giving an opportunity to realize my dream. I trust, God willing, the book will live up to his expectations.

It is absolutely essential to note that there are many books available on statistical theory as well as its applications. However, it is equally true that books dedicated to the requirements of scientists working in the field of "Veterinary and Animal Science" are only a few. It is also argued that when the underlying methodology is same, there is no need of a separate publication for animal science workers. I prefer agree to disagree with that logic.

It is in the fitness of things to note that most of the animal science workers may not have requisite background in mathematics and/or statistical theory to understand the various formulae that are being used during the statistical analysis of data. This poses two problems; the first being the difficulty in understanding the very basis of the analytical procedure and secondly, difficulty in interpreting the results obtained in relation to the aim of the experiment.

That the examples cited in many of the books mostly correspond to the fields other than "Veterinary and Animal Science" further limits the utility of such books to Animal Science workers. The availability of ready-made packages for statistical analysis of data has only worsened the situation because the animal science workers can easily "analyze" their data but interpretation becomes tougher than before. Knowledge of actual analytical procedures enables an Animal Science worker not only to understand the statistical treatment but also to "feel" the data and the results.

In view of the above, it is believed that there exists a latent hope/expectation among the community of animal scientists for a book which can enumerate the various statistical methods, with as little statistical theory as possible and with specific examples from the field of "Animal Science". The latter aspect is believed to make the reader more familiar with what is being read thereby facilitate easy understanding of the contents.

It is obvious therefore, that such a task had better be taken up by an Animal Science worker himself; but is undoubtedly, a tough and challenging task, to tell the least, probably never attempted before by a veterinarian. Hence, this humble attempt to present an animal scientist's thoughts on "when" and "how" to apply statistical tools and draw inference(s) while processing Animal Science data.

Readers while going through this publication, will definitely, and rightly too, feel that too many examples from the field of poultry science are given; I must confess that, having been in the field for nearly three decades, such a bias is totally involuntary and all but expectable. It is also true that examples in my field of specialization are easy to conceive, present and discuss. I hope such an indulgence will be acceptable.

Technical terms are used with no explanation(s) assuming that an animal scientist doesn't need them. Proof for formulae are not discussed primarily because it is not mandatory that an animal scientist should be in the know of them but not due to their non-availability; many books dedicated to mathematical statistics elaborately deal with those details.

All steps in calculations are shown only in those cases where the calculations are likely to be complicated for an animal scientist; otherwise, final result is given. Exercises are not included mainly to reduce the bulk of the book and also because, for each of the tests, an example is discussed with calculations.

The "joy" of analyzing the data manually and interpreting the results thereafter is unique and it need not be "bartered" for the "convenience" offered by a computer; hopefully, most readers would subscribe to this view. To prove the point, all calculations in this book are undertaken on a Scientific Calculator (with "Statistics" mode facility).

Only those statistical tables which are frequently used are given as appendices; others can be accessed in many publications; this is to facilitate location of the tables by the users.

I am sure; this publication will delight both Dr PV Rao and Mr Suneel Gomber equally and immensely.

My special thanks are due to my mother (for having opened my babe eyes into the field of basic mathematics), guardian Dr SK Susheela Bai who has been and continues to be my guiding force, teachers of mathematics during my primary and secondary Schooling who inspired me develop 'Love' towards Mathematics (which has only become more intense over the years) while laying a firm foundation of the subject in me and to Mr Krishnaswamy, who taught a course each on "Differential Calculus" and "Integral Calculus" during B.V.Sc program. I take this opportunity to thank my teachers Mr Guruswamy and Mr Gurusiddappa during BVSc Program at UAS, Bangalore, Mr Rajender Singh and Mr Singhal during MVSc at IVRI, Izatnagar and Dr

Nageshwara Rao and Dr Eshwar Reddy during PhD at APAU, Hyderabad who gave me insights into the vast ocean of statistics and without whose teaching material I wouldn't have dared chase such a dream.

I thank the Dean and one and all at Rajiv Gandhi College of Veterinary and Animal Sciences, Puducherry, who are directly or indirectly helpful in this endeavor; especially Dr N.K. Maity, Professor and Head, Department of Veterinary Pharmacology and Toxicology, Dr A. Bhattacharya, Professor and Head, Department of Veterinary Public Health, Dr S. Venugopal, Assistant Professor, Department of APM, Mr R. Ganesan, Assistant Professor (Statistics), Department of Animal Genetics and Breeding, Dr K. Rajkumar, Assistant Professor, Department of Veterinary Epidemiology and Dr S. Venkatesa Perumal, Assistant Profesor, Department of Veterinary Biochemistry.

I am thankful to my parents-in-law, brothers-in-law, brothers, sister, wife and children who have, as always been, stood by me while preparing this book.

PV Sreenivasaiah
Department of Avian Production and Management
Rajiv Gandhi College of Veterinary and Animal Sciences
Puducherry 605 009

E-mail: prof.pvs@gmail.com
Website: http://www.prof-pvs.i8.com
Puducherry
February 28, 2007

Contents

Symbols and Abbreviations

a/α	Type-I error, intercept, average effect of gene	e	Base of natural log
$\approx$	Approximately equal to	EMCP	Expectation mean cross-products
AM	Arithmetic mean	EMS	Expectation mean square
A^c/B^c	Complement of A/B	E(X)	Expectation of X
ANOVA	Analysis of variance	!	Factorial
ANACOV	Analysis of covariance	f	Frequency
ANR	Average number at risk	F	F statistic/inbreeding co-efficient
AR	Attack rate		
Arcsin	$\sin^{-1}$	GM	Geometric mean
β	Type-II error	$\geq$	Greater than or equal to
β/b	Regression coefficient	h^2	Heritability, in narrow sense
β_1/sk	Coefficient of skewness		
β_2	Coefficient of kurtosis	H_A	Alternate hypothesis
bp	Base pairs	H_0	Null hypothesis
BV	Breeding value	HM	Harmonic mean
cM	Centi-Morgan	HR	Hazard ratio
χ^2	Chi-square	HW Equilibrium	Hardy–Wienberg equi-librium
C–Chart	Control chart		
CI	Cumulative incidence	IBD	Identity by descent
CIR	Cumulative incidence rate	IR	Incidence rate
Cl	Clearance rate	IRR	Incidence rate ratio
CoV	Covariance	ITC	Internal time component
CR	Chain relative, correlated response	∞	Infinity
		$\cap$	Intersection of sets
CRD	Completely randomized design	k	Constant term, assigned variable
C_T	Top-down concordance	κ	Kappa statistic
CV	Coefficient of variation	$\leq$	Less than or equal to
Δ	Small change	LCLM	Lower critical limit-mean
λ	Constant (orthogonal coefficients)	LD_{50}	Lethal dose$_{50}$, median (semi-) lethal dose
d/δ	Deviation, difference, dose-factor	LOD	Logarithm of odds
		LSD	Least significant diffe-rence
$\sim$	Distributed		
DMR	Duncan's multiple range	LR	Link relative

μ	Population mean (normal distribution)	RBD	Randomized block design
m	Mean (poisson variate)	ROC	Receiver–operator characteristic
mu	Map unit	RR	Relative risk
υ	Degrees of freedom	r_e	Environmental correlation
M	Morgan		
MCP	Mean cross-products	r_g	Genetic correlation
MD	Mean deviation	r_I	Intra-class correlation coefficient
MSS	Mean sum of squares		
MSS_E/MSS_e	Mean sum of squares, error	r_p	Phenotypic correlation
		r_s	Spearman's rank r
MSS_e^p	Mean sum of squares, error (pooled)	R^2/r^2	Coefficient of determination or correlation index
MSS_e^w	Mean sum of squares, error (weighted)	ssu	Secondary sample units
		s/σ	Standard deviation
$|\ |$	Modulus	SAR	Secondary attack rate
^nC_r	Combination of n items r at a time	se	Standard error
		s^2/σ^2	Variance
N_e	Effective population size	SCP	Sum of cross products
^nP_r	Permutation of n items r at a time	SD/S	Selection differential
		se	Standard error
NR	Non-recombinants	Σ	Summation
In	Natural logarithm	S_n	Sensitivity
$\neq$	Not equal to	S_p	Specificity
n	Number of observations, sample size, assigned variable	SPC	Statistical process control
		SS	Sum of squares
OR	Odds ratio	θ	Recombination fraction (frequency)
OR_{MH}	Mentel–Haenszel odds ratio	t	Student's t statistic
		$t\frac{1}{2}$	Half-life
ξ	Orthogonal coefficient	T	Kendall's rank r
psu	Primary sample units	$\cup$	Union of sets
p	Probability of success (occurrence)	UCLM	Upper critical limit-mean
		UCLR	Upper critical limit-range
π	Pi, a constant	V(A)	Additive genetic variance
PR	Prevalence ratio	V(D)	Variance due to dominance or dams within sire
PV	Predictive value		
q	Probability of non-occurrence $(1-p)$	V(E)	Environmental variance
		V(EP)	Variance due to epistasis
QD	Quartile deviation	V(P)	Phenotypic variance
Q_i	ith quartile	V(S)	Sire component of variance
QTL	Quantitative trait locus		
ρ/r	Correlation coefficient	VE	Vaccine efficacy
R	Response to selection, repeatability, recombinants	x	Independent variable
		$\bar{x}$ or $\bar{X}$	Mean
R_{XY}	Male'cot's coefficient of parentage	y	Dependent variable
		z	Fisher's z for r
		Z	Normal deviate
R–Chart	Range chart	ZIR	Zoonosis incidence ratio

Introduction

It is generally agreed that, regardless of the field of work, scientific data has to be collected after deciding the statistical treatment the data is likely to be subjected to subsequently and not *vive versa*. The problem(s)/variable(s) for investigation, type of data expected, Statistic(s) to be computed, number of observations needed, accuracy and reliability desired have to be decided before the start of investigation/collection of data so that the statistical inference becomes not only acceptable but also reproducible. This greatly facilitates not only the analysis part but also renders the interpretation most relevant ensuring high reproducibility of the conclusions (Statistical inference) drawn thereon. After all, reliability of conclusion(s) is cardinal for any experiment whether it is in the field of animal science or otherwise.

In simple terms, **design of the experiment, and the analytical procedures should be decided as a prerequisite for collection of the experimental data.**

1. POPULATION *VERSUS* SAMPLE

Population also referred to as **Universe** encompasses all possible measurement concerning the variable in question. It is not possible to obtain determinations on or from each and every subject and hence, a **Sample** is considered from which determinations are obtained and conclusions are drawn in respect of the population.

Since the entire Population can't be included in most of the studies, statistical inference depends primarily on data obtained from samples. This follows that computation of a statistic depends on the type of data, number of variables under study and number of samples involved, etc.

For example, if average milk production of Jersey cattle is the variable in question, it is not possible to get data from all Jersey cattle in the entire World. Therefore, a herd of Jersey cattle available for the scientist serves as a sample from which average milk production of Jersey cattle will be calculated. Hence, Sample is a subset of population.

There are several methods of sampling; but, general assumption the most statistical procedures assume is that a sample is drawn satisfying the following conditions:
1. Each member of the population has an equal and independent chance of being selected
2. Selection of any member does not influence selection of any other member

A sample drawn in the above fashion is referred to as **random sample**. Although assigning each member of a population a unique number and then using random numbers to draw random sample is most ideal, on most occasions, at least in veterinary and animal science studies, it is not feasible.

However, if the variable in question is extremely rare, it is reasonable to consider obtaining all the measurements from the population itself. For instance, study involving seriously endangered species of animals.

2. PARAMETER VERSUS STATISTIC

A population is described by measuring its **parameters** and **statistic** refers to the estimate of population parameter by utilizing a sample; the former is usually denoted by Greek alphabets (like μ, σ, ρ, β, etc.) and the latter by Latin letters.

It is evident from the discussions above that Statistic obtained from different samples of the same population need not be identical; needless to state that the researcher is interested to obtain a Statistic as close to the Parameter as possible from the sample; in other words, the **best** estimate.

2.1. Properties of a Good Estimator

2.1.1. Unbiasedness
Let us consider that it is required to know the average weight at hatch of WL chicks. It will be ideal to have as many chicks as possible because if the number is very small, there is all likelihood that few extreme values will influence the Statistic and renders it far different from the parameter. That means, when the sample size is small, the statistic under-or over-estimates the parameter. On the other hand, if the sample size is large, the differences will be minimized to yield an **unbiased** statistic.

2.1.2. Reliability
If the statistic is close to the parameter, it simply means that the statistic is **precise** in estimating the population value and hence it is **reliable/efficient**.

2.1.3. Consistency
If the sample size is increased, the statistic tends to become closer to the parameter and such a Statistic is referred to as **consistent** statistic.

3. TYPES OF DATA

As far as biological data is concerned, many investigations are quantitative involving numerical facts which fall into the following types:

3.1. Data on Ratio Scale
This type of data includes lengths, weights, volumes, capacities, number of items and lengths of time which are characterized by:
1. A constant size interval between any two adjacent units on the measurement scale
2. There exists a zero point on the measurement scale and there is a physical significance to this zero

3.2. Data on an Interval Scale

Data on interval scale (like temperature scales) are characterized by:

1. A constant size interval between any two adjacent units on the measurement scale
2. There is no true zero

A well known example of this category is that water at $80\,°C$ is twice as hot as that at $40\,°C$. However, same water at $176\,°F$ ($80\,°C$) is not twice as hot as that at $104\,°F$ ($40\,°C$)!!

Similarly, time of the day and time of the year are referred to as **circular scales** which have an arbitrary zero point.

3.3. Data on Ordinal Scale

Ordinal scale data include ranks, grades etc. In fact, data on ratio and interval scale may have to be expressed on ordinal scale when exact measurements are not made. For instance, weight of one animal recorded as "more" or "less" than the other because exact weight on ratio scale is not available. Obviously, quantitative comparisons are impossible. In spite of this fact, several procedures are applicable to ordinal data.

3.4. Data on Nominal Scale

Data on nominal scale, as the name indicates, consist of characters like color, comb shape, wool types, male/female, taxonomic classification etc. which can be classified only on **quality** rather than numerical measurement. Such data are also referred to as **attribute** and statistical methods applicable to ratio, interval and ordinal scales are generally not applicable to this type of data. Methods suitable to attributes are also available; for example, χ^2 test.

3.5. Continuous and Discrete Data

The most commonly encountered types of data; former indicating a variable that could assume any conceivable value within any observed range and the latter only certain values. Ratio-, interval- and ordinal-scale data may be either continuous or discrete whereas, the nominal-scale data is always discrete.

The continuous variables are generally considered to follow normal distribution and the discrete data to follow binomial or poisson or other specifically described distribution. Depending on the number of variables in question, number of samples under consideration, type of data and its underlying distribution along with other conditions actually determine the statistic to be computed for arriving at scientific inference(s).

4.   COMMON NOTATIONS USED

By far the most commonly used notation/symbol is $\sum$ (called "sigma"). It means "adding or summation". It should, at least theoretically or under classical situation,

have a subscript and a superscript thus: $\sum_{i=1}^{n} x_i$ which means, adding of x_i's where the

subscript i takes values from 1 up to n; in other words, $x_1 + x_2 + x_3 + ...x_n$. However, even if such subscripts and superscripts are not indicated, they are assumed depending on the context. In this publication, the classical form is used in Chapters "Central tendency" and "Dispersion" to make the reader familiar with the meaning of the symbol; in subsequent Chapters, they are omitted.

It is also possible that $> 1 \sum$'s are employed (especially in statistical analysis of quantitative genetics data in the field of animal breeding). For example, $\sum_{i=1}^{s} \sum_{j=1}^{d} \sum_{k=1}^{p} x_{ijk}$ which means that x_{ijk} refers to kth observation under jth classification which, in turn, is a classification under ith group; k takes values from 1, 2, 3 ... p, j takes values from 1, 2, 3 ... d and i takes values from 1, 2, 3 ... s. If i refers to sires, j refers to dams and k refers to progenies, the above symbol indicates the summation of all p progenies under each of the d dams under each of the s sires; in simple terms, total of pds observations. It should be noted that understanding the symbol begins from the right-hand side and progresses towards left-hand side. The logic is extendable for all situations.

Note: The other "sigma" denoted by "σ" refers to population standard deviation as indicated above.

2

Central Tendency

If a poultry farmer is asked to tell the average weight of broilers produced, he would give a value; say 2 kg at 6 weeks. It does not mean that all the birds weigh exactly 2 kg but, most weights fall around 2 kg. In other words, weights of broilers tend towards a central value of 2 kg; hence, the term **central tendency**.

Most commonly used measure of central tendency, as in the above case, is **arithmetic mean** or simply **mean** or **average**. The other methods of measuring central tendency include **median, mode,** etc.

1.   ARITHMETIC MEAN (AM)

1.1.   Ungrouped Data

If $x_1, x_2, x_3, x_i \dots x_n$ represent 1st, 2nd, 3rd, ith ….. nth observation, then mean is the ratio of sum of the observations to the number of observations; i.e. $\overline{X} = \dfrac{\sum\limits_{i=1}^{n} x_1}{n}$ or

simply $\overline{X} = \dfrac{\sum x_i}{n}$ where, x_i represents ith observation where i takes value 1, 2, 3 …. n.

1.1.1.   Example

The following are the day old body weight of broiler chicks: 42, 41, 38, 45, 40, 43, 40, 42, 46 and 40 g. The mean of this set of observations is $417 \div 10 = 41.7$ g.

If each of the x_i is repeated f_i times, then $\sum\limits_{i=1}^{n} x_i = \sum\limits_{i=1}^{n} f_i x_i$ and $n = \sum\limits_{i=1}^{n} f_i$; therefore,

$$\overline{X} = \frac{\sum\limits_{i=1}^{n} f_i x_i}{\sum\limits_{i=1}^{n} f_i}$$

1.2. Grouped Data

1.2.1. Without Classes

1.2.1.1. Example

If in the **Example 1.1.1** above, chicks weighing 38, 40, 41, 42, 43, 45 and 46 g are recorded 3, 6, 8, 16, 20, 10 and 2 times, it is obvious that there were $3 + 6 + 8 + 16 + 20 + 10 + 2 = 65$ chicks weighing a total of $(38 \times 3 + 40 \times 6 + 41 \times 8 + 42 \times 16 + 43 \times 20 + 45 \times 10 + 46 \times 2) = 2756$ g. Hence, the mean of this set of observations is $2756 \div 65 = 42.4$ g.

1.2.2. With Classes

When the number of observations is very large, it may be necessary and/or convenient to group the data into **classes** wherein each class represents a small range of values (class width) whose **frequency** can be counted and are presented in the form of a **frequency distribution table**.

1.2.2.1. Example

The following table gives the frequency distribution of weights of Japanese quail eggs.

Egg weight class (g)	Class value (x_i) (g)	No of eggs (frequency, f_i)	$f_i x_i$ (g)
6.0–7.0	6.5	5	32.5
7.0–8.0	7.5	15	112.5
8.0–9.0	8.5	30	255.0
9.0–10.0	9.5	50	475.0
10.0–11.0	10.5	110	1155.0
11.0–12.0	11.5	70	805.0
12.0–13.0	12.5	40	500.0
13.0–14.0	13.5	25	337.5
14.0–15.0	14.5	5	72.5
Total		350	3745.0

Hence, mean $= 3745.0 \div 350 = 10.70$ g.

In a frequency distribution table, the following have to be noted:

1. Class value (class midpoint or class mark) represents all the observations within the intervals (limits) of the class; that means, eggs weighing 6.0 to 6.9 g will be considered to be 6.5 g eggs (7.0 g egg will be counted for the next class) and so on based on the assumption that there is equal number of observations on either side of class value within each class interval. Therefore, smaller the class interval (1.0 g in the above example) more accurate will be the mean determined.

2. The classes are mutually exclusive in the sense that an observation is counted under only one class.

3. If the upper limit of one class the same as the lower limit of the subsequent class (**exclusive class**), then if an observation is equal to the upper limit of any class, it is counted for the immediate next class as seen in the above example. Alternatively, if the upper limit of one class is different from the lower limit of the subsequent class, it is referred to as **inclusive class**.

4. If one of the limits of any class is lacking, it is called as an **open-end class**; obviously, such a class is generally expected as the first or the last class in a frequency distribution.

5. Under special circumstances, to avoid unwieldy frequency distribution, it is also possible to form class intervals of varying width.

It is generally agreed that in a frequency distribution the number of classes and width of the class are determined arbitrarily depending on the nature, type and range in the data obtained. However, if one is particular of a formula for this purpose, considering that there are N number of observations, the number of classes (k) can be obtained by: $k = 1 + 3.322 \log N$; in the above example, it works out to be 9.45 or 9. Obviously, the class width is calculated by (highest value – lowest value) $\div$ k or Range $\div$ number of classes; in the above example, it is $(15.0 - 6.0) \div 9 = 1.0$.

(**Note:** The above formula for calculation of number of classes ensures that there will be at least 4 classes even when there are only 10 observations and only 20 classes when there are 1 m observations.)

With the advent of modern computers, it is possible to enter the above 350 observations individually in less time than that required for setting up the frequency table. Undoubtedly, the mean value so obtained will be more accurate. But, there is a distinct advantage of the frequency distribution table which the direct entry of individual observations can not provide; that is about the way the values are distributed around the mean value. Even without graphical representation of the data, it is possible to visualize the following by a closer inspection of the frequency distribution table:

1. Frequency increases from a lower class value towards the mean value and then again decreases.
2. If plotted on a graph paper, it would give a bell-shaped curve
3. Maximum number of observations are around the mean value

1.1.1.1. Short-cut method

Calculation of mean can be simplified the origin of each of the values/class mark. This would facilitate calculations.

1.1.1.1.1 Without classes

In the **Example 1.2.1.1** above, if 38 g (an arbitrary value, k) are subtracted from each of the values, we get the following:

Original value, g (x_i)	$x_i - k = d_i$	f_i	$f_i (x_i - d) = f_i d_i$
38	0	3	0
40	2	6	12
41	3	8	24
42	4	16	64
43	5	20	100
45	7	10	70
46	8	2	16
Total		65	286

The mean value is obtained by $\overline{X} = k + \dfrac{\sum\limits_{i=1}^{n} f_i d_i}{\sum\limits_{i=1}^{n} f_i} = 38 + \dfrac{286}{65} = 42.4\ \text{g}$

1.2.2.2.2 With classes

In the **Example 1.2.2.1**, if 10.5 g (an arbitrary value, k) are subtracted from each of the class marks representing a class width of w (1.0 g in this example), the resultant table will be as follows:

Egg weight class (g)	Class value (x_i) (g)	$d_i = x_i - k$ (Frequency, f_i)	No of eggs	$f_i d_i$ (g)
6.0–7.0	6.5	−4	5	−20
7.0–8.0	7.5	−3	15	−45
8.0–9.0	8.5	−2	30	−60
9.0–10.0	9.5	−1	50	−50
10.0–11.0	10.5	0	110	0
11.0–12.0	11.5	1	70	70
12.0–13.0	12.5	2	40	80
13.0–14.0	13.5	3	25	75
14.0–15.0	14.5	4	5	20
Total			350	70

The mean value is obtained by the formula

$$\overline{X} = k + w \left(\dfrac{\sum\limits_{i=1}^{n} f_i d_i}{\sum\limits_{i=1}^{n} f_i} \right) = 10.5 + 1.0 \left(\dfrac{70}{350} \right) = 10.7\ \text{g}$$

In both the examples above, it can be noticed that the calculations get simplified to a great deal the change of origin.

Note: Use of frequency distribution (histogram) in feed manufacturing is discussed in Chapter "**Statistics in specific veterinary fields**".

1.1.1. Weighted Arithmetic Mean

Arithmetic mean gives equal importance to each and every observation/class value. However, it is possible that different classes may have differing relative importance (referred to as **weight**).

1.1.2. Pooling of means

If $\overline{X}_i$ are the means of N_i observations ($i = 1, 2, 3, \ldots n$), then pooled mean, $\overline{X}_P = \dfrac{\sum\limits_{i=1}^{n} N_i X_i}{\sum\limits_{i=1}^{n} N_i}$

Note: Care has to be exercised while pooling of means; the means pooled should belong to related groups. For instance, egg weights of chicken and Japanese quails can not be pooled but those of groups of each of those species can be pooled separately.

2. MEDIAN

2.1. Discrete Data

Median refers to the central/middle value in a distribution. In other words, if all the values are arranged in an ascending/descending order (or as per their magnitude), median is that value which will have equal number of observations on its either sides.

Considering n as total number of observations, when n is odd median is the value of $[(n + 1) \div 2]$th observation. When n is even, median is obtained by the average of $[(n \div 2) - \frac{1}{2}]$th and $[(n \div 2) + \frac{1}{2}]$th terms.

2.2. Continuous Data

In case of continuous data, it is not possible to exactly locate the median value because the frequencies lose their individuality due to continuity. Therefore, it is necessary to find out a particular point on the curve which will have half of the frequencies on either side. Hence, median refers to value pertaining to $(n \div 2)^{th}$ frequency and is calculated by the formula:

$$\text{Median } = L_m + w\left(\frac{Z - f_{cum}}{f_m}\right) \text{ or } L_m + (Z - f_{cum})\frac{L_u - L_m}{f_m}$$

where, L_m and L_u are the lower and upper limit of the class which includes $(n \div 2)$th term (median class), f_{cum} is the cumulative frequency of the class preceding the median class, $Z = (n \div 2)$, f_m is the frequency of the median class and w is the width of the median class.

If cumulative frequency is calculated from bottom of the table upwards,

$$\text{Median } = L_m - w\left(\frac{Z - f_{cum}}{f_m}\right) \text{ or } L_m - (Z - f_{cum})\frac{L_u - L_m}{f_m}$$

In the **Example 1.2.2.1**, the calculation of median is shown below:

Egg weight class (g)	Class value (x_i) (g)	No of eggs (Frequency, f_i)	Cumulative frequency (from top)	Cumulative frequency (from bottom)
6.0–7.0	6.5	5	–	350
7.0–8.0	7.5	15	20	345
8.0–9.0	8.5	30	50	330
9.0–10.0	9.5	50	100	300
10.0–11.0	10.5	110	210	250
11.0–12.0	11.5	70	280	140
12.0–13.0	12.5	40	320	70
13.0–14.0	13.5	25	345	30
14.0–15.0	14.5	5	350	–

Median class is the one that contains $(350 \div 2) = 175$th observation and it refers to Class $10.0 - 11.0$ g. Hence, median of the above distribution is: $10.0 + 1.0[(175 - 100) \div 110]$ or $11.0 - 1.0[(175 - 140) \div 110] = 10.68$ g.

(**Note:** if the cumulative frequencies shown in the last two columns of the above table are plotted graphically, value on the x-axis corresponding to the point of intersection refers to median. Such cumulative frequency lines are popularly referred to as **less than** and **more than 0 gives**, respectively.)

2.3. A Special Note on Use of Median

2.3.1. Pharmacology/Toxicology

In therapeutic/toxicological study of drugs/toxins, the concept of median/percentiles is commonly employed. An example shown below will outline the statistical treatment of the data obtained:

2.3.1.1. Example

The following are the results of testing toxicity of varying levels of nicotine on a group of 10 rats for each level. The number of rats dying after the experimental period is tabulated below and we have to find out the lethal dose (LD_{50} or **semi-lethal dose** or **median lethal dose**) of nicotine to kill 50% of rats. Generally, dose is increased/decreased by a constant factor for different groups; in this example, the dose is increased by a factor of 2 from 10 to 20, 20 to 40 and so on.

Dosage, mg/kg	Number of deaths	% death
10	0	0
20	2	20
40	4	40
80	10	100
160	10	100

The data is plotted with log of dosage on the x-axis and % death on the y-axis; log dose corresponding to 50% death is obtained and its antilog is the dosage referred to as LD_{50} **or median/semi-lethal dose**.

On the same lines, Median Effective Dose (LD_{50}) is calculated with % effectively treated on the y-axis; the ratio of LD_{50} to ED_{50} is called the **Therapeutic Index (TI)**. It is obvious that any drug should have least toxicity (i.e. a very high LD_{50}) and effective at a very low dose in treating the ailment (i.e. a very low ED_{50}). In other words, TI should be as large as possible to ensure that the drug in question both safe and effective.

2.3.2. Microbiology/Immunology

The same concept as described above is extended for estimation of Tissue-Culture Infection Dosage ($TCID_{50}$), Egg Infection Dosage (EID_{50}), Egg Lethal Dose (ELD_{50}) and Plaque Forming Units (pfu).

3. MODE

Mode is the value which occurs most frequently in the set of data.

3.1. Discrete Data

In the **Example 1.2.1.1**, mode was 43 g and if > 1 values exhibit the same modal frequency, then the mode is said to be ill-defined.

However, it should be noticed that the frequencies on either side of mode are not very different from the modal frequency. Under such circumstances, it is preferred to calculate mode by developing grouping and analysis tables.

3.1.1. Grouping Table

Column 1: Indicates the frequencies
Column 2: Frequencies grouped in twos
Column 3: Same as column 2 but first frequency is left out
Column 4: Frequencies group in threes
Column 5: Same as column 4 but first frequency is left out
Column 6: Same as column 4 but first two frequencies are left out
In each of the columns, highest frequency is highlighted.

Grouping table						
Chick weight (g)	Frequency (Column 1)	Column 2	Column 3	Column 4	Column 5	Column 6
38	3	9		17		
40	6		14		30	
41	8	24				
42	16		36	46		44
43	20	30			32	
45	10		12			
46	2					

3.1.2. Analysis Table

By use of analysis table, number of times that each of the chick weights has appeared as modal frequency in the grouping table is noted. It is the modal frequency corresponds to a cell formed by combination of 2/3 cells, each of such cells is considered to contain the modal frequency.

Analysis table							
Column ↓	Chick weight (g)						
	38	40	41	42	43	45	46
1					1		
2					1	1	
3				1	1		
4				1	1	1	
5					1	1	1
6			1	1	1		
Total			1	3	6	3	1

It can be seen that 43 g has appeared maximum number of times in the modal frequency and hence, it is the mode.

3.2. Continuous Data

In continuous data, the actual magnitude of the variable can be found out by preparing grouping and analysis tables as described above. Mode can also be calculated by using the following formula (ignoring signs):

$$\text{Mode} = L_{md} + w\left(\frac{\left|f_{md} - f_{pmd}\right|}{\left|f_{md} - f_{pmd}\right| + \left|f_{md} - f_{smd}\right|}\right)$$

$$\text{or} \quad L_{md} + w\left(\frac{f_{md} - f_{pmd}}{2f_{md} - f_{pmd} - f_{smd}}\right)$$

where, L_{md} is the lower limit of modal class, w is the width of the modal class, f_{pmd}, f_{md} and f_{smd} is the frequency of pre-modal, modal and class succeeding modal class, respectively.

In **Example 1.2.2.1**, by visual inspection, 10.0 – 11.0 g class is the modal class. However, the actual weight which has occurred most frequently is

$$\text{Mode} = 10.0 + 1.0\left(\frac{\left|110 - 50\right|}{\left|110 - 70\right| + \left|110 - 50\right|}\right)$$

$$\text{or} \quad 10.0 + 1.0\left(\frac{110 - 50}{220 - 50 - 70}\right) = 10.6 \text{ g}$$

(**Note:** If a histogram is developed on the frequency distribution table, and two lines are drawn diagonally from each upper corner of the modal class bar to the upper corner of the adjacent bar on either side, the value on the x-axis corresponding to the point of intersection of the two lines so drawn to is the modal value)

3.3. Relationship between Mean, Median and Mode

In a symmetric distribution (normal distribution), all the three values coincide. In other words, if mean = median = mode, the distribution is called **symmetric** else the distribution is referred to as **asymmetric (Skewed)**.

In moderately skewed distributions,

Mode = Mean – 3 (Mean – Median) or Mode = 3 Median – 2 Mean

Median = Mode + ⅔ (Mean – Mode).

In **Example 1.2.1.1**, Mean = 10.70 g, Median = 10.68 g and Mode = 10.6 g; hence, it appears reasonable to say that the distribution of egg weights in Japanese quails is Normal (*see* Chapter "Dispersion" for further details on this aspect).

In any case, on most occasions, normality of the distribution is assumed and hence, comparison of mean, median and mode is rarely carried out on Animal science data.

4. GEOMETRIC MEAN (GM)

If a set of data contains n observations, geometric mean is the nth root of the product of observations. When n is excessively large, logarithm is employed to simplify the calculations. The ceometric mean is generally employed to estimate the average annual % increase in population, prices, sales etc. because each value is a % of the preceding value and not the first value.

For discrete data, geometric mean can be calculated as: $\sqrt[n]{x_1 x_2 x_3 \ldots x_n}$

or $anti\log\left(\dfrac{\log x_1 + \log x_2 + \log x_3 + \ldots + \log x_n}{n}\right) = anti\log\left(\dfrac{\sum\limits_{i=1}^{n}\log x_i}{n}\right)$. For discrete series,

geometric mean $= anti\log\left(\dfrac{\sum\limits_{i=1}^{n} f_i \log x_i}{\sum\limits_{i=1}^{n} f_i}\right)$ and for continuous series, geometric mean $=$

$anti\log\left(\dfrac{\sum\limits_{i=1}^{n} f_i \log m_i}{\sum\limits_{i=1}^{n} f_i}\right)$, where, m_i are the class values of the ith class.

4.1. Examples

4.1.1. Example

The percentage increase in egg price during 1976 to 1985 is 2.82, 4.35, 0.56, 0.08, 2.37, 9.87, 6.48, 11.56, 0.62 and 1.23, respectively. In this case, the price during 1976 has increased by 2.86% of that of 1975 during 1977 by 4.35% of that of 1976 and so on. Therefore, **the average increase in price is not the arithmetic mean** (39.94 ÷ 10) = 3.994 % **but it is the geometric mean** which is calculated as follows:

Geometric mean = antilog [(log 2.82 + log 4.35 + log 0.56 + … log 1.23) ÷ 10] which is 1.93 %.

Geometric mean is also popularly used in

1. Calculating averages involving microbial numbers which generally run in 10^x scale.
2. In determining annual % change.

4.1.2. Example

Population of improved layers in India increased from 40 m during 1977 to 325 m during 2000. In other words, in 23 years between 2000 and 1977, increase in layer population was 712.5% or 30.98%, if calculated with the logic of Arithmetic mean. But, it must be considered that the growth is comparable to compound interest and not simple interest and hence, Arithmetic mean will not be correct.

Let us check this out: If the layer population had increased at a rate (r) of 30.98% annually from 40 m during 1977, it should have reached a figure of $40 \times [1 + (30.98 \div 100)]^{23} = 19850.65$ m. Obviously, this is not correct. Hence, the calculations are made as follows:

$P_{2000} = P_{1977} \times [1+(r \div 100)]^{23}$; hence $r = 100 \times 100 \times \left[23\sqrt{(325 \div 40)} - 1 \right] = 9.54\%$ where, P_{2000} and P_{1977} represent layer population during 2000 and 1977, respectively.

4.2. Weighted Geometric Mean

Analogous to weighted arithmetic mean, weighted geometric mean can be calculated as follows:

Geometric mean $= \sqrt[n]{x_1^{w_1} x_2^{w_2} x_3^{w_3} \dots x_4^{w_4}}$; on logarithmic scale it becomes

$$antilog\left(\frac{w_1 \log x_1 + w_2 \log x_2 + w_3 \log x_3 + \dots w_n \log x_n}{w_1 + w_2 + w_3 + \dots w_n} \right)$$

or $antilog\left(\dfrac{\sum\limits_{i=1}^{n} w_i \log x_i}{\sum\limits_{i=1}^{n} w_i} \right)$

5. HARMONIC MEAN (HM)

If reciprocal of each of the observations is used to compute arithmetic mean and again reciprocal is taken for such an arithmetic mean, the resultant value is the harmonic mean of the observations. In short, Harmonic mean is the reciprocal of the arithmetic mean of the reciprocals.

Harmonic mean $= \dfrac{n}{\left(\dfrac{1}{x_1} + \dfrac{1}{x_2} + \dfrac{1}{x_3} + \dots \dfrac{1}{x_n} \right)} = \dfrac{n}{\sum\limits_{i=1}^{n} \dfrac{1}{x_i}}$

On the same lines, for discrete series, harmonic mean $= \dfrac{n}{\sum\limits_{i=1}^{n} \dfrac{f_i}{x_i}}$ and for continuous

series, hornonic mean $= \dfrac{n}{\sum\limits_{i=1}^{n} \dfrac{m_i}{x_i}}$ where, m_i is the mid-value (class mark) of the respective class.

5.1. Weighted Harmonic Mean

Similar to weighted arithmetic and geometric means, weighted harmonic mean is calculated thus:

Weighted harmonic mean $= \dfrac{\sum\limits_{i=1}^{n} w_i}{\left(\dfrac{w_1}{x_1} + \dfrac{w_2}{x_2} + \dfrac{w_3}{x_3} + \dots \dfrac{w_n}{x_n} \right)} = \dfrac{\sum\limits_{i=1}^{n} w_i}{\sum\limits_{i=1}^{n} \dfrac{m_i}{x_i}}$

Harmonic mean is of limited use in the field of veterinary and animal sciences. It can be employed to compute rate of increase in profits in an animal enterprise, average sale price of animal products and the like.

5.1.1. Example

A large commercial hatchery makes 1st profit of Rs 1 m at a rate of Rs 0.4 m p.a. 2nd Rs 1 m at a rate of Rs 0.5 m p.a. and 3rd Rs 1 m at a rate of Rs 0.9 m p.a. To find the average rate for obtaining Rs 1 m as profit, harmonic mean has to be calculated.

If Arithmetic mean is calculated, it works out to be $(0.4 + 0.5 + 0.9) \div 3 = $ Rs 0.6 m p.a. If harmonic mean is calculated, it will be

$$\text{Harmonic mean} = \frac{3}{\left(\dfrac{1}{0.4} + \dfrac{1}{0.5} + \dfrac{1}{0.9}\right)} = 0.53 \text{ m p.a.}$$

Let us check which is more appropriate:

As per the data, 1st Rs 1 m profit is achieved @ Rs 0.4 m p.a., that means in 2½ years; the 2nd Rs 1 m @ Rs 0.5 m p.a., that means in 2 years and the 3rd Rs 1 m @ Rs 0.9 m p.a., which means in 1.11 years. Hence, a total profit of Rs 3 m is realized in 5.61 years or @ $(3 \div 5.61) = $ Rs 0.53 m p.a. which clearly indicates that harmonic mean is more appropriate.

5.2. Relationship between AM, GM and HM

For the same set of data $AM \geq GM \geq HM$

6. AVERAGES

Analysis of chronological data (time series, quantitative data arranged in the order of their occurrence), includes identification of one or many of the following:

1. Secular (long-term) movements—tendency to increase or decrease; for instance, replacement of bullock-carts by automobiles has caused a long-term change, in opposite directions, reductions in the production, supply and demand of bullock-carts and increments in the production of automobiles.
2. Seasonal movements—changes observed during a 12 month period; seasonal variation in demand for eggs and consequent slump in the prices during summer is a well-known phenomenon in India.
3. Cyclical movements—changes due to booms/depressions; drastic reductions in demand and prices of poultry products during the recent outbreak of Avian Influenza is an example of changes due to depression.
4. Irregular/erratic movements—unpredictable changes; that effects of tsunami on various aspects of animal health and production fall into this category.

Further details on analysis of chronological data are given in a separate chapter. However, moving average and progressive average are used for studying certain trends.

6.1. Moving Average

An arithmetic average value is calculated for a pre-determined number (say odd numbers like 3, 5, 7, etc.) of periods (say weeks, months, years, etc.) and is considered to represent that trend for the period in question located at the middle of the period. If the predetermined number is even, the moving average is considered to represent the last period. This method is useful for studying Secular variations.

6.1.1. Example

Price of layer mash from 1975 to 1990 is tabulated below. Let us find out 3-year and 5-year moving averages and note the effect of calculating moving average.

Year	Price (Rs/Ton)	Moving average (Rs/Ton)		Short-term fluctuation			
				Multiplicative model*		Additive model**	
		3-year	5-year	3-year	5-year	3-year	5-year
1975	1274	–	–	–	–	–	–
1976	1224	1320.0	–	92.73	–	–96.0	–
1977	1462	1382.3	1394.4	105.77	104.85	79.7	67.6
1978	1461	1491.3	1489.0	97.97	98.12	–30.3	–28.0
1979	1551	1586.3	1630.8	97.77	95.11	–35.3	–79.8
1980	1747	1743.7	1733.0	100.19	100.81	3.3	14.0
1981	1933	1884.3	1860.8	102.58	103.88	48.7	72.2
1982	1973	2002.0	1996.6	98.55	98.82	–29.0	–23.6
1983	2100	2101.0	2111.6	99.95	99.45	1.0	–11.6
1984	2230	2217.3	2180.8	100.57	102.26	12.7	49.2
1985	2322	2277.0	2244.0	101.98	103.48	45.0	78.0
1986	2279	2296.7	2343.4	99.23	97.25	–17.7	–64.0
1987	2289	2388.3	2486.6	95.84	92.05	–99.3	–197.6
1988	2597	2610.7	–	99.48	–	–13.7	–
1989	2946	–	–	–	–	–	–

* (Column 2 ÷ respective moving average)* 100
** (Column 2 – respective moving average)

The above table clearly demonstrates that moving averages (especially, 3-year average is) reduce the influence of fluctuations and hence, the overall trend becomes smooth. Further, the data in the table are annual values and therefore, the fluctuations recorded indicate only cyclical variation.

6.2. Progressive Average

An arithmetic average value is calculated by including all previous values up to the period in question; the progressive average for the first period the same as the value corresponding to the first period. Therefore, progressive average for the last period will be same as the arithmetic mean of all the observations.

Progressive average for the data shown in **Example 4.1.2** is shown below.

Year	Price (Rs/Ton)	Progressive average (Rs/Ton)
1975	1274	1274.0
1976	1224	1249.0
1977	1462	1320.0
1978	1461	1355.2
1979	1551	1394.4
1980	1747	1453.2
1981	1933	1521.7
1982	1973	1578.1
1983	2100	1636.1
1984	2230	1695.5
1985	2322	1752.4
1986	2279	1796.3
1987	2289	1834.2
1988	2597	1888.7
1989	2946	1959.2

7. POSITIONAL MEASURES

7.1. Quartiles

When the entire data is divided into four equal parts (quarters), each of them is called **quartile** also referred to as **quantile**. They are respectively designated first (Q_1), Second (Q_2), and Third (Q_3) quartiles. Obviously, Q_2 is the median. The first and third quartile can be calculated employing $(n \div 4)$ and $(3n \div 4)$ for Z in the formula for the median along with values of the corresponding classes in the frequency distribution. In **Example 1.2.2.1**, Q_1 and Q_3 are 9.38 g and 11.75 g, respectively.

(**Note:** For discrete data, n is replaced by $n + 1$)

7.2. Deciles and Percentiles

While the quartiles divide the data into four equal parts, deciles divide into 10 and percentiles into 100 parts. The calculation of Deciles and Percentiles is on the same basis of quartiles; the value of Z in the formula for median is changed to $D \times (n \div 10)$ or $P \times (n \div 100)$ where D and P refer to the decile and percentile numbers, respectively. Median is the D_5 or P_{50} value. For data in **Example 1.2.2.1**, P_{10} and P_{90} are 8.5 and 12.875 g, respectively.

(**Note:** For discrete data, n is replaced by $n + 1$)

8. SELECTION OF A SUITABLE MEASURE OF CENTRAL TENDENCY

Arithmetic mean	Very commonly used measure but not when other measures are more appropriate as listed below.
Median	1. For open-end grouped distribution 2. When very high and very low values are likely to affect the mean value 3. Estimation of ED_{50}, EC_{50}, LD_{50} and TI in toxicological studies 4. Estimation of $TCID_{50}$, EID_{50}, ELD_{50} and pfu in micrbiological studies
Mode	1. Describe qualitative data like consumer preference of a particular animal product 2. Discrete series like number of dairy animals per household
Geometric mean	1. For ratios and percentages 2. For microbial numbers 3. Construction of index number
Harmonic mean	1. To compare value of one variable with a constant quantity of another like time required to realize a fixed amount of profit 2. Quantity purchased/sold per unit amount
Moving and progressive averages	1. For time series 2. In livestock economics

9. TRANSFORMATION OF DATA

In case of certain data, transformation (also referred to as **variance stabilizing transformation**) becomes essential and the measures of central tendency are computed on the transformed scale and later on retransformed back to the original scale. They will be dealt in a separate Chapter.

3

Dispersion

Study of measures of central tendency (*see* Chapter 2) brings out the following three points:
1. The data is spread around a central value
2. There may be same central value for data with different degrees of spread and consequently
3. Measure of spread is a necessity.

This aspect will be discussed in this chapter.

1. VARIANCE AND STANDARD DEVIATION

This is by far the most commonly used measure of dispersion.

A simple method of measuring the spread would be to find out how much each of the observations $(x_1, x_2, x_3, \ldots x_i)$ is deviating from the mean and find an average of it. That is, average of all deviations about the mean or **average deviation**. In other words, Average deviation = $\Sigma(x_i - \text{Mean}) \div n$

It is evident that, if the mean value is correct, numerator of the above equation will always be zero because, mean being the central value, there will be equal deviations on either sides of it (+ and –) and hence, for any data, average deviation is zero. It follows that average deviation can't serve as an indicator of spread of values around the mean.

Therefore, to make the –ve values +ve, all the values are squared so that the resultant mean value of the squared deviations has to be referred to as **mean squared deviation** or **variance**, denoted s^2.

When mean is known, one of the values in any set of data can be deduced if all other values are given. Hence, out of 'n' observations, only $(n - 1)$ observations can contribute to variability. Therefore, the denominator in the equation for variance is often changed to **degrees of freedom, $(n - 1)$**; this is especially important when $n \leq 10$, in particular and $n \leq 30$, in general. This is also attributable to the fact that the ratio $(1/x)$ rapidly reduces as $x \to 10$; but as n becomes larger, the difference between the reciprocals of n and $(n - 1)$ becomes negligible. Therefore, when $n > 30$, denominator for calculation of s^2 can be 'n' itself.

To undo the squaring of the deviation values, square root is taken for the mean squared deviation (variance) to obtain the **standard deviation** denoted **sd**.

2. COEFFICIENT OF VARIATION

It may be often necessary to compare variability of means whose expected maximum and minimum values differ widely; for instance, body weights of calves *Vs* body weight of Japanese quails. Under such circumstances, sd as a percentage of its mean value (referred to as **coefficient of variation**, designated **CV** is more appropriate than absolute values of sd. Obviously, CV = 100 × (sd ÷ Mean).

3. STANDARD ERROR

If several samples are drawn from the population and mean value of each of the samples is considered as an observation, the set of means will have its own mean (mean of means) and sd (sd of mean of means, also called **standard error** designated **se**). Hence, it is not possible to calculate se from a sample set of observations; however, it is shown mathematically that se $\approx$ sd $\div \sqrt{n}$

4. COMPUTATIONS

Computational (machine) formula for calculation of variance is:

$$s^2 = \frac{\displaystyle\sum_{i=1}^{n} x_i^2 - \frac{\left(\displaystyle\sum_{i=1}^{n} x_i\right)^2}{n}}{(n-1)}$$

Discussions above pertain to calculations with individual observations; however, other situations are considered at a later part of this chapter. Let us continue with the concepts on dispersion.

4.1. Examples

4.1.1. Example

The following data refers to number of eggs produced by three flocks of WL layers (number of layers same in all the flocks):

Days	1	2	3	4	5	6	7	8	9	10
Flock 1	44	50	38	49	42	50	46	39	58	54
Flock 2	52	48	38	43	48	45	48	45	45	58
Flock 3	40	54	41	38	53	40	51	58	55	40

If arithmetic mean and **range** (difference between the highest and the lowest value) in the above flocks are as follows:

	n	Σx_i	Mean	Highest	Lowest	Range
Flock 1	10	470	47	58	38	20
Flock 2	10	470	47	58	38	20
Flock 3	10	470	47	58	38	20

Hence, on the basis of mean and range, the above flocks are indistinguishable. But, close scrutiny of the individual observations indicates that the flocks differed in distribution of values (dispersion) around the mean. The variance (s²), standard deviation (sd), CV and se of the three flocks were as follows:

	Σx_i^2	s²	sd	CV	se
Flock 1	22462	41.33	6.43	13.68	2.03
Flock 2	22348	28.67	5.35	11.39	1.69
Flock 3	22640	61.11	7.82	16.63	2.47

It is now clear from the above table that Flock 2 birds were more consistent because the values of s², sd and CV were the lowest followed by Flock 1 and Flock 2, in that order. Corresponding values of se also indicate that the mean of the Flock 1 was a better estimate of population mean, μ.

4.1.2. Example

The following table gives the growth rate (g/week) of broilers and calves:

	Mean	sd	CV
Broilers	200	30	15
Calves	4000	400	10

Apparently, it can be noticed that the growth rate of calves showed higher variability as indicated by sd value; but, it is not actually true because, the mean growth rate of calves was also higher. Therefore, CV was calculated which clearly indicated that, actually, variability in broiler growth was higher.

Note: As mentioned earlier, evaluation of dispersion in case of discrete/continuous series both by direct and by deviation method are considered below. Since the basis is the same; only formulae are listed below:

1. For a frequency distribution table, with notations as explained in Chapter

$$\text{Central tendency, } s^2 = \frac{\sum_{i=1}^{n} f_i x_i^2 - \dfrac{\left(\sum_{i=1}^{n} f_i x_i\right)^2}{n}}{\left(\sum_{i=1}^{n} f_i - 1\right)}$$

2. If, on the same lines as explained in Chapter **"Central tendency"**, an arbitrary value (which may be even the mean itself) can be subtracted from x_i's and/or the resultant value is divided by a constant but arbitrary value to obtain corresponding deviations (d_i's); then,

$$s^2 = \frac{\sum_{i=1}^{n} d_i^2 - \dfrac{\left(\sum_{i=1}^{n} d_i\right)^2}{n}}{(n-1)}$$

3. Similarly, if d_i's are calculated in a frequency table,

$$s^2 = \dfrac{\displaystyle\sum_{i=1}^{n} f_i d_i^2 - \dfrac{\left(\displaystyle\sum_{i=1}^{n} f_i d_i\right)^2}{n}}{\left(\displaystyle\sum_{i=1}^{n} f_i - 1\right)}$$

Let us take the **Example 1.2.2.1** (from Chapter **Central tendency**) and calculate s^2 by different methods described above.

Egg weight class (g)	Class value (x_i) (g)	No of eggs (f_i)	$f_i x_i$ (g)	$f_i x_i^2$	d_i $(x_i - 10.5)$	$f_i d_i$	$f_i d_i^2$
6.0–7.0	6.5	5	32.5	211.25	−4	−20	80
7.0–8.0	7.5	15	112.5	843.75	−3	−45	135
8.0–9.0	8.5	30	255.0	2167.50	−2	−60	120
9.0–10.0	9.5	50	475.0	4512.50	−1	−50	50
10.0–11.0	10.5	110	1155.0	12127.50	0	0	0
11.0–12.0	11.5	70	805.0	9257.50	1	70	70
12.0–13.0	12.5	40	500.0	6250.00	2	80	160
13.0–14.0	13.5	25	337.5	4556.25	3	75	225
14.0–15.0	14.5	5	72.5	1051.25	4	20	80
Total		350	3745.0	40977.50		70	920

$s^2 = [40977.50 - (3745)^2 \div 350] \div 349 = 2.596$ g^2 (Case 1)

$s^2 = [920 - (70)^2 \div 350] \div 349 = 2.596$ g^2 (Case 3)

The same will be applicable to Case 2 as well. It is very important and interesting that s^2 (and obviously therefore s) is unaffected by change of origin and/or scale. Further, s^2 is expressed in square of the unit whereas, s in same as that of measurement. Standard deviation, $s = 1.611$ g.

4. Shephard's correction for grouping: It is obvious from the formula for central tendency (Chapter 2) and dispersion that class – value (mid – value) is assumed to repeat to a tune of the corresponding frequency; which introduces an error called "**Grouping error**". This can be corrected by subtracting $\dfrac{1}{12} w^2$ (where w is the class width) from s^2; in **Example 1.2.2.1** (from Chapter "**Central tendency**"), the corrected $s^2 = 2.596 - (1 \div 12) \times 1^2 = 2.513$.

5. Pooling of s^2/s: If $\overline{X}_P$ is the pooled mean (*see* Chapter **Central tendency**), $\overline{X}_i$ and s_i^2 are the corresponding means and variances of the related groups, then pooled variance, $S_P^2 = \left(\dfrac{\displaystyle\sum_{i=1}^{n} N_i s_i^2 + \sum_{i=1}^{n} N_i d_i^2}{\displaystyle\sum_{i=1}^{n} N_i}\right)$ where and pooled standard deviation

5. OTHER MEASURES OF DISPERSION

Other measures for estimating dispersion are not commonly used at least by Veterinary and Animal Science workers. Hence, only formulae are listed below:

1. Range: This is the simplest method of estimating dispersion and is the difference between the highest and the lowest value in the set of data.
2. Coefficient of range is the ratio of range to the sum of the lowest and highest values.
3. Inter-quartile range or Quartile deviation (QD): This is calculated as ½ of the difference between Q_3 and Q_1 (see Chapter **Central tendency** for computation of Q_1 and Q_3) and **semi-inter-quartile range** is ½ of quartile deviation.
4. Coefficient of quartile deviation is the ratio of quartile deviation to sum of Q_1 and Q_3.
5. Percentile range: This is similar to quartile deviation by replacing Q_3 and Q_1 with P_{90} and P_{10}, respectively. On the same lines under quartile deviation, **semi-inter-percentile range** and **coefficient of percentile deviation** can be calculated. See Chapter **Central tendency** for calculation of percentiles.
6. Mean Deviation (MD): As discussed under Variance above, sum of deviations from the mean will always be zero and hence MD is calculated as the average of deviations from mean, ignoring signs; in case of a frequency distribution, it will be the average of product of frequency with its corresponding deviation from mean (ignoring signs).

In statistical notation it can be represented thus: $\text{MD} = \dfrac{\sum\limits_{i=1}^{n}|d_i|}{n}$ or $\dfrac{\sum\limits_{i=1}^{n}f_i|d_i|}{\sum\limits_{i=1}^{n}f_i}$; in Normal

Distribution, QD < MD < s and generally, QD = ⅔ s and MD = 0.8 s or QD : MD : s = 10 : 12 : 15

7. Coefficient of MD: It is calculated as the ratio of MD to either Median or Mean.
8. Diversity indices (Zar, 2003): In case of nominal data, if the set can be considered a random sample, then the Shannon-Wiener diversity index or Shannon-Weaver

diversity index can be calculated thus: $H' = -\sum\limits_{i=1}^{k} p_i \log p_i$

where, k is the number of categories, p_i is the proportion of observations found in category i. This index is useful while studying nesting patterns, reproductive behavior etc. species like wild birds. For instance, if most of the nests are located at a specific type of site, diversity is less; on the contrary, if they are distributed uniformly at several types of sites, the diversity is very high. With sample size n

and frequency of observations in category i is f_i, $H' = \dfrac{n\log n - -\sum\limits_{i=1}^{k} p_i \log p_i}{n}$. Further,

$H'_{max} = \log k$ and evenness or homogeneity or relative diversity, $J' = \dfrac{H'}{H'_{max}}$;

consequently, $(1 - J')$ is a measure of dominance or heterogeneity.

If the set of data can not be considered a random sample, then information-theoretic

diversity, $H = \dfrac{\log\left(\dfrac{n!}{\prod\limits_{i=1}^{k} f_i!}\right)}{n} = \dfrac{\log\dfrac{n!}{f_1!f_2!\ f_3!\ ....f_k!}}{n}$ which can be simplified by

logarithms to $H = \dfrac{\log n! \ -\sum\limits_{i=1}^{k}\log f_i!}{n}$.

In this case also $H_{max} = \dfrac{\log n! - (k-d)\log c! - d\log(c+1)!}{n}$ and $J = \dfrac{H}{H_{max}}$. However,

with data on domestic animals, diversity indices are not common.

9. Graphic method (Lorenz curve): This method was originally used to measure distribution of wealth and income. However, it can be adapted for studying distribution of profits, production of livestock products, etc.

5.1. Example

Let us assume the following data on income from dairy farming and draw a Lorenz curve. The cumulative % values with % diaries on x-axis and % income from diary on the y-axis. The Lorenz curve is shown in Fig. 3.1 which clearly shows that line corresponding to number of dairy farms in South India was farther from the diagonal (line of equal distribution) and hence, it is reasonable to conclude that, as per the data, number of dairy farms in South India showed greater inequalities.

| | | | | | | Income in Rs ('000) | | |
| Income from dairy | Number of dairies | | Cumulative | | | Cumulative, % | | |
	South India	North India	Income from dairy	Dairies in South India	Dairies in North India	Income from dairy	Dairies in South India	Dairies in North India
150	45	80	150	45	80	7.50	6.00	6.67
200	150	100	350	195	180	17.50	26.00	15.00
250	250	275	600	445	455	30.00	59.33	37.92
300	175	475	900	620	930	45.00	82.67	77.50
350	80	220	1250	700	1150	62.50	93.33	95.83
400	40	40	1650	740	1190	82.50	98.67	99.17
350	10	10	2000	750	1200	100.00	100.00	100.00

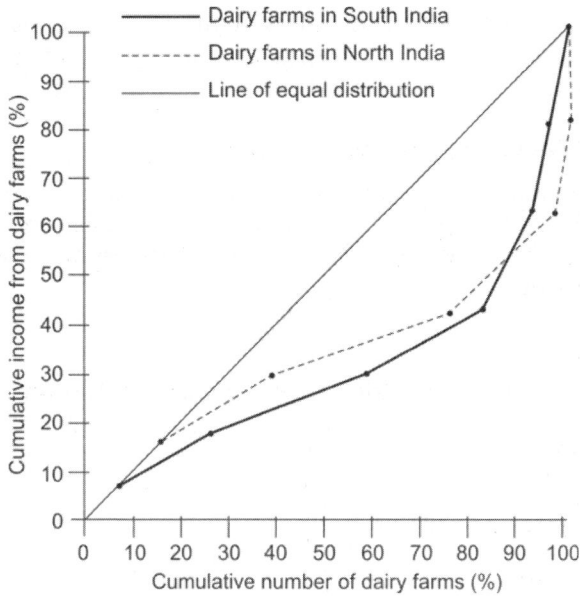

Fig. 3.1: Lorenz curve

6. CHARACTERIZING A DISTRIBUTION

At the beginning of this Chapter, we saw three sets of data having the same mean and range but still differed; it was enumerated with the concept of variance and standard deviation. Similarly, it is also possible that sets of data can have the same mean and standard deviation but still differ; but the differences may be discernible when they are graphically presented. Two types of differences can be expected; one symmetry of the curve and height of the curve.

6.1. Symmetry and Skewness

If the variable is perfectly normally distributed (Normal distribution will be discussed in Chapter "**Continuous probability distributions**"), the resultant curve of frequency against magnitude of the variable will be **symmetric**. In other words, a perpendicular from the peak of the distribution to the x-coordinate will cut off equal areas on either sides or the value of the variable referring to the peak is the **mean** and since it is placed exactly at the center, it is the **median** and since it refers to peak of the curve (highest frequency), it is the **mode** as well. Therefore, **in a symmetric or normal distribution, mean = median = mode**.

Obviously, if the three measures of central tendency are not equal, the curve will be asymmetric or **skewed**; if peak of the curve is to the left of the mean value, it is positively skewed and *vice versa*. Measure of symmetry is therefore referred to as **skewness/ coefficient of skewness**.

6.2. Height of the Curve and Kurtosis

If most of the frequencies are very close to the mode (mean), when plotted, the curve appears sharper at the peak frequency than a symmetric distribution (referred to as leptokurtic). On the other hand, if the modal frequency by itself is slightly more than the frequencies on either side, such a curve gives a flat look (referred to as **platykurtic**). The Normal Distribution is **mesokurtic**. Kurtosis measures **bulginess** of the curve.

6.3. Measuring Skewness and Kurtosis

It is not a general practice to calculate skewness and kurtosis on Animal science data; usually, Normal Distribution is assumed and statistical analyses performed. Hence, only formulae are given below with calculation of skewness and kurtosis by using the data presented in Example 2.3.

6.3.1. Skewness

(Formulae of Quartiles and Percentiles given in Chapter "**Central tendency**")

6.3.1.1. Absolute measure

Absolute Sk = Mean – Mode

or Absolute $Sk = Q_3 + Q_1 - 2$ Median

6.3.1.2. Relative measures

1. Karl – Pearson's Coefficient of Skewness, $Sk_P = \dfrac{\overline{X} - \text{Mode}}{s}$. In moderately skewed

    distributions, Mode = 3 Median – 2 Mean; therefore, $Sk_P = \dfrac{3(\overline{X} - \text{Median})}{s}$. Sk_P is

    the commonly used measure.
2. Bowley's Coefficient of Skewness (Quartile measure of skewness),

    $Sk_B = \dfrac{Q_3 + Q_1 - 2 \text{ Median}}{Q_3 - Q_1}$

3. Kelly's Coefficient of Skewness, $Sk_K = \dfrac{P_{90} + P_{10} - \text{Median}}{P_{90} - P_{10}}$ where P_i's refer to

    percentiles.

6.3.1.3. Calculations

Data given in **Example 1.2.2.1** (Chapter "**Central Tendency**")

Egg weight class (g)	Class value (x_i) (g)	f_i	d_i $(x_i - k)$	$f_i d_i$	$f_i d_i^2$	$f_i d_i^3$	$f_i d_i^4$
6.0–7.0	6.5	5	–4	–20	80	–320	1280
7.0–8.0	7.5	15	–3	–45	135	–405	1215
8.0–9.0	8.5	30	–2	–60	120	–240	480
9.0–10.0	9.5	50	–1	–50	50	–50	50
10.0–11.0	10.5	110	0	0	0	0	0
11.0–12.0	11.5	70	1	70	70	70	70
12.0–13.0	12.5	40	2	80	160	320	640
13.0–14.0	13.5	25	3	75	225	675	2025
14.0–15.0	14.5	5	4	20	80	320	1280
Total		350		70	920	370	7040

The arithmetic mean, median and mode for the above data was 10.70, 10.68 and 10.60 g, respectively; standard deviation, s was 1.611 g. Hence,

$$Sk_p = \frac{10.68 - 10.70}{1.611} = 0.01 \text{ or } \frac{3(10.70 - 10.68)}{1.611} = 0.01;$$

$$Sk_B = \frac{11.75 + 9.38 - 2(10.68)}{11.75 - 9.38} = -0.10 \text{ and } Sk_K = \frac{12.875 + 8.5 - 10.68}{12.875 - 8.5} = 2.50$$

Sk_p can also be calculated by using moments about the mean. The 1st moment about

the origin (mean) designated μ_1 is $\dfrac{\sum\limits_{i=1}^{n}(x_i - \overline{X})}{n}$, which is always zero, the 2nd moment

is $\dfrac{\sum\limits_{i=1}^{n}(x_i - \overline{X})^2}{n}$, designated μ_2, which is the variance, the 3rd moment is $\dfrac{\sum\limits_{i=1}^{n}(x_i - \overline{X})^3}{n}$,

designated μ_3, the 4th moment is $\dfrac{\sum\limits_{i=1}^{n}(x_i - \overline{X})^4}{n}$, designated μ_4 and so on. For a fre-

quency distribution, they will be, $\dfrac{\sum\limits_{i=1}^{n}f_i(x_i - \overline{X})}{\sum\limits_{ni=1}^{n}f_i}$, $\dfrac{\sum\limits_{i=1}^{n}f_i(x_i - \overline{X})^2}{\sum\limits_{ni=1}^{n}f_i}$, $\dfrac{\sum\limits_{i=1}^{n}f_i(x_i - \overline{X})^3}{\sum\limits_{ni=1}^{n}f_i}$ and

$\dfrac{\sum\limits_{i=1}^{n}f_i(x_i - \overline{X})^4}{\sum\limits_{ni=1}^{n}f_i}$, respectively. With change in origin, the moments can be calculated by

replacing $(x_i - \overline{X})$ with $(x_i - k) = d_i$ in the respective equations followed by multi-plication with the class width, w_i; they are designated μ_1', μ_2', μ_3' and μ_4', respecti-vely. They are converted to actual moments as follows: $\mu_1 = \mu_1'$; $\mu_2 = \mu_2' - (\mu_1')^2$; $\mu_3 = \mu_3' - 3\mu_1'\mu_2' + 2\mu_1'^3$ and $\mu_4 = \mu_4' - 4\mu_1'\mu_3' + 6\mu_1'^2\mu_2' - 3\mu_1'^4$.

Finally, Skewness, designated β_1 is given by $\dfrac{\mu_3^2}{\mu_2^3}$

In **Example 1.2.2.1** (Chapter "Central tendency"), $\mu_1, \mu_2, \mu_3, \mu_4$ and β_1 are 0.500, 2.379, –2.6365, 21.9318 and 0.516, respectively. Hence, the distribution is slightly skewed.

6.3.2. Kurtosis

Kurtosis, designated β_2, is given by $\dfrac{\mu_4}{\mu_2^2}$; Normal distribution will have a kurtosis value of 3. In **Example 1.2.2.1** (Chapter "**Central tendency**"), $\beta_2 = 3.875$; hence the distribution is slightly leptokurtic. (If β_2 is < 3, the distribution is platykurtic.)

[**Note:** After calculating mean, median and mode (see Chapter **Central Tendency**), it appeared that the distribution was normal; the same is evident after calculating skewness and kurtosis. Hence, it is reasonable to assume normal distribution for the data for further statistical analyses.]

4

Probability

1. INTRODUCTION

Let us assume that for formulating a certain ration, 2 energy sources and 6 protein sources are available. If the ration has to contain one energy source and a protein source, we need to find out number of possible ways to make it; It is clear that there are 2 (k_1) and 6 (k_2) ways for choosing energy and protein source, respectively. When chosen together, each of the energy sources can be combined with 6 possible ways of protein source; that means, totally $2 \times 6 = 12$ ways or $k_1 k_2$ ways. This can be extended to any number of objects.

An important example is the triplet codes in DNA formed by 3 nitrogen bases; at each position of the triplet, any one of the 4 nitrogen bases (Adenine, Cytosine, Guanine and Thymine) can occupy; i.e. for each location in the triplet, there are 4 possible alternatives or $k_1 = 4$, $k_2 = 4$ and $k_3 = 4$. Therefore, the number of triplet codons $= 4 \times 4 \times 4$ or $4^3 - 64$.

1.1 Permutation (Zar, 2003)

Arrangement of objects in a particular sequence (linear arrangement) is permutation.

1.1.1 Example

Suppose a cow (C), a horse (H) and a sheep (S) have to be arranged linearly; First position can be occupied by any one of the three animals (C or H or S). If 1st position is occupied by C, there only 2 ways to fill the 2nd position (H or S) and after the second position is occupied, there is only one way to fill the 3rd (if 2nd is H, third will be S else if the 2nd is S, the 3rd has to be H). In other words, $k_1 = 3$, $k_2 = 2$ and $k_3 = 1$; hence, total permutations possible is $k_1 \times k_2 \times k_3 = 3 \times 2 \times 1 = 6$.

To generalize, if there are n positions to be filled with n objects, total permutations, $^nP_n = n(n-1)(n-2)...(3)(2)(1)$; the right-hand side of the equation is denoted mathematically with a **sign '!' called 'Factorial' meaning a product of all integers from 1 to n**. Hence, $^nP_n = n!$. It should be noted that $0! = 1$

1.1.2 *Example*

If there are fewer than n positions (say r positions) to permute n objects, then $^nP_r = \dfrac{n!}{(n-r)!}$. To illustrate this, let us consider that there are only two positions to be filled by a cow (C), a horse (H), a pig (P) and a sheep (S); for each of the animals in 1st position ($k_1 = 4$), there are only 3 alternatives ($k_2 = 3$). Therefore, total permutations possible is $4 \times 3 = 12$. Let us check this with the formula; $^4P_2 = \dfrac{4!}{(4-2)!} = \dfrac{4!}{2!}$

$$= \frac{(1)(2)(3)(4)}{(1)(2)} = 12$$

Suppose in **Example 1.1.2**, there are 2 H's, one C and one S, it is easy to note that presence of 2 H's are indistinguishable as to whether the linear arrangement is 1st H, 2nd H or 2nd H and 1st H; hence, number of permutations of 4 animals will not be $4! = 24$ but only 12. Mathematically, it can be represented thus: If n_i represents number of like individuals in category i, then $^nP_{n_1,n_2...n_i} = \dfrac{n!}{n_1!n_2!...n_i!}$; in the above example,

$$^4P_{1,2,1} = \frac{4!}{1!\ 2!\ 1!} = 12$$

1.2 Combination

Let us consider **Example 1.1.2** and write down various permutations possible: CH, CP, CS, HC, HP, HS, PC, PS, PH, SC, SH and SP. It is clear that CH and HC, CP and PC, CS and SC, HP and PH, HS and SH and PS and SP are different only in order of arrangement; i.e. only 6 arrangements are possible. If order of arrangement is not important, the number of combinations can be calculated as follows: $^nC_r = \dfrac{n!}{r!(n-r)!}$;

in **Example 1.1.2**, it will be $^4C_2 = \dfrac{4!}{2!(4-2)!} = \dfrac{4!}{2!\ 2!} = 6$

1.3 Sets

1.3.1 *Example*

A collection of items is referred to as a **set**; say, for example, animals in a livestock farm. Each of the items (animals, in this case) is called an **element**. The animals may include buffaloes (B), cows (C), dogs (D), fowls (F), Goats (G), Horse (H) etc. If another set contains same elements (not necessarily same number or sequence of elements), the two sets are said to be **equal sets**.

Suppose, we classify the above set into ruminants and non-ruminants; we get two **subsets**; B, C and G under ruminants and D, F and H under non-ruminants. It is clear that a subset is also a set and its elements are elements of a larger set. If a set/subset is used for experiment, it is referred to as **outcome set**. For example, if one uses ruminant set, and draws two animals, the possible outcomes are: BB, BC, BG, CC, CB, CC, GG, GB and GC.

It can be noted that each of the outcomes itself is a set and hence, subset of the outcome set is called **event**; in the above example, occurrence of BB, BC, CB and CC is an event. Further characterization of an event is possible depending on the nature of the event and the experiment in question. For instance, in the above case, drawing one buffalo can be an event which includes BC, BG, CB and GB; in the same way, the event could be drawing both of same kind which will then include events BB, CC and GG.

Further, in the **Example 1.3.1**, subsets ruminants and non-ruminants **complementary to each other**; it means, when ruminants are defined, the rest of the animals in the set are, obviously, non-ruminants and *vice versa*.

Let us consider another situation; for example, in a livestock farm, one is interested to know the possibility (probability) of drawing at least two ruminants; it means that it includes the possibility of drawing B or C or G two at a time. Naturally, if possibility values are available for drawing B, C and G, they have to be added to get the desired possibility; hence, such situations are referred to as **union of events**.

2. CONCEPT OF PROBABILITY

Ratio of frequency of an event (occurrence of an event, favorable cases) to that of total number of events (total number of events, total number of cases) is called **probability (relative frequency) of the event**. It is obvious that the numerator can't be < 0 and the denominator < numerator. Therefore, **probability of an event varies between 0 and 1 or $0 \leq$ probability ≤ 1**.

Assuming n eggs are incubated, we say that c number of chicks may hatch out; in other words, we are talking of **likelihood** or we are **predicting** certain outcome. Here, hatching chicks is a **favorable outcome** and total number of eggs incubated is total number of **equally likely outcomes**. That means, each egg incubated (of n eggs) has an equal chance of hatching. Then, **probability of hatching is the ratio of c to n**. In statistical terms, we say that probability is the ratio of number of favorable cases to total number of equally likely cases.

2.1 Example

Let us now consider one egg being incubated; the chance of the egg hatching is ½ and hence, the chance that it does not hatch is also ½. In this case, the egg can either hatch or not hatch; but not both or occurrence of one event is precluding occurrence of the other; such events are called **mutually exclusive** events. Further, events having only two possible outcomes are also called **binomial events**.

2.2 Addition Rule—Mutually Exclusive Events

When an egg is incubated, there are only two possibilities; it hatches or doesn't; but both can't occur simultaneously. Such events which mutually preclude the occurrence of the other event are referred to as **mutually exclusive events**. In this case, the probability of the egg hatching is ½ and that of not hatching is also ½. But, note that the probability of **egg hatching or not hatching is 1** because, one of them must occur and it precludes the other event.

Therefore, in general, **if A and B are two mutually exclusive events, then P(A or B) = P(A) + P(B) or P(A$\cup$B) = P(A) + P(B)**.

2.2.1 Addition Rule—Special Case

Suppose we need to know the probability of selecting a grass-eating animal or a ruminant among the animals listed above i.e. B, C, D, F, G and H (one animal each available in the set), then the probability of selecting a ruminant (B or C or G) is (3 ÷ 6) = . Probability of selecting a grass-eating animal (B or C or G or H) is (4 ÷ 6) = $\frac{2}{3}$. If we apply the addition rule mentioned above and calculate the probability of selecting a grass-eating animal or a ruminant, we get ($\frac{1}{2}$ + $\frac{2}{3}$) > 1 which is incorrect. This is because, the probability of B, C and G are appearing on both occasions; in other words, the events are **intersecting**.

Hence, the actual probability of selecting a grass-eating animal or a ruminant is equal to probability of selecting grass eating animal + probability of selecting a ruminant − **probability of selecting a ruminant and a grass-eating animal = $\frac{1}{2}$ + $\frac{2}{3}$** − $\frac{1}{2}$ = $\frac{2}{3}$. In this particular example, ruminants are virtually a subset of grass-eating animals and therefore, probability of selecting a grass-eating animal or a ruminant is simply the probability of the larger set i.e. $\frac{2}{3}$.

Hence, **in general, for two intersecting events A and B, P(A or B) = P(A) + P(B) − P(A and B) or P(A ∪ B) = P(A) + P(B) − P(A ∩ B) or by substituting P(A ∩ B) = P(A) × P(B), P(A ∪ B) = P(A) + P(B)[1 − P(A)]**. As the number of intersecting events increase, number and levels of intersections also increase. For example, for 3 intersecting events A, B and C, P(A or B or C) = P(A) + P(B) + P(C) − P(A and B) − P(A and C) − P(B and C) − P(A and B and C) and so on.

2.3 Multiplication Rule—Independent Events

2.3.1 Example

If we consider 2 eggs kept for hatching, it is obvious that the outcome from the first egg does not affect/influence that from the other; this is referred to as **independent events**. In this case, the following 4 events are possible (equally likely):

1. Both eggs hatch
2. First hatches and the second doesn't
3. First does not hatch but the second does
4. Both do not hatch

It is clear that out of total of 4 possible outcomes, that both eggs hatch is likely once; i.e. Probability of both eggs hatching (favorable outcome) is $\frac{1}{4}$; on the same lines probability that both don't hatch is also $\frac{1}{4}$; at least one of them hatches is $\frac{1}{4}$ + $\frac{1}{4}$ = $\frac{1}{2}$. Also note that the total probability = $\frac{1}{4}$ + $\frac{1}{4}$ + $\frac{1}{2}$ = 1 and probability of hatching or not hatching for each of the eggs is $\frac{1}{2}$.

Let us consider the 1st event of both eggs hatching; probability of each egg hatching is $\frac{1}{2}$ whereas, both hatching together is $\frac{1}{4}$ or $\frac{1}{2}$ × $\frac{1}{2}$. The same is true for the 4th event above. But, the 2nd and 3rd events differ only in order of occurrence and are mutually exclusive; hence, probability of at least one egg hatching is $\frac{1}{4}$ + $\frac{1}{4}$ = $\frac{1}{2}$. This aspect will be utilized in Chapter 6 for introducing probability distributions.

To generalize, **if two events A and B are independent, then P(A and B) = P(A) × P(B) or P(AB) = P(A) × P(B)**.

This can be extended for any number of eggs; but the number of equally likely outcomes increases as well as favorable outcomes increase making it difficult to calculate the probabilities of each of the favorable outcome.

Hence, let us generalize the above into algebraic form. Let probability of success (hatching) be p and probability of failure (not hatching) be q. The following are evident from the above discussions:

1. $p = q = \frac{1}{2}$ or $p + q = 1$ when the events are mutually exclusive (binomial) events and number of trials (n) is 1. Further, one of the mutually exclusive events does occur. Therefore, if A and B are mutually exclusive events, $P(A \cup B) = P(A) + P(B)$; the symbol '$\cup$' is read as 'Union'. This logic is extendable to any number of mutually exclusive events.

2. If events are binomial and independent, $n > 1$, the probability of different combinations of events can be obtained by expanding the binomial $(q + p)^n$ which is generalized as $^nC_r q^r p^{(n-r)}$ where coefficient of each of the terms, refers to number of combinations of r items at a time out of n items; r taking the values 0, 1, 2, 3 ... n. In the above example, considering 2 eggs, $(q + p)^2 = {}^2C_0 q^0 p^2 + {}^2C_1 q^1 p^1 + {}^2C_2 q^2 p^0$

   $= p^2 + 2pq + q^2$ representing probability of 2, 1 and 0 number of chicks hatching (success), respectively. Substituting $p = q = \frac{1}{2}$ in the above, we get the probabilities as ¼, ½ and ¼ which is same as calculated above. The equation is extendable to any n; obviously, as n increases, number of terms in the expanded equation increases. For instance, for $n = 3$, the probability of 3, 2, 1 and 0 success is given by the terms obtained by the expansion of the binomial $(q + p)^3 =$

   $^3C_0 q^0 p^3 + {}^3C_1 q^1 p^2 + {}^3C_2 q^2 p^1 + {}^3C_3 q^3 p^0 = p^3 + 3p^2 q + 3pq^2 + q^3$ which on substitution of $p = q = \frac{1}{2}$ yields probability of ⅛, ⅜, ⅜ and ⅛, respectively for 3, 2, 1 and 0 successes.

3. All binomial events are mutually exclusive but not *vice versa*; for instance, from a tray of 8 eggs (one egg each from 8 different species), the probability of picking egg of any one species is ⅛ and picking of an egg of one species precludes picking up of egg from any other species. Since there are 8 possible outcomes, the events are mutually exclusive although not binomial. In this case, $p = \frac{1}{8}$ and $q = (1 - \frac{1}{8}) = \frac{7}{8}$ because, $p + q = 1$. Therefore, it can be generalized that if p is the probability of success and q that of failure of a binomial/mutually exclusive event, the probability of getting r successes out of n trials can be obtained by $^nC_r p^r q^{(n-r)}$.

4. If two events A and B are independent, $P(A \text{ and } B) = P(A) + P(B)$. Mathematically, $P(A \cap B) = P(A) \ P(B)$; the symbol '$\cap$' is read as 'intersection'.

2.4 Conditional Probability—Bayes' Theorem

Conditional probability refers to probability of an event given a sample information. Hence probabilities without sample information are often referred to as *unconditional or priori or prior* **probabilities** and those after revision considering sample information are called *conditional or posteriori or posterior* **probabilities**.

2.4.1 Example

In a poultry farm, Leghorn (WL) layers producing 70% of daily egg production are known to produce 2% under-sized eggs whereas Cornish (WC) layers producing the remaining 30% of eggs lay 8% under-sized eggs. If an undersized egg is drawn at random, we want to know the probability that it is produced by WL or WC.

In this case, probability that an egg is produced by WL (A_1) = 0.70 and that produced by WC (A_2) = 0.3. Let us assume that the probability of drawing an under-sized egg as B. Further, probability that an egg is defective and produced by WL, $P(B/A_1)$ is 0.02; similarly $P(B/A_2)$ is 0.08. Note that addition information is available in this case which helps compute **conditional probabilities** as follows:

Event	Probability			
(1)	*Priori* (2)	Conditional (3)	*Joint* (4) = (2 × 3)	*Posteriori* 4 ÷ P(B)
A_1	0.70	0.02	0.014	0.3684
A_2	0.30	0.08	0.024	0.6316
Total	1.00		P(B) = 0.038	1.0000

It is now evident that the probability that the under-sized egg is that of WL is only 36.84% although they are contributing more eggs and the probability that the under-sized egg is from WC is 63.16%.

From the above table, we get the following formulae:

$$P(A_1/B) = \frac{P(A_1 \text{ and } B)}{P(B)}; \quad P(A_2/B) = \frac{P(A_2 \text{ and } B)}{P(B)} \quad \text{where}$$

$$P(A_1 \text{ and } B) = P(A_1) \times P(B/A_1), \quad P(A_2 \text{ and } B) = P(A_2) \times P(B/A_2)$$

and $P(B) = P(A_1 \text{ and } B) + P(A_2 \text{ and } B)$.

In general, if A_1, A_2, A_3 ... A_n are n mutually exclusive and collectively exhaustive events, and B is another event (whose probability is > 0), then

$$P(A_i/B) = \frac{P(B/A_i) \times P(A_i)}{\sum_{i=1}^{n} P(B/A_i) \times P(A_i)}. \text{ The following generalizations are listed without}$$

proofs and the reader can refer to more theoretical books for the same.

1. For any two events A and B, **if A^c represents complement of A** (i.e. A not occurring), **P(B) = P(B/A) × P(A) + P(B/A^c) × P(A^c)** (Rosner, 2000).
2. **Total probability rule**: In general, if A_1, A_2, A_3 ..... A_n are n mutually exclusive and exhaustive events, the unconditional probability of B, i.e. P(B), will be the weighted average of the conditional probabilities of B given A_i[P(B/A_i)] as follows:

$$P(B) = \sum_{i=1}^{n} P(B/A_i) * P(A_i)$$

3. MATHEMATICAL EXPECTATION

A variable is considered random (Stochastic) variable if its value is determined through a random experiment/trial. If it takes only integer values, as in case of number of animals in a farm or number of chicks hatched, etc., then, it is referred to as **discrete**

random variable; alternatively, if a random variable takes all values within a range like weight of broilers, milk production, etc., it is called **continuous random variable**. If $X_1, X_2, X_3 \ldots X_n$ are n discrete random variables with probability value of $p_1, p_2, p_3 \ldots$

p_n, respectively, with the condition that $\sum_{i=1}^{n} p_i = 1$, then the mathematical expectation,

$E(X) = \sum_{i=1}^{n} p_i X_i$. Let us take an example:

3.1 Example

A farmer can sell an average of 2500 eggs per day during summer months and 15000 eggs during other seasons. If probability of a particular day being hot is 0.4 and that it will be cool is 0.6, let us find out the expected sale of eggs on that day:

Given are X_1 = 2500, X_2 = 15000, p_1 = 0.4 and p_2 = 0.6; therefore,

E(X) = 0.4 × 2500 + 0.6 × 12000 = 10000 eggs are **expected** to be sold.

4. APPLICATIONS

4.1 Screening Tests

Symptom(s) is(are) used to for diagnosis of a disease and hence, can be considered for purposes of Statistics as a 'screening test'. Ideally, **predictive value (PV)** of any screening test (symptom/s included) should be as high as possible in either case; that means, a screening test should be able to identify either the presence of the disease or absence of the disease to be useful under practical situations.

Therefore, the following criteria are also measured:

4.1.1 Terminologies

4.1.1.1 Sensitivity

Sensitivity of a screening test (symptom) is the **probability** that the symptom is present given that the person has the disease. If A = symptom and B = disease, predictive vale positive, **PV⁺ = P(B/A) and P(A/B) = Sensitivity.**

4.1.1.2 Specificity

Specificity of a screening test (symptom) is the **probability** that the symptom is not present given that the person does not have the disease. If A = symptom and B = disease, predictive vale negative, **PV⁻ = P(Bᶜ/Aᶜ) and P(Aᶜ/Bᶜ) = Specificity;** where ᶜ **indicates the complement of the respective events.**

4.1.1.3 False positive ad false negative

If the screening test indicates presence of a disease when the disease is not actually present, it is called **false positive** and *vice versa*.

Any screening test to be effective in predicting (diagnosing) a disease must have both sensitivity and specificity as high as possible.

4.1.1.4 Prevalence

Prevalence of a disease is the **probability** of the animal currently having the disease regardless of the duration of actually having it. It is calculated as a simple ratio of number of animals having the disease to that of total number of animals in the population under study.

2.1.1.5 Incidence

(Cumulative) incidence of a disease is the **probability** that an animal, not suffering earlier with the disease, will develop the disease over a specified period of time.

4.1.2 Estimation of PV

If A = symptom/Screening test, B = disease, and probability of the disease in reference population = P(B), we know from the above that $PV^+ = P(B/A)$. Designating P(B) as x, and substituting sensitivity for P(A/B) and specificity for $P(A^c/B^c)$ in the Bayes' rule, we get

$$P(B/A) = PV^+ = \frac{P(A/B) \times P(B)}{P(A/B)P(B) + P(A/B^c)P(B^c)}$$

$$= \frac{\text{Sensitivity} \times x}{\text{Sensitivity} \times x + (1 - \text{Specificity})(1-x)}; \text{ similarly,}$$

$$P(B^c/A^c) = PV^- = \frac{\text{Specificity} \times (1-x)}{\text{Specificity} \times (1-x) + (1 - \text{Sensitivity}) \times x}$$

Therefore, it can be noted that predictive value (either positive or negative) is a function of sensitivity, specificity and probability of the disease in the reference population. Let us take an example to elucidate the concept of PV of a test:

4.1.2.1 Example

Tuberculin test which is used to diagnose TB in animals. Let us assume that it identifies 60% of diseased and 35% of normal animals as positive and that 8% of milch animals in the population do have TB.

Given: Sensitivity = 0.60, Specificity = 1 – 0.35 = 0.65, x = 0.08; therefore,

PV^+ = (0.60 × 0.08) ÷ [(0.60 × 0.08) + (0.35 × 0.92)] = 0.1297 and

PV^- = (0.65 × 0.92) ÷ [(0.65 × 0.92) + (0.40 × 0.08)] = 0.9492 which indicates that the Tuberculin test is more efficient to predict absence rather than presence of TB in milch animals. In other words, it is not reliable for diagnosis of presence of TB in milch animals.

4.2 Risk Analysis

Details of risk analysis are given in Chapter "**Statistics in specific veterinary fields**" and hence, only definitions are given below:

4.2.1 Risk Difference and Ratio

If P_x is the probability of developing disease in exposed animals and p_y in unexposed animals, then, **risk difference** is the difference and **risk ratio** is the ratio between the two probabilities (p_y as denominator).

4.2.2 Odds Ratio

In general, if p is the probability of success, ratio of p to $(1 - p)$ is referred to as odds in favor of success.

If p_f odds in favor of disease in exposed animals and p_g is that in unexposed group, odds ratio is the ratio of the former to the latter.

4.3   Animal Genetics

Qualitative (Mendelian) Genetics has several applications of probability concepts; the details are given in Chapter "**Statistics in specific veterinary fields**".

5

Discrete Probability Distributions

If $X_1, X_2, X_3 \ldots X_n$ are n discrete random variables with probability value of $p_1, p_2, p_3 \ldots$ p_n, respectively, with the condition that $\sum_{i=1}^{n} p_i = 1$, then the distribution of the random variable is said to be defined with a probability function, $\sum_{i=1}^{n} P(X_i) = \sum_{i=1}^{n} p_i = 1$. If frequency in the observed distribution table is replaced by the corresponding probability, probability distribution is obtained; if it is based on the observed data, it is referred to as **observed frequency distribution**; alternatively, if it is based on the mathematically derived (expected) frequencies, it is called **theoretical (expected) probability (frequency) distribution**.

The expected probability of hatching of two eggs discussed in Chapter "Probabilty" falls under the theoretical probability distribution with the probability function $\sum_{i=1}^{n} P(X_i) =$ ¼ + ½ + ¼ = 1. If the random variable is discrete, as in this case, the probability function is called **probability mass function**; if it is continuous, it is called **probability density function**.

The popular theoretical distributions are:
I. Discrete distributions
  1. Binomial (Bernoulli) distribution
  2. Negative binomial distribution
  3. Multinomial distribution
  4. Poisson distribution
  5. Hyper-geometric distribution
II. Continuous distribution
  1. Normal distribution
  2. Student's t distribution
  3. χ^2 distribution
  4. F distribution

Of the discrete distributions, binomial and poisson distributions are more popular than the rest.

1. BINOMIAL DISTRIBUTION

As discussed in Chapter **"Probability"**, if p is the probability of success and q that of failure of a binomial/mutually exclusive event, the probability of getting r successes out of n trials can be obtained by $^{n}C_{r}p^{r}q^{(n-r)}$. It is easy to calculate the value of coefficients of each of the terms by evaluating the respective $^{n}C_{r}$ (*see* Appendix 5.1 for details). Otherwise Pascal's triangle can also be used as a ready reckoner; Pascal's triangle up to $n = 10$ is reproduced below:

n							Pascal's triangle Binomial coefficients							Sum
1							1	1						2
2						1	2	1						4
3					1	3	3	1						8
4				1	4	6	4	1						16
5			1	5	10	10	5	1						32
6		1	6	15	20	15	6	1						64
7	1	7	21	35	35	21	7	1						128
8	1	8	28	56	70	56	28	8	1					256
9	1	9	36	84	126	126	84	36	9	1				512
10	1	10	45	120	210	252	210	120	45	10	1			1024

Construction of Pascal's triangle:

1. First and last terms are always unity
2. Subsequent terms are obtained by adding the two terms on either side in the row above it. For example, consider the last row; 2nd term is obtained by adding 1st and the 2nd terms $(1 + 9 = 10)$ of the preceding row which lie on its either side; similarly, 3rd term $= (9 + 36) = 45$ and so on.

It can be seen from the above coefficients that if $p = \frac{1}{2}$, the binomial distribution is symmetric; if $p > \frac{1}{2}$, the distribution will be skewed to the left and *vice versa*.

Mean of the binomial distribution is given by np and variance by npq. With a large n, and neither p nor q approaching zero, binomial variable (X) can be approximated (standardized) to a Normal variable by $z = \dfrac{X - np}{\sqrt{npq}}$.

1.1. Example

In a dairy farm, there is a possibility that 40% of workers develop allergy to animal odors. If there are 6 workers, we are interested to know the probability that not more than 2 of them would develop allergy.

Obviously, we have to estimate probability of 0, 1 and 2 persons developing allergy given $p = 0.40$, $q = 0.60$, $n = 6$ and $r = 0$, 1 and 2; i.e. to add the first 3 terms of the expansion $(q + p)^6$ or $q^6 + 6pq^5 + 15p^2q^4 = 0.5443$ suggesting that half of the workers are likely to show allergy.

1.2. Example

An exporting firm receives eggs and accepts a batch of eggs when a sample of 6 eggs drawn contains not more than 1 defective egg. It is also known that 3% defective eggs are expected in consignments. We have to estimate the probability that a sample is accepted.

The data given are: $p = 0.03$, $n = 6$ and $r = 0$ and 1. If $r > 1$, the consignment is rejected. Hence, we need to add first two terms of $(q + p)^6$ or $q^6 + 6pq^5 = 0.9875$ indicating that on 98.75% occasions, the consignment will be accepted.

1.3. Fitting a Binomial Distribution

Fitting a Binomial distribution is not a common practice by animal science workers. Even if it is required, p (or q) and n will be available. With those, it is easy to calculate each of the terms of the expansion $(q + p)^n$ for number (frequency) of successes (r) taking values 0, 1, 2 ... n. Value obtained for each of the terms is the *expected frequency* for the respective number of successes. If *actual frequencies* are available, the **goodness of fit** of the distribution can be tested (*see* Chapters "**Tests of hypothesis**" for details).

1.3.1. Example

A whole-sale dealer of eggs recorded the following number of broken eggs in cartons received. Further, probability of eggs being broken is 10%. Hence, in this case, $p = 0.1$ ($q = 0.9$) and $n = 5$; we need to find the expected frequency of 0, 1, 2, 3, 4 and 5 broken eggs. They are calculated by evaluating $^5C_r p^r q^{(n-r)}$ for $r = 0, 1, 2, 3, 4$ and 5; they are shown in 3rd row.

No of defective eggs	0	1	2	3	4	5	Total
No of samples	40	34	18	3	3	2	100
Expected probability*	0.5905	0.3281	0.0729	0.0081	0.0004	0.0000	1.0000
Expected No of samples (Whole No)**	59	33	7 ***	1***	–	–	100

* To nearest 4 decimal places

** Calculated as a product of expected probability and total number of samples

*** Pooled for calculation of χ^2 to make expected frequency > 5

$\chi^2 = 46.649$ which is > 3.841, the table value of $\chi^2_{0.05, 1}$ (Appendix 4); hence, the observed frequencies do not appear to follow Binomial distribution (see Chapter "**Tests of Hypotheses**" for details of χ^2 goodness of fit test).

The mean, variance and standard deviation of the above distribution will be np, npq and $\sqrt{npq}$ which will be 10, 9 and 3 samples, respectively.

As indicated in the beginning of the chapter, the 2nd row shows **observed** and the 4th row the **expected** frequency (probability) distribution.

Standard tables giving exact binomial probabilities for different values of p, n and r are available (not provided in this publication) to facilitate fitting of distribution.

2. POISSON DISTRIBUTION

Poisson distribution is distribution of rare events (i.e. $p \rightarrow 0$); for instance, hen laying a 4-yolked egg, a cow calving a triplet of calves, a case of traumatic pericarditis in a cow, etc. Hence, the distribution is otherwise referred to as law of improbable events and recommended when $n \geq 20$ and $p \leq 0.1$. In other words, if $n \rightarrow \infty$ and $p \rightarrow 0$, binomial event becomes a Poisson event.

The probability of r successes of a Poisson event with m being the mean of the poisson distribution and e, the base of the natural logarithm, $P(r) = \dfrac{e^{-m}m^r}{r!}$; mathematical derivation of this equation from binomial expansion can be obtained from relevant books on Mathematical Statistics. Variance of the Poisson distribution is also m (it is understandable that being a distribution of rare events, variability will also be high).

2.1. Applications

Poisson distribution is useful in study of incidence of a disease, microbiological studies on bacterial growth, etc. While studying incidence of a disease, the following assumptions are made:

1. P(death) directly proportional (α) to time interval; from time 0 to time t, which is made of several small intervals, denoted Δt during which interval death occurs. That means, P(death) = $\lambda\Delta t$, where λ is an unknown constant. Hence, it follows that (a) P(no death) during $\Delta t = 1 - \lambda\Delta t$, (b) P($>$ 1 death) during $\Delta t = 0$ and mean, $m = \lambda t$ where λ is the expected number of events per unit time (Δt) and m is the expected number of events over the given time t.

2. Number of deaths per unit time is constant throughout t; therefore, t should neither be too large nor too small.

3. Death occurring in one Δt has no bearing on the preceding or the succeeding Δt; that is, death during any of the Δt's is independent of one another. This condition is clearly violated during an epidemic and hence, Poisson distribution is invalid for epidemics.

Note: The meaning of t changes depending on the variable; for example, if we are dealing with growth of bacterial colonies on an agar plate, t will mean total area available for bacteria and so on.

2.1.1. Example

Suppose number of dogs dying due to rabies in a year is a Poisson event with a mean of 9. Let us find out the probability distribution of deaths due to rabies over a 6-month period.

Given m for 1 year as 9 (λt where $t = 1$ year); therefore, for 6 months, $m = 4.5$. Since only m is required to calculate expected values, the following table gives expected probabilities for $r = 0, 1, 2, 3, 4, 5$ and ≥ 6 months by substituting relevant values in the formula $P(r) = \dfrac{e^{-m}m^r}{r!}$.

Month	0	1	2	3	4	5	≥ 6	Total
Probability*	0.0111	0.0500	0.1125	0.1687	0.1898	0.1708	0.2971	1
Frequency**	–	–	1	1.5	2	1.5	3	9

* To nearest 4 decimal places

** Calculated as a product of expected probability and total number of deaths

2.1.2. Example

Let us assume that an agar plate of diameter 7 cm [area (A) 154 cm²] is available and P(bacterial colony at any point) is low (Poisson variable) and that of finding in any two points is independent, the number of bacterial colonies on the agar plate becomes a Poisson variable. Clearly, in this case, $t = A = 154$ cm²; if we assume that P(a colony in a small area) $= \lambda \Delta A$ with $\lambda = 0.05$ colonies/cm², we get $m = \lambda A = 0.05 \times 154 = 7.7$. Let us find out the expected distribution of 0, 1, 2, 3, 4, 5 and > 5 bacterial colonies (these are r values).

Colonies, r	0	1	2	3	4	5	≥ 6	Total
Probability*	0.0005	0.0035	0.0134	0.0345	0.0663	0.1021	0.7797	1

* To nearest 4 decimal places

2.2. Fitting a Poisson Distribution

The procedure is similar to that of binomial distribution with change in formula to the one shown above for calculating expected frequencies.

The mean, variance and standard deviation of poisson distribution will be m, m and $\sqrt{m}$ which, in the above example, will be 7.7, 7.7 and 2.7749 colonies/cm², respectively.

2.2.1. Example

The number of resistant colony of *E.coli* with respective frequency is given below:

No. of resistant colonies (r_i)	No. of Petri dishes (f_i)	$\Sigma f_i r_i$	$f_i \left(\dfrac{e^{-m} m^r}{r!} \right)$
0	98	0	94.65
1	40	40	43.50
2	8	16	10.02 *
3	3	9	1.50 *
4	1	4	0.30 *
Totals	150	69	149.97 **

* Pooled for calculation of χ^2 to make expected frequency > 5

** Difference in total due to approximation error

$\chi^2 = 0.433$ which is < 3.841, the table value of $\chi^2_{0.05, 1}$ (Appendix 4) hence, the observed frequencies appear to follow Poisson distribution (*see* Chapter "**Tests of hypotheses**" for details of χ^2 goodness of fit test).

Standard tables giving exact poisson probabilities for different values of m and r are available to facilitate fitting of distribution. The probabilities so obtained are multiplied with corresponding frequencies to get expected frequencies.

Poisson distribution is widely used on data concerning cancer, occupational health, etc. in human beings; the same analogy can be applied in animals as well.

3.   NEGATIVE BINOMIAL DISTRIBUTION

Suppose we have incubated 10 eggs and first 3 eggs didn't hatch; but we are interested in finding the probability that the 4th egg hatches. This event is made of two sub-events (i) probability of k failures and $(r - 1)$ success out of $(r + k - 1)$ trials and (ii) probability of success in the $(r + k)$th trial. The requisite probability can be calculated as $^{r+k-1}C_k p^r q^k$; i.e. probability of $(r + k)$ trials to occur so that rth success to happen or, in the present case, waiting till 4 eggs to hatch/not hatch so that 4th egg hatches. The distribution of k, for a given r and p; the latter being same for each trial, is called negative Binomial distribution which is also referred to as contagious or clustered distribution. Examples where this distribution is likely to be used in animal science are tick infestation in animals, bacterial clumps in a microscopic field, etc.

4.   MULTINOMIAL DISTRIBUTION

As the name indicates, unlike 'bi'nomial having only two possible outcomes, 'Multi'nomial distribution refers to > 2 possible outcomes (say k types of equally probable outcomes) for an event. If $E_1, E_2, E_3 ..., E_k$ are the k events with probability of E_i being p_i (same for each trial) such that $\Sigma p_i = 1$, then the probability of $n_1, n_2, n_3 ..., n_k$ outcomes of types $E_1, E_2, E_3 ..., E_k$ in a total of $n_1 + n_2 + n_3 ... + n_k = n$ independent trials

is given by $\dfrac{n!}{n_1! n_2! n_3! ... n_k!}\left[p_1^{n_1} p_2^{n_2} p_3^{n_3} ... p_k^{n_k} \right]$.

4.1. Example

Suppose coat color in cattle is controlled by a single pair of genes; dominant homozygote (RR) being red, recessive homozygote (rr) being white and the heterozygote (Rr) being Roan in color; and Roan individuals are mated, we need to know the probability of obtaining 6 red, 9 roan and 6 white progeny. The required

probability is given by $\dfrac{20!}{6! 9! 6!}\left[0.25^6\ 0.50^9\ 0.25^6 \right]$ = 0.0015 (for calculation of proba-

bilities of RR, Rr and rr among the progeny, *see* Chapter "**Statistical in specific veterinary fields**").

5.   HYPERGEOMETRIC DISTRIBUTION

Let us consider a hypothetical example of a clinical trial of a new vaccine against a disease which gave the following results:

		Vaccination		Total
		Done	**Not done**	
Disease	Occurred	a	b	R_1
	Did not occur	c	d	R_2
	Total	C_1	C_2	N

Probability that the vaccine is ineffective is given by $\dfrac{C_1!\,C_2!\,R_1!\,R_2!}{N!}\left[\dfrac{1}{a!\,b!\,c!\,d!}\right].$

5.1. Example

Let us consider that in a study on effectiveness of a new vaccine, 25 animals were considered of which 10 were vaccinated and the rest left unvaccinated. If none of the vaccinated and 12 of the unvaccinated animals showed the disease, let us calculate the effectiveness of the vaccine.

		Vaccination		Total
		Done	**Not done**	
Disease	Occurred	0	12	12
	Did not occur	10	3	13
	Total	10	15	25

In this example, a = 0, b = 12, c = 10, d = 3 as laid-out above, and hence, the probability

that vaccine is ineffective = $\dfrac{12!\,13!\,10!\,15!}{25!}\left[\dfrac{1}{0!\,12!\,10!\,3!}\right]$ = 0.0001 indicating that the

vaccine was indeed effective with a probability of (1 – 0.0001) = 0.9999 or 99.99%.

Hyper-geometric distribution is also frequently used in studies on wild birds (population, catching, nesting, etc.).

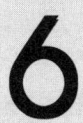

6

Continuous Probability Distributions

1. NORMAL DISTRIBUTION

Binomial distribution tends to become a continuous distribution as $p \to \frac{1}{2}$ and $n \to \infty$. That is, if the sample size is large and expected frequency for both "success" and "failure" is intermediate, the distribution of expected probabilities will tend to be continuous, symmetric and bell-shaped. Similarly, as value of $m \to \infty$, Poisson distribution (since n is already very large) also tends to become a continuous distribution. The continuous distribution is commonly referred to as **Normal distribution** and also as normal probability distribution or Normal frequency curve or Gaussian distribution or Gaussian Law of Error.

In case of Binomial distribution it can be shown that even if p and q are not equal (i.e. $p = q = \frac{1}{2}$), with a large n itself, the distribution becomes Normal.

1.1 Example

Let us find out binomial probabilities for hatching of 10 eggs; i.e. $n = 10$, $r = 0, 1, 2, 3 \ldots$ 10 and $p = q = \frac{1}{2}$. As indicated in the Chapter **"Probability"**, the above can be obtained by expansion of the binomial equation $(p + q)^{10}$. The expected frequencies are as follows:

r	^nC_r	$p^r q^{(n-r)}$	$^nC_r p^r q^{(n-r)}$
0	1		0.0010
1	10		0.0098
2	45		0.0439
3	120		0.1172
4	210		0.2051
5	252	0.000977*	**0.2461**
6	210		0.2051
7	120		0.1172
8	45		0.0439
9	10		0.0098
10	1		0.0010
Total	1024		1.0001

1. $p = q = \frac{1}{2}$; hence, $p^r q^{(n-r)} = p^{10}$ or $(\frac{1}{2})^{10} = 0.000977$ for all cases
2. Values approximated to 4 decimal places; hence the total is 1.0001

If the above probabilities are plotted with r on x-axis and $^nC_r p^r q^{(n-r)}$ on the y-axis, and the points are joined by a smooth curve, a symmetric, bell-shaped curve results. It is also easy to visualize that as n increases, the probabilities assume all values within a range and hence become a continuous variable. Mean of the above distribution (np) = 5, variance (npq) is 2.5 and standard deviation 1.5811. It can also be seen that mode is also 5 as is the median.

It is very important to note that not **all bell-shaped curves are normal and only** **that curve whose height (y_i) at x_i is given by** $y_i = \dfrac{1}{\sigma\sqrt{2\pi}} e^{-\frac{1}{2}\left(\frac{x_i-\mu}{\sigma}\right)^2}$ **is the normal curve** **where μ is the mean, σ is the standard deviation with mathematical constants e (base of natural logarithm, 2.7183) and π (ratio of circumference to diameter of a circle, 3.1428). The y_i, the height of the curve, is usually called normal density and it is not a frequency** (*see* Fig. 6.1).

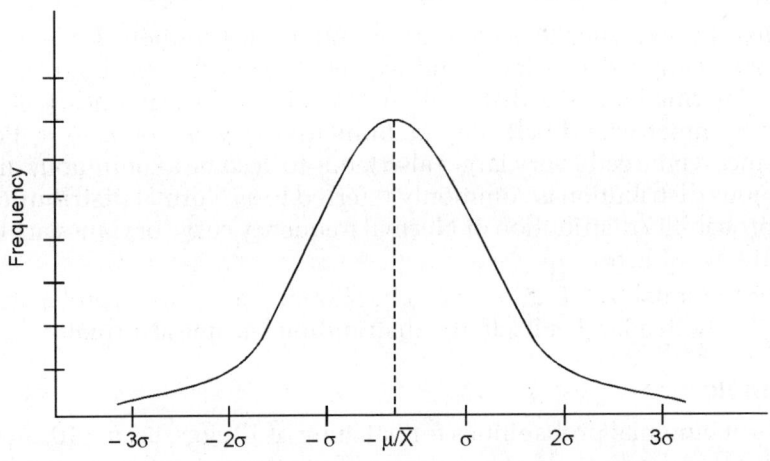

Fig. 6.1: Normal distribution

The equation clearly reveals that infinite number of normal curves is possible for a given μ depending on σ and *vice versa*. Therefore, it is rather impossible to develop standard tables for all possible normal distributions. This problem is solved by changing origin and/or scale (referred to as **Z scale**) to obtain a normal distribution curve with $\mu = 0$ and $\sigma = 1$; such a normal curve with mean 0 and unit standard deviation is called **standardized or standard normal curve on Z scale** (*see* Fig 6.2)

The formula for converting x-scale to Z-scale is obviously $z = \dfrac{x-\mu}{\sigma}$ (called **Z-transformation**) and replacing this in the density function we get density function for a standard normal curve as $y_i = \dfrac{1}{\sigma\sqrt{2\pi}} e^{-\frac{z_i^2}{2}}$. Standard table giving area under standard normal curve, called **Z–table** is available for calculations (*see* Appendices 1 and 2).

In the **Example 1.2.2.1** (Chapter "**Central tendency**"), $\overline{X}$ =10.70 g and s = 1.611 g. Let us now find out the number of eggs weighing between 8 g and 12 g by use of Z-table (Appendix 1):

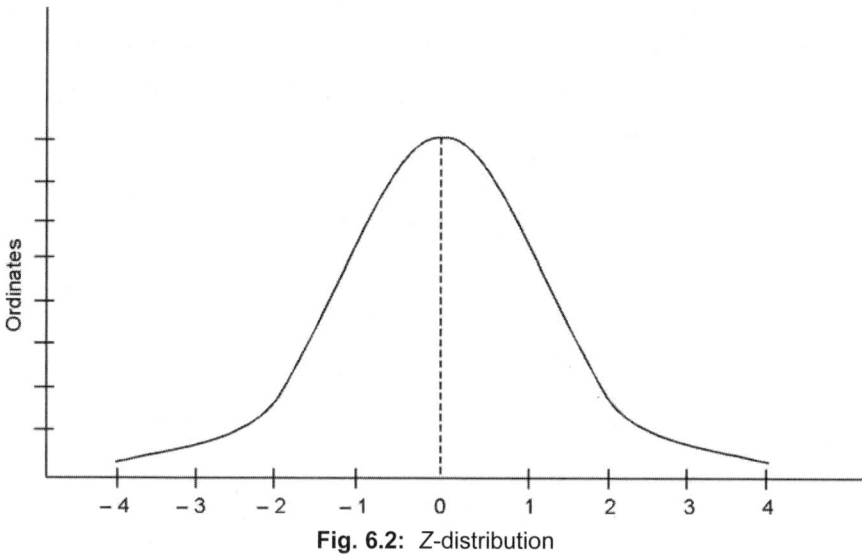

Fig. 6.2: Z-distribution

Given: $\mu = 10.70$ g, $\sigma = 1.611$ g, $x_1 = 8$ g and $x_2 = 12$ g. Hence, area between x_1 and x_2 is the required solution. Converting x values to corresponding Z values by the formula

$Z = \dfrac{x - \mu}{\sigma}$, we get $Z_1 = -1.676$ and $Z_2 = 0.807$. From Appendix 1, we get corresponding

area as 0.4535 or 45.35% and 0.2910 or 29.10%, respectively (*see* Fig. 6.3); hence, totally 74.45% of eggs are weighing between 8 g and 12 g. Since total eggs were 350, 260.575 (or 261) eggs are expected to weigh in this range. Actually 260 eggs were weighing between 8 and 12 g.

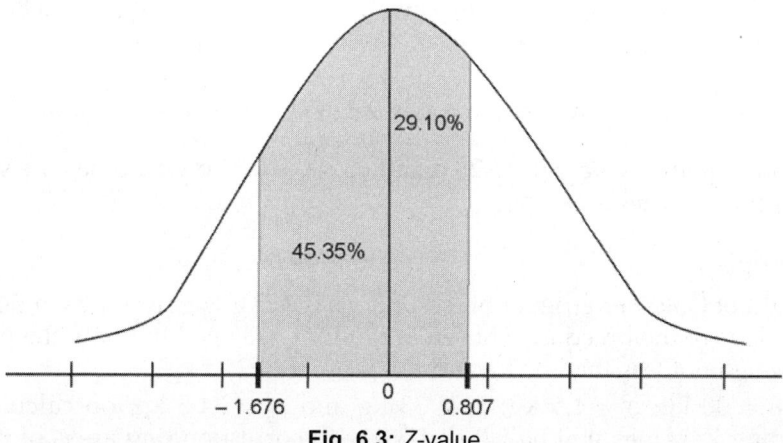

Fig. 6.3: Z-value

Let us calculate the egg weight range, on either side of $\overline{X}$, that will contain 80% of eggs in the above example:

Given: $\mu = 10.70$ g, $\sigma = 1.611$ g, $Z_1 + Z_2 = 0.8$ or 0.4 on either side of mean ($= 0$). From table given in Appendix 1, locating 0.4 in the body of the table, we get the Z-values as

– 1.28 and + 1.28 (*see* Fig 6.4). Since $Z = \dfrac{x-\mu}{\sigma}$, $x = \mu - Z\sigma$ and $\mu + Z\sigma$. Replacing $\mu = 10.70$ g and $\sigma = 1.611$ g, we get the sesired solution; i.e. 80% of eggs are likely to weigh between 8.64 g and 12.76 g.

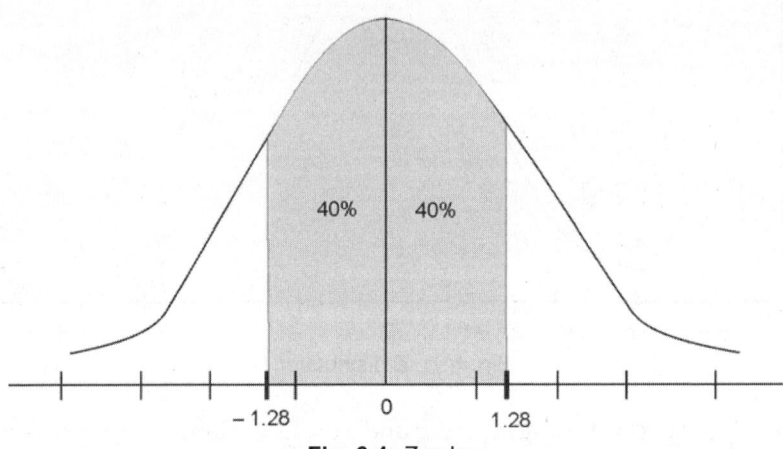

Fig. 6.4: Z-value

1.2 Example

A large flock of white leghorn layers produce 10 % of eggs < 45 g and 20% eggs > 60 g. Assuming egg weight follow Normal distribution, let us deduce mean and standard deviation of the eggs produced by the flock: (*see* Appendix 1 for Z table).

Assuming mean = μ and standard deviation = σ, since 10% of eggs were below 45 g, 40% of eggs must be weighing between μ and 45 g; the corresponding Z–value for 40% = –1.28. Similarly, since 20% of eggs weigh > 60 g, 30% of eggs must be weighing between μ and 60 g; the corresponding Z – being 0.84 (*see* Fig 6.4).

Since $Z = \dfrac{x-\mu}{\sigma}$, it follows that $x = \mu + Z\sigma$. Replacing x and Z values, we get 2 simultaneous equations: $45 = \mu - 1.28\,\sigma$ and $60 = \mu + 0.84\,\sigma$ which has the solution as $\mu = 54.06$ g and $\sigma = 7.08$ g.

1.3 Example

Adult weight of Golden Retriever breed of dogs is 30 kg with a standard deviation of 1.5 kg. If 2 dogs of the breed are chosen at random, we need to know the probability that they weigh not less than 33 kg and not more that 34.5 kg.

Given: $\mu = 30$ kg, $\sigma = 1.5$ kg, $x_1 = 33$ kg and $x_2 = 34.5$ kg; on calculation, the corresponding Z–values will be 2.0 and 3.0 with corresponding areas of 0.4772 and 0.4987 (*see* Fig 6.5). In other words, 47.72% dogs weigh between 30 and 33 kg whereas 49.87% weigh between 30 and 34.5 kg; the latter includes the former also. Therefore, probability of dogs weighing between 33 and 34.5 kg = (0.4987 – 0.4772) = 0.0215 or 2.15%.

Utility of standard normal curve (standard normal deviate, **Z**) will also be discussed in Chapter **"Tests of hypotheses"**

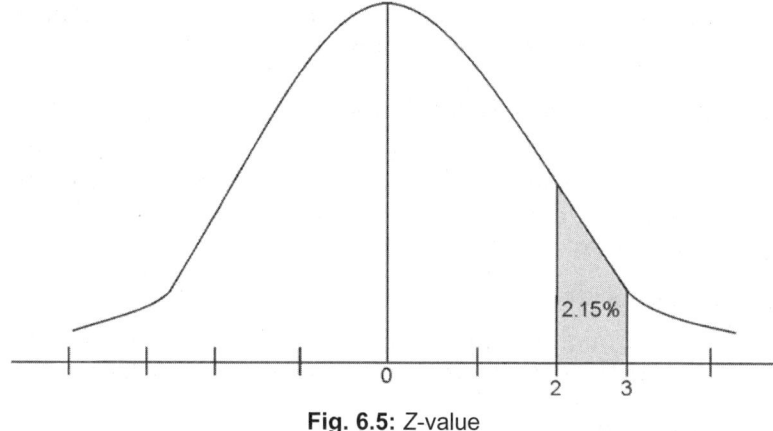

Fig. 6.5: Z-value

Mean, variance and standard deviation of normal distribution are $\overline{X}$, σ^2 and σ, respectively. μ_3, μ_4, β_1(coefficient of skewness) and β_2(Coefficient of kurtosis) are 0, $3\sigma^4$, 0 and 3, respectively.

1.4 Why is Normal Distribution so Important?

1.4.1 Central Limit Theorem

As sample size (n) increases, the distribution of means of samples from not only Normal distribution but also from any population (distribution) tends to become Normal; in other words, distribution of sample means, regardless of the nature of the distribution of the population, tends to be Normal. Central limit theorem is applicable to median and standard deviation also.

Further, if all possible samples, each of size n are drawn from any population (whose variance is σ^2) is given by (σ^2/n); it is, obviously, the variance of mean of means or simply **variance of mean**. The square root of variance of means or standard deviation of mean of means or simply standard deviation of means is popularly referred to as **standard error of mean** or **standard error** (*see* Chapter **"Dispersion"** also).

1.4.2 Limits for Population Values

With the assumption that the variable is normally distributed, it is very easy to find the limits for population values as follows (*see* Fig 6.1):

Limits	Z value *	% of measurements
$\mu \pm 0.67\ \sigma$	±0.67	50.00
$\mu \pm 1.00\ \sigma$	±1.00	68.27
$\mu \pm 1.96\ \sigma$	±1.96	95.00
$\mu \pm 2.00\ \sigma$	±2.00	95.44
$\mu \pm 2.24\ \sigma$	±2.24	97.50
$\mu \pm 2.58\ \sigma$	±2.58	99.00
$\mu \pm 2.81\ \sigma$	±2.81	99.50
$\mu \pm 3.00\ \sigma$	±3.00	99.73
$\mu \pm 3.29\ \sigma$	±3.29	99.90

* Area under standard normal curve

The above property is extremely useful to characterize the population, testing of hypotheses, etc. They will be discussed in subsequent chapters.

1.4.3 Simplified Calculation Procedures

As discussed already, as n increases, it is generally acceptable to assume Normal distribution which saves the laborious calculations needed for discrete distributions. In certain situations, it may not be possible to obtain any solution without assuming normality of distribution.

1.4.3.1 Z–transformation

As discussed above through examples, converting Normal variable into standard Normal variable makes it extremely easy to calculate area/ordinates of the distribution.

1.4.4 Nature of Distribution of Variables

It is generally accepted that most, though not all, variables in nature are normally distributed and hence, assumption of normality is a necessity with little possibility of incorrect inference.

1.5 Fitting a Normal Distribution

Generally, fitting of normal distribution to animal science data is not a common practice. If one is interested, the procedure is as follows:

In the **Example 1.2.2.1** (Chapter "**Central tendency**"), $\overline{X}$ =10.70 g and s = 1.611 g.

Considering each of the class limits as x_i's, we can calculate $z_i = \dfrac{x_i - \overline{X}}{s}$ and find out

the corresponding expected proportions, p_U and p_L; the difference between the latter two gives the expected proportion for the class interval and when multiplied by the total frequency, we get the expected frequency. The following table gives the details:

Egg weight class (g)	No of eggs (f_i)	$Z_i = \dfrac{x_i - \overline{X}}{s}$		$p_i = \lvert Z_U - Z_L \rvert$	Expected frequency ($f_e = p_i \times \Sigma f_i$)
		Z_L	Z_U		
6.0–7.0	5	−2.92	−2.30	0.0089	3.12
7.0–8.0	15	−2.30	−1.68	0.0358	12.53
8.0–9.0	30	−1.68	−1.06	0.0981	34.34
9.0–10.0	50	−1.06	−0.43	0.1890	66.15
10.0–11.0	110	−0.43	0.19	0.2417**	84.60
11.0–12.0	70	0.19	0.81	0.2157	75.50
12.0–13.0	40	0.81	1.43	0.1326	46.41
13.0–14.0	25	1.43	2.05	0.0562	19.67
14.0–15.0	5	2.05	2.67	0.0164	5.74
Total	350			0.9944***	348.06***

** $p_i = Z_U + Z_L$ because of change from left to right of $Z = 0$.

*** Difference due to approximation

$$\chi^2 = \sum_{i=1}^{k} \frac{f_i^2}{f_e} - \sum_{i=1}^{k} f_i = 18.092$$ on (k-1-m) d.f, where k = No. of classes (9), m = No. of

parameters fit (2); i.e. on 6 d.f. The calculated value is > table value of χ^2 (Appendix 4); hence, the sample data is not likely to have come from a Normal distribution whose $\overline{X}$ =10.70 g and s = 1.611 g.

1.6 Testing Normality of Distribution

Methods are developed for testing normality of population distribution. They are not discussed here for the following reasons:
1. The methods are laborious and time-consuming but still not adequate.
2. It is not generally necessary because assumption of normality will not distort conclusions to an extent that warrants testing for normality.
3. Validity of central limit theorem obviates any shortcoming(s) due to assumption of normality of distribution.

Coefficient of skewness (β_1) and kurtosis (β_2) serve as quick measures of normality of a distribution on many occasions. In **Example 1.2.2.1** (Chapter "**Central tendency**"), skewness (β_1) and kurtosis are 0.516 and 3.875 as against the standard values of 0 and 3 for normal distribution, respectively. Hence, the distribution is slightly skewed and slightly leptokurtic.

2. STUDENT'S t DISTRIBUTION

Mr W.S. Gosset under pen-name "Student" published the distribution of ratio of deviation of sample mean from population mean (i.e. ($\overline{X}$ - μ)) to the standard error of the sample mean (i.e. $s/\sqrt{n}$). It can be easily recognized that the computation of t values is similar to those of Z, save the non-availability of σ which is replaced by s. Thus, this distribution is of great value for statistical inference from small samples. The t distribution is symmetric and dependent on degrees of freedom, υ; as υ increases, t – distribution → Z–distribution. Appendix 3 gives table values for calculations involving the distribution.

3. CHI-SQUARE (χ^2) DISTRIBUTION

If $x_1, x_2, x_3 \ldots, x_n$ are randomly drawn from a normal population, χ^2 is the distribution of their respective $[(n-1)s^2 \div \sigma^2]$ on $(n-1)$ degrees of freedom (υ). It is also a distribution of sum of squares of independent standard normal deviates; i.e. $\chi^2 = Z_1^2 + Z_2^2 + Z_3^2 \ldots + Z_n^2$.

χ^2 distribution is a continuous but non-symmetric or non-central which is dependent on degrees of freedom, υ. Appendix 4 gives table values for calculations involving the distribution.

4. F-DISTRIBUTION

This is the distribution of variance ratio consisting of family of distributions which are dependent on the degrees of freedom of variances in both numerator and denominator; the former designated υ_1 and the latter υ_2. This distribution, similar to χ^2 distribution, is also continuous but non-symmetric or non-central. Appendix 5 gives table values for calculations involving the distribution.

7

Tests of Hypotheses
(For One and Two Samples)

An experiment is conducted obviously to draw conclusion(s) (**Statistical inference**) about the selected variable in a sample or a population; on most occasions, the latter may not be possible. Further, before going in for statistical maneuvers, the statistician will assume (hypothesize) certain inferences whose validity will have to be ascertained by suitable statistical procedures. These procedures (tests) are referred to as **Tests of hypotheses**. In addition, the confidence with which the inferences are drawn is equally important while drawing conclusion on any hypothesis. This aspect, which is an integral part of testing hypotheses, is referred to as **Tests of significance**.

Therefore, statistical inference can be classified into the following two main categories:

1. Statistical inference about a population, called **Hypothesis testing which includes tests of significance**
2. Statistical inference about the reliability/suitability/acceptability of a Statistic calculated from a sample as an estimate of an unknown Parameter–referred to as **Estimation**.

1. HYPOTHESIS TESTING

1.1 Setting-up Hypotheses

A hypothesis is an assumption made about a population for further confirmation by proper statistical procedures. For instance, a flock of WL produce at an average of 295 eggs per annum (sample mean, $\overline{X}$) and we would like to know whether the sample is a subset of (drawn from) a population of WL whose μ is 308 eggs.

It is universally accepted to make two hypotheses namely

1. Null hypothesis designated $\mathbf{H_0}$ which always assumes that there is no difference between sample and population; whatever difference exists is due to **chance** primarily due to sampling. In the above example, it means that the flock is actually from the same population but during sampling, birds to the left of μ are selected; but, are close enough to the μ to consider it as a representative of μ. Hence, Null hypothesis is also referred to as **hypothesis of no difference**. Further, H_0 in this case will be $\mu = \overline{X}$.

2. Alternate hypothesis designated H_A which can vary depending on the experimental conditions but always counters the H_0. Let us consider some of the H_A possible: (i) $\mu \# \overline{X}$, (ii) $\mu < \overline{X}$ and (iii) $\mu > \overline{X}$.

1.2 Setting-up Level of Significance

Now, another factor comes into picture; the confidence with which the scientist can accept or reject H_0. This is referred to as **level of significance**. In the above example, let us assume that level of significance is 5%; it means the experimenter is having a risk of rejecting H_0 (i.e. $\mu = \overline{X}$) when it is actually true (incorrect rejection). In other words, the conclusion is likely to be true 95 times out of 100 such samples. The probability (0.05 in this case) of incorrect rejection of H_0 is called **Type-I error (α)**. It is a common practice to fix α at 5% (0.05) or 1% (0.01).

Conversely, it is also possible that H_0 is accepted when it is actually false; this is also referred to as **Type-II error (β)**. A good statistical tool (test) should be able to effectively detect inconsistency of H_0 and hence **$(1 - \beta)$** is often referred to as **power of test** (probability of correct rejection of H_0). The following table summarizes the above discussion:

	H_0 **is True**	H_0 **is False**
Reject H_0	Type-I error (α)	No error $(1 - \beta)$
Accept H_0	No error	Type-II error (β)

1.2.1 α Vs β

Ideally, for any test both α and β should be as low as possible. But, it is clear from the above table that for a test to be very powerful, level of significance has to be increased from the usual 95% or 99% ($\alpha = 0.05$ or 0.01) to 99.9% or even 99.99% ($\alpha = 0.1$ or 0.01); in other words, to reduce β, α has to be increased and *vice versa*.

However, it is equally obvious that accepting H_0 when it is false is more serious (β) than rejecting when it is true (α). Hence, it is a universal practice to fix α or level of significance or size of rejection (critical) region; generally, α is fixed at 5% or 1% (probability 0.05 or 0.01) which also means that chance of accepting a true H_0 is 95% or 99% (probability 0.95 or 0.99).

1.2.2 Interpretation

Interpretation of the calculated value of the statistic *vis-à-vis* table value is summarized below:

Condition, ignoring sign	Interpretation at given Level of significance (α)
Calculated value < Table value *	The observed difference is likely to be due to sampling fluctuation; H_0 may be accepted
Calculated value ≥ Table value *	The observed difference is not likely to be due to sampling fluctuation; H_0 may not be accepted

* *see* Appendices

1.2.2.1 Single-tailed test *vs* two-tailed test

Assuming that we are interested to test sample $\overline{X}$ as an estimator of population $\overline{X} = \mu$; i.e. $H_0: = \mu$. The following HA are possible:

1. $H_A: \overline{X} \# \mu$; in this case, it does not specify whether $\overline{X} < \mu$ or $\overline{X} > \mu$; therefore, it is necessary that, rejection region must be set at both ends or tails of the curve equally, halving the level of significance (α). Hence, the name **Two-tailed test**. σ is the standard deviation of the sample (*see* Fig. 7.1).

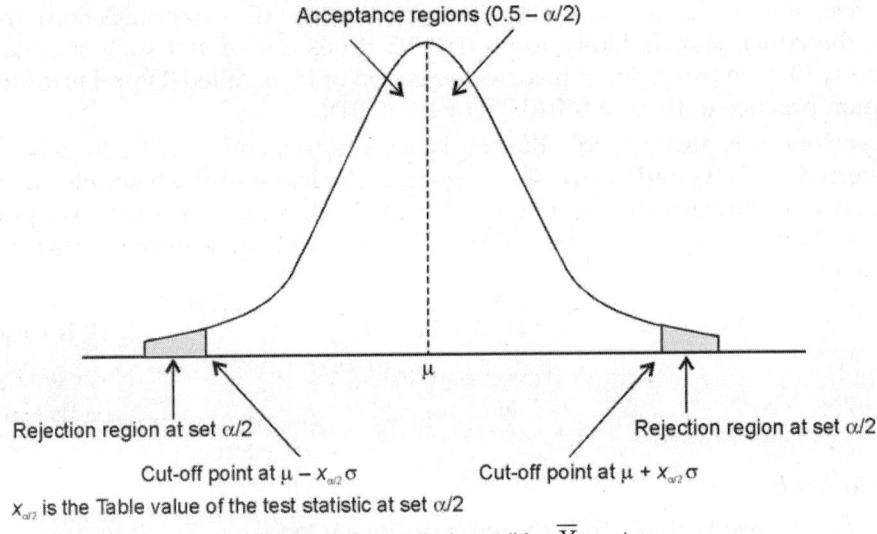

Fig. 7.1: Two-tailed test ($H_A: \overline{X} \neq \mu$)

2. $H_A: \overline{X} > \mu$ or $\overline{X} < \mu$; In this case, either the right-hand side or the left-hand side of the curve are involved, respectively. Hence, the name **Single-tailed test**. σ is the standard deviation of the sample (*see* Fig. 7.2).

1.2.2.2 Statistical *vis-à-vis* practical significance

When sample size is very large, the denominator of the variance (standard deviation) increases thereby reducing the magnitude of s^2; since variance forms a part of the denominator in all tests of hypotheses, even very small differences between the means (which forms the numerator) results in higher value of the calculated statistic making it **statistically significant**. The converse is true with very small samples; resulting in large differences not detected statistically to be true difference. It is generally agreed that when the calculated value of the test statistic is < the table value at set α (usually 0.05 or occasionally, 0.01) merely indicates that the H_0 is likely to be true; on the other hand, if calculated value of the test statistic is > the table value, **it is reasonable to state H_0 is rejected**. In addition, practical utility/importance of the difference that is detected significant or otherwise has to be kept in mind while making a conclusion. Readers desirous of more information on this aspect are advised to refer to other publications dedicated to **statistical decision theory**.

Hence, it is apt to state **sample means are significantly different but not population means are significantly different** because, the latter can only be **practically different or not different**. Samples drawn from population are only *suggestive* whether the population means are different or not. As a general rule, if the sample size is large enough (say about 30) and observed difference is of practical value, it must be considered important and to accept H_0, under such circumstance, should be with a cautious note.

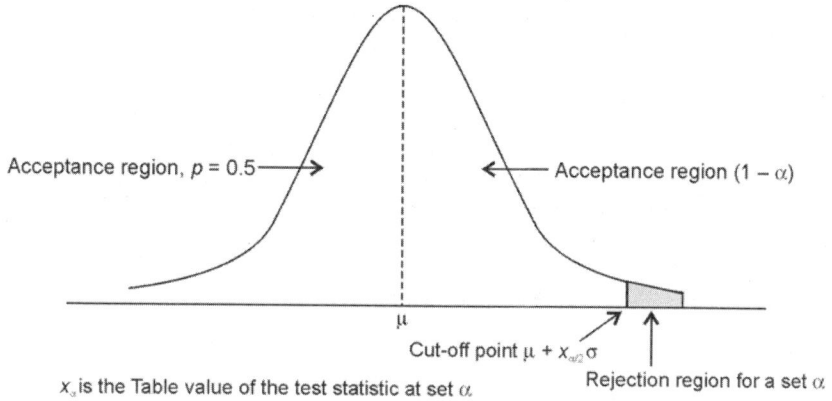

Fig. 7.2: One-tailed test ($H_A: > \mu$)

Generally, value of **x** for two-tailed test is 1.96 and 2.58 for an α of 0.05 and 0.01, respectively; the corresponding values for the single-tailed test are 1.645 and 2.227.

1.2.3 Power of a Test

Any test of significance is expected to reject H_0 whenever it is false; in other words, the test should be powerful enough to detect inconsistency of H_0. $(1 - \beta)$ is the area of the distribution curve of mean under H_A left over after it is intersected by the distribution curve of mean under H_0.

Let us revisit the **Example 1.2.2.1** (Chapter "**Central tendency**") on weight of Japanese quail eggs and run a test of significance with $H_0 : \mu = 10.80$ g and $H_A: \mu \#$ 10.80 g (i.e. a two-tailed test). The $= 10.70$ g, $s = 1.611$g and $n = 350$; the Z-test is as follows with α set at 0.05 for which table value of $Z_{0.975} = 1.96$:

1. Converting ($\overline{X} - \mu$) into a standard normal deviate (Z) by $z = \dfrac{\overline{X} - \mu}{s / \sqrt{n}} = \dfrac{\sqrt{n}(\overline{X} - \mu)}{s}$.

Since $s \div \sqrt{n} = 0.086$, we get the calculated value of Z as $(10.70 - 10.80) \div 0.086 = -1.161$. Since the calculated value < table value, H_0 is acceptable. From Appendix 6.1, the corresponding probability for $Z = 0$ to 1.161 is obtained as 0.355. Hence, the total area (probability) contained in two tails $= 2 \times (0.5 - 0.355) = 0.29$ or the probability that H_0 is not rejected $= 0.29$.

2. It is also easy to calculate the mean values on either side of distribution under H_0 which will indicate the cut-off point for the rejection region by calculating the minimum value for ($\overline{X} - \mu$) to yield a Z value ± 1.96 $\left(\overline{X} - \mu\right) = z\left(\dfrac{s}{\sqrt{n}}\right)$ which will be 0.17 g in the present example; therefore, the cut-off points will be 10.80 ± 0.17 g or 10.63 g on the left-hand side and 10.97 g on the right-hand side of the curve (Fig 7.3).

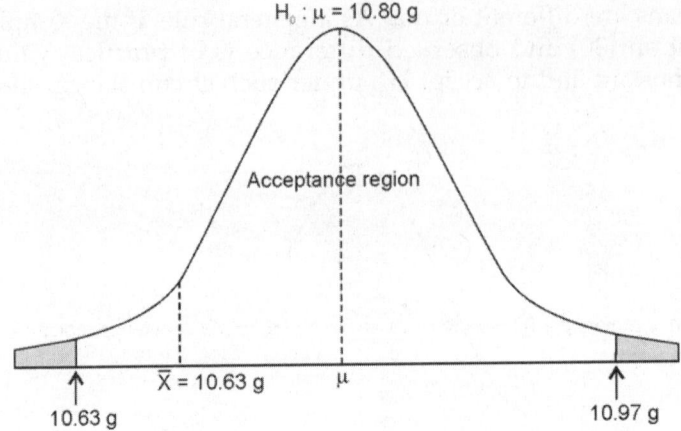

Fig. 7.3: Test for $\overline{X} = \mu$

3. Now, let us calculate whether these cut-off points are relevant for the curve under H_A: $\mu = 11.00$ g. The corresponding values of Z are $(10.63 - 11.00) \div 0.086 = -4.30$ (whose probability as per Appendix 1 is zero) and $(10.97 - 11.00) \div 0.086 = -0.349$ whose probability is 0.14 to the left and 0.50 to the right of the mean; hence, the total probability that the entire distribution lies to the right of 10.97 g is 0.64 or power of test is 0.64.

The distribution curves under H_0 ($\mu = 10.70$ g) and H_A ($\mu = 11.00$ g) are drawn below (Fig 7.4).

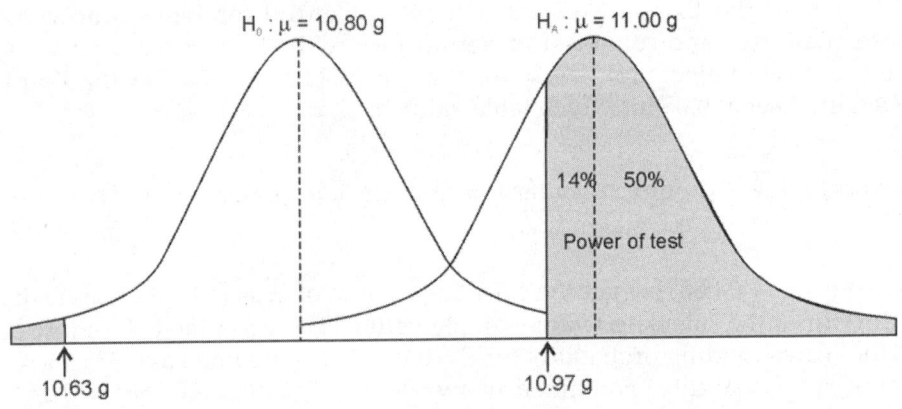

Fig. 7.4: Power of test-schematic representation

Power of test $(1 - \beta)$ is directly proportional to α, n and difference between means under H_0 and H_A. It is inversely proportional to s. In any case, for a given α, larger sample size increases power of test. Therefore, with higher sample size alone, power of test can be considerably increased.

1.3 Sample Size

1.3.1 For Estimating μ at a Set Precision

If s^2 is the sample estimate of variance of a normal population and d is the half the required confidence interval, then sample size can be calculated by the formula

$n = \dfrac{s^2 t^2_{(1-\alpha/2,\upsilon)}}{d^2}$. If population size N, is known, the value of n obtained can be used to

calculate revised sample size, $m = \dfrac{n}{1+(n-1)/N}$.

1.3.2 For Testing Mean of a Normal Distribution

Sample size required is directly proportional to variance (σ^2 or s^2) and power of test $(1 - \beta)$; and inversely proportional to level of significance (α) and the numerator of the test statistic/criterion ($\overline{X}_0$ or $\mu_0 - \overline{X}_1$ or μ_1, as the case may be). Without going into mathematical derivation, sample size required to perform a one–tailed test on H_0: $\mu = \mu_0$ Vs H_A: $\mu = \mu_1$ (i.e. $\mu < \mu_0$ or $\mu > \mu_0$) at a significance level α and probability of

detecting a significant difference or power of test = $(1 - \beta)$ is $n = \dfrac{\sigma^2 \left(Z_{(1-\beta)} + Z_{(1-\alpha)} \right)^2}{\left(\mu_0 - \mu_1 \right)^2}$

and for a two–tailed test it will be $n = \dfrac{\sigma^2 \left(Z_{(1-\beta)} + Z_{(1-\alpha/2)} \right)^2}{\left(\mu_0 - \mu_1 \right)^2}$.

In **Example 1.2.2.1** (Chapter "**Central tendency**"), let us assume that μ_0 = 10.80 g and σ = 1.50 g. Let μ_1 = 11.00 g, α = 0.05 and β = 0.20; table values (two–tailed test) of $Z_{(1-\beta)}$ = 0.84, $Z_{(1-\alpha/2)}$ = 1.96. Hence, n = 441; the same for one – tailed test will be 347 (because $Z_{(1-\alpha)}$ = 1.645). The actual sample size was 350; it is for this reason that the power of the two – tailed test, as per the calculation, was only 0.64.

Note: If population values are not available, sample values with corresponding values of the statistic employed (usually Student's t, along with degrees of freedom, υ) have to be replaced in the above formulae.

1.3.3 For a Set Confidence Interval, L

Without going into mathematical derivation, sample size required so that the two–tailed $100 \times (1 - \alpha)$ confidence interval does not exceed wider than L, is approximately obtained by: $n = 4Z^2_{(1-\alpha/2)} s^2 \div L^2$ with usual notations. In **Example 1.2.2.1** (Chapter "**Central tendency**"), where s = 1.611 g and Z = 1.96, if L = 0.5 g, n = 160; hence, the actual sample size (350) is adequate for the purpose and in fact, L can be narrowed down further.

The above formula can be rearranged to obtain the confidence interval that can be set with a known n as $L = \sqrt{4Z^2_{(1-\alpha/2)} s^2 \div n}$; in the present example, it suggests that L can be reduced to 0.338 when n = 350.

1.3.3.1 For a set minimum detectable difference, δ

Sample size required to detect $\overline{X}_0$ or $\mu_0 - \overline{X}_1$ or μ_1, as the case may be, is approximately given by: $n = \dfrac{s^2}{\delta^2}\left(t_{(1-\alpha,\upsilon)} + t_{(1-\beta,\upsilon)}\right)^2$ for one-tailed test; for two-tailed test, $t_{(1-\alpha,\upsilon)}$ is replaced by $t_{(1-\alpha/2,\upsilon)}$. If population variance is known, Z values can replace t values.

Suppose in **Example 1.2.2.1** (Chapter "**Central tendency**"), assuming a sample size of 20 may be required (for locating table values of t), $\delta = 0.5$ g, $\alpha = 0.05$ and $\beta = 0.10$, with s being 1.611 g, $t_{(0.975, 19)} = 2.093$ and $t_{(0.9, 19)} = 1.328$, $n = 35.5$ (for two-tailed test); using this value for sample size, the calculations are redone and repeated (iteration) till no more reduction in n is obtained. The lowest value so obtained is the sample size required for detecting the desired δ. The same conditions hold good for one-tailed test as well with suitable table values of t at $(1-\alpha)$ level of significance.

By rearranging the above formula as $\delta = \sqrt{\dfrac{s^2}{n}}\left(t_{(1-\alpha,\upsilon)} + t_{(1-\beta,\upsilon)}\right)$ we can obtain the minimum detectable difference when n is known; in the above example, if $n = 350$, $\delta = 0.294$ g in a two-tailed test.

2. ESTIMATION

Estimation means the use of data obtained from sample(s) for predicting unknown but true population parameter(s). Two types of estimates are possible:

1. Point estimate—a single value predicting the population parameter; for instance, mean, median, standard deviation etc.
2. Interval estimate—gives a range of values within which the population parameter will assume a value; considering μ, interval estimate will be $x_1 < \mu < x_2$.

Properties (requirements) of a good estimate have been discussed in Chapter "Introduction".

2.1 Point Estimates

2.1.1 Normal Distribution

2.1.1.1 For mean, variance and standard error

If the underlying distribution is even approximately Normal with mean μ variance σ^2, based on the validity of Central Limit Theorem (*see* Chapter "**Probability distributions**"), for a large sample, sample mean is the valid estimate of μ, s^2 its σ^2 and $(s \div \sqrt{n})$ its Standard error.

2.1.2 Binomial Distribution

2.1.2.1 For mean, variance and standard error

For a random Binomial variable with parameter p (probability of success) and sample size n, Mean, variance and standard error is $\hat{p}, \hat{p}\hat{q}/n$ and $\sqrt{\hat{p}\hat{q}/n}$, respectively and for number of successes out of n binomial trials, mean, variance and standard error is $n\hat{p}, n\hat{p}\hat{q}$ and $\sqrt{n\hat{p}\hat{q}}$, respectively.

2.1.3 Poisson Distribution

The mean, variance and standard deviation of Poisson distribution will be m, m and $\sqrt{m}$, respectively.

2.2 Interval Estimates

2.2.1 Normal Distribution

2.2.1.1 Mean

2.2.1.1.1 When σ is known

Under this condition, the sample mean ($\overline{X}$) is converted into standard normal deviate (Z) (see Chapter **"Probability distributions"**). Since 95% of the Z values will be between ± 1.96 (two-tailed), it follows that ($\overline{X}$ - μ) = ± 1.96 (σ ÷ $\sqrt{n}$) or 95% confidence limits for μ will be μ ± 1.96 (σ ÷ $\sqrt{n}$). It is however necessary to note that, on most practical situations, μ and/or σ will be unknown. In general, $\mu \pm Z_{(1+\alpha/2)}$(σ ÷ $\sqrt{n}$) will give 100 × (1 + α) % confidence limits for μ.

In **Example 1.2.2.1** (Chapter **"Central tendency"**), let us assume that μ = 10.80 g and σ = 1.50 g. Since n = 350, 95% confidence intervals for μ are 10.64 g and 10.96 g.

2.2.1.1.2 When σ is not known

In this case, the sample mean ($\overline{X}$) is converted into Student's t values (t) (see Chapter **"Probability distributions"**) by replacing σ by s in the formula for calculation of Z. The Student's t distribution is a family of distributions depending on the degrees of freedom (designated υ). Hence, it follows that ($\overline{X}$ - μ) = $\pm t_{\upsilon, (1-\alpha/2)}$ (s ÷ $\sqrt{n}$) or 100 × (1 – α)% confidence limits for μ will be $\pm t_{\upsilon, (1-\alpha/2)}$ (s ÷ $\sqrt{n}$). Table values at known υ and set α can be obtained from standard table (Appendix 3).

Note:
1. Since confidence intervals involve either halves of the curve (two-tailed), table value corresponding to probability ½ α is taken.
2. When n exceeds 30, table value of t will be same as that of Z.

In **Example 1.2.2.1** (Chapter **"Central tendency"**), it is calculated that that $\overline{X}$ = 10.70 g and s = 1.61 g. Since n = 350, 95% confidence intervals for mean are 10.53 g and 10.87 g.

2.2.1.2 Variance

The χ^2 distribution is used for this purpose (see Chapter **"Probability distributions"**) which is also a family of distributions decided solely by degrees of freedom, υ. 100 × (1 – α)% confidence limits for σ² is as follows:

$$\left[\frac{(n-1)s^2}{\chi^2_{n-1,1-\alpha/2}}, \frac{(n-1)s^2}{\chi^2_{n-1,\alpha/2}} \right]$$ (details of

mathematical proof can be obtained from books dedicated to Mathematical Statistics). Table values of χ^2 are available in Appendix 4.

2.2.2 Binomial Distribution

For a binomial parameter, p, $100 \times (1 - \alpha)\%$ confidence limits are $\sum_{r=x}^{n} {}^{n}C_r p^r q^{(n-r)}$ and

$\sum_{r=0}^{x} {}^{n}C_r p^r q^{(n-r)}$ with usual meaning for notations. (details of mathematical proof can be obtained from books dedicated to Mathematical Statistics).

2.2.3 Poisson Distribution

For a poisson parameter, m, $100 \times (1 - \alpha)\%$ confidence limits are $1 - \sum_{r=0}^{n-1} \dfrac{e^{-m} m^r}{r!}$ and

$\sum_{r=0}^{n} \dfrac{e^{-m} m^r}{r!}$ with usual meaning for notations. (details of mathematical proof can be obtained from books dedicated to Mathematical Statistics).

3. TESTS OF SIGNIFICANCE

3.1 One Sample Tests

3.1.1 For Mean of a Normal Distribution

Minimum detectable difference (δ) in one sample tests can be estimated by the formula

$\delta = \sqrt{\dfrac{s^2}{n}} \left(t_{(1-\alpha,\upsilon)} + t_{(1-\beta,\upsilon)} \right)$ for one-tailed test; for two-tailed test, $t_{(1-\alpha,\upsilon)}$ is replaced by $t_{(1-\alpha/2,\upsilon)}$. If population variance is known, Z values can replace t values and σ^2 for s^2.

In **Example 1.2.2.1** (Chapter "**Central tendency**"), $s = 1.611$ g; if $n = 20$, $\alpha = 0.05$ and $\beta = 0.10$, for two-tailed test, $t_{(0.975, 19)} = 2.093$, $t_{(0.9, 19)} = 1.328$ and $\delta = 1.23$ g.

It is equally interesting that by rearranging above formula it is possible to estimate $t_{(1-\beta, \upsilon)}$ which can be use to get probability for β and then the power of the test $(1 - \beta)$.

$t_{(1-\beta,\upsilon)} = \dfrac{\delta}{\sqrt{\dfrac{s^2}{n}}} - t_{(1-\alpha/2,\upsilon)}$ and in the above example, if $\beta = 1.0$ g, $t_{(1 - \beta, \upsilon)} = 0.683$ whose

probability is > 0.25 (Appendix 3); by considering 0.683 as a normal deviate, the corresponding Z value (Appendix 1) of 0.251 is obtained. Hence, $\beta = 0.251$ and $(1 - \beta) = 0.749$ or 74.90%.

3.1.1.1 With known σ^2

3.1.1.1.1 Two-tailed test

3.1.1.1.1.1 Procedure

H_0: $\overline{X} = \mu$; σ known $\qquad H_A$: $\overline{X} \# \mu$

Test statistic: $Z = \dfrac{\overline{X} - \mu}{\sigma / \sqrt{n}}$ at α level of significance

Conclusion: if $|Z_{calc}| < Z_{(1-\alpha/2)}$, accept H_0; if $|Z_{calc}| \geq Z_{(1-\alpha/2)}$, reject H_0

3.1.1.1.1.2 Example

Day-old chick weight in a sample of 10 broilers was 38.75 g. Test whether the mean weight is consistent with population value of 40 g with a standard deviation of 2 g. Level of significance (α) = 0.05

Given: $\overline{X}$ = 38.75 g and σ = 2 g, n = 10 and μ = 40 g

Calculated value of $Z = -1.98$, Table value of $Z_{0.975} = 1.96$

Conclusion: H_0 may be rejected

3.1.1.1.2 One–tailed test

3.1.1.1.2.1 Procedure

H_0: $\overline{X} = \mu$; σ known H_A: $\overline{X}$ # μ

Test statistic: $Z = \dfrac{\overline{X} - \mu}{\sigma / \sqrt{n}}$ at α level of significance

Conclusion: if $|Z_{calc}| < Z_{(1-\alpha/2)}$, accept H_0; if $|Z_{calc}| \geq Z_{(1-\alpha/2)}$, reject H_0

3.1.1.1.2.2 Example

Day-old chick weight in a sample of 10 broilers was 38.75 g.. Test whether the mean weight is consistent with population value of 40 g with a standard deviation of 2 g. Level of significance (α) = 0.05 (same as in case of two-tailed test).

Given: $\overline{X}$ = 38.75 g and σ = 2 g, n = 10 and μ = 40 g

Calculated value of $Z = -1.98$, Table value of $Z_{0.95} = 1.645$

Conclusion: H_0 may be rejected

3.1.1.2 With unknown σ^2

3.1.1.2.1 Two-tailed test

3.1.1.2.1.1 Procedure

H_0: $\overline{X} = \mu$; σ not known H_A: $\overline{X}$ # μ

Test statistic: $Z = \dfrac{\overline{X} - \mu}{s / \sqrt{n}}$ at α level of significance

Conclusion: if $|t_{calc}| < t_{(n-1),(1-\alpha)}$, accept H_0; if $|t_{calc}| \geq t_{(n-1),(1-\alpha)}$, reject H_0

3.1.1.2.1.2 Example

Day-old chick weight in a sample of 10 broilers was 38.75 g with a standard deviation of 2 g. Test whether the mean weight is consistent with population value of 40 g.

Given: $\overline{X}$ = 38.75 g and s = 2 g, n = 10 and μ = 40 g

Calculated value of t = –1.98, Table value of $t_{9, 0.975}$ = 2.26

Conclusion: H_0 may be accepted

3.1.1.2.2 One-tailed test

3.1.1.2.2.1 Procedure

H_0: $\overline{X}$ = μ; σ not known $\qquad$ H_A: $\overline{X}$ < μ

Test statistic: $Z = \dfrac{\overline{X} - \mu}{s/\sqrt{n}}$ at α level of significance

Conclusion: if $|t_{calc}| < t_{(n-1),(1-\alpha)}$, accept H_0; if $|t_{calc}| \geq t_{(n-1),(1-\alpha)}$, reject H_0

3.1.1.2.2.2 Example

Day-old chick weight in a sample of 10 broilers was 38.75 g with a standard deviation of 2 g. Test whether the mean weight is consistent with population value of 40 g (same as in case of two-tailed test).

Given: $\overline{X}$ = 38.75 g and s = 2 g, n = 10 and μ = 40 g

Calculated value of t = –1.98, Table value of $t_{9, 0.95}$ = 1.83

Conclusion: H_0 may not be accepted

Note: The same example is used for all conditions to demonstrate the difference due to change in the test statistic from Z to Student's t.

3.1.2 For Variance of a Normal Population

3.1.2.1 Procedure

H_0: s^2 = σ^2; H_A: s^2 > σ^2 (one-tailed); Test statistic: $\chi^2_{(calc)} = \dfrac{(n-1)s^2}{\sigma^2}$ is distributed as $\chi^2_{(1-\alpha),(n-1)}$; α for table value of χ^2 depends on H_A (one- or two-tailed; α or $\alpha/2$, respectively).

3.1.2.2 Example

In **Example 1.2.2.1** (Chapter "**Central tendency**"), if n = 20, let us test whether value of s(1.611 g) obtained is indistinguishable from the population σ of 1.50 g at α = 0.05.

χ^2_{calc} = 21.92 which is lesser than the Table value of 30.14 for a p = 0.95 at $(n-1)$ or υ = 19; therefore, H_0 may be accepted indicating that the sample variance is likely to be a true representative of its population value.

3.1.3 For Coefficient of Variation, Skewness and Kurtosis

These are not generally applied by animal science workers. If one is interested to perform such tests, book on mathematical statistics will provide the requisite methods.

3.1.4 For Correlation and Regression Coefficients

Testing for association between variables will be discussed in chapter "Association between variables".

3.1.5 *For a Binomial Proportion*

3.1.5.1 Normal–theory method

In this method Binomial distribution is approximated by Normal distribution which is generally applicable when $np_0 q_0 \geq 5$ where p_0 and q_0 are population proportions. Due to simplicity of procedure, this method is popularly practiced.

3.1.5.1.1 *Procedure*

$H_0: p = p_0; H_A: p \# p_0$ (two-tailed); Test statistic: $Z_{(calc)} = \dfrac{p - p_0}{\sqrt{\dfrac{p_0 q_0}{n}}}$; if Z_{calc} is $< Z$ tabulated at

$(1 - \alpha)$ [or $(1 - \alpha/2)$, as the case may be] level of significance, H_0 is acceptable; else, it is likely to be rejected.

3.1.5.1.2 *Example*

From a survey of 10,000 cattle, 200 freemartins were recorded. Let us find out whether this proportion is more than the population proportion of 0.018 for freemartins.

Given: $n = 10,000$, $p_0 = 0.018$, $p = (200 \div 10000) = 0.02$.

$H_0: p = p_0; H_A: p > p_0$ (one–tailed test)

Test statistic, $Z_{calc} = 1.504$ is less than 1.645 (table value of $Z_{0.95}$).

Conclusion: Sample proportion of 0.018 is consistent with the population proportion of 0.02.

3.1.5.2 Exact method

As the name suggests, the exact Binomial proportion, where x is the observed number of events, is calculated as follows:

If $p \leq p_0$, $p = 2\left(\sum\limits_{r=x}^{n} {}^nC_r p_0^r q_0^{(n-r)} \right)$ and If $p > p_0$, $p = 2\left(\sum\limits_{r=x}^{n} {}^nC_r p_0^r q_0^{(n-r)} \right)$. The calculations in

this method are rather cumbersome although standard binomial tables do facilitate the process. Hence, this method is not commonly employed in the field of Animal Science.

3.1.6 *For a Poisson Distribution*

3.1.6.1 Critical value method

If p_i is the probability of the event in ith individual in a population, X is the total

number of events, then the expected number of events $\mu_0 = \sum\limits_{i=1}^{n} p_i$. A two-tailed $100 \times$

$(1 - \alpha)$ confidence interval is set for the observed μ. The event being rare, if this interval (c_1, c_2) contains μ_0, then the H_0 that $\mu = \mu_0$ is accepted. In other words if $(c_1 \leq \mu_0 \leq c_2)$, H_0 is accepted. Table for Poisson expectation of μ is available to facilitate the process.

3.1.6.2 *p*-value method

As in case of Binomial proportion, exact Poisson proportion can be calculated as follows and compared with the population proportion:

If $p < p_0$, $p = 2\left(\sum\limits_{r=0}^{x} \dfrac{e^{-m}m^r}{r!}\right)$ and If $p \geq p_0$, $p = 2\left(1 - \sum\limits_{r=0}^{x-1} \dfrac{e^{-m}m^r}{r!}\right)$ where, x is the number of successes actually recorded.

3.2 Two-sample Tests

Unlike one-sample tests where statistic computed on a sample drawn from a large population is compared with the known/assumed parameter of the population, in two-sample tests, the unknown parameters of two different populations are compared.

3.2.1 Paired Samples

If two observations are made on the same experimental subject over space and time, such observations are called "Paired observations" and samples "Paired samples". For example: suppose we are interested to find the effect of a particular drug on blood pressure of dogs; then, a sample of dogs of same breed, age and nutritional status, etc. is selected and blood pressure recorded individually. The test drug is given and on the same animals blood pressure is recorded after a known period of time and compared with their respective previous value. It is clear that each observation made earlier has a corresponding observation made later on the same experimental subject; hence, the data becomes paired data. Care has to be exercised especially on uncontrollable factors such as age, climate, etc. on the variable while considering data as paired.

The advantages of pairing include 1) most of the factors other than the test factor (factors innate to an individual) remain same for each of the experimental subjects on both occasions and 2) cost of experimentation is considerably reduced because the same individual gives both 'before' and 'after' values.

Pairing described above is referred to as **Self–pairing** when the same individual is observed 'before' and 'after' application of treatments as is commonly employed in pathology, pharmacology, parasitology and clinical subjects; however, pairing can also involve two individuals of the same parents on whom two different treatments are applied (**Natural–pairing**) or assigned by the experimenter based on certain criteria like body weight, age, etc. (**assigned–pairing**).

3.2.1.1 Test for difference between means (mean difference)

3.2.1.1.1 Procedure

Let μ_0 be the population mean and d_i's are the deviations of ith pair of observation with mean μ_0 and variance σ^2_0; the latter, on most occasions, unknown but approximated by s^2_d.

H_0: $\mu_0 = 0$, that means, the pair (treatments) do not differ

H_A: $\mu_0 \neq 0$ (two-tailed) or H_A: $\mu_0 < 0$ or > 0 (one-tailed)

Statistic: under H_0, $t = \dfrac{\bar{d} - \mu_0}{s_d/\sqrt{n}} = \dfrac{\bar{d}}{s_d/\sqrt{n}}$ where, $s_d = \sqrt{\dfrac{\sum\limits_{i=1}^{n} d_i^2 - \dfrac{\left(\sum\limits_{i=1}^{n} d_i\right)^2}{n}}{n-1}}$ with n pairs of observations. If $|t| \leq t_{(n-1),(1-\alpha/2)}$ (two-tailed) or $t \leq -t_{(n-1),(1-\alpha)}$ (one–tailed, $H_A: \mu_0 < 0$) or (one-tailed, $H_A: \mu_0 > 0$), H_0 may be accepted; else, H_0 is liable to be rejected.

3.2.1.1.2 Example

Let us consider that an experiment is conducted on WL layers to test the efficacy of a particular feed ingredient in reducing cholesterol levels in egg yolk. The following table gives the changes (mg/100 g) in the egg of test birds after treatment. We need to know whether the treatment was effective or not.

Bird	1	2	3	4	5	6	7	8	9	10	11	12
Change (d_i)	2	-5	-13	-16	-7	4	1	-1	-6	-11	-12	-8

Given: $n = 12$, $\Sigma d_i = 72$, $\Sigma d_i^2 = 886$, $\bar{d} = 6$ mg/100 g, $s_d = 6.42$ mg/100 g, $H_0: \mu = 0$, $H_A = \mu \# 0$ (two-tailed) or $\mu > 0 / \mu < 0$ (one-tailed); $\alpha = 0.05$

Statistic: $t = \dfrac{\bar{d}}{s_d/\sqrt{n}} = \dfrac{6}{6.42/\sqrt{12}} = 3.237$ on $\upsilon = 11$. Table value of t on $\upsilon = 11$ (degrees

of freedom) is 2.201 (two-tailed) and 1.796 (one-tailed).

Conclusion: $t_{calc} > t_{table}$ in either case; hence, H_0 is does not appear to be consistent and hence may be rejected. Therefore, the treatment appears to be effective in reducing egg yolk cholesterol levels.

3.2.1.2 Testing paired sample by ranking: Wilcoxon paired–sample test

This is a non-parametric test. The following example describes the test:

3.2.1.2.1 Example

The following are the difference between clutch size of daughter from that of their respective dams ($d_i = C_D - C_d$). Test H_0: Clutch size is same among dams and daughters at $\alpha = 0.05$.

	1	2	3	4	5	6	7	8	9	10	Total (+'s) T_+	Total (−'s) T_-
d_i		-3	4	7	6	-3	-1	8	-2	4	5	
Rank of $|d_i|$		3.5	5.5	9	8	3.5	1	10	2	5.5	7	
Signed Rank of $|d_i|$	-3.5	5.5	9	8	-3.5	-1	10	-2	5.5	7	45	10

Note: Last row is the product of sign of the 2nd row and value of the 3rd row

If calculated T_+ and/or $T_- \leq$ table value of $T_{\alpha, \upsilon = n}$, H_0 may be rejected; otherwise, H_0 can be accepted. In the above example, table value of $T_{0.05, 10} = 8$ which is < both T_+ and T_-; hence, H_0 may be accepted.

Note:

1. The Wilcoxon T distribution values are not provided in this publication since this test is not a routine one for animal science workers; analogous to other tests, one- or two-tail alternatives depending on H_A is possible in this test also.

2. One-sample median test, Normal approximation as well as approximation to t distribution is possible; since this test is not very common for animal scientists, the reader is advised to refer other books on mathematical statistics for details.

3.2.1.3 Test for nominal scale data: McNemar's test

If the paired data is nominal and dichotomous (two possible values), this test is applicable. Hence, wherever experimental results, which are nominal in nature, before and after a treatment or procedure is available, this test can be applied

3.2.1.3.1 Example

Two anti-fungal creams were tried on dogs afflicted with a certain fungal disease of skin. The results are given below in a 2 × 2 contingency table. We need to know whether the creams yielded similar relief or not at $\alpha = 0.05$. χ^2 test with Yates' correction for continuity is conducted subject to the condition that $(x_{12} + x_{21}) \geq 10$; if $(x_{12} + x_{21}) < 10$, a Binomial test is recommended.

H_0: Proportion of dogs showing relief is same for both the creams
H_A: Proportion of dogs showing relief is not same for both the creams

Cream B ↓	Cream A	
	Relieved	Not relieved
Relieved	18 (x_{11})	5 (x_{12})
Not relieved	14 (x_{21})	13 (x_{22})

$$\chi^2 = \frac{(|x_{12} - x_{21}| - 1)^2}{x_{12} + x_{21}} = 3.368$$ which is < table value of $\chi^2_{0.05,\,1} = 3.841$. Therefore, it is

reasonable to accept H_0.

It is interesting to note that χ^2 calculated is similar to square of normal deviate, Z

where, $Z = \dfrac{(|x_{12} - x_{21}| - 1)}{\sqrt{x_{12} + x_{21}}}$; in fact, this can as well be used.

McNemar's test can be extended to a $r \times r$ contingency table also; in which case,

$$\chi^2 = \sum_{i=1}^{r} \sum_{j>i} \frac{(|x_{ij} - x_{ji}|)^2}{x_{ij} + x_{ji}}$$ on $\upsilon = {}^r C_2$; when $r = 3$, $\upsilon = 3$, when $r = 4$, $\upsilon = 6$ and so on.

Accordingly, number of pairs for the numerator and denominator will be same as r.

3.3.1.3.2 McNemar's test for correlated proportions—exact test

In the above example, considering off-diagonal values (x_{12} and x_{21}) as discordant pair, denoted n_D, diagonals as concordant, denoted n_C, and x_{21} as type A discordat pair, denoted n_A, when $n_D < 20$, Normal theory test may not be valid. Then, the following probabilities are calculated:

1. If $n_A < n_D/2$, $p = 2 \times \displaystyle\sum_{k=0}^{n_A} {}^{n_D}C_k \left(\frac{1}{2}\right)^{n_D}$

2. If $n_A > n_D/2$, $p = 2 \times \displaystyle\sum_{k=n_A}^{n_D} {}^{n_D}C_k \left(\frac{1}{2}\right)^{n_D}$

3. If $n_A = n_D/2$, $p = 1.000$

In the above example, n_A, n_D and n_C are 14, 19 and 31, respectively; hence, $n_A > n_D/2$;

therefore, $p = 2 \times \sum\limits_{k=14}^{19} {}^{19}C_{14}\left(\dfrac{1}{2}\right)^{19} = 0.044 + 0.015 + 0.004 + 0.001 + 0.0001 + 0.000004 = 0.064$

3.2.1.4 Effect of treatment order: Gart's test

It is not uncommon that > 1 treatments may be required to treat a particular ailment. Under such circumstances, order in which the treatments are given also is important. Such effects can be tested by this method.

3.2.1.4.1 Example

Treatments A and B were considered in an experimental set-up. 20 dogs were given treatment A followed by treatment B; another 20 dogs were subjected to the reverse order of treatment. From results tabulated below, it is required to test 1) whether the two treatments have the same effect or not and 2) whether the order of medication has any effect or not at $\alpha = 0.05$.

Effect of treatment:

H_0: The two medications have similar effect

H_A: The two medications don't have similar effect

	Order of treatments		Total
	A, then B	B, then A	
Response with treatment A	15 (a)	8 (b)	23 (R_1)
Response with treatment B	5 (c)	12 (d)	17 (R_2)
Total	20 (C_1)	20 (C_2)	40 (n)

$$\chi^2 = \frac{n\left[|ad - bc| - \dfrac{n}{2}\right]^2}{R_1 R_2 C_1 C_2} = 3.683 \text{ which is} < \text{table value of } \chi^2_{0.05, 1} = 3.841. \text{ Therefore, it is}$$

reasonable to accept H_0.

Effect of order of treatment:

H_0: The orders of medication have similar effect

H_A: The orders of medication don't have similar effect

	Order of treatments		Total
	A, then B	B, then A	
Response with treatment A	15 (a)	12 (b)	27 (R_1)
Response with treatment B	5 (c)	8 (d)	13 (R_2)
Total	20 (C_1)	20 (C_2)	40 (n)

$$\chi^2 = \frac{n\left[|ad - bc| - \dfrac{n}{2}\right]^2}{R_1 R_2 C_1 C_2} = 0.456 \text{ which is} < \text{table value of } \chi^2_{0.05, 1} = 3.841. \text{ Therefore, it is}$$

reasonable to accept H_0.

3.2.2 *Independent Samples*

3.2.2.1 Testing equality of variances

Testing means of two independent samples slightly differs depending on whether the variances are equal or not. Hence, it is necessary that variances have to be tested for equality (homogeneity). The ratio of variances (larger to the smaller) follows **F distribution** which is also referred to as **variance ratio**. The table values of F are located by υ for larger variance as column and υ of smaller variance as the row for a set $(1 - \alpha)$ or $(1 - \alpha/2)$, for one- and two-tailed tests, respectively. As in case of Z, t and χ^2 tests, if

$F_{calc} > F_{table}$, H_0 $(\sigma_1^2 = \sigma_2^2)$ is liabe to be rejected. If H_0 is accepted pooled $s^2 = \dfrac{\upsilon_1 s_1^2 + \upsilon_2 s_2^2}{\upsilon_1 + \upsilon_2}$

3.2.2.1.1 *Example*

Data on feed consumption (g) of WL chicks reared in cages and on deep-litter is given below. We need to test H_0: $s^2_c = s^2_{dl}$

Bird	1	2	3	4	5	6	7	8	9	10	n	Σx	Σx^2	s^2
Cages	42	34	35	35	38	28	40	33	36	36	10	357	12879	3.860
Deep-litter	50	53	60	55	62	58	55				7	393	22167	4.140

$F = s^2_{dl} \div s^2_c = 1.073$ which is < 3.374, table value of $F_{0.05, 6, 9}$; hence, H_0 may be accepted. Further, pooled $s^2 = (9 \times 3.86 = 6 \times 4.14) \div (9 + 6) = 4.583$

3.2.2.2 With equal variances

3.2.2.2.1 *Known σ^2*

3.2.2.2.1.1 *Procedure*

Assuming that $\overline{X}_1$ and $\overline{X}_2$ with mean μ_1 and μ_2, and variances σ^2/n_1 and σ^2/n_2, respectively, as the samples are independent, $\overline{X}_1 - \overline{X}_2$ is also normally distributed with mean $(\mu_1 - \mu_2)$ and variance $\dfrac{\sigma^2}{\left(\dfrac{1}{n_1} + \dfrac{1}{n_2}\right)}$. If σ^2 is known, $\dfrac{\overline{X}_1 - \overline{X}_2}{\sigma\sqrt{\dfrac{1}{n_1} + \dfrac{1}{n_2}}}$ will be a Standard Normal Variate (Z).

H_0: $\mu_1 = \mu_2$; H_A: $\mu_1 \# \mu_2$ (two–tailed) or $\mu_1 < \mu_2/\mu_1 > \mu_2$ (one–tailed)

If $Z_{calc} < Z_{table}$ at a set $(1 - \alpha/2)$ (two–tailed)/$(1 - \alpha)$ (one–tailed), H_0 may be accepted; else, H_0 is liable to be rejected.

3.2.2.2.1.2 *Example*

Data on egg production of 100 WL layers reared in cages and on deep-litter is given below: $(\sigma^2 = 2.25$ eggs^2 or $\sigma = 1.5$ eggs)

Bird	1	2	3	4	5	6	7	8	9	10	n	Σx	Mean
Cages	82	84	85	85	88	88	90	93	96	96	10	887	88.700
Deep-litter	90	93	90	95	92	98	95				7	653	93.286

$H_0: \mu_1 = \mu_2; H_A: \mu_1 \,\#\, \mu_2$

Statistic $Z = \dfrac{\bar{X}_c - \bar{X}_{dl}}{\sigma\sqrt{\dfrac{1}{n_1} + \dfrac{1}{n_2}}} = \dfrac{88.700 - 93.286}{1.5\sqrt{\dfrac{1}{10} + \dfrac{1}{7}}} = 6.204$ which is > 1.96, the table value of

$Z_{0.05}$; hence, H_0 may not be accepted.

3.2.2.2.2 *Unknown σ^2*

3.2.2.2.2.1 *Procedure*

A pooled estimate of variance of two independent samples is calculated as

$s^2 = \dfrac{(n_1 - 1)s_1^2 + (n_2 - 1)s_2^2}{n_1 + n_2 - 2}$ and statistic $t = \dfrac{\bar{X}_1 - \bar{X}_2}{s\sqrt{\dfrac{1}{n_1} + \dfrac{1}{n_2}}}$ on $\upsilon = (n_1 + n_2 - 2)$. If

$|t| \le t_{(n_1 + n_2 - 2),\,(1-\alpha/2)}$ (two-tailed) or $t \le -t_{(n_1 + n_2 - 2),\,(1-\alpha)}$ or $|t| \le t_{(n_1 + n_2 - 2),\,(1-\alpha/2)}$ (two-tailed) or $t \le -t_{(n_1 + n_2 - 2),\,(1-\alpha)}$ (one-tailed, $H_A: \mu_0 > 0$), H_0 may be accepted; else, H_0 is liable to be rejected.

Note: If $n_1 = n_2 = n$, the denominator simplifies to $s\sqrt{\dfrac{2}{n}}$ and $\upsilon = 2 \times (n - 1)$.

3.2.2.2.2.2 *Example*

If (one – tailed, $H_A: \grave{\imath}_0 < 0$) or

Bird	1	2	3	4	5	6	7	8	9	10	n	Σx	Mean	s^2
Cages	42	34	35	35	38	28	40	33	36	36	10	357	35.70	3.860
Deep-litter	50	53	60	55	62	58	55				7	393	56.14	4.140

Let us consider the example under 3.2.2.1.1 concerning data on feed consumption (g) of WL chicks reared in cages and on deep-litter which is reproduced below:

The variances were found to be homogenous and pooled $s^2 = 4.583$. Let us test H_0: $\bar{X}_c = \bar{X}_{dl}$; $H_A: \bar{X}_c \neq \bar{X}_{dl}$ (two–tailed)

Statistic $t = \dfrac{\bar{X}_c - \bar{X}_{dl}}{s\sqrt{\dfrac{1}{n_1} + \dfrac{1}{n_2}}} = 20.44 \div 1.055 = 19.374$ which is > 1.753, the table value of

$t_{0.05,\,15}$; hence, H_0 may not be accepted.

3.2.2.3 With unequal variances (Satterthwaite's approximation)

3.2.2.3.1 *Procedure*

With unequal variances, the test statistic t can not be accurately derived. However, t is approximated as $t = \dfrac{\bar{X}_1 - \bar{X}_2}{\sqrt{\dfrac{s_1^2}{n_1} + \dfrac{s_2^2}{n_2}}}$; and $\upsilon \neq n_1 + n_2 - 2$ but it is computed as nearest integer of the ratio $\upsilon = \dfrac{\left(\dfrac{s_1^2}{n_1} + \dfrac{s_2^2}{n_2}\right)^2}{\dfrac{\left(\dfrac{s_1^2}{n_1}\right)^2}{(n_1-1)} + \dfrac{\left(\dfrac{s_2^2}{n_2}\right)^2}{(n_2-1)}}$.

$H_0: \mu_1 = \mu_2$; $H_A: \mu_1 \neq \mu_2$ (two-tailed) or $\mu_1 < \mu_2 / \mu_1 > \mu_2$ (one–tailed)

If $|t| \leq t_{\upsilon,(1-\alpha/2)}$ (two-tailed) or $t \leq -t_{\upsilon,(1-\alpha)}$ (one–tailed, $H_A: \mu_0 < 0$) or $t \geq t_{\upsilon,(1-\alpha)}$ (one–tailed, $H_A: \mu_0 > 0$), H_0 may be accepted; else, H_0 is liable to be rejected.

3.2.2.3.2 *Example*

Data on growth rate (g) of broilers reared in cages and on deep-litter is given below:

Bird	1	2	3	4	5	6	7	8	9	10	n	Σx	Σx^2	s^2
Cages	82	54	75	75	58	68	80	73	76	56	10	697	49519	10.209
Deep-litter	59	57	60	61	62	58	55	56			8	468	27420	2.449

$F = s^2_c \div s^2_{dl} = 4.168$ which is > 3.677, table value of $F_{0.05,\,9,7}$; hence, H_0 may not be accepted.

Hence, degrees of freedom for t – test will be revised (from $10 + 8 - 2 = 16$) to

$$\upsilon = \frac{\left(\dfrac{10.209}{10} + \dfrac{2.449}{8}\right)^2}{\dfrac{\left(\dfrac{10.209}{10}\right)^2}{9} + \dfrac{\left(\dfrac{2.449}{8}\right)^2}{7}} = 1.760995 \div 0.129192 = 13.631 \approx 14 \text{ and}$$

Statistic $t = \dfrac{\bar{X}_1 - \bar{X}_2}{\sqrt{\dfrac{s_1^2}{n_1} + \dfrac{s_2^2}{n_2}}} = (69.7 - 58.5) \div 1.152 = 9.722$ which is > 1.761, the table value

of $t_{0.05,\,14}$. Therefore H_0 is liable to be rejected.

3.2.2.4 Difference between variances from two correlated populations

Suppose measurements of shank length and body weight are made on two separate samples, the samples can easily be considered independent; but, if both measurements are made on the same individual, the variables are likely to be correlated. Under such situations, if F is the Ratio of greater to lesser variance, n is the umber of pairs of observations and r is the correlation coefficient between the variables, then statistic

$$t = \frac{(F-1)}{2\sqrt{\dfrac{F(1-r^2)}{(n-2)}}} = \frac{(F-1)\sqrt{(n-2)}}{2\sqrt{F(1-r^2)}} \text{ on } \upsilon = (n-2).$$

Note: Association between variables will be dealt in a separate chapter.

3.2.2.5 Test for difference between two CVs

It may be required to test whether the two samples came from populations with same CV or not. It is possible to test by use of F test (variance ratio) with variances of the logarithms of the data when the underlying distributions are, at least, nearly Normal.

That means $F = \dfrac{\left(s_{\log}^2\right)_{Larger}}{\left(s_{\log}^2\right)_{Smaller}}$.

It can also be tested by statistic $Z = \dfrac{V_1 - V_2}{\sqrt{\left(\dfrac{V_P^2}{n_1 - 1} + \dfrac{V_P^2}{n_2 - 1}\right)\left(0.5 + V_P^2\right)}}$

where, $V_P^2 = \dfrac{(n_1 - 1)V_1 + (n_2 - 1)V_2}{(n_1 - 1) + (n_2 - 1)}$, the pooled CV.

3.2.2.5.1 Example

The following table gives egg weight–chick weight relationship in Japanese quails. We need to test the following hypothesis:

H_0: The intrinsic variability of egg and chick weights are same in Japanese quail eggs; i.e. $\dfrac{\sigma_{egg\ wt}}{\mu_{egg\ wt}} = \dfrac{\sigma_{chick\ wt}}{\mu_{chick\ wt}}$

H_A: The intrinsic variability of egg and chick weights are not same in Japanese quail eggs; i.e. $\dfrac{\sigma_{egg\ wt}}{\mu_{egg\ wt}} \# \dfrac{\sigma_{chick\ wt}}{\mu_{chick\ wt}}$

	Egg weight (g)	Log of egg weight	Chick weght (g)	Log of chick weight
	6.0	0.7782	4.0	0.6021
	7.0	0.8451	4.5	0.6532
	8.0	0.9031	4.9	0.6902
	9.0	0.9542	5.5	0.7404
	10.0	1.0000	6.0	0.7782
	11.0	1.0414	6.7	0.8261
	12.0	1.0792	7.1	0.8513
	13.0	1.1139	8.0	0.9031
	14.0	1.1461	8.5	0.9294
	15.0	1.1761	9.1	0.9590
Totals, g	105	10.0373	64.3	7.9330
Sum of squares, g²	1185	10.2326	440.87	6.4256
υ	9	9	9	9
Means, g	10.5	1.0037	6.43	0.7933
Variances, g²	9.1667	0.0175	3.0468	0.0147
CVs	0.2883	0.1319	0.2715	0.1528

Statistic F = (0.0175 ÷ 0.0147) = 1.190 which is < 3.179, the table value $F_{0.05, 9, 9}$; hence H_0 may be accepted.

Alternatively, V_P = (9 × 0.2883 + 9 × 0.2715) ÷ 18 = 0.2799 and the statistic

$$Z = \frac{0.2883 - 0.2715}{\sqrt{\left(\frac{0.2799^2}{9} + \frac{0.2799^2}{9}\right)(0.5 + 0.2799^2)}} = 0.1674 \text{ which is} < 1.96, \text{ the table value of } Z_{0.05};$$

hence, H_0 can be accepted.

3.2.3 Sample Size Determination

3.2.3.1 To detect a difference of δ between two means

Minimum sample size required to detect a difference of δ between two means is given by $n \geq \frac{2s^2}{\delta^2}\left(t_{\alpha,\upsilon} + t_{\beta,\upsilon}\right)^2$ where s^2 is the pooled variance. For instance, if n = 100 (per sample), α = 0.05, β = 0.90, s^2 = 0.52 and δ = 0.50, then, $t_{0.05, 198}$ = 1.972 and $t_{0.10, 198}$ = 1.286. Therefore, $n \geq 44.2$ (or say, 45).

On occasions when samples can not have equal size and one of them is fixed at n_1, then to obtain a desired n, $n_2 = (nn_1) \div (2n_1 - n)$. Assuming n_1 = 30 in the above case, n_2 = 88.

3.2.3.2 Minimum detectable difference

By rearranging the equation above, we get $\delta \geq \sqrt{\frac{2s^2}{n}}\left(t_{\alpha,\upsilon} + t_{\beta,\upsilon}\right)$ where s^2 is the pooled variance. With n = 100, in the above case, δ = 0.332.

3.2.4 Categorical Data—Binomial Proportions

3.2.4.1 Normal theory method

Used when sample size is large enough to make assumption of Normal approximation of Binomial distribution reasonably valid. Hence, $H_0: p_1 = p_2$ where p_1 and p_2 are sample proportions and p and q are population values. In other words, we assume that p_1 and p_2 are Normally distributed with mean p and variance pq/n_1 and pq/n_2, respectively.

The statistic calculated is obviously the Standard Normal Deviate, $Z = \dfrac{|p_1 - p_2|}{\sqrt{pq\left(\dfrac{1}{n_1} + \dfrac{1}{n_2}\right)}}$.

The conclusions depending on one- or two-tailed alternatives are similar to those explained in other Z tests.

If p and q, the population proportions are not available, then p is approximated as $p = \dfrac{n_1 p_1 + n_2 p_2}{n_1 + n_2} = \dfrac{x_1 + x_2}{n_1 + n_2}$ and $q = (1 - p)$ where x's indicate observed number of events in 1st and 2nd sample, respectively. Further, a correction factor for continuity, a factor

$\left(\dfrac{1}{2n_1}+\dfrac{1}{2n_2}\right)$ can be added (if $p_1 < p_2$) or subtracted (if $p_1 \geq p_2$) from the numerator of

the statistic $Z = \dfrac{|p_1 - p_2| \pm \left(\dfrac{1}{2n_1}+\dfrac{1}{2n_2}\right)}{\sqrt{pq\left(\dfrac{1}{n_1}+\dfrac{1}{n_2}\right)}}$; The conclusions depending on one– or two–

tailed alternatives are similar to those explained in other Z tests.

3.2.4.1.1 Example

Let us consider a hypothetical example; before the outbreak of Avian Influenza, 400 persons out of 500 were consuming eggs which later on reduced to 50 out of 400. We have to test H_0: The proportion of egg consumers remained the same against H_A: The proportion of egg consumers reduced (one-tail test).

In this case, $p_1 = (400 \div 500) = 0.8,\ p_2 = (50 \div 400) = 0.125,\ p = (400 + 50) \div (500 + 400)$

$= 0.5$ and therefore, $q = 0.5$. Further, $\left(\dfrac{1}{2n_1}+\dfrac{1}{2n_2}\right) = 0.00225$ (this value is subtracted

since $p_1 > p_2$.

$Z = (0.675 - 0.00225) \div 0.034 = 19.787$ which is > 1.645, the table value; hence, H_0 is liable to be rejected and that the data is suggestive of reduction in egg consumption due to outbreak of Avian Influenza.

3.2.4.2 Contingency table (2 × 2) method

3.2.4.2.1 Example: No confounding

Suppose an extension worker collects data on income status of dairy farmers on two occasions and classifies them into high- and low-income groups. The data is tabulated as follows:

Second visit ↓	First visit High	Low	Total
High	28 (a)	5 (b)	33 (R_1)
Low	22 (c)	15 (d)	37 (R_2)
Total	50 (C_1)	20 (C_2)	70 (N)

H_0: The proportion of high-income groups are same in both visits

H_A: The proportion of high-income groups are not same in both visits

If each of the observations is represented as x_{ij}, where the subscript 'i' refers to row number and 'j' refers to column number to indicate that the observation belongs to ith row and jth column, and $R_{i.}$ indicates total of ith row, C_j, the total of jth column and

N, the overall total, then the expected frequencies $E_{ij} = \dfrac{R_i C_j}{N}$. In the above example,

$x_{11} = 28$, $x_{12} = 5$, $x_{21} = 22$, $x_{22} = 15$, $R_1 = 33$, $R_2 = 37$, $C_1 = 50$. $C_2 = 20$ and $N = 50$. The expected value of each of the cells is as follows (note that the totals will not change for either row or column):

Second visit ↓	First visit		Total
	High	Low	
High	23.6	9.4	33
Low	26.4	10.6	37
Total	50	20	70

If observed values are denoted O_{ij} and expected values as E_{ij}, then the statistic χ^2 (on $\upsilon = 1$) can be calculated as $\sum_i \sum_j \dfrac{(O_{ij} - E_{ij})^2}{E_{ij}}$; however, a continuity correction of ½ is

subtracted (Yates' correction) to get the final formula as $\sum_i \sum_j \dfrac{\left(|O_{ij} - E_{ij}| - \dfrac{1}{2}\right)^2}{E_{ij}}$

summation indicating all the cells.

It is obvious that the above formula is cumbersome for computation; hence, the computational formula is $\chi^2 = \dfrac{N\left(|ad - bc|^2 - \dfrac{N}{2}\right)^2}{R_1 R_2 C_1 C_2}$; In the above example,

$\chi^2 \dfrac{70\left(|28 \times 15 - 5 \times 22| - \dfrac{70}{2}\right)^2}{33 \times 37 \times 50 \times 20} = 4.336$ which is > 3.841, the table value of $\chi^2_{0.5,\,1}$; hence, H_0 may not be accepted.

Note: Computational formula for χ^2 without Yates' correction can be derived as $\chi^2 = \sum_i \sum_j \dfrac{O_{ij}^2}{E_{ij}} - N$.

3.2.4.2.2 With confounding (Mantel–Haenszel test)

If a factor other than the variable(s) under study is related to the variable(s), then the factor so involved is called a **Confounding variable** and its effect(s) has(have) to be controlled to obtain true inference(s) about the variable(s) in test. If the effect of the confounder is same (either positive or negative), it is said to be a **positive confounder**; on the contrary, if the effects are opposite on the variable(s), positive on either of them and negative on the other, then it is said to be a **negative confounder**. If the confounder itself is causally related to either of the variables, it is said to be in the **causal pathway** between the variables. For instance, relationship of a disease to exposure based on nutritional status (say a particular vitamin/mineral/other nutrient level) as demonstrated by increased severity of coccidiosis in poultry due to **higher** levels of Vit A.

Under such conditions, the following procedure outlines the Mantel–Haenszel test (H_0: Disease and exposure are not associated):

1. Separate 2 × 2 contingency tables are constructed for each level/degree/**strata** (k) of the confounding variable(s); i.e. k number of 2 × 2 tables designated:

		Exposure		
		Yes	No	Totals
Disease	Yes	a_i	b_i	$a_i + b_i$
	No	c_i	d_i	$c_i + d_i$
	Totals	$a_i + c_i$	$b_i + d_i$	n_i

where $O_i = a_i$, $E_i = [(a_i + b_i)(a_i + c_i) \div n_i]$ and variance of O_i is given by

$$V_i = \frac{(a_i + b_i)(c_i + d_i)(a_i + c_i)(b_i + d_i)}{n_i^2 (n_i - 1)}$$

2. Observed frequency (O), Expected frequency (E) and Variance (V) are computed as

$$\sum_{i=1}^{k} O_i, \ \sum_{i=1}^{k} E_i \ \text{and} \ \sum_{i=1}^{k} V_i, \ \text{respectively.}$$

3. Then, if **V ≥ 5**, $\chi_{MH}^2 = \dfrac{\left(|O - E| - \dfrac{1}{2}\right)^2}{V}$ is calculated and tested against table value of χ^2

on $\upsilon = 1$ and set α.

Note: Common odds ratio (OR) for k contingency tables (2 × 2) formed can be calculated as

$$OR_{MH} = \frac{\sum_{i=1}^{k}(a_i d_i \div n_i)}{\sum_{i=1}^{k}(b_i c_i \div n_i)}$$

3.2.4.3 Case of R × 2 contingency table

3.2.4.3.1 Example—no confounding

The following hypothetical data pertains to frequency of age at first calving in normal and foot- and mouth disease (FMD)—affected cows. We need to test for association between disease history and age at first calving.

Age at first calving (years)	Disease history		Total
	FMD-affected	Normal	
1.5	1	25	26
2.0	2	35	37
2.5	7	28	35
3.0	15	8	23
3.5	28	1	29
≥ 4.0	32	1	33
Totals	85	98	183

At the outset, it is necessary to check number of the expected frequencies < 5; none of the cells in the above table has expected frequency < 5 although the observed frequency is < 5 for 3 cells. Further, none of the cells has an observed frequency < 1. Therefore, a two-tail χ^2 test can be formed with H_0: The disease history and age at first calving are not associated.

Calculation of χ^2 value for R × 2 contingency table can be simplified as

$$\chi^2 = \frac{N^2}{C_1 C_2}\left[\sum_{i=1}^{R}\frac{O_{i1}^2}{R_i} - \frac{C_1^2}{N}\right]$$ on $\upsilon = (R-1)$; the term $\sum_{i=1}^{R}\frac{O_{i1}^2}{R_i}$ is calculated as $(1^2 \div 26) + (2^2 \div 37) + \ldots + (32^2 \div 33)$ and the rest of the terms are easy to compute.

For the above data, $\chi^2 = 120.259$ which is > 11.07, the table value of $\chi^2_{0.05,\,5}$. Therefore, H_0 is liable to be rejected indicating that FMD is associated with age at first calving; inspection of the frequencies indicated that FMD delays age at first calving.

Note: Observed values in the 2nd column can as well be used to obtain the same χ^2 value with the

above formula modified as follows: $\chi^2 = \frac{N^2}{C_1 C_2}\left[\sum_{i=1}^{R}\frac{O_{i2}^2}{R_i} - \frac{C_2^2}{N}\right]$.

3.2.4.3.2 Case of 2 × C contingency table: No confounding

This case is similar to the R × 2 contingency table being transposed. Obviously, the

formulae change as $\chi^2 = \frac{N^2}{R_1 R_2}\left[\sum_{j=1}^{C}\frac{O_{1j}^2}{C_j} - \frac{R_1^2}{N}\right]$ when the 1st row frequencies are used for

calculation and $\chi^2 = \frac{N^2}{R_1 R_2}\left[\sum_{j=1}^{C}\frac{O_{2j}^2}{C_j} - \frac{R_2^2}{N}\right]$ when 2nd row frequencies are used; for either

of them, $\upsilon = (C-1)$.

3.2.4.4 Testing homogeneity of Binomial proportion: R × 2 table (no confounding)

If the observed frequencies in the 1st column refers to number of successes and the 2nd column to number of failures, probability of success for the ith row (p_i's) can be

calculated as $\frac{O_{i1}}{R_i}$ and corresponding probability of failure as $\frac{O_{i2}}{R_i}$ or $(1-p_i)$. With this

information, χ^2 on $\upsilon = (R-1)$ can be calculated as follows (H_0: Binomial proportions are same in all the rows):

1. Calculate pooled probability of success, $P = (C_1 \div N)$ and $Q = (1-P)$ or as $(C_2 \div N)$.

2. χ^2 on $\upsilon = (R-1)$ is given by $\frac{1}{PQ}\left[\sum_{i=1}^{R}O_{i1}p_i - C_1 P\right]$.

3. χ^2 on $\upsilon = (R-1)$ is also given by $\frac{1}{PQ}\left[\sum_{i=1}^{R}O_{i2}q_i - C_2 Q\right]$ if 2nd column is used.

4. If $\chi^2_{calc} >$ table value of $\chi^2_{(1-\alpha/2),\,(R-1)}$, H_0 may be rejected.

Note: If the observed frequencies are in the form of 2 × C table, probability of success for the jth

column (p_j's) can be calculated as $\frac{O_{1j}}{C_j}$ and corresponding probability of failure as $\frac{O_{2j}}{C_j}$ or $(1-p_j)$.

Pooled probability of success, $P = (R_1 \div N)$ and $Q = (1-P)$ or as $(R_2 \div N)$. Then, χ^2 on $\upsilon = (C-1)$ can be calculated as $\dfrac{1}{PQ}\left[\displaystyle\sum_{j=1}^{C}O_{1j}p_j - R_1P\right]$ or $\dfrac{1}{PQ}\left[\displaystyle\sum_{j=1}^{C}O_{2j}q_j - R_2Q\right]$

3.2.4.4.1 Example

Let us consider the example under 3.2.4.3.1; by transposing the data we get the following table and let us test H_0: The Binomial proportions are homogenous in all columns:

Disease status	Age at first calving (years)						Totals
	1.5	2.0	2.5	3.0	3.5	≥ 4.0	
FMD (O_{1j}'s)	1	2	7	15	28	32	85 (R_1)
Normal	25	35	28	8	1	1	98
Totals (C_j's)	26	37	35	23	29	33	183 (N)
p_j's*	0.038	0.054	0.200	0.652	0.966	0.970	0.464 (P)

* Calculated as ($O_{1j} \div C_j$) $P = R_1 \div N$ Since $P = 0.464$, $Q = 0.536$

Therefore, χ^2 ($\upsilon = 5$) $= 120.521$ which is > 11.07, the table value of $\chi^2_{0.05,\,5}$; hence, H_0 may be rejected.

3.2.4.4.2 Test for trend in Binomal proportion (2 × C table): No confounding

In this test, any trend (increasing/decreasing) trend in Binomial proportions over C groups (groups forming columns) will be evaluated (H_0: There is no trend in Binomial proportions over the groups). It is clear that a modification in calculation of χ^2 in a 2 × C contingency table is made. As described above, probability of success for the jth column (p_j's) can be calculated as $\dfrac{O_{1j}}{C_j}$ and corresponding probability of failure as $\dfrac{O_{2j}}{C_j}$ or $(1 - p_j)$. Pooled probability of success, $P = (R_1 \div N)$ and $Q = (1 - P)$ or as $(R_2 \div N)$. Considering O_{1j} as the observed value corresponding to the jth column of the 1st row, C_j as the total of jth column, R_1 as the total of 1st row and N as the total frequencies, the following quantities are computed:

$$A = \left(\sum_{j=1}^{C}O_{1j}\times j\right) - \frac{R_1\left(\sum_{j=1}^{C}C_j\times j\right)}{N} \text{ and } B = PQ\left[\left(\sum_{j=1}^{C}C_j\times j^2\right) - \frac{\left(\sum_{j=1}^{C}C_j\times j\right)^2}{N}\right].$$

Finally, $\chi^2 = A^2/B$ on $\upsilon = 1$. If the calculated value of the statistic is > table value on 1 degree of freedom and $(1 - \alpha)$, H_0 may be rejected. Further, if $A > 0$, the proportions increase with increasing score and *vice versa*.

3.2.4.4.2.1 Example

Let us consider the example under 3.2.4.3.1; by transposing the data we get the following table showing all the notations used for calculation of A and B:

Disease status ↓	Age at first calving (years)						Totals
	1.5	2.0	2.5	3.0	3.5	≥ 4.0	
FMD (O_{1j}'s)	1	2	7	15	28	32	85 (R_1)
Normal	25	35	28	8	1	1	98
Totals (C_j's)	26	37	35	23	29	33	183 (N)
p_j's *	0.038	0.054	0.200	0.652	0.966	0.970	0.464 (P)
j values	1	2	3	4	5	6	

* Calculated as $(O_{1j} \div C_j)$ $P = R_1 \div N$ Since $P = 0.464$, $Q = 0.536$

Therefore, A = 418 – [(85*640) ÷ 183] = 120.732, B = (0.464 × 0.536) × [2770 – (640² ÷ 183)] = 132.248 and χ^2 = (120.732² ÷ 132.248) = 110.219 which is > 3.841, the table value of $\chi^2_{1, 0.05}$; hence. H_0 may be rejected. Further, since A > 0, it is reasonable to conclude that the binomial probabilities exhibited an increasing trend as is evident by their values also.

3.2.4.4.3 Test for trend in binomial proportion (2 × C table): With confounding

(Mantel–extension test)

As the name indicates, this test is an extension of Mantel–Haenszel (MH) test outline above as **Example 3.2.4.2.2**. An outline of the test is given below (H_0: Average score with or without disease in a stratum is same):

		Exposure				Totals
		1	2	....	k	
Disease	Present	p_{i1}	p_{i2}	....	p_{ik}	P_i
	Absent	q_{i1}	q_{i2}	....	q_{ik}	Q_i
	Totals	T_{i1}	T_{i2}	....	T_{ik}	N_i
	Score	x_1	x_2	....	x_k	

Similar to Mantel–Haenszel test, $O_i = \sum\limits_{i=1}^{k} p_{ij}x_j$, $E_i = \dfrac{P_i}{N_i}\left(\sum\limits_{i=1}^{k} T_{ij}x_j\right)$ and

$$V_i = \dfrac{P_i Q_i \left[N_i \sum\limits_{i=1}^{k} T_{ij}x_j^2 - \sum\limits_{i=1}^{k} T_{ij}x_j \right]}{N_i^2 (N_i - 1)}$$

are observed score, expected score and variance of O_i, respectively. Then, considering that there are s number of contingency tables, Observed frequency (O), Expected frequency (E) and Variance (V) are computed as $\sum\limits_{i=1}^{s} O_i$, $\sum\limits_{i=1}^{s} E_i$

and $\sum\limits_{i=1}^{s} V_i$, respectively. Finally, Then, if **V ≥ 5**, $\chi^2_{TR} = \dfrac{\left(|O - E| - \dfrac{1}{2}\right)^2}{V}$ is calculated and

tested against table value of χ^2 on $\upsilon = 1$ and set α.

3.2.4.5 Association in R × C contingency tables

A table with R rows and C columns is called a R × C contingency table. If O_{ij} represents the observed frequency of the ith row and jth column, R_i and C_j represent totals of ith row and jth column and N, the total frequencies ($\sum_i R_i$ or $\sum_j C_j$ or $\sum_i \sum_j O_{ij}$); then the

expected frequencies are calculated as $E_{ij} = \dfrac{R_i C_j}{N}$.

After computing the expected frequencies, c² on $\upsilon = (R-1) \times (C-1)$ is calculated as

$$\sum_i \sum_j \frac{\left(O_{ij} - E_{ij}\right)^2}{E_{ij}} = \sum_i \sum_j \frac{O_{ij}^2}{E_{ij}} - N \text{ and compared with the table value as a two-tail test.}$$

This test needs the following two conditions satisfied:
1. Number of cells with $E_{ij} < 5$ should be $< (R \times C \div 5)$ and
2. No cell should have $E_{ij} < 1$.

3.2.4.5.1 Example

The following are the hypothetical data; we have to test the following H_0: There is no association between fungal creams and relief levels

Anti-fungal cream		Relief levels				Totals
		High	Medium	Low	Very low	(R$_i$'s)
1	Observed	24	20	22	34	100
	Expected	25.60	23.60	23.47	27.33	
2	Observed	43	31	32	39	145
	Expected	37.12	34.22	34.03	39.63	
3	Observed	32	30	28	35	125
	Expected	32.00	29.50	29.33	34.17	
4	Observed	52	42	36	50	180
	Expected	46.08	42.48	42.24	49.20	
5	Observed	41	54	58	47	200
	Expected	51.20	47.20	46.93	54.67	
Totals (C$_j$'s)	192	177	176	205	750 (N)	

Calculated $\chi^2 = 12.223$ which is < 21.026, the table value of $\chi^2_{0.05, 12}$; hence, H_0 is acceptable. However, with different genetic groups and testing of segregation ratios involved, this test is extended further to partition χ^2 values as per rows and calculate $\chi^2_{Heterogeneity}$; this is enumerated in Chapter "**Statistics in Specific Veterinary fields**". However, the concept of $\chi^2_{Heterogeneity}$ is outlined on next page:

H_0's:
1. Each of the treatments is producing same relief levels
2. All the treatments are homogenous in producing relief

Anti-fungal cream		High	Medium	Low	Very low	Total (R_i's)	χ^2 on $\upsilon = 3$ Calc	Table
			Relief levels					
1	Observed	24	20	22	34	100		
	Expected	25.60	23.60	23.47	27.33		2.369	7.815
2	Observed	43	31	32	39	145		
	Expected	37.12	34.22	34.03	39.63		1.366	7.815
3	Observed	32	30	28	35	125		
	Expected	32.00	29.50	29.33	34.17		0.089	7.815
4	Observed	52	42	36	50	180		
	Expected	46.08	42.48	42.24	49.20		1.701	7.815
5	Observed	41	54	58	47	200		
	Expected	51.20	47.20	46.93	54.67		6.699	7.815
					χ^2_{Total} on $\upsilon = 15$		12.223	24.996
Totals (C_j's)	Observed	192	177	176	205	750 (N)		
	Expected	187.50	187.50	187.50	187.50			
					χ^2_{Pooled} on $\upsilon = 3$		3.035	7.815
					$\chi^2_{Heterogeneity}$ on $\upsilon = 12$		9.188	21.026

It is evident from the above that all calculated values of χ^2 are < respective tabulated values at $\alpha = 0.05$. Hence, the null hypotheses are acceptable.

3.2.4.6 Fisher's exact test

When sample size is small, Normal approximation of Binomial proportion may not be valid. Under such conditions, this test is used.

3.2.4.6.1 *Example*

Let us consider a hypothetical example of fat levels in broiler diet and death due to fatty-liver kidney syndrome (FLKS). The layout will be as follows:

Cause of death ↓	Fat in diet		Total
	High	Low	
Not FLKS	8 (a)	5 (b)	13 (R_1)
FLKS	2 (c)	1 (d)	3 (R_2)
Total	10 (C_1)	6 (C_2)	16 (N)

Assuming that the marginal totals are fixed the exact probability of observing the table with cells a, b, c and d can be calculated as: $\Pr(a,b,c,d)$
$$= \frac{(a+b)!(c+d)!(a+c)!(b+d)!}{n!a!b!c!d!} = \frac{R_1!R_2!C_1!C_2!}{n!a!b!c!d!} \text{ ; for the above example, } \Pr(a, b, c, d) = 0.482$$

With the marginal totals fixed, it is easy to visualize that many 2×2 tables are possible by altering the value of 'a' i.e. observation x_{11}. In the above example, only four 2×2 tables are possible which are shown below.

7	6	13
3	0	3
10	6	16

(A)

8	5	13
2	1	3
10	6	16

(B)

9	4	13
1	2	3
10	6	16

(C)

10	3	13
0	3	3
10	6	16

(D)

The probabilities for the above tables A, B, C and D are calculated as 0.214, 0.482, 0.268 and 0.036, respectively. This follows **hypergeometric distribution** (*see* Chapter "**Probability distributions**").

Note: Sum of the probabilities above = 1.000

The observed table is (B) and the following hypotheses can be tested:

1. $H_0: p_1 = p_2; H_A: p_1 \# p_2;$
   Probability = $2 \times$ min [Pr($a = 7$) + Pr($a = 8$), Pr($a = 8$) + Pr($a = 9$) + Pr($a = 10$), 0.5]. That means Probability = $2 \times$ min (0.696, 0.786, 0.5) = 1.000
2. $H_0: p_1 = p_2; H_A: p_1 < p_2;$
   Probability = [Pr($a = 7$) + Pr($a = 8$)] = 0.696
3. $H_0: p_1 = p_2; H_A: p_1 > p_2;$
   Probability = [Pr($a = 8$) + Pr($a = 9$) + Pr($a = 10$)] = 0.786

The above procedure can be generalized as follows:

After developing all possible 2×2 contingency tables (say k tables), of which table a is the one which is actually observed, with cell x_{11} taking the value 0 to k,

1. To test $H_0: p_1 = p_2; H_A: p_1 \# p_2, p - \text{value} = 2 \times \text{min}[\text{Pr}(0) + \text{Pr}(1) + ... + \text{Pr}(a), \text{Pr}(a) + \text{Pr}(a+1) + \text{Pr}(a+2) + ...+ \text{Pr}(k), 0.5]$
2. To test $H_0: p_1 = p_2; H_A: p_1 < p_2, p - \text{value} = \text{Pr}(0) + \text{Pr}(1) + ... + \text{Pr}(a)$
3. To test $H_0: p_1 = p_2; H_A: p_1 > p_2, p - \text{value} = \text{Pr}(a) + \text{Pr}(a+1) + \text{Pr}(a+2) + ... + \text{Pr}(k)$

Since the probabilities on either side are high, probability of getting a table as extreme as the one observed or even more extreme that that is considerably high; therefore, it appears that fat in diet and death due to FLKS are associated.

3.2.4.7 Matched–pair data (McNemar's test)

See Section 3.2.1.3 for details.

3.3 Non-parametric Methods

Dealt as a separate Chapter

3.4 Others

3.4.1 χ^2 Goodness of Fit

By utilizing data in **Example 1.2.2.1** (Chapter "**Central tendency**"), the procedure for fitting a Normal distribution as well as χ^2 goodness of fit is already demonstrated under section 1.5 in Chapter "**Continuous probability distributions**". It is worth listing the procedure again (H_0: The sample has come from a Normal population):

1. Parameters of the probability model were estimated by using the data available; in the instant case, $\mu = 10.70$ g and $\sigma = 1.611$ g (i.e. Number of parameters, designated $m = 2$).

2. Utilizing the above values, the probabilities and subsequently expected frequency for each group (number of groups, designated $k = 9$) is computed.

3. Then, $\chi^2_{(k-m-1)}$, α is given by $\sum_{i=1}^{k}\frac{(O_i-E_i)^2}{E_i} = \sum_{i=1}^{k}\frac{O_i^2}{E_i} - \sum_{i=1}^{k}O_i = 18.092$ which is > 12.59, the table value of $\chi^2_{6,\,0.05}$. Hence, H_0 may not be accepted.

The same concept can be extended for testing the goodness of fit in case of other distributions like Binomial ($m = 1$), Poisson ($m = 1$), etc.

Note: χ^2 distribution has many more applications in animal genetics and breeding; they are dealt separately in Chapter "**Statistics in Specific Veterinary fields**".

3.4.2 The Kappa Statistic (κ)

3.4.2.1 Example

Suppose an extension worker has conducted two independent surveys on the same individuals, but at different times, regarding dairy farming as the main source of income or otherwise and is tabulated below:

II Survey ↓	I Survey Dairy	Not dairy	Totals	Row probabilities $(R_i \div N)$
Dairy	170 (a)	125 (b)	295 (R_1)	0.454 (a_1)
Not dairy	80 (c)	275 (d)	355 (R_2)	0.546 (a_2)
Totals	250 (C_1)	400 (C_2)	650 (N)	
Column probabilities ($C_i \div N$)	0.385 (b_1)	0.615 (b_2)		

Observed concordance, $p_o = (a + d) \div N = 0.685$ and expected concordance, $p_e = \Sigma a_i b_i = 0.511$ indicating that 51.1 % concordance is expected if the individuals are responding independently regarding their main source of income.

The Kappa statistic can be used to measure reproducibility between surveys reporting on a categorical variable and is calculated as follows based on H_0: $\kappa = 0$ and H_A: $\kappa > 0$ (one-tailed test):

$$\kappa = \frac{p_o - p_e}{1 - p_e} \text{ with } se(\kappa) = \sqrt{\frac{1}{n(1-p_e)^2}\left[p_e + p_e^2 - \sum_{i=1}^{c}\{a_i b_i (a_i + b_i)\}\right]} \text{ where } c = \text{number of}$$

columns/rows and $Z = \kappa \div se(\kappa.)$ is a Normal deviate.

In the above example, $\kappa = 0.356$, $se(\kappa) = 0.039$ and $Z = 9.128$ which is > 1.645, the table value of Z at $\alpha = 0.05$. Hence, H_0 can be rejected indicating that there was a good reproducibility between two surveys.

3.4.3 Kolmogorov–Smirnov Goodness of Fit

3.4.3.1 For discrete ordinal data

3.4.3.1.1 Example

Five recipes ($k = 5$) were used to prepare feeds for dogs with graded levels of chicken meat (levels A, B, C, D and E) to enhance palatability, flavor and consequent acceptability. When fed, 13, 18, 12, 10 and 7 dogs liked the above feed, respectively. We need to test the H_0: All feeds were equally acceptable by the dogs against H_A: There was a graded increase in acceptability of feed analogous to chicken content.

| | Feed (with increasing levels of chicken meat) | | | | | n |
	A	B	C	D	E	
O_i	13	18	12	10	7	60
$E_i(H_0)$	12	12	12	12	12	60
Cumulative O_i	13	31	43	53	60	
Expected Cumulative O_i	12	24	36	48	60	
$|d_i|$	1	7	13	5	0	

d_{max} = maximum $|d_i|$ = 13 which is > 9, the table critical value of $d_{max, 5, 60}$. Hence, H_0 may be rejected.

Note: Standard tables of Kolmogorov–Smirnov critical d_{max} values are not provided in this publication; they can be obtained from other publications; for instance Zar (2003).

3.4.3.2 For continuous data

3.4.3.2.1 Example

Suppose distribution of ticks in an old poultry farm was studied over the entire height of walls (maximum height, x_{max} = 3.0 m) and following were recorded; we need to test H_0: Ticks are distributed uniformly up to a height of 3 m:

i	Height in m (x_i)	f_i	Cumulative f_i	Relative f_i^*	Expected relative f_i^{**}	D_i ***	D_i' ****
1	0.4	2	3	0.100	0.133	0.033	0.133
2	0.8	8	10	0.333	0.267	0.066	0.167
3	1.2	7	17	0.567	0.400	0.167	0.067
4	1.6	10	27	0.900	0.533	0.367	0.034
5	2.0	1	28	0.933	0.667	0.266	0.233
6	2.4	1	29	0.967	0.800	0.167	0.133
7	2.8	1	30	1.000	0.933	0.067	0.034

* Cumulative frequency ÷ n

** $x_i \div x_{max}$

*** |Relative f_i – Expected relative f_i|

**** |Relative f_{i-1} – Expected relative f_i| $n = \Sigma f_i = 30$

The test statistic, D = max [(max D_i), (max D_i')] = (0.367, 0.233) = 0.367 on $\upsilon = n$ (i.e. 30) and at set α. Table value of $D_{0.05, 30}$ = 0.2417 which is < calculated value and hence, H_0 may be rejected.

Note: Standard tables of Kolmogorov–Smirnov critical D values are not provided in this publication; they can be obtained from other publications; for instance Zar (2003).

3.4.4 Three-dimensional Contingency Tables

3.4.4.1. Example

In a survey on occurrence of newcastle disease, the following data (hypothetical) were recorded:

Observed frequencies	Disease present Location I	Location II	Disease absent Location I	Location II	Species totals
Species-1	$20\ (O_{111})$	$40\ (O_{121})$	$80\ (O_{112})$	$60\ (O_{122})$	$R_1 = 200$
Species-2	$40\ (O_{211})$	$80\ (O_{221})$	$60\ (O_{212})$	$70\ (O_{222})$	$R_2 = 250$
Disease totals	$T_1 = 180$		$T_2 = 270$		Grand total
Location totals	$C_1 = 200$		$C_2 = 250$		$= 450\ (N)$

We would like to test H_0: There is no association between Species, Location and Disease in the population from which the samples are drawn or, in other words, there are no two- or three-way interactions among the variables.

3.4.4.1.1 Overall association

Let us designate species (rows) by r (1, 2, ... i), location (columns) by c (1, 2, ... j) and disease (tiers) (present, absent) by t (1, 2, ... k) and each of the frequencies O_{ijk} and corresponding expected frequencies as E_{ijk} which are calculated as $E_{ijk} = \dfrac{S_i L_j D_k}{N^2}$ and

$$\chi^2_{RCT} = \sum_{i=1}^{r}\sum_{j=1}^{c}\sum_{k=1}^{t}\frac{\left(O_{ijk}-E_{ijk}\right)^2}{E_{rct}}$$ at set α and on $\upsilon = (rct - r - c - t + 2)$. The expected frequencies

for the example are as follows ($\upsilon = 4$):

Expected frequencies	Disease present Location I	Location II	Disease absent Location I	Location II
Species-1	$35.56\ (E_{111})$	$44.44\ (E_{121})$	$53.33\ (E_{112})$	$66.67\ (E_{122})$
Species-2	$44.44\ (E_{211})$	$55.56\ (E_{221})$	$66.67\ (E_{212})$	$83.33\ (E_{222})$

The calculated $\chi^2 = 35.210$ which is > 9.488, the table value of $\chi^2_{0.05,\ 4}$; hence, H_0 may be rejected.

Since H_0 is rejected, it is necessary to test all interactions to find out the exact dependency/independency of the variables.

3.4.4.1.2 Independence of species (rows) from location (column) and disease (tiers)

Expected frequencies	Disease present Location I	Location II	Disease absent Location I	Location II	Species totals
Species-1	$26.67\ (E_{111})$	$53.33\ (E_{121})$	$62.22\ (E_{112})$	$57.78\ (E_{122})$	$R_1 = 200$
Species-2	$33.33\ (E_{211})$	$66.67\ (E_{221})$	$77.78\ (E_{212})$	$72.22\ (E_{222})$	$R_2 = 250$
Location and disease totals $(CT)_{jk}$'s	$(CT)_{11} = 60$	$(CT)_{12} = 120$	$(CT)_{21} = 140$	$(CT)_{22} = 130$	Grand total $= 450\ (N)$

H_0: Species are independent of location and disease; the expected frequencies are calculated as $E_{ijk} = \dfrac{R_i(CT)_{jk}}{N}$ and χ^2 at a set α and $\upsilon = (rct - ct - r + 1) = 3$ in this example. χ^2 is calculated by the formula shown under section **3.4.4.1.1**. The calculated value of $\chi^2_{CT} = 16.079$ which is > 7.815, the table value of $\chi^2_{0.05,\,3}$; hence H_0 is rejected which indicates that there is interaction between species, locations and disease.

3.4.4.1.3 Independence of location (column) from species (rows) and disease (tiers)

The calculations are similar to the above but with suitable modifications in the table and formula as shown below:

Expected frequencies	Disease present		Disease absent		Location totals
	Species-1	Species-2	Species-1	Species-2	
Location-I	26.67 (E_{111})	53.33 (E_{121})	62.22 (E_{112})	57.78 (E_{122})	$C_1 = 200$
Location-II	33.33 (E_{211})	66.67 (E_{221})	77.78 (E_{212})	72.22 (E_{222})	$C_2 = 250$
Species and disease totals $(RT)_{ik}$'s	$(RT)_{11} = 60$	$(RT)_{12} = 120$	$(RT)_{21} = 140$	$(RT)_{22} = 130$	Grand total $= 450$ (N)

H_0: Locations are independent of species and disease; the expected frequencies are calculated as $E_{ijk} = \dfrac{C_j(RT)_{ik}}{N}$ and χ^2 at a set α and $\upsilon = (rct - rt - c + 1) = 3$ in this example.

χ^2 is calculated by the formula shown under section **3.4.4.1.1**. Since $(CT)_{jk} = (RT)_{ik}$, the expected values for both **3.4.4.1.2** and **3.4.4.1.3** are same and hence, the calculated value of $\chi^2_{RT} = 16.079$ which is > 7.815, the table value of $\chi^2_{0.05,\,3}$; hence H_0 is rejected.

3.4.4.1.4 Independence of diseses (tiers) from species (rows) and locations (columns)

The calculations are similar to the above but with suitable modifications in the table and formula as shown below:

Expected frequencies	Species-1		Species-2		Disease totals
	Location-I	Location-II	Location-I	Location-II	
Disease present	40.00 (E_{111})	40.00 (E_{121})	40.00 (E_{112})	60.00 (E_{122})	$T_1 = 180$
Disease absent	60.00 (E_{211})	60.00 (E_{221})	60.00 (E_{212})	90.00 (E_{222})	$T_2 = 270$
Species and location totals $(RC)_{ij}$'s	$(RC)_{11} = 100$	$(RC)_{12} = 100$	$(RC)_{21} = 100$	$(RC)_{22} = 150$	Grand total $= 450$ (N)

H_0: Diseases are independent of species and locations; the expected frequencies are calculated as $E_{ijk} = \dfrac{T_k(RC)_{ij}}{N}$ and χ^2 at a set α and $\upsilon = (rct - rc - t + 1) = 3$ in this example.

χ^2 is calculated by the formula shown under section **3.4.4.1.1**. The calculated value of $\chi^2_{RC} = 67.778$ which is > 7.815, the table value of $\chi^2_{0.05,\,3}$; hence H_0 is rejected.

Hence, the hypothetical data revealed presence of all the two-way interactions and the three–way interaction between species, locations and disease occurrence.

Note: The procedure is extendable to R × C × T contingency tables. For multi-dimensional contingency tables log–linear models are used.

3.4.5 Animal–time Data

The analyses of animal–time data, like incidence density, survival, etc. are dealt under "**Veterinary Epidemiology**" in Chapter "**Statistics in specific veterinary fields**".

3.5   Summary

The summary of tests of hypotheses outlined above is given below:

One-sample tests			
Condition (s)			**Test**
Normal distribution or Central limit theorem valid	Concerns mean	σ known	Z-test
		σ not known	t–test
	Concerns σ		χ^2 test *
Binomial distribution	Normal approximation valid		Normal theory methods
	Normal approximation not valid		Exact method
Poisson distribution	Poisson test		
Other distributions	Concerned distribution tests or non-parametric tests		

Two-sample tests					
Condition(s)					**Test**
Normal distribution	Concerns means	Samples paired		Paired t test	
		Samples independent		Equal variances	t test
				Unequal variances	t test
		Concerns variances			F test *
			2 × 2 contingency table	No confounding	χ^2 test
				With confounding	Mantel–Haenszel test
				Trends, no confounding	χ^2 test
Binomial distribution	Independent samples	All expected frequencies ≥ 5	2 × k contingency table	Trends, with confounding	Mantel extension test
				No trends, only association	Heterogeneity χ^2 test
			R × C table		χ^2 test
		All expected frequencies not ≥ 5			Fisher's exact test

(Contd.)

(Contd.)

	Samples not independent		McNemar's test
Animal–time data	Incidence rate constant over a period	No confounding	Test for incidence rate
		With confounding	Test for stratified person–time data
	Incidence rate not constant over a period		Survival analysis methods (log–rank test)
Others			Non-parametric methods
* Very sensitive to non-Normality			*Adapted from* Rosner, 2000

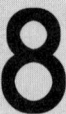

8

Non-Parametric Methods

(For Two Samples)

It is in the fitness of things to note that the methods of estimation and hypotheses testing explained in the earlier chapters are on data which generally represent a population which follows a defined distribution and described mathematically by parameters; be it normal, binomial poisson or others. Hence, such procedures and tests are referred to as "**parametric methods**". On the other hand, if sample size is small with underlying distribution not defined and **central limit theorem** being inapplicable, defining a distribution and the parameters does not arise. Such methods on small samples with no defined underlying distribution are referred to as "**non-parametric methods**".

Classification of data is outlined in Chapter "**Introduction**"; and it is easy to visualize that for **cardinal or ordinal data**, especially the latter, allotting numeric values and assuming central limit theorem appears to be too erroneous. This follows that estimation and hypothesis testing methods have to be different for such data. However, cardinal data can be subjected to parametric tests if underlying distribution can be defined and central limit theorem is applicable.

1. THE SIGN TEST

This test is applied to paired samples when (1) no quantitative measurement is employed and/or not possible, (2) that the underlying distribution is normal is doubtful and (3) as a quick substitute for t-test.

1.1 Quick Test Procedure (Snedecor and Cochran, 1994)

Suppose a taste panel (consisting 10 panelists) gave the following preferences on two chicken preparations (+ sign indicating preference to the product over the other product):

Judge	1	2	3	4	5	6	7	8	9	10
Product A	+	−	+	−	+	+	+	+	+	−
Product B	−	+	−	+	−	−	−	−	−	+

H_0: Same number of panelists preferred each of the products.

It is apparent that 7 out of 10 panelists preferred product A to product B. If r of n panelists gave one sign, approximate normal deviate, Z (corrected for continuity) is given by $Z = \dfrac{(|2r - n| - 1)}{\sqrt{n}} = 0.949$ which is < 1.96, the value of Z at $= 0.05$ (Appendix 1).

Alternatively, $Z^2 = \chi^2$; that means $\chi^2 = \dfrac{(|2r - n| - 1)^2}{n} = 0.900$ which is also < 3.841, the table value of $\chi^2_{0.05, 1}$ (Appendix 4). Hence, H_0 appears to be acceptable.

1.2 Normal Theory Method

1.2.1 Example

As a hypothetical example let us consider that two treatments (A and B) to alleviate hyper-pigmentation of abdominal skin in dogs were tried; each ointment applied to left and right sides at random to all the dogs. After a certain period treatment, the two portions were observed and the data were recorded into the following categories:

1. Treatment A is more effective than treatment B
2. Treatment B is more effective than treatment A
3. Both are equally effective

We would like to test H_0: Treatments A and B are equally effective or the difference between treatments was 0 (*see* Chapter "**Tests of hypotheses**" for meaning and basis of H_0).

A convenient way is when the degree of improvement can be put on a quantitative scale; say a number depending on degree of reduction in pigmentation. Let us designate the values as a_i and b_i for ith dog under treatment A and B, respectively. Obviously, the difference between the treatments will be $(a_i - b_i)$ designated d_i and H_0: $d = 0$ where d represents the population **median (or 50th percentile)** of the underlying distribution of d_i's. It is important to note that although an underlying distribution is mentioned, there is no numeric value for actual d_i's; instead it will be 0 or > 0 or < 0.

Further, dogs with $d_i = 0$ will be excluded since they are not useful in determining superiority of either of the treatments. Hence, let us assume that, of all the dogs under test (100), n dogs (80) had $d_i \# 0$ out of which n_G number of dogs (65) had $d_i > 0$ and n_L number of dogs (15) had $d_i < 0$. If n_G is large, treatment A is preferable and *vice versa*.

With the above discussion, we have to now test H_0: Probability that d_i will be non–zero $= \frac{1}{2}$ by assuming that normal approximation to Binomial is valid under the condition that $n \geq 20$ which also means that $npq \geq 5$ or $(\frac{1}{4})n \geq 5$.

To test H_0: $d = 0$ where d represents the population **median (or 50th percentile)** Vs d $\# 0$ where $n \geq 20$ and n_G number of dogs having $d_i > 0$; two following quantities are calculated (Z is the table value of standard normal deviate at set α, two-tail given in Appendix 1):

1. $U = \dfrac{1}{2}(n+1) + Z_{1-\alpha/2}\sqrt{n/4} = 49.265$ and

2. $L = \dfrac{1}{2}(n+1) - Z_{1-\alpha/2}\sqrt{n/4} = 31.735$

In this example $\alpha = 0.05$ which represents the upper and lower critical points in the Z–distribution. Hence, if $n_G > U$ or $n_G < L$, H_0 is rejected. Since $n_G = 65$ in the example, H_0 is rejected and treatment A appears to be superior to treatment B.

1.3 Exact Method

Employed when $n < 20$; the exact Binomial probabilities are calculated instead of Normal approximation. Let us consider the same **Example 1.2.1** with reduced number of dogs to 18 of which $n_G = 10$, $n_L = 6$ and 2 dogs had d_i's $= 0$. Therefore, $n = (18 - 2) = 16$, and $n_G > (\frac{1}{2})n$ which necessitates testing of H_0: $p = \frac{1}{2}$ Vs H_A: $p \# \frac{1}{2}$.

In this case, we have to calculate the actual Binomial probability of n_G is calculated

as $2\left[\sum_{r=10}^{16} {}^{16}C_r \left(\frac{1}{2}\right)^{16}\right]$ i.e. cumulative probability of $n_G \geq 10$ out of 16 dogs showing

differential response to the treatments. This value works out to be 0.4544 which is quite high and therefore, H_0 is liable to be rejected.

Note: Tables of exact binomial proportions (not provided in this publication but available in many others as for instance, Zar, 2003) greatly facilitate calculations.

2. THE WILCOXON SIGNED-RANK TEST

This test is similar to paired t-test (*see* **Section 3.2.1** in Chapter "**Tests of hypotheses**"), but non-parametric.

2.1 Example

Suppose the same experiment discussed under Section **1.2.1** was conducted and the effect of treatments was ranked on a scale of 1 to 6; with 1 given to no improvement and 6 to maximum improvement. The observed frequencies are as follows: $d_i > 0$

	Positive ($d_i > 0$)		Negative($d_i < 0$)		$(f_P + f_N)$ *	Ranks	
Scale	d_i	f_P	d_i	f_N		Range	Average
6	6	5	−6	0	5	76–80	78.0
5	5	10	−5	0	10	66–75	70.5
4	4	16	−4	0	16	50–65	57.5
3	3	14	−3	2	16	34–49	41.5
2	2	12	−2	5	17	17–33	25.0
1	1	8	−1	8	16	1–16	8.5
Total		65 (n_G)		15 (n_L)	80 (n)		281.0

* Values wherein absolute values of d_i's are same for both 'positive' and 'negative' columns which are referred to as 'Tied values'.

Note: Maximum numerical difference possible on the scale used is +6 in favor of treatment A and –6 in favor of treatment B; similarly, the lowest differences possible are +1 and –1, respectively. Accordingly, d_i's vary between 1 and 6 for treatment A and –1 to –6 for treatment B.

We need to test H_0: $d = 0$ where d represents the population **median (or 50th Percentile)** Vs $d \# 0$. The procedure is to find sum of signed-ranks in which treatment A is better which is given by $(5 \times 78) + (10 \times 70.5) + \ldots + (8 \times 8.5) = 2964$ Vs the expected signed-rank sum, E(signed-rank sum) which is $n \times (n + 1) \div 4 = 1620$; since the observed signed-rank sum is > expected signed-rank sum, H_0 is not tenable ($n =$ number of non-zero differences; 80 in this example).

In addition, since $n > 16$, normal approximation can be made and variance of signed-rank sum calculated as $n \times (n + 1) \times (2n + 1) \div 24$ which has to be corrected for 'ties' by

subtracting $\sum_{i=1}^{k}\left(t_i^3 - t_i\right) \div 48$ where k is the number of ties and t_i refers to number of

differences with the same absolute value i.e. $(f_P + f_N)$; in the present example, Variance $= [80 \times 81 \times 161 \div 24] - [\{(5^3 - 5) + (10^3 - 10) + (16^3 - 16) + (16^3 - 16) + (17^3 - 17) + (16^3 - 16)\}$ $\div 48] = (43470 - 380.125) = 43089.875$ and sd (signed-rank sum) $= \sqrt{(variance)} = 207.581$.

Finally, a value $T = \dfrac{\left(\left|\text{Signed-Rank sum} - E\,(\text{Signed-Rank sum})\right| - \dfrac{1}{2}\right)}{sd\,(\text{Signed-Rank sum})}$ is calculated

and tested against Standard Normal Deviate, Z at set α. In this example, $T = (2964 \div 207.581) = 14.278$ which is > 1.96, the table value of Z at $= 0.05$ (Appendix 1); hence, H_0 is rejected and concluded that treatment A is better than treatment B.

Note: To test H_0: treatment B is better than treatment A, calculate signed-rank sum by considering f_N with average ranks; this yields a signed-rank sum of $(2 \times 41.5) + (5 \times 25) + (8 \times 8.5) = 276$ which is $<$ E(signed-rank sum) of 1620 indicating that H_0 is not acceptable. Further computations are, obviously, unnecessary.

3. THE WILCOXON RANK–SUM TEST

This test is similar to t-test (*see* **Section 3.2.2** in Chapter "**Tests of hypotheses**"), but non-parametric.

3.1 Example

The following hypothetical data refers to volume of erythrocytes (μ ml) from normal and triploid avians from two independent samples:

Volume of erythrocytes, μ ml										n	Σx	$\overline{X}$
Normal	247	236	268	254	248	251	260	244	238	254	10	2500	250
Normal* 1.5 @	370.5	354	402	381	372	376.5	390	366	357	381	10	3750	375
Triploid	380	390	377	392	397	374					6	2310	385

@ Calculated from 1st row based on H_0

It is required to test H_0: Triploid birds have 1.5 times the normal erythrocyte volume.

Ranks are assigned pooling data from both Normal*1.5 and triploid birds which are shown below (for ties, the method described in Chapter "**Central tendency**" is used):

	Ranks									Total
Normal* 1.5	13	16	1	6.5	12	10	4.5	14	15	6.5 98.5 (R_1)
Triploid	8	4.5	9	3	2	11				37.5 (R_2)

Number of observations in normal* 1.5 and triploid birds are $n_1 = 10$ $n_2 = 6$, respectively and total observations are $N = 16$. Average of the combined sample = $(n_1 + n_2 + 1) \div 2 = 8.5$, and under H_0, the following are computed:

$E(R_1) = n_1(n_1 + n_2 + 1) \div 2 = 85$ and variance $(R_1) = n_1 n_2(n_1 + n_2 + 1) \div 12 = 85$. Under the assumption that at least Normal*1.5 group has an underlying distribution as approximately Normal (since size = 10), further calculations are as follows:

$$T = \frac{\left[\left| R_1 - E(R_1) \right| - \frac{1}{2} \right]}{\sqrt{var(R_1)}} = 1.410 \text{ which is} < 1.96, \text{ table value of } Z \text{ at} = 0.05 \text{ (Appendix 1);}$$

hence, H_0 appears to be acceptable.

Note: If ties are noticed in the ranks, then, variance (R_1) is calculated as

$$\left(\frac{n_1 n_2}{12} \right) \left[n_1 + n_2 + 1 - \frac{\sum_{i=1}^{k} t_i^3 - t_i}{(n_1 + n_2)(n_1 + n_2 - 1)} \right]$$

where t_i's refer to frequencies having same rank and k, the number of ties. In the above example, frequencies are not available.

4. MANN-WHITNEY TEST

4.1 Mann-Whitney Test: Testing of Ranks (Zar, 2003)

This test is considered synonymous to Wilcoxon Rank-sum test and hence, the same example which was considered under **section 3.1** is taken for this test also.

4.1.1 Example

Volume of erythrocytes (µ ml) from normal and triploid avians are given below. We need to test whether volume of triploid cells is 1.5 times that of normal cells or not.

	Volume of erythrocytes, µ ml										n	Σx	$\overline{X}$
Normal	247	236	268	254	248	251	260	244	238	254	10	2500	250
Normal* 1.5 @	370.5	354	402	381	372	376.5	390	366	357	381	10	3750	375
Triploid	380	390	377	392	397	374					6	2310	385

@Calculated from 1st row based on H_0

H_0: Triploid birds have 1.5 times the normal erythrocyte volume

H_A: Triploid birds do not have 1.5 times the normal erythrocyte volume

	Ranks									Total
Normal* 1.5	13	16	1	6.5	12	10	4.5	14	15	6.5 98.5 (R_1)
Triploid	8	4.5	9	3	2	11				37.5 (R_2)

After assigning ranks, ascertain that $R_1 + R_2 = N(N + 1) \div 2$. When ranks are tied, procedure used for calculation of median (*see* Chapter "**Central tendency**") is used.

$n_1 = 10$ $n_2 = 6$ and $N = 16$; since $n_1 > n_2$, the Mann–Whitney statistic is calculated as follows: $U' = n_2 n_1 + \dfrac{n_2(n_2 + 1)}{2} - R_2$ and $U = n_1 n_2 - U'$. In this example, $U' = 43.5$ and $U = 16.5$. $U_{0.05, 10, 6} = 49$; since calculated value is < table value, H_0 may be accepted.

When $n_1 < n_2$, the Mann–Whitney statistic is calculated as follows:

$$U' = n_1 n_2 + \frac{n_1(n_1 + 1)}{2} - R_1 \text{ and } U = n_1 n_2 - U'$$

Note: Mann-Whitney tables are not provided in this publication since this test is not a routine one for animal science workers; analogous to other tests, one- or two-tail alternatives depending on H_A is possible in this test also. Since no parameter is involved, this is a non-parametric test.

4.1.2 Normal Approximation

Generally for Mann–Whitney test, size of the larger sample will be < 40 and that of smaller one < 20. However, for large n_1 and n_2, the U-distribution (discrete distribution) can be subjected to Normal approximation by (including correction for continuity)

$Z_c = \dfrac{|U - \mu_U| - 0.5}{\sigma_U}$ where $\mu_U = \dfrac{n_1 n_2}{2}$ and $\sigma_U = \sqrt{\dfrac{n_1 n_2(N + 1)}{12}}$. If tied ranks were preset

(t_i = number of ties in a group of tied values) and normal approximation is done, then,

$\sigma_U = \sqrt{\dfrac{n_1 n_2}{N^2 - N} \dfrac{N^3 - N - \sum t}{12}}$, where $\sum t = \sum (t_i^3 - t_i)$ is recommended.

4.2. Difference between Two Medians: Median Test

H_0: Two samples are from populations having the same median

H_A: The medians of the two populations are not equal

4.2.1 Procedure

An overall median for pooled data of both samples is calculated. Then, a 2 × 2 contingency table is set-up by counting the number of observations in each of the samples falling and not falling above the overall median. A χ^2 test is run with/without Yates' correction for continuity depending on expected frequencies and conclusion drawn regarding validity of H_0.

4.2.1.1 Example

Let us assume that two samples of size 20 and 25, respectively (dogs recovering from a disease graded A, B, C, D and E, in a descending order of recovery) had an overall median of C. When each of the samples was compared with the overall median, 12 and 10 were found to get A or B, respectively while the rest were of C, D or E grade. Now, it is necessary to test the above hypotheses with this sample data.

	Sample 1	Sample 2	Total
> Median (A/B)	12 (*a*)	10 (*b*)	22 (R$_1$)
≤ Median (C/D/E)	8 (*c*)	15 (*d*)	23 (R$_2$)
Total	20 (C$_1$)	25 (C$_2$)	45 (*n*)

$$\chi^2 = \frac{n\left(|ad - bc|^2\right)}{R_1 R_2 C_1 C_2} = 1.779 \; Vs \text{ table value of } 3.841 \text{ on } \upsilon = 1 \text{ and } \alpha = 0.05 \text{ (Appendix 4).}$$

Hence, H$_0$ appears to be acceptable.

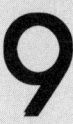

9

Association Between Variables I

(Simple Linear Regression and Correlation)

Many characters in nature, both qualitative as well as quantitative, are apparently associated; for instance, age and body weight, duration of cooking and acceptability of a product, age at sexual maturity and egg production, age at first calving and birth weight of calf, egg weight and chick weight, orientation of egg and hatchability, etc; the list is virtually inexhaustible. Further, it is also interesting to note that associations are broadly of two types, *viz.* 1) when one of them increases the other also increases and vice versa which is referred to as **positive association** like that between egg weight and chick weight and 2) when one of them increases the other decreases and vice versa which is referred to as **negative association** like that between age at sexual maturity and egg production. There may be several underlying causes for apparent association; they include physical, chemical (biochemical) or biological (including genetic).

1.   REGRESSION *Vis-à-vis* CORRELATION

Let us consider the association between egg weight (x) and chick weight (y) in more detail; it is easy to notice that y depends on x and not *vice versa*; hence, x is referred to as **independent variable** and y, the **dependent variable**. It is also necessary to note that in an association between variables, it is not mandatory that one of them must be dependent on the other; for instance, between °C and °F, neither of them is dependent on the other, but there is a mathematical relationship between them. In certain circumstances, though, it will not be proper to designate a variable dependent as for instance in case of length of fore-limb *vs* that of hind-limb.

When an association between variables doesn't specify dependency (or independency), **correlation** between them **is calculated to assess intensity and direction of association**. On the other hand, if dependency is identified, **regression can be calculated to assess not only intensity and direction, but also functional relation of association**. Hence, correlation has no units and ranges between −1 and +1 whereas, regression has units (that of dependent variable per unit of independent variable) and can take any value between −∞ and +∞; as in case of egg weight – chick weight association, g/g of egg weight and so on.

Note: It is a common practice to designate dependent variable as y and independent variable as x.

1.1 Example

Let us take up a very common case: Day-old chicks require a brooding temperature of 95 °F in the beginning which has to be reduced at a rate of 5 °F per week for a period of generally 4 weeks. Suppose, the brooder is provided with a Centigrade thermometer; then what should be the reduction in the centigrade scale?

If we apply the formula $C = (5 \div 9) \times (F - 32)$, the result indicates that the temperature on Celsius scale has to be reduced by (–) 15 °C! per week which is impossible to implement. There are two ways of solving the riddle:

1.1.1 Solutions

1.1.1.1 Solution 1

$$C_1 = \frac{5}{9}(x - 32) \text{ converts } x°F \text{ into Celsius scale} \qquad \text{(Equation 1)}$$

$$C_2 = \frac{5}{9}(x + y - 32) \text{ converts } (x + y)°F \text{ into Celsius scale} \qquad \text{(Equation 2)}$$

Obviously, difference of y °F on Celsius scale is given by (Equation 2 – Equation 1) $= \frac{5}{9}y$; or in simple terms, the difference on the Celsius scale is $(5 \div 9)$ times that on the Fahrenheit scale.

1.1.1.2 Solution 2

To make it easy to understand, let us consider the equation for converting °C to °F; i.e.

$F = \frac{9}{5}C + 32$ or $32 + \frac{9}{5}C$ which is same as the equation of a straight line ($y = c + mx$) or linear regression ($y = a + bx$) where 'c or a' (as the case may be) represents **intercept or value of y when $x = 0$** and 'm or b' (as the case may be) represents **change in the value of y per unit change in x** referred to as "**Slope or Regression Coefficient**".

In simple terms, when °C = 0, °F = 32 and for every 1°C increase or decrease, °F will increase or decrease by $(9 \div 5)$; or $\Delta F = \frac{9}{5}\Delta C$. By rearranging, $\Delta C = \frac{5}{9}\Delta F$ which is same as obtained under Solution 1.

Therefore, the following points are worth a special mention:
1. The relationship between °C and °F is a straight line (linear) and
2. The association is positive; indicating that a change in one scale brings about a uniform change in the other; in other words, if one increases, the other also increases and *vice versa*.

Several other types of relationship are possible and commonly encountered relationships can be graphically represented as follows:

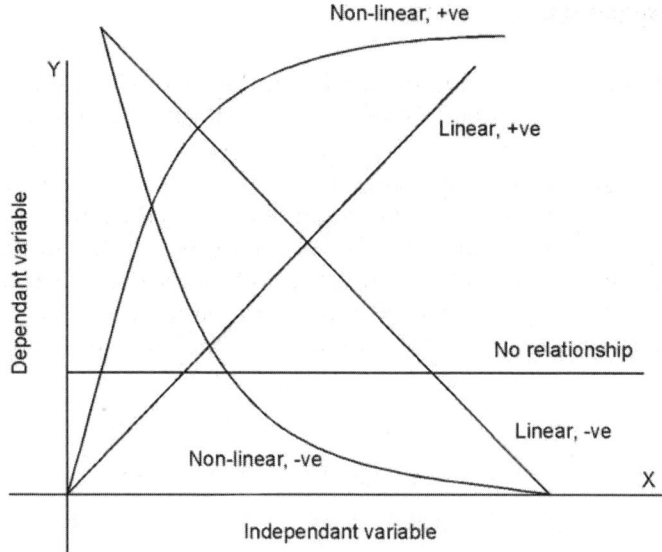

Fig. 9.1

Caution: It is in the fitness of things to note that if calculations are made between annual cattle population and annual literacy in India since Independence, it is possible to obtain highly significant association!; but it can't be used to conclude that increase in literacy is due to increased cattle population! Such associations, if calculated, can best be called *nonsense association*. Therefore, utmost care should be exercised before proceeding into analysis of association between two variables.

2. MODELS OF EXPERIMENTAL DESIGN

2.1.1 Fixed-Effect Model (Model I)

Suppose a scientist is conducting an experiment to test the effect of four different floor–space allowances on growth rate of broilers. Since levels are specifically chosen, it is referred to as fixed–effect model. In this model H_0 will specify the means while stating equality as in this example, H_0: $\mu_1 = \mu_2 = \mu_3 = \mu_4$

2.1.2 Random-Effect Model (Model II)

Consider an experiment to find the effect of diurnal variation on certain hormone levels in layers; in this case, the diurnal variation is not controlled by the experimenter but comes as random variable; hence, this model is the random-effect model. In random–model, H_0 will be: there is no effect of diurnal variation on the hormone levels in layers.

2.1.3 Mixed-Model (Model III)

If an experiment has both fixed and random effects, it is referred to as mixed-model; For instance known sires are mated to random group of dams and the progeny values are considered as the criterion for analysis. This will be discussed in Chapter "**Analysis of variance**".

3.   LINEAR REGRESSION

For calculation of regression, x variable can be random- or a fixed-effect and forms the *abscissa* whereas y variable, a random-effect, which forms the *ordinate* while plotting as a graph.

Simple linear regression is represented as $y_i = \alpha + \beta x_i$ where α and β represent parameters (constants). Since a perfect straight line which the equation predicts is not likely in a population, more so in case of biological traits, another factor referred to as 'residual' or 'error (ε_i)' comes into picture necessitating a modification in the above equation to $y_i = \alpha + \beta x_i + \varepsilon_i$; the error refers to the deviation of the values the equation predicts from the actual values with an assumption that $\Sigma \varepsilon_i = 0$.

3.1   Example

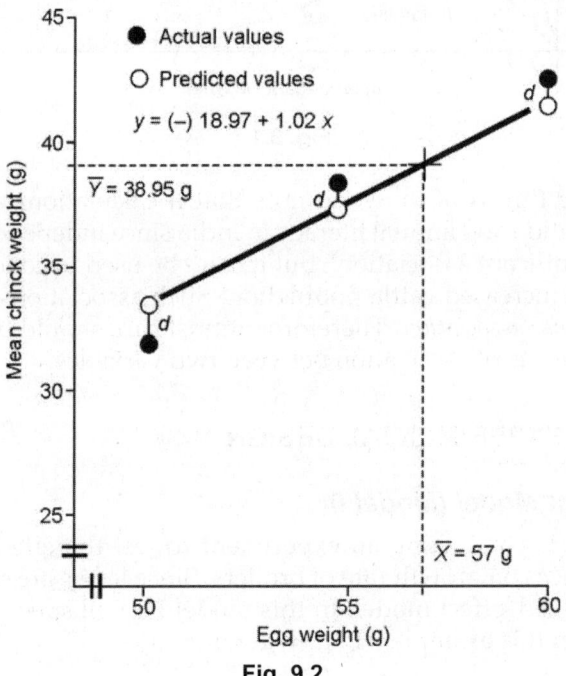

Fig. 9.2

A hypothetical data of chick weight (y) as function of egg weight (x) was used to fit a linear regression equation (procedure will be dealt under Section **3.2** in this Chapter). The figure above shows that the actual values (y) lie on either side of the predicted values (y') represented by the straight line in such a way that sum of the deviations {d_i's, $(y_i - y_i')$} above (positive) and below (negative) the line will be zero in other words *error* (residual) *sum of squares*, $\sum_{i=1}^{n}(y_i - y_i')^2$, is minimized ($n$ = number of pairs of observations).

It is ideal that all values in the population are available for estimating α and β; but, it is equally true that, on most occasions it is not possible. Hence, a sample of n observations are used to estimate α and β; the estimates are a, the intercept b_{yx}, the regression coefficient of y on x and e_i, the error component.

3.2 Fitting a Linear Regression Equation

Certain assumptions must be satisfied in order that tests of hypotheses be carried out and confidence limits be set for the calculated b_{yx} from the sample data; they are as follows:

3.2.1 Assumptions

1. For every value of x, there is a Normal distribution of y and a Normal distribution of e_i. In other words, e_i's are Normally distributed with mean 0 and variance s^2.
2. S_y^2 at all points of x, is homogenous.
3. Mean values of y fall on the predicted line indicating linear relationship between x and y.
4. Values of y are drawn at random from the population and independent of one another.
5. There is no (or negligible) error in the measurement of x or error in measurement of x is at least considerably less than in that of y.

Note: If assumptions 1, 2 and 3 are in violation, they can be corrected by suitable transformation of data (*see* Chapter "**Transformations**"); weighted regression analysis is sometimes resorted to if Assumption 2 is violated.

The concept of a, b_{yx} and part of Assumptions 1 and 2 are graphically represented below:

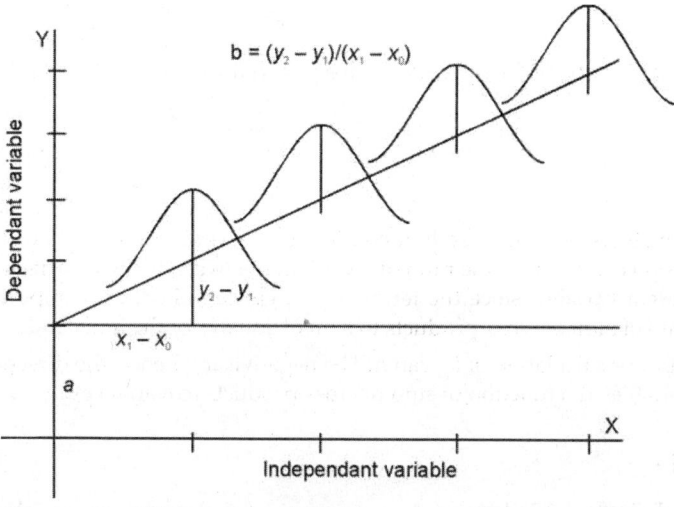

Fig. 9.3

3.2.2 Computation

For calculation of a and b_{yx} values, the following are calculated:

1. Corrected sum of squares x, $SS_x = \sum_{i=1}^{n} x_i^2 - \dfrac{\left(\sum_{i=1}^{n} x_i\right)^2}{n}$ (*see* Chapter "**Dispersion**")

2. Corrected sum of cross-products between x and y, designated scp_{xy} by the formula

$$SCP_{xy} = \sum_{i=1}^{n} x_i y_i - \frac{\left(\sum_{i=1}^{n} x_i\right)\left(\sum_{i=1}^{n} y_i\right)}{n} ;$$ this is similar to calculation of corrected sum of

squares x except that instead of squaring each value of x, it is multiplied with the

corresponding value of y and then added to get $\sum_{i=1}^{n} x_i y_i$

3. Regression coefficient (slope) is the ratio of corrected sum of cross-products between the variables to the corrected sum of squares of the independent variable; i.e.

$$b_{yx} = \frac{SCP_{xy}}{SS_x}$$

4. For running test of hypothesis, corrected sum of squares of y, $SS_y = \sum_{i=1}^{n} y_i^2 - \frac{\left(\sum_{i=1}^{n} y_i\right)^2}{n}$

is required (see Chapter "**Dispersion**") and $se(b) = \sqrt{var\left(b_{yx}\right)} = \sqrt{\frac{SS_y - b_{yx}\left(SCP_{xy}\right)}{SS_x\left(n-2\right)}} =$

$\sqrt{\frac{MSS_e}{SS_x}}$; the meaning of MSS_e and ss_x are given along with ANOVA for regression

coefficient.

Note:

1. If the numerator and denominator is divided by υ i.e. $(n-1)$, Covariance$_{xy}$ and s_x^2 are obtained; in fact, the regression coefficient is the ratio of covariance between the two variables to the variance of the independent variable; since the terms $(n-1)$ get cancelled, the computations formula is given as the ratio of sum of cross-products to sum of squares of the independent variable.

2. The denominator for calculation of b_{yx} can not be negative and hence, the direction of association between the variables is a function of sum of cross-products (covariance).

3.2.2.1 Example

Daily milk yield (kg) of 12 dams (x) and mean of 6 daughters per dam (y) is given below (hypothetical) from which we have to calculate a, b_{yx}, test the significance of b_{yx} (H_0: b = 0) and set confidence intervals for b:

$\bar{x} = 6.2417$ kg, $\bar{y} = 6.40$ kg, $SS_x = 31.5292$ kg^2, $SCP_{xy} = 30.77$ kg^2, $b_{yx} = \frac{SCP_{xy}}{SS_x} = 0.9759$ kg/kg,

$a = \bar{y} - b_{yx}\bar{x} = 0.3087$ kg; $y = 0.3086 + 0.9759x$, $SS_y = 30.9200$ kg^2, $se(b_{yx}) = 0.0532$ kg;

Sl No	Dam (x)	Daughter (y)	x^2	y^2	xy	$\hat{y}$ *
1	5.3	5.5	28.09	30.25	29.15	5.48
2	3.1	3.6	9.61	12.96	11.16	3.33
3	8.2	7.8	67.84	60.84	63.96	8.31
4	8.0	8.5	64.00	72.25	68.00	8.12
5	6.5	6.3	42.25	39.69	40.95	6.65
6	6.3	6.7	39.69	44.89	42.21	6.46
7	3.8	3.6	14.44	12.96	13.68	4.02
8	7.1	7.3	50.41	53.29	51.83	7.24
9	7.7	8.0	59.29	64.00	61.60	7.82
10	4.6	4.9	21.16	24.01	22.54	4.80
11	6.6	6.7	43.56	44.89	44.22	6.75
12	7.7	7.9	59.29	62.41	60.83	7.82
Totals	74.9	76.8	499.03	522.44	510.13	76.80

* Predicted values from the regression equation for corresponding x_i values; Residual sum of squares, $\sum_{i=1}^{n}(y_i - \hat{y}_i)^2 = 0.8892$ kg²

Note: It is not advisable to predict values of y_i's for value of x outside the range of observed values of x which are used computing the regression equation because, on either side of the range, it is not certain whether the association between x and y is linear or not; if linear, whether the magnitude of association is same or not. If one is certain that the association continues to be the same beyond the range, then extrapolation will not be erroneous.

3.2.2.1.1 Testing significance of regression coefficient

3.2.2.1.1.1 Student's t-test

$t = \dfrac{b_{yx} - \beta}{se(b_{yx})}$ on $v = (n-2)$ and set α; since H_0 states $\beta = 0$, $t = \dfrac{b_{yx}}{se(b_{yx})} = (0.9759 \div 0.0532)$

$= 18.352$ which is > 2.228, the table value of $t_{0.05, 10}$; therefore, H_0 is liable to be rejected.

3.2.2.1.1.2 Analysis of variance (ANOVA) method

Details of ANOVA will be discussed in a separate Chapter. However, testing for significance of b_{yx} by ANOVA is as follows:

Source	v	Sum of squares	Mean sum of squares	F ratio**
Total	$n-1$	SS_y	$SS_y \div v = MSS_T$	–
Linear regression	1	$SS_b = b_{yx}*SCP_{xy}$	$SS_b \div v = MSS_b$	$MSS_b \div MSS_e$
Residual	$n-2$	$SS_e = SS_y - SS_b$	$SS_e \div v = MSS_e$	–

** Relevant only if $F > 1$, on $v = 1$ and $(n-2)$ for greater and smaller MSS, respectively

In **Example 3.2.2.1**, the ANOVA table will be as follows:

Source	υ	Sum of squares	Mean sum of squares	F ratio[@]
Total	11	$SS_y = 30.9200$		–
Linear regression	1	$SS_b = 30.0824$	$MSS_b = 30.0824$	337.247**
Residual	10	$SS_e = 0.8916$	$MSS_e = 0.0892$	–

[@] Relevant only if F > 1, on $\upsilon = 1$ and $(n - 2)$ for greater and smaller MSS, respectively

Calculated value of F ratio is > table value of $F_{0.05, 1, 10}$; hence, H_0 can be rejected.

Note:

1. Generally '*' is placed on the calculated F value if it is significant only at $\alpha = 0.05$ and '**' is placed when it is significant at $\alpha = 0.01$.

2. Proportion of total variation in the dependent variable contributed by its association with the independent variable is referred to as **Coefficient of Determination (R^2 or r^2)** is obviously the ratio of ss_b to ss_y; i.e. $30.0824 \div 30.92 = 0.9729$ or 97.29%. The quantity r is the correlation coefficient which will be discussed later in this Chapter.

3. It also follows that $(1 - r^2)$ is the Coefficient of non-determination or the variation in y_i's not due to the regression; which is 2.81% in the above example.

4. When υ for greater variance is unity (1), $\sum_{i=1}^{n}(y_i - \hat{y}_i)^2$ =Residual sum of squares and $t^2 = F$; the latter is applicable to both Table and calculated values at a set α; the small difference noticed in the above example is only due to decimal approximation error.

3.2.2.1.2 Setting confidence intervals

3.2.2.1.2.1 For regression coefficient

If the standard error of a Statistic is known, the general formula for confidence intervals for the Statistic is as follows:

Confidence interval = Statistic $\pm t_{\alpha, \upsilon}$*Standard error of the statistic; the two-tailed table value of t is located. In the above example, the 5% confidence intervals will be $0.9759 \pm 2.228*0.0532 = 0.9759 \pm 0.1185$ kg. In simple terms, it can be stated that b lies within the limits of 0.8574 kg and 1.0944 kg; and this has a chance of being wrong being only 5%.

3.2.2.1.2.2 For estimated values of dependent variable

Standard error of the predicted values $\left(s_{\hat{y}}\right)$ is given by $s_{\hat{y}} = \sqrt{MSS_e\left(\dfrac{1}{n} + \dfrac{(x_i - \bar{x})^2}{SS_x}\right)}$ with

usual meaning for all notations. With the availability of $s_{\hat{y}}$, hypothesis testing is possible for the estimated values of y. For instance, $s_{\hat{y}}$ for the predicted y value at Sl No 6 ($x =$

6.5 kg, $y = 6.3$ kg and $\hat{y} = 6.46$ kg) is $\sqrt{0.0892\left(\dfrac{1}{12} + \dfrac{(6.3 - 6.2417)^2}{31.5292}\right)} = 0.0863$ kg. Now

we can test H_0: Population mean of daughters from a dam producing 6.5 kg is ≤ 6.5 kg (one–tail test) by calculating $t = \dfrac{6.46 - 6.5}{0.0863} = -0.463$ which is > -2.268, the table value

of $t_{0.05, 10}$; hence, H_0 is acceptable.

3.2.2.2 Predicting independent variable (inverse prediction)

Rarely though, it may be required to predict the value of independent variable for a known value of dependent variable. By rearranging the linear regression equation we can calculate $\hat{x}_i$ for a specified value of y_i thus: $\hat{x}_i = \dfrac{y_i - a}{b_{yx}}$ and if $k = b_{yx}^2 - t_{\alpha,(n-2)}^2$

$\operatorname{var}(b_{yx})$, confidence limits can be obtained by solving $\bar{x} + \dfrac{b_{yx}(y_i - \bar{y})}{k} \pm$

$\dfrac{t}{k}\sqrt{MSS_e\left[\dfrac{(y_i - \bar{y})^2}{SS_x} + k\left(1 + \dfrac{1}{n}\right)\right]}$. If there are multiple values of y_i's (m) for each value of

x_i, then $\hat{x}_i = \dfrac{\bar{y}_i - a}{b_{yx}}$ and confidence limits of can be obtained by $\bar{x} + \dfrac{b_{yx}(\bar{y}_i - \bar{y})}{k} \pm$

$\dfrac{t}{k}\sqrt{MSS_e^w\left[\dfrac{(\bar{y}_i - \bar{y})^2}{SS_x} + k\left(\dfrac{1}{m} + \dfrac{1}{n}\right)\right]}$ where $\bar{y}_i = \dfrac{\sum\limits_{j=1}^{m} y_{ij}}{m}$, $\bar{y} = \dfrac{\sum\limits_{i=1}^{n}\sum\limits_{j=1}^{m} y_{ij}}{nm}$, $k = b_{yx}^2 - t_{\alpha,(n+m-3)}^2$

$\operatorname{var}(b_{yx})$, and $MSS_e^w = MSS_e + \dfrac{\sum\limits_{j=1}^{m}(y_{ij} - \bar{y}_i)^2}{(n+m-3)}$.

In the above example, let us find the value of x for $y = 7$ kg; in other words, what could be the dam's production if daughter's production is 7 kg? Predicted value will be $(7.0 - 0.3087) \div 0.9759 = 6.86$ kg, with 95% confidence intervals 6.2417 +

$\dfrac{0.9759(7.0 - 6.40)}{0.9154} \pm \dfrac{2.228}{0.9154}\sqrt{0.0892\left[\dfrac{(7.0 - 6.4)^2}{31.5292} + 0.9154\left(1 + \dfrac{1}{12}\right)\right]} = 6.8814 \pm 0.0.7280$ kg;

i.e. between 6.1534 and 7.6094 kg.

3.2.2.3 Linear regression with multiple values of dependent variable

Instances wherein multiple values of dependent variable is available for each value of independent variable are not uncommon in animal science data. For example, it is common that many broilers of the same age (independent variable) are weighed and often, the same birds are weighed at different ages with the corresponding values of each of the birds being recorded. One way is to calculate mean value of the dependent variable at each point of independent variable and carry-on the regression analysis as described above. In fact it augurs well with one of the assumptions for linear regression is the presence of a normally distributed population of y_i's at each value of x. However, precious information on the variability of y_i's at each value of x is lost in the process.

Alternatively, independent variable may be assumed to be repeating (replicating) and y_i's are considered individually instead of a mean value representing them. This procedure helps use the entire information (variability) available in the data.

3.2.2.3.1 Example

Data in the table below is a hypothetical one on the body weight of broilers; equal frequency at each point of x is chosen; but, the procedure is valid for unequal frequencies as well. We need to fit a linear regression equation and test H_0's: 1) Population regression is linear and if it is true, 2) $\beta = 0$

Age in weeks (x_i)	Body weights, kg (y_i)	$\sum_{j=1}^{n_i} x_{ij}$	$\sum_{j=1}^{n_i} y_{ij}$	$\sum_{j=1}^{n_i} x_{ij}^2$	$\sum_{j=1}^{n_i} y_{ij}^2$	$\sum_{j=1}^{n_i} x_{ij} y_{ij}$
1	0.10,0.12,0.14,0.08	4	0.44	4	0.0504	0.44
2	0.23,0.28,0.22,0.20,0.30	10	1.23	20	0.3097	2.46
3	0.54,0.60,0.70	9	1.84	27	1.1416	5.52
4	1.00,1.30,1.40,0.90,0.95	20	5.55	80	6.3625	22.20
5	1.50,1.70,1.65,1.60	20	6.45	100	10.4225	32.35
6	2.00,2.20,1.75,2.50,1.90	30	10.35	180	21.7625	62.10
Totals		93	25.86	411	40.0492	125.07

$\bar{x} = 3.5769$ wks, $\bar{y} = 0.9946$ kg, $SS_x = 78.3462$ wks², $SCP_{xy} = 32.5708$ wk kg, $b_{yx} = \dfrac{scp_{xy}}{ss_x} = 0.4157$ kg/wk, $a = \bar{y} - b_{yx}\bar{x} = -0.4923$ kg/wk; $y = -0.4923 + 0.4157x$, $SS_y = 14.3284$ kg², $se(b_{yx}) = 0.0205$ kg/wk

It can be noticed that $\sum_{i=1}^{6}\sum_{j=1}^{n_i} x_{ij} = 93$, $\sum_{i=1}^{6}\sum_{j=1}^{n_i} y_{ij} = 25.86$, $\sum_{i=1}^{6}\sum_{j=1}^{n_i} x_{ij}^2 = 411$, $\sum_{i=1}^{6}\sum_{j=1}^{n_i} y_{ij}^2 = 40.0492$

and $\sum_{i=1}^{6}\sum_{j=1}^{n_i} x_{ij} y_{ij} = 125.07$ in the above example. Further computations are indicated in the table itself.

The following sums of squares have to be computed for further analyses and tests of hypotheses:

1. Total sum of squares, $SS_y = \sum_{i=1}^{6}\sum_{j=1}^{n_i} y_{ij}^2 - \dfrac{\left(\sum_{i=1}^{6}\sum_{j=1}^{n_i} y_{ij}\right)^2}{\sum_{i=1}^{6} n_i} = 40.0492 - 25.7208 = 14.3284$

on $\upsilon = \sum_{i=1}^{6} n_i - 1 = 26 - 1 = 25.$

2. Sum of squares **between (among)** ages $SS_g = \sum_{i=1}^{6} \dfrac{\left(\sum_{j=1}^{n_i} y_{ij}\right)^2}{n_i} - \dfrac{\left(\sum_{i=1}^{6}\sum_{j=1}^{n_i} y_{ij}\right)^2}{\sum_{i=1}^{6} n_i}$ on $\upsilon = (6-1)$

= 5; i.e. $[(0.44^2 \div 4) + (1.23^2 \div 5) \ldots + (10.35^2 \div 5)] - (25.86^2 \div 26)] = 39.4651 - 25.7208$
= 13.7443 kg² on $\upsilon = 5$.

3. Sum of squares **within** ages $SS_w = (SS_y - SS_g) = 11.3941 - 11.2769 = 0.5841$ on $\upsilon =$

$$\sum_{i=1}^{6} n_i - 1 - \upsilon \text{ for among ages} = 26 - 1 - 5 = 20$$

Sum of squares between ages SS_g comprises of two quantities:

a. Sum of squares due to regression, $SS_b = b_{yx} \times SCP_{xy} = 13.5397$ on $\upsilon = 1$

b. Sum of squares due to deviation from linearity $SS_d = (SS_g - SS_b) = 13.7443 - 13.5397 = 0.2046$ on $\upsilon = (5 - 1) = 4$.

Now, the ANOVA table can be laid-out:

Source	υ	Sum of squares	Mean sum of squares	F ratio [@]
Total	25	$SS_y = 14.3284$		-
Between ages	5	$SS_g = 13.7443$		
Linear regression	1	$SS_b = 13.5397$	$MSS_b = 13.5397$	$MSS_d \div MSS_r$ [#] = 411.541**
Deviation from linearity	4	$SS_d = 0.2046$	$MSS_d = 0.0512$	$MSS_d \div MSS_w$ = 1.753[NS]
Within groups	20	$SS_w = 0.5841$	$MSS_w = 0.0292$	

[@] Relevant only if F > 1, on $\upsilon = 1$ and $(n - 2)$ for greater and smaller MSS, respectively

[#] MSS_r (residual mean sum of squares) $= (SS_d + SS_w) \div (\upsilon_d + \upsilon_w) = (0.2046 + 0.5841) \div (4 + 20) = 0.0329$

Coefficient of determination, $r^2 = (13.5397 \div 14.3284) = 0.9450$ or 94.50%

** Value greater than the table value even at $\alpha = 0.01$

[NS] Value less than the table value at $\alpha = 0.05$

Now, to test H_0: 1) population regression is linear and if it is true, calculated value of F (1.753) for deviations from linearity is < 3.51, the table value of $F_{0.05,\,4,20}$; hence, H_0 is acceptable and β is linear.

To test H_0: 2) β = 0, the calculated value 411.541 for linear regression is > 5.72 as well as 9.55, the table value of $F_{0.05,\,1,20}$ and $F_{0.01,\,1,20}$; hence, H_0 is not acceptable and β > 0.

Note: If H_0: (1) Population regression is linear is not accepted, H_0: (2) β = 0 is tested using F ratio calculated as $(MSS_b \div MSS_w)$ on respective υ's.

3.2.2.4 Linear regression from a bi-variate frequency table

This is analogous to calculation of b_{yx} from frequency distribution table.

3.2.2.4.1 Example

A hypothetical example of milk yield (kg) and their corresponding fat content (%) are tabulated below.

Fat content (%), y_i $\downarrow$	Milk yield (kg), x_i					
	4	8	12	16	20	Σf_y
3	1	4	8	26	22	61
4	5	10	27	25	18	85
5	30	18	30	14	11	103
6	26	12	18	10	7	73
7	15	8	6	3	2	34
Σf_x	77	52	89	78	60	356 (N)

$\Sigma f_x = \Sigma f_y = N = 356$; $\Sigma f_x x_i = 77 \times 4 + 52 \times 8 + \ldots + 60 \times 20 = 4240$ kg; $\Sigma f_y y_i = 61 \times 3 + 85 \times 4 + \ldots + 34 \times 7 = 1714$ %; $\Sigma f_x x_i^2 = 77 \times 16 + 52 \times 64 + \ldots + 60 \times 400 = 61344$ kg²; $\Sigma f_y y_i^2 = 61 \times 9 + 85 \times 16 + \ldots + 34 \times 49 = 8778$ %²; $\Sigma f_i x_i y_i = 1 \times 4 \times 3 + 4 \times 8 \times 3 + \ldots + 2 \times 20 \times 7 = 19324$ kg%;

$SS_x = \sum f_i x_i^2 - \dfrac{\left(\sum f_i x_i\right)^2}{N} = 10845.1236$ kg²; $SS_y = \sum f_i y_i^2 - \dfrac{\left(\sum f_i y_i\right)^2}{N} = 525.7640$ %²; $SCP_{xy} =$

$\sum f_i x_i y_i - \dfrac{\left(\sum f_i x_i\right)\left(\sum f_i y_i\right)}{N} = -1089.9326$ kg%

Following calculation of SCP_{xy}, SS_x and SS_y, the rest of computation is same as shown under **Section 3.2.2**. Hence, $b_{yx} = -0.1005$, $se(b_{yx}) = 0.0104$; $t = 9.663$ (on $\upsilon = 354$ or ∞) which is > 1.960, the table value of $t_{0.05, \infty}$; hence, H_0 ($\beta = 0$) may be rejected. Testing of H_0 can be carried–out by ANOVA procedure also to get $SS_b = MSS_b = 109.5382$; $SS_e = 416.2258$; $MSS_e = 1.1758$ and $F = 93.1606$ on $\upsilon = 1$ and 354 (or ∞) at set α (0.05) which is also $>$ table value of F at corresponding υ and α. Again, it can be noticed that $F = t^2$ when υ for the numerator is unity. Hence, it is reasonable to conclude that fat % reduces as milk yield increases.

3.2.2.5 Linear regression through origin

As the name indicates, the straight line when plotted starts at coordinates (0, 0); in other words, the intercept, $a = 0$ and $y_i = bx_i$; the calculations, with usual meaning for notations, will be as follows (see Section **3.2.2**):

$$SCP_{xy} = \sum_{i=1}^{n} x_i y_i - \dfrac{\left(\sum_{i=1}^{n} x_i\right)\left(\sum_{i=1}^{n} y_i\right)}{n} \, , \quad SS_x = \sum_{i=1}^{n} x_i^2 - \dfrac{\left(\sum_{i=1}^{n} x_i\right)^2}{n} \, , \quad b_{yx} = \dfrac{SCP_{xy}}{SS_x} \, , \text{ total sum of}$$

squares $= SS_y = \sum_{i=1}^{n} y_i^2 - \dfrac{\left(\sum_{i=1}^{n} y_i\right)^2}{n}$, sum of squares due to regression, $SS_b = b_{yx} \times SCP_{xy}$

on $\upsilon = 1$, residual sum of squares, $SS_e = SS_y - SS_b$ on $\upsilon = (n-1)$ because the intercept is not calculated. With these values, ANOVA can be run as already described. If t–test has to be run, $se(b_{yx})$ is calculated as $se(b) = \sqrt{var\left(b_{yx}\right)} = \sqrt{\dfrac{SS_y - b_{yx}\left(SCP_{xy}\right)}{SS_x\left(n-2\right)}} = \sqrt{\dfrac{MSS_e}{SS_x}}$

and to test H_0: $\beta = 0$, **on $\beta = (n-1)$** and set α.

3.2.2.5.1 Inverse prediction when intercept = 0

As discussed under section **3.2.2.2**, we can calculate $\hat{x}_i$ for a specified value of y_i thus:

$\hat{x}_i = \dfrac{y_i}{b_{yx}}$ and if $k = b_{yx}^2 - t_{\alpha,(n-2)}^2 \, \text{var}\left(b_{yx}\right)$, confidence limits can be obtained by solving

$\bar{x} + \dfrac{b_{yx} y_i}{k} \pm \dfrac{t}{k} \sqrt{MSS_e \left(\dfrac{y_i^2}{SS_x} + k \right)}$. If there are multiple values of y_i's (m) for each value of

x_i, then $\hat{x}_i = \dfrac{\bar{y}_i}{b_{yx}}$ and confidence limits of $\hat{x}_i$ can be obtained by $\bar{x} + \dfrac{b_{yx} \bar{y}_i}{k} \pm$

$\dfrac{t}{k} \sqrt{MSS_e^w \left(\dfrac{\bar{y}_i^2}{SS_x} + \dfrac{k}{m} \right)}$ where $\bar{y}_i = \dfrac{\sum\limits_{j=1}^{m} y_{ij}}{m}$, $\bar{y} = \dfrac{\sum\limits_{i=1}^{n}\sum\limits_{j=1}^{m} y_{ij}}{nm}$, $k = b_{yx}^2 - t_{\alpha,(n+m-2)}^2 \, \text{var}\left(b_{yx}\right)$, and

$$MSS_e^w = \dfrac{MSS_e + \sum\limits_{j=1}^{m}\left(y_{ij} - \bar{y}_i\right)^2}{(n+m-2)}.$$

3.2.2.6 Effect of coding

It may be necessary to change the origin and/or scale to facilitate computations (*see* Chapters "**Central tendency**" and "**Dispersion**"); Let us assume that x_i's were multiplied by k_x and a_x is added to each of them (i.e. $x_i = k_x x_i + a_x$) ; the corresponding values for y_i's being k_y and a_y (i.e. $y_i = k_y y_i + a_y$). With the constants being added or subtracted to x and/or y, the slope b_{yx} remains unaltered. If constants are coefficients, then b_{yx} on coded scale will be $b_{yx}\left(\dfrac{k_y}{k_x}\right)$ which can be brought back to original scale by

multiplying the coded b_{yx} with $\left(\dfrac{k_x}{k_y}\right)$. Coding will not alter value of r^2 and calculated values of t and F.

The above procedure is particularly useful when converting results on °C scale to °F scale and *vice versa*.

3.3 Comparing > 1 Slopes

3.3.1 Two Slopes

Extending the concept of t–statistic, for difference between two regression coefficients, b_1 and b_2, $t = \dfrac{(b_1 - b_2)}{se(b_1 - b_2)}$ on $\upsilon = (n_1 + n_2 - 4)$ where the denominator, $se(b_1 - b_2) =$

$\sqrt{\text{var}(b_1) + \text{var}(b_2)}$ and pooled residual mean sum of squares is obtained as the ratio

of sum of the residual mean squares to the sum of their υ's i.e. $MSS_e^p = \dfrac{MSS_e^{b_1} + MSS_e^{b_2}}{\upsilon_e^{b_1} + \upsilon_e^{b_2}}$;

the denominator will be $(n_1 + n_2 - 4)$.

Let us consider **Example 3.2.2.1** as first set of data; therefore, $b_1 = 0.9759$ kg, var (b_1) $= 0.0028$ kg², $MSS_e^{b_1} = 0.0892$ and $v_e^{b_1} = 10$. As a second set of data, let us consider a similar example with a different dam–daughter values as follows (only final values listed):

3.3.1.1 Example

Sl No	Dam (x)	Daughter (y)
1	8.3	7.5
2	6.1	6.6
3	11.2	10.8
4	11.0	11.5
5	9.5	9.3
6	10.3	10.7
7	6.8	5.6
8	10.1	9.3
9	11.7	12.0
10	8.6	7.9
11	9.6	9.7
12	8.7	· 8.9
Totals	111.9	109.8

$\bar{x} = 9.325$ kg, $\bar{y} = 9.15$ kg, $ss_x = 32.3625$ kg², $SCP_{xy} = 35.545$ kg², $b_{yx} = \dfrac{SCP_{xy}}{SS_x} =$ 1.0983 kg/kg, $a = \bar{y} - b_{yx}\bar{x} = -1.0916$ kg; $y = -1.0916 + 1.0983x$, $ss_y = 71.16$ kg², $se(b_{yx})$ $= 0.1045$ kg.

From the above, the following are required for testing the two slopes: $b_2 = 1.0983$ kg/kg, var $(b_2) = 0.0109$ kg², $MSS_e^{b_2} = 0.3531$ and $v_e^{b_2} = 10$.

$$H_0: b_1 = b_2; \ t = \frac{0.9759 - 1.0983}{\sqrt{0.0028 + 0.0109}} = -1.046 \text{ which is} < 2.086, \text{ the table value of } t_{0.05,\ 20};$$

this gives a scope for pooling the slopes by the formula $b_p = \dfrac{b_1 SS_{x_1} + b_2 SS_{x_2}}{SS_{x_1} + SS_{x_2}}$

$$= \frac{\left(SCP_{xy}\right)_1 + \left(SCP_{xy}\right)_2}{SS_{x_1} + SS_{x_2}} = \frac{30.770 + 35.545}{31.5292 + 32.3625} = 1.0379 \text{ kg/kg. Since } se(b_1 - b_2) =$$

$\sqrt{\text{var}(b_1) + \text{var}(b_2)} = se(b_1 + b_2)$, $se(b_p) = \sqrt{\text{var}(b_1) + \text{var}(b_2)} = 0.1170$ kg/kg.

Note: If H_0 is accepted, the lines are likely to be parallel to one another; if H_0 is rejected, i.e. $b_1 \# b_2$, the lines are intersecting; then, coordinates of the point of intersection of the two lines can be obtained by

$x_{int} = \dfrac{a_2 - a_1}{b_2 - b_1}$ and $y_{int} = a_1 + b_1 x_{int}$ or $y_{int} = a_2 + b_2 x_{int}$

3.3.1.2 Comparing two elevations

In the above example, H_0 was accepted; this situation gives another scope for testing elevations (vertical position when plotted on a graph paper) of the two lines (**Examples 3.2.2.1** and **3.3.1.1**) by the calculating the following (H_0: The elevations of the regression lines are same):

1. Pooled $SS_x = SS_{x_1} + SS_{x_2} = 63.8917$

2. Pooled $SS_y = SS_{y_1} + SS_{y_2} = 102.08$

3. Pooled $SCP_{xy} = SCP_{xy_1} + SCP_{xy_2} = 66.315$

4. Pooled $b_{yx} = \dfrac{\text{Pooled } SCP_{xy}}{\text{Pooled } SS_x} = 1.0379$

4. Pooled $SS_e = \text{Pooled } SS_y - \dfrac{\left(\text{Pooled } SCP_{xy}\right)^2}{\text{Pooled } SS_x} = 33.2498$

5. Pooled $\upsilon = n_1 + n_2 - 3 = 21$ and

6. MSS_e for Pooled $b_{yx} = \dfrac{\text{Pooled } SS_e}{\text{Pooled } \upsilon} = 1.5833$; then, the elevations are tested by

computing $t = \dfrac{(\bar{y}_1 - \bar{y}_2) - \text{Pooled } b_{xy}(\bar{x}_1 - \bar{x}_2)}{\sqrt{MSS_e \text{ for Pooled } b_{yx}\left[\dfrac{1}{n_1} + \dfrac{1}{n_2} + \dfrac{(\bar{x}_1 - \bar{x}_2)^2}{\text{Pooled } SS_x}\right]}} = 0.637$ which is < 2.080,

the table value of $t_{0.05,\,21}$; hence, H_0 is acceptable.

Note: Alternatively, Analysis of Covariance (ANCOVA) can be employed; but, the procedure requires more computations (*see* Chapter "**Analysis of Covariance**" for details).

3.3.2 More Than Two Slopes

To compare > 2 slopes, numerator and denominator, and mean sums of squares for ANOVA are calculated for each of the regression lines as described under **Section 3.2.2.1.1.2**; they are tabulated and denoted as follows:

	SS_x	SS_y	SCP_{xy}	MSS_e	υ_e
Regression 1	xx_1	yy_1	xy_1	e_1	$n_1 - 2$
Regression 2	xx_2	yy_2	xy_2	e_2	$n_2 - 2$
Regression k	xx_k	yy_k	xy_k	e_k	$n_k - 2$
Pooled regression				Column total (e_p)	Column total $\upsilon_p = \Sigma n_i - 2k$
Common regression	Column total (xx_c)	Column total (yy_c)	Column total (xy_c)	$e_c = (xy_c)^2 \div xx_c$	$\upsilon_c = \Sigma n_i - k - 1$
Total regression	$xx_t{}^*$	$yy_t{}^{**}$	$xy_t{}^{***}$	$e_t = (xy_t)^2 \div xx_t$	$\upsilon_t = n_i - 2$

*, ** and *** Computed combining data of all 'k' samples; see below for formulae

$$ * \ xx_t = \sum_{j=1}^{k}\sum_{i=1}^{n_i} x_{ij}^2 - \frac{\left(\sum_{j=1}^{k}\sum_{i=1}^{n_i} x_{ij}\right)^2}{\sum_{j=1}^{k} n_{ij}} , \ ** \ yy_t = \sum_{j=1}^{k}\sum_{i=1}^{n_i} y_{ij}^2 - \frac{\left(\sum_{j=1}^{k}\sum_{i=1}^{n_i} y_{ij}\right)^2}{\sum_{j=1}^{k} n_{ij}} , \text{and} $$

$$ *** \ xy_t = \sum_{j=1}^{k}\sum_{i=1}^{n_i} x_{ij} y_{ij} - \frac{\left(\sum_{j=1}^{k}\sum_{i=1}^{n_i} x_{ij}\right)\left(\sum_{j=1}^{k}\sum_{i=1}^{n_i} y_{ij}\right)}{\sum_{j=1}^{k} n_{ij}} $$

To test $H_0: \beta_1 = \beta_2 = \ldots = \beta_k$, statistic $F = \dfrac{\left(\dfrac{e_c - e_p}{k-1}\right)}{\dfrac{e_p}{\upsilon_p}}$ on $\upsilon_1 = (k-1)$ and $\upsilon_2 = \upsilon_p$. If H_0 is

acceptable, common regression coefficient, b_c can be computed as the ratio of xy_c to xx_c whose values are available in the above table.

Note: Comparison of multiple slopes is not generally encountered; therefore, only procedure is outlined. It is for the same reason further tests on multiple elevations and multiple comparisons are not discussed; however, they can be obtained from other publications; for instance, Zar (2003). In any case, H_0: k population regressions (β's) and α's are identical can be tested by calculating

$$ F = \dfrac{\left(\dfrac{e_t - e_p}{2(k-1)}\right)}{\dfrac{e_p}{\upsilon_p}} \text{ on } \upsilon_1 = 2 \times (k-1) \text{ and } \upsilon_2 = \upsilon_p. $$

4. SIMPLE LINEAR (PRODUCT–MOMENT) CORRELATION

Basic differences between correlation and regression are outlined in **Section 1** above. Simple product–moment correlation is also referred to as **Pearson's Correlation Coefficient** and is designated r.

4.1 Computations and Testing Hypotheses About r

Correlation coefficient between variables x and y (r_{xy} and denoted by r henceforth) is calculated as the ratio of sum of cross products to the geometric mean of the sum of squares, i.e. $r = \dfrac{SCP_{xy}}{\sqrt{SS_x SS_y}}$ with usual meaning for the notations. Analogous to regression coefficient, numerator and each of the denominators can be divided by $(n-1)$, to get covariance and variances which can be used to replace SCP and SS terms in the above equation. However, the term $(n-1)$ gets cancelled and hence, the above formula is actually employed.

As discussed in **Section 3.2.2.1.1**, coefficient of determination (r^2) determines the variability in dependent variable which is attributable to its association with dependent variable; since it is the square of r, it is also called as **Correlation index**. Obviously,

$(1-r^2)$ estimates deviation and standard error of r is estimated as $\sqrt{\dfrac{(1-r^2)}{(n-2)}}$ on $\upsilon = (n-2)$

and set α. It should be noted that r is calculated when there is dependency among the variables is difficult to define.

Let us revisit the **Example 3.2.2.1**; with the assumption that dependency can not be defined between dam and daughter values; the computed values are as follows: $\sum\limits_{i=1}^{n} x_i$

$= 74.9 \text{ kg}, \ \bar{x} = 6.2417 \text{ kg}, \ \sum\limits_{i=1}^{n} y_i = 76.8 \text{ kg}, \ \bar{y} = 6.40 \text{ kg}, \ \sum\limits_{i=1}^{n} x_i^2 = 499.03 \text{ kg}^2, \ SS_x = 31.5292 \text{ kg}^2,$

Crude Sum of Cross Products $= 510.13$, $SCP_{xy} = 30.77 \text{ kg}^2$, $\sum\limits_{i=1}^{n} y_i^2 = 522.44 \text{ kg}^2$, $SS_y =$

30.9200 kg^2; Therefore, $r = \dfrac{30.77}{\sqrt{31.5290 \times 30.92}} = 0.9855$, $r^2 = 0.9712$ or 97.12% and standard error of r is 0.0537.

To test H_0: Population correlation coefficient, $\rho = 0$, $t = r \div se(r) = 18.364$ which is > 2.228, the table value of $t_{0.05, 10}$; hence H_0 may not be accepted.

Alternatively, $F = \dfrac{1+|r|}{1-|r|}$ on $\upsilon = (n-2)$ for both numerator and denominator and set α. In this example, $F = 136.93$ which is > 3.72, the table value of $F_{0.05, 10, 10}$; hence, H_0 can be rejected.

4.1.1 Fisher's z Transformation

When Normality of distributions of x and y variables is assumed, the above procedure is satisfactory to test H_0: $\rho = 0$ (two-tailed); however, if H_0 assumes an existence of $\rho > 0$, assumption of underlying distribution as normal is not reasonable. Hence, to test H_0: $\rho = $ a specified value (say ρ'), both ρ and ρ' are converted to z values by the

formula $z = 0.5\ln\left(\dfrac{1+r}{1-r}\right)$ or $z = 1.1513\log\left(\dfrac{1+r}{1-r}\right)$ on $\log_{10}$ scale; this is followed by

calculation of normal deviate, $Z = \dfrac{z_r - z_\rho}{\sqrt{\dfrac{1}{n-3}}} = (z_r - z_\rho)\sqrt{n-3}$ on $\rho = (n-3)$, where the

denominator represents the standard error of the numerator.

In the **Example 3.2.2.1**, let us test H_0: $\rho = 0.8$; $z_r = 2.4598$, $z_\rho = 1.0986$ and $Z = 2.239$ which is > 1.96, the table value of $Z_{0.05}$; hence, H_0 may be rejected.

4.1.2 Confidence Intervals

Confidence intervals at set α can be determined as follows:

1. Lower limit $(L_L) = \dfrac{(1+F_\alpha)r+(1-F_\alpha)}{(1+F_\alpha)+(1-F_\alpha)r}$ and

2. Upper limit $(L_U) = \dfrac{(1+F_\alpha)r-(1-F_\alpha)}{(1+F_\alpha)-(1-F_\alpha)r}$

The limits of $r = 0.9855$ are 0.9471 and 0.9961 as calculated by the above formulae.

4.1.3 Determination of Sample Size

For a defined power of test (β) and a specified ρ' (non-zero value) to test H_0: $\rho = 0$ is truly false and $\rho = \rho'$, sample size required is given by $n = \left(\dfrac{Z_\beta + Z_\alpha}{z_{\rho'}}\right)^2 + 3$ where Z_α is table value of Z (single-tail), Z_α is table value of Z (single- or two-tailed) and $z_{\rho'}$ is the fisher's z value for ρ' value.

4.1.4 Correlation from a bi-variate Frequency Table

Let us revisit the **Example 3.2.2.4** above wherein all preliminary calculations are made in a bi-variate frequency table of milk yield Vs fat content of milk; the values are

$SS_x = \sum f_i x_i^2 - \dfrac{\left(\sum f_i x_i\right)^2}{N} = 10845.1236$ kg²; $SS_y = \sum f_i y_i^2 - \dfrac{\left(\sum f_i y_i\right)^2}{N} = 525.7640$ %²;

$SCP_{xy} = \sum f_i x_i y_i - \dfrac{\left(\sum f_i x_i\right)\left(\sum f_i y_i\right)}{N} = -1089.9326$ kg% and $N = 356$. Therefore, $r = -0.4564$; se $(r) = 0.0473$; $t = 9.649$ which is > 1.96, the table value of $t_{0.05,\ \infty}$; Hence, H_0 ($\rho = 0$) may be rejected.

4.1.5 Relationship between b and r from a Sample

Simple linear regression and correlation coefficients are related to one another through the following equations:

1. $b_{yx} = r\sqrt{\dfrac{SS_y}{SS_x}}$ and $b_{xy} = r\sqrt{\dfrac{SS_x}{SS_y}}$

2. $r = \sqrt{b_{yx}b_{xy}}$

3. $r = \sqrt{\dfrac{MSS_b}{SS_x}}$ or $r = \sqrt{\dfrac{b_{yx}SCP_{xy}}{SS_x}}$

4.2 Testing of Hypothesis about Two *r*'s

This test can be one- or two-tailed depending on H_A. In any case, to test H_0: $\rho_1 = \rho_2$, both *r*'s (which are estimates of corresponding ρ's) are transformed by the Fisher's transformation into z_1 and z_2 values and the Standard Normal Deviate is calculated by

the formula $Z = \dfrac{z_1 - z_2}{\sqrt{\dfrac{1}{n_1 - 3} + \dfrac{1}{n_2 - 3}}}$ which, if $n_1 = n_2 = n$, simplifies into

$$Z = 0.7071 \times (z_1 - z_2) \times (n - 3)$$

Let us consider *r*'s from **Examples 3.2.2.1 and 3.3.1.1**; the values are as follows (H_0: $\rho_1 = \rho_2$):

Example	r	z	(n – 3)
3.2.2.1	0.9855	2.4598	9
3.3.1.1	0.7407	0.9520	9

Hence Z = 9.5955 which is > 1.96, the table value of $Z_{0.05}$; hence, H_0 may be rejected and the samples are not likely to be of the same population.

Note: If H_0 is not rejected, pooled *r* can be computed first by obtaining pooled value of Fisher's z value by $z_p = \dfrac{(n_1 - 3)z_1 + (n_2 - 3)z_2}{(n_1 - 3) + (n_2 - 3)}$ which is then retransformed to *r* value by $z = \dfrac{e^{2z} - 1}{e^{2z} + 1}$ on Natural

logarithms and by $z = \dfrac{10^{0.8686z} - 1}{10^{0.8686z} + 1}$ on $\log_{10}$ scale. If $n_1 = n_2$, then the formula for pooled Fisher's z

value condenses to $z_p = \dfrac{z_1 + z_2}{2}$.

Note:

1. Suppose H_0 was acceptable in the above case, since $n_1 = n_2$, $z_p = 1.7059$ and pooled *r* = 0.9362 (calculated by the formula given above).

2. To test H_0: $\rho_1 - \rho_2 = \rho'$ where $\rho \neq 0$, the numerator for the normal deviate test can be modified as $\left| z_1 - z_2 \right| - z_{\rho'}$.

3. Standard tables are available for both transformation of *r* to z and retransformation of z to *r*; but, they are not reproduced in this publication because both transformation to z values and retransformation to *r* values can be easily performed on an electronic calculator itself.

4.3 Hypothesis About > 2 *r*'s

4.3.1 All *r*'s Together

4.3.1.1 Fisher's z transformation

Let us assume k samples of size $n_1, n_2, n_3, \ldots n_k$ have yielded an *r* value each and we have to test H_0: $\rho_1 = \rho_2 = \rho_3 = \ldots = \rho_k$, then

1. Each of the *r*'s is subjected to Fisher's z transformation to obtain $z_1, z_2, z_3, \ldots z_k$, respectively

2. $\chi^2 = \sum\limits_{i=1}^{k}(n_i-3)z_i^2 - \dfrac{\left[\sum\limits_{i=1}^{k}(n_i-3)z_i\right]^2}{\sum\limits_{i=1}^{k}(n_i-3)}$ on $\rho = (k-1)$ and set α.

3. If H_0 is acceptable, pooled z is calculated as $z_p = \dfrac{\sum\limits_{i=1}^{k}(n_i-3)z_i}{\sum\limits_{i=1}^{k}(n_i-3)}$ and retransformed to

   r value by use of standard the formula given under **Section 4.2**.
4. If H_0 is acceptable at Step 2 above, we can further test another H_0: $\rho = 0$ by the

   Method of Neyman and Paul (*from* Zar, 2003) as follows: $Z = \dfrac{\sum\limits_{i=1}^{k}n_i r_i}{\sqrt{\sum\limits_{i=1}^{k}n_i}}$ at a set α either

   as one– or two–tail test depending on the nature of H_A.
5. If at Step 4, H_0: $\rho = \rho'$ where $\rho' \# 0$ can be tested by the Standard Normal Deviate at a set α.

4.3.1.1.1 Example

A hypothetical example is given to illustrate the procedure of testing and pooling of r's (H_0: $\rho_1 = \rho_2 = \rho_3$):

i	r_i	z_i	z_i^2	n_i	$n_i - 3$	$(n_i-3) \times z_i$	$(n_i-3) \times z_i^2$
1	0.40	0.4236	0.1794	23	20	8.4720	3.5880
2	0.45	0.4847	0.2349	28	25	12.1175	5.8725
3	0.50	0.5493	0.3017	33	30	16.4790	9.0510
Totals					75	37.0685	18.5115

$\chi^2 = 0.191$ which is < 5.99, the table value of $\chi^2_{0.05, 2}$; hence, H_0 is acceptable. Therefore, $z_p = 0.4942$ and pooled r $(r_p) = 0.4575$.

However, z–transformation is known to introduce bias which needs corrections; but Paul's hypothesis testing is accepted to be a better alternative to correction formula given by two statisticians, including Fisher; the same is given below:

4.3.1.2 Paul's hypothesis testing (with correction for bias) for > 2 r's

The test statistic is calculated by the formula $\chi_P^2 = \sum\limits_{i=1}^{k} \dfrac{n_i\left(r_i - r_p\right)^2}{\left(1 - r_i r_p\right)^2}$ on $\upsilon = k-1$. In **Example**

4.3.1.1.1, $\chi_p^2 = 0.1139 + 0.0025 + 0.1002 = 0.2166$ which is also < 5.99, the table value of $\chi^2_{0.05, 2}$; hence, H_0 is acceptable. Therefore, $z_p = 0.4942$ and pooled r $(r_p) = 0.4575$.

4.3.2 Multiple Comparisons with Two r's at a Time

If H_0: $\rho_1 = \rho_2 = \rho_3 = \ldots = \rho_k$ is rejected, then it may be necessary to make multiple comparisons with two r's at a time in order to specify which of the r's is different from one another. Under such circumstances, which is rare in Animal Science, a Tukey–test

can be run by calculating $q = \dfrac{z_i - z_j}{\sqrt{\dfrac{1}{2}\left(\dfrac{1}{n_i - 3} + \dfrac{1}{n_j - 3}\right)}}$ where z_i and z_j are the Fisher's z

values for the two r's on n_i and n_j observations, respectively on $\upsilon = k - 1$ and set α. If n_i

$= n_j = n$, the formula condenses to $q = \dfrac{z_i - z_j}{\sqrt{\dfrac{1}{n - 3}}}$ (Denominator indicates standard error

of the difference between r's).

Application of the above procedure to **Example 4.3.1.1.1** is shown in the following table:

Comparison (ri Vs rj)	$z_i - z_j$	$\sqrt{\dfrac{1}{2}\left(\dfrac{1}{n_i - 3} + \dfrac{1}{n_j - 3}\right)}$	q	$q_{0.05, \infty, 3}$	H_0
3 Vs 1	0.1257	0.1921	0.6423	3.314	Acceptable
3 Vs 2	0.0646	0.1875	0.3445	3.314	Acceptable
2 Vs 1	0.0611	0.1990	0.3070	3.314	Acceptable

Note: Table values of q distribution are not given in this publication and the same are available in several other publications (as, for instance, Zar, 2003).

5. RANK CORRELATION

5.1 Spearman's Rank Correlation (r_s)

If the bi-variate population can't be considered to be Normally distributed, then ranking of x_i's and y_i's and calculation of Rank correlation coefficient is the alternative to product–moment correlation coefficient. Spearman's r_s is the most popularly used rank correlation coefficient. If there is (are) tie (ties) among ranks, average ranks are allotted (*see* **Section 3.1** Chapter "**Non-parametric methods**"). A hypothetical example below will demonstrate the procedure for calculation of r_s:

5.1.1 Example

Acceptability of milk (x_i) and butter (y_i) of 10 cows (n) is ranked below; it is required to test whether the ranks are correlated (**concordance**) or not.

	1	2	3	4	5	6	7	8	9	10	Total
x_i	3	8	1	6.5**	2	10	4.5*	9	4.5*	6.5**	
y_i	2	6***	3	6***	1	9	6***	8	10	4	
d_i	1	2	-2	0.5	1	1	-1.5	1	-5.5	1.5	
d_i^2	1	4	4	0.25	1	1	2.25	1	30.25	2.25	47.0

*, ** and *** indicate tied ranks d_i = (rank of x_i – rank of y_i)

If there are no ties among ranks, $r_s = 1 - \dfrac{6 \sum\limits_{i=1}^{n} d_i^2}{n^3 - n}$; but, if there are ties, as in the above

example, $r_s = \dfrac{\left[\left(\dfrac{n^3 - n}{6} \right) - \sum\limits_{i=1}^{n} d_i^2 - \sum t_x - \sum t_y \right]}{\sqrt{\left[\left(\dfrac{n^3 - n}{6} \right) - 2\sum t_x \right] \left[\left(\dfrac{n^3 - n}{6} \right) - 2\sum t_y \right]}}$ where $\sum t_x = \dfrac{\sum (t_i^3 - t_i)}{12}$ and

$\sum t_y = \dfrac{\sum (t_j^3 - t_i)}{12}$ where t_i and t_j are the number of tied value in x and y variables,

respectively.

In the above example, t_i = 2, t_j = 1; hence, Σt_x = 0.5 and Σt_y = 0. Consequently, r_s = 102.5 ÷ 149.4992 = 0.6856. (Assuming that there are no ties in the above example, r_s = 0.6867)

To test H_0: ρ = 0, critical values of r_s for the given n and set α (see Appendix 6) are located; if calculated value is > table value, H_i may be rejected. In the given example, critical value of r_s for n = 10 and α = 0.05 is 0.564 and hence, H_0 may be rejected.

When $n \geq 10$ and r_s (ps) ≤ 0.9, Fisher z transformation can be employed to test r_s as described under **Sections 4.2** and **4.3**. However, standard error of z is estimated as

$\sqrt{\dfrac{1.060}{n-3}}$ instead of $\sqrt{\dfrac{1}{n-3}}$.

Note:

1. When there are no ties, calculation of r_s either by the procedure of the product moment correlation by considering ranks themselves as x_i and y_i values or by taking d_i values will yield the same result. However, if there are ties, it is advisable to follow the method enumerated above.

2. On the same lines, r_s can be tested by t–test described for product–moment correlation itself; but, accuracy may be reduced especially if the sample size is low.

5.2 Kendall's Rank Correlation Coefficient (τ)

This is another measure of degree of concordance; the procedure is as follows:

1. Arrange the ranks for x_i's (or y_i's) in an ascending order
2. Bring the ranks of corresponding y_i's (or x_i's as the case may be)
3. Starting from left–hand side, for each of the y_i's (or x_i's as the case may be) count the number of smaller ranks in y_i's (or x_i's as the case may be) to the right of the value in question.
4. Add all such numbers of smaller ranks and designate it as Q.

5. Then $\tau = 1 - \dfrac{4Q}{n(n-1)}$

In **Example 5.1.1**, the calculations will be as follows:

	3	5	1	7	9	4	10	2	8	6	Total
x_i	1	2	3	4.5*	4.5*	6.5**	6.5**	8	9	10	
y_i	3	1	2	6***	10	6***	4	6***	8	9	
Q	2	0	0	1	5	1	0	0	0	0	9

*, ** and *** indicate tied ranks $di = (\text{rank of } x_i - \text{rank of } y_i)$

Hence, $\tau = 0.60$.

Note: τ can be tested by t-test described for product–moment correlation itself; but, accuracy may be reduced in the process especially if the sample size is low.

5.3   Weighted Rank Correlation

5.3.1   Two Groups

5.3.1.1   Example

A hypothetical data is given below regarding the ranking of importance of six control measures against Avain Influenza in chicken reared at backyard and reared indoors. It is necessary to find out whether H_0: The same control measures are useful to control the disease in birds reared by two systems is valid or not (one-tail test).

Control measures	Rank		Savage number (S_i)@		$(S_i)_1 * (S_i)_2$
	Backyard	**Indoor**	**Backyard**	**Indoor**	
1	3	6	0.950	0.167	0.15865
2	1	4	2.450	0.617	1.51165
3	4	3	0.617	0.950	0.58615
4	6	2	0.167	1.450	0.24215
5	2	5	1.450	0.367	0.53215
6	5	1	0.367	2.450	0.89915

@ $S_i = \sum_{j=i}^{n} \frac{1}{j}$; in this example, $n = 6$; hence, for Rank 3, $S_3 = \frac{1}{3} + \frac{1}{4} + \frac{1}{5} + \frac{1}{6} = 0.950$

Top–down correlation, when there are no ties among the ranks to test agreement of

the top ranks is given by: $r_T = \dfrac{\sum_{i=1}^{n} (S_i)_1 (S_i)_2 - n}{(n - S_1)}$ = –0.5831 which is < critical value 0.810

for $n = 6$ and $\alpha = 0.05$ (Appendix 7). Hence, H_0 is acceptable; in any case, the negative sign of the correlation does indicate the necessity of caution to be exercised while adopting control measures to the two groups. But, when $n > 30$, the test statistic is the

Standard Normal Deviate calculated as $Z = \dfrac{r_T}{\sqrt{n-1}}$ and tested as per usual procedure.

Note:

1. For tied ranks, Savage are taken as the average of the Savage scores of the ranks tied; for instance, if ranks 4, 5 and 6 are tied, all the three are allotted a Savage score of $(S_4 + S_4 + S_6) \div 3$.

2. Rank correlation (r_s) calculated as described under **Section 5.1.1** is –0.7143 which is < 0.886, the critical value of r_s for $n = 6$ and $\alpha = 0.05$ (*see* Appendix 6).

3. To test agreement at the bottom (instead of at the top as done above), larger Savage scores have to be allotted to larger ranks.

5.3.2 *More than Two Groups (Kendall's Coefficient of Concordance)*

5.3.2.1 Example

Let us consider that deboned meat from ten broilers ($n = 10$) was used to prepare three different products ($m = 3$) and the Panelists ranked the products. The ranks, suitably corrected for ties, are given below:

Bird	Products (Ranks)			$\sum_{j=1}^{m} R_j$	$\sum_{j=1}^{n} R_j^2$
	1	**2**	**3**		
1	2	1	1	4.0	16.00
2	7.5	7	8	22.5	506.25
3	3.5	3	2	8.5	72.25
4	5	4.5	3	12.5	156.25
5	9	8	9	26.0	676.00
6	3.5	4.5	5.5	13.5	182.25
7	7.5	6	5.5	19.0	361.00
8	10	10	7	27.0	729.00
9	1	2	4	7.0	49.00
10	6	9	10	25.0	625.00
				$\sum_{i=1}^{n}\sum_{j=1}^{m} R_{ij} = 165.0$	$\sum_{i=1}^{n}\sum_{j=1}^{m} R_{ij}^2 = 3373.00$

H_0: There is no association between ranks of different products.

In the absence of ties, Kendall's coefficient of concordance, W is calculated as

$$W = \frac{\sum_{i=1}^{n}\sum_{j=1}^{m} R_{ij}^2 - \dfrac{\left(\sum_{i=1}^{n}\sum_{j=1}^{m} R_{ij}\right)^2}{n}}{\dfrac{m^2\left(n^3 - 1\right)}{12}} = 0.8682.$$ Test statistic for W is Friedman's χ^2 which is given

by $\chi_r^2 = m \times (n - 1) \times W$ on $\upsilon = (n - 1)$ and set α. For n up to 6 and m up to 15, table values of χ_r^2 are given in Appendix 8; for other values of m and n, Appendix 4 is valid.

In the above example, $\chi_r^2 = 23.441$ which is > 16.919, the table value of $\chi_{0.05,\,9}^2$; hence, H_0 is not acceptable.

However, since there are 2, 1 and 1 ties, in product 1, 2 and 3, respectively (totally 4 ties, $t = 4$), correction factor for ties and W are calculated as follows: $\sum_{k=1}^{t} t_k = \sum_{k=1}^{t} \left(n_k^3 - n_k \right)$ where n_k is the number of birds involved in the kth tie. In the example, all the 4 ties are involving 2 birds each; hence, $\sum_{k=1}^{t} t_k = 4 \times (2^3 - 2) = 24$, and $W = \dfrac{\sum\limits_{i=1}^{n}\sum\limits_{j=1}^{m} R_{ij}^2 - \dfrac{\left(\sum\limits_{i=1}^{n}\sum\limits_{j=1}^{m} R_{ij} \right)^2}{n}}{\dfrac{m^2\left(n^3 - 1\right) - m\sum\limits_{k=1}^{t} t_k}{12}}$

$= 0.8752$. Corrected $\chi_r^2 = 23.630$ which is also > 16.919, the table value of $\chi^2_{0.05,\,9}$; hence, H_0 is not acceptable.

5.3.3 Top–down Concordance (C_T)

This is extension of the procedure given in **Example 5.3.1.1** on two groups; and the Top–down concordance (C_T) is calculated as follows: $C_T = \dfrac{\sum\limits_{i=1}^{n}\left(\sum\limits_{j=1}^{m} S_j \right)^2 - m^2 n}{m^2 \left(n - S_1 \right)}$ with test

statistic χ^2 (denoted χ_T^2) $= m \times (n - 1) \times C_T$ on $\upsilon = (n - 1)$ and set α.

Let us calculate C_T for the **Example 5.3.2.1** illustrated above.

Bird	Products (Savage numbers)			$\sum\limits_{j=1}^{m} S_j$	$\left(\sum\limits_{j=1}^{m} S_j \right)^2$
	1	2	3		
1	1.929	2.929	2.929	7.787	60.637369
2	0.408	0.479	0.336	1.223	1.495729
3	1.263	1.429	1.929	4.621	21.353641
4	0.846	0.971	1.429	3.246	10.536516
5	0.211	0.336	0.211	0.758	0.574564
6	1.263	0.971	0.746	2.980	8.880400
7	0.408	0.646	0.746	1.800	3.240000
8	0.100	0.100	0.479	0.679	0.461041
9	2.929	1.929	1.096	5.954	35.450116
10	0.646	0.211	0.100	0.957	0.915849

$\sum\limits_{i=1}^{n}\sum\limits_{j=1}^{m} R_{ij} = 30.005$ $\sum\limits_{i=1}^{n}\left(\sum\limits_{j=1}^{m} S_j \right)^2 = 143.545225$

H_0: There is no association between ranks of different products.

Test statistic $C_T = \dfrac{143.545225 - 3^2 \times 10}{3^2 \times (10 - 2.929)} = 0.8414$ and $\chi_T^2 = 22.718$ which is > 16.919, the table value of $\chi^2_{0.05,\,9}$; hence, H_0 is not acceptable.

Note: Similar to that under **Section 5.3.1**, to test agreement at the bottom (instead of at the top as done above), larger Savage scores have to be allotted to larger ranks.

5.4 Correlation for Nominal Data (Contingency Coefficients)

5.4.1 Example

Suppose 12 cases of Theileriosis in cattle was studied in relation to the presence of a external parasite and the following data was recorded:

Animal No.	1	2	3	4	5	6	7	8	9	10	11	12
Disease	+	+	−	+	+	−	−	+	−	−	+	+
Parasite	+	−	+	+	+	+	−	−	−	+	+	−

With the above data, it is necessary to know whether H_0: There is no association between disease and presence of parasite is valid or not. This can be achieved by the following 3 methods [in addition to Binomial test (H_0: $p = ½$) or sign test or Fisher's exact test; *see* Chapters "**Test of hypotheses**" and "**Non–parametric methods**" for details]:

5.4.1.1. Cramer or Φ (phi/fy/fee) coefficient

Of the three methods, this method is more frequently used. The data can be rearranged into a 2 × 2 contingency table as follows:

Parasite ↓	Disease		Total
	Present	**Absent**	
Present	4 (*a*)	3 (*b*)	7 (R_1)
Absent	3 (*c*)	2 (*d*)	5 (R_2)
Total	7 (C_1)	5 (C_2)	12 (*N*)

For the above data, χ^2 can be calculated as described under **Section 3.2.1.4.1** of

Chapter "**Test of hypotheses**" which is then used to calculate $\phi_1 = \sqrt{\dfrac{\chi^2}{n}}$; this statistic

ranges between 0 and 1 (χ^2 is calculated without correction for continuity).

In the above example, $\chi^2 = \dfrac{n(ad-bc)^2}{R_1 R_2 C_1 C_2} = 0.0098$ and $\Phi_1 = 0.0286$. Alternatively,

$\phi_2 = \dfrac{(ad-bc)}{\sqrt{C_1 C_2 R_1 R_2}} = -0.0286$ can be considered as a correlation coefficient. If "+" is allotted

a numerical value 0 and "−" as 1, then $a = 0$, $b = 3$, $c = 3$ and $d = 0$ with an $r = -0.257$ is obtained by the above formula. For a contingency table larger than 2 × 2,

$\phi_1 = \sqrt{\dfrac{\chi^2}{n(k-1)}}$, where k is smaller one of the number of rows or columns. The sign of

the statistic indicates nature of association.

Significance of ϕ_1 can be assessed by significance of the contingency table itself as described under **Section 3.2.1.4.1** of Chapter "**Test of hypotheses**" and in this example, H_0 is acceptable.

5.4.1.2 Yule coefficient of association (Q)

This can be calculated as $Q = \dfrac{ad - bc}{ab + bc} = -0.333$; the sign of the statistic indicates nature of association.

5.4.1.3 Ives and Gibbons' correlation coefficient (r_n)

Correlation coefficient r_n is calculated as $\dfrac{(a+d)-(b+c)}{(a+d)+(b+c)} = \dfrac{(a+d)-(b+c)}{N}$; in the above example, it works out to be 0.

Note: Testing of both r_n and Q is not described since they are not commonly employed on Animal science data; however, they can be obtained from other publications.

5.5   Intra-class Correlation (r_I)

As the name indicates, this correlation refers to association between members within a "class" or "group" as we come across in Animal breeding; for instance, we are testing differences between genetic groups under the assumptions that sampling is random from a bivariate population (Model II ANOVA) and homogeneity of variances (*see* Chapter "**One-factor analysis of variance**" for details). Rarely, even twins may form the members of each group. Then, it is necessary to know whether the members of the same group have association among themselves or not before testing the differences between groups.

5.5.1   Equal Observations per Group

The association described above, referred to as **Intra–class correlation** designated r_I, is calculated as $r_I = \dfrac{MSS_g - MSS_e}{MSS_g + (n-1)MSS_e}$ an estimate of population parameter ρ_I where MSS_g and MSS_e are mean sum of squares due to groups and error, respectively. To test H_0: $\rho_I = 0$, statistic F is calculated as $F = \dfrac{MSS_g}{MSS_e}$ and checked for significance by the usual procedure. Alternatively, F–test can be done first followed by calculation of r_I by the formula $r_I = \dfrac{F-1}{F+1}$.

5.5.1.1 Example

Hypothetical example of average daily lactation yields (kg) of 10 pairs of twin cows is given below ($k = 10$, $n = 2$) :

Twin No.	1	2	3	4	5	6	7	8	9	10	Sum	Crude SS
Yields	12.5	8.5	13.0	8.0	9.5	10.8	16.4	13.0	9.0	10.6	111.3	1299.71
(kg)	13.5	8.0	11.5	8.3	9.4	11.2	15.7	12.9	8.8	10.0	109.3	1251.53
Totals	26.0	16.5	24.5	16.3	18.9	22.0	32.1	25.9	17.8	20.6	220.6	2551.24

H_0: $\rho_1 = 0$. Computation of ANOVA is pre-requisite (*see* Chapter "**Analysis of Variance**" for details) which yielded the following results:

Source	v	SS	MSS = SS ÷ v
Total	19	118.022	
Twins (Groups)	9	115.692	12.8547
Error	10	2.330	0.2330

Hence, $r_1 = 0.9644$ and F = 55.170 which is > 3.78, the table value of $F_{0.05,\,9,10}$; therefore, H_0 is liable to be rejected.

5.5.2 Unequal Observations per Group

On most occasions than not, Animal scientist encounters unequal group frequencies. Under such circumstances, weighted n can be calculated by the formula

$$n = \frac{\displaystyle\sum_{i=1}^{k} n_i - \frac{\displaystyle\sum_{i=1}^{k} n_i^2}{\displaystyle\sum_{i=1}^{k} n_i}}{k-1}.$$

5.5.3 Hypothesis testing (H_0: $\rho_1 = 0$)

5.5.3.1 When $n = 2$ in all groups

Procedure is similar to testing r with Fisher's z transformation with k in place of n.

Further, $se(z_1) = \sqrt{\dfrac{1}{k - \dfrac{3}{2}}}$; standard error of difference between two z_1's is given by

$$se(z_1 - z_2) = \sqrt{\frac{1}{k_1 - \dfrac{3}{2}} + \frac{1}{k_2 - \dfrac{3}{2}}}.$$

5.5.3.2 When $n > 2$ in any group(s)

In this case, Fisher's $z_1 = 0.5 \ln \dfrac{1+(n-1)r_1}{1-r_1}$ where n is the weighted n and r_1 is first

converted to r' by the formula $r' = \dfrac{nr_1}{2+(n-2)r_1}$ before applying the above formula to obtain z_I. After reconverting z_I to r' by the formula given under **Section 4.2**, the latter may be converted to r_I by the formula $r_I = \dfrac{-2r'}{(n-2)r'-n}$. Further,

$$se(z_I) = \sqrt{\dfrac{n}{2(n-1)(k-2)}} \; ; \text{standard error of difference between two } z_I\text{'s is given by}$$

$$se(z_1 - z_2) = \sqrt{\dfrac{\dfrac{n}{k_1-2} + \dfrac{n}{k_2-2}}{2(n-1)}} \; .$$

5.6 Concordance Correlation (r_c)

Suppose a new instrument has been developed to estimate a particular constituent, be it in a laboratory or elsewhere, it is necessary to test whether the new equipment (or sometimes new set of the same instrument) is performing the same as the first one or not. Such testing can be done by calculating r_c, the concordance correlation coefficient. This Statistic can be used even for evaluating new procedures for estimation of a particular constituent in place of existing normal procedures and the like.

5.6.1 Procedure

The calculation of r_c requires the same preliminary steps as that of product – moment correlation, r, after which the following formulae are used to compute r_c, and setting-up confidence intervals (after Fisher's z transformation):

$$r_c = \dfrac{2SCP_{xy}}{SS_x + SS_y + (n-1)(\bar{x}-\bar{y})^2}, \quad r = \dfrac{SCP_{xy}}{\sqrt{SS_x SS_y}}, \quad u = \dfrac{(n-1)(\bar{x}-\bar{y})^2}{\sqrt{SS_x SS_y}} \quad \text{and} \quad se(z_c) =$$

$$\sqrt{Var(z_c)} = \sqrt{\dfrac{\dfrac{(1-r^2)r_c^2}{(1-r_c^2)r^2} + \dfrac{4r_c^2(1-r_c)}{r(1-r_c^2)^2} - \dfrac{2r_c^4 u^2}{r^2(1-r_c^2)^2}}{n-2}} \; . \text{ With this, 95\% confidence intervals}$$

can be set for Fisher's z values as $z \pm 1.96 \times se(r_c)$; the lower and upper limits of Fisher's z values can be retransformed to r_c values by using the formula given under **Section 4.2**.

Note: Standard error of difference between two r_c's = $\sqrt{Var(z_1) \times Var(z_2)}$

5.6.1.1 Example

Two colorimeters (x and y) were used to estimate protein content (%) in 10 ($n = 10$) broiler starter rations. The results are tabulated below:

Feed No.	1	2	3	4	5	6	7	8	9	10
Protein content, %, x_i's	23.2	23.5	23.0	24.0	22.0	21.0	23.0	22.5	24.0	23.1
Protein content, %, y_i's	23.8	24.1	24.0	25.0	22.7	21.6	23.9	23.0	24.4	24.0

$$\sum_{i=1}^{n} x_i = 229.3, \sum_{i=1}^{n} x_i^2 = 5265.35, \sum_{i=1}^{n} y_i = 236.5, \sum_{i=1}^{n} y_i^2 = 5601.67, \sum_{i=1}^{n} xy = 5430.71, SS_x =$$

$$7.501, SS_y = 8.445, SCP_{xy} = 7.765, r = 0.9756, r_c = 0.7535, u = 0.5862, z_c = 0.5In\left(\frac{1+0.7535}{1-0.7535}\right)$$

$$= 0.9810, \text{ se } (z_c) = \sqrt{\frac{0.161705 + 1.356611 - 1.245850}{8}} = 0.1845, 95\% \text{ confidence intervals}$$

for $z_c = 0.9810 \pm 0.1845$; therefore, lower limit of $z_c = 0.7965$ and upper limit of $z_c = 1.1655$ with corresponding values of r_c being 0.6620 and 0.8228, respectively. To test the H_0: There is no concordance between the values obtained by the two colorimeters, Student's t value is calculated as the ratio of z to se (z); in this example it is 5.317which is > 2.306, the table value of $t_{0.05, 8}$; hence, H_0 can be rejected and concluded that there is concordance between the results from the two colorimeters.

Note: Coding has no effect either on any of the correlation coefficients of the Fisher's z values.

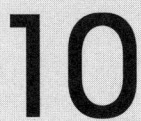

10

Association Between Variables II

(Multiple Linear Regression and Correlation)

Quite often, though not always as a rule, more than two factors (variables) are found associated to one another; take for example, growth as dependent variable on age, temperature, humidity, nutrition status, genetic make-up, space allowance for the animal, etc. It is possible to study association of these variables two at a time; but, it will be cumbersome, especially as the number of variables increases. In addition, such an analysis assumes that only one of the factors is associated at a time with the dependent variable whereas, any or many of the factors may be influencing the dependent variable simultaneously and there may be several interrelationships among the independent variables themselves.

Analogous to simple linear regression, the following assumptions are made:

1. Dependent variable (y) is assumed to have come at random from a Normally distributed population of y's existing in the population of observed combination of independent variables.

2. At all combinations of independent variables, s_y^2 is homogenous.

3. Values of y are drawn at random from the population and independent of one another.

4. Error (e_j, the variance of deviations of y_j from the regression of y on all the independent variables) is normally and independently distributed with mean 0 and variance s_{yx}^2

5. There is no correlation between independent variables.

6. There is no (or negligible) error in the measurement of x's or error in measurement of x's is at least considerably less than in that of y.

Note:

1. Nominal or dichotomous or binomial data do not follow normal distribution and hence, multiple regression can not be fit to such data; however, **logistic regression** is applicable to such data as well as to situations where the dependent variable has > 2 discrete possible values (polytomous or multinomial variable).

2. If the variables are not functionally related to one another or none of the variables can be defined as dependent, the association is referred to as **multiple correlation**.

3. Since more than 2 variables are considered in a normal population, we can also refer the population as **multi-variate normal population**.

1. MULTIPLE REGRESSION EQUATION

Calculation of a multiple regression equation necessitates matrix inversion which is not only tedious but also requires high accuracy; hence, generally, computers are used for computation. However, general procedure is described so that it will easy to understand the results (computer output).

1.1 Computation

1.1.1 Sums and Sum of Squares

Let us assume that there are m independent variables with n observations in each of them, sum and sum of squares for all x_{ij}'s ($i = 1, 2, 3.... m$; $j = 1, 2, 3....n$) and y_i are computed as is done for simple linear correlation or regression coefficient:

1. Sums $\sum_{j=1}^{n} x_{ij} = \sum x_{1j}, \sum x_{2j}, \sum x_{3j} ... \sum x_{mj}$, designated $\sum x_1, \sum x_2, \sum x_3, ... \sum x_m$; and $\sum_{i=1}^{n} y_i$

   designated $\sum y$.

2. Crude sums of squares $\sum_{j=1}^{n} x_{ij}^2 = \sum x_{1j}^2, \sum x_{2j}^2, \sum x_{3j}^2, ... \sum x_{mj}^2$, designated $\sum x_1^2$,

   $\sum x_2^2, \sum x_3^2, ... \sum x_m^2$ and designated $\sum y^2$

3. Crude sum of cross products between all combination of two independent variables at a time (out of m variables) over all the n observations; these are designated $\sum x_1 x_2$, $\sum x_1 x_3, ... , \sum x_{(m-1)} x_m$ and

4. Crude sum of cross products separately between y_i and each of the x_{im} values designated $\sum x_1 y, \sum x_2 y, \sum x_3 y ..., \sum x_m y$.

5. The above values are utilized to compute corrected sums and sum of cross-products as described in Chapter "**Association between variables I**"; i.e. $SS(x_i) =$

   $$\sum x_i^2 - \frac{(\sum x_i)^2}{n}, \quad SS(y) = \sum y^2 - \frac{(\sum y)^2}{n}, \quad SCP(x_1 x_2) = \sum x_1 x_2 - \frac{(\sum x_1)(\sum x_2)}{n},$$

   $$SCP(x_1 x_3) = \sum x_1 x_3 - \frac{(\sum x_1)(\sum x_3)}{n}, \quad \dots$$

   $$SCP(x_{(m-1)} x_m) = \sum x_{(m-1)} x_m - \frac{(\sum x_{(m-1)})(\sum x_m)}{n} \quad \text{and}$$

   $$SCP(x_m y) = \sum x_m y - \frac{(\sum x_m)(\sum y)}{n}.$$

6. The values @ 5 above are arranged as a symmetric matrix with $SS(x_m)$ forming the diagonals and SCP's involving corresponding x's as off–diagonals to get an ($m \times m$) matrix as shown below:

7.
$$\begin{bmatrix} SS(x_1) & SCP(x_1x_2) & \cdots & SCP(x_1x_m) \\ SCP(x_2x_1) & SS(x_2) & \cdots & SCP(x_2x_m) \\ \cdot & \cdot & \cdots & \cdot \\ \cdot & \cdot & \cdots & \cdot \\ \cdot & \cdot & \cdots & \cdot \\ SCP(x_mx_1) & SCP(x_mx_2) & \cdots & SS(x_m) \end{bmatrix}$$; this can be used to develop a **product-moment correlation matrix** designated by r_{ik} where i and k takes values from 1 to m by dividing the corresponding $SCP(x_ix_k)$ by the geometric mean of the $SS(x_i)$ and $SS(x_k)$.

8.
$$\begin{bmatrix} r_{11} & r_{12} & \cdots & r_{1m} \\ r_{21} & r_{22} & \cdots & r_{2m} \\ \cdot & \cdot & \cdots & \cdot \\ \cdot & \cdot & \cdots & \cdot \\ \cdot & \cdot & \cdots & \cdot \\ r_{m1} & r_{m2} & \cdots & r_{mm} \end{bmatrix}$$; diagonal elements being equal to unity because it represents correlation with itself.

9. The SS/SCP matrix @ 7 above is inverted (procedure beyond the scope of this publication) to get $(m \times m)$ inverse matrix shown below:

10.
$$\begin{bmatrix} C_{11} & C_{12} & \cdots & C_{1m} \\ C_{21} & C_{22} & \cdots & C_{2m} \\ \cdot & \cdot & \cdots & \cdot \\ \cdot & \cdot & \cdots & \cdot \\ \cdot & \cdot & \cdots & \cdot \\ C_{m1} & C_{m2} & \cdots & C_{mm} \end{bmatrix}$$

11. In case of computation of multiple correlation, terms involving y will not be available because there is no "dependent" variable.

1.1.2 Multiple Regression Equation

On the same lines of simple linear regression, multiple regression equation can be written as $y_j = \alpha + \beta_1 x_{1j} + \beta_2 x_{2j} + \beta_3 x_{3j} + \ldots + \beta_m x_{mj} + \varepsilon_j$ or $y_j = \alpha + \sum_{i=1}^{m} \beta_j x_{ij} + \varepsilon_j$ where m is the number of independent variables and j assumes the value $1, 2, 3, \ldots n$. For sample data, $\hat{y}_j = a + \sum_{i=1}^{m} b_j x_{ij}$. At least $(m + 2)$ data points are required to fit multiple regression equation which will be done so as to minimize $\sum_{j=1}^{n} (y_j - \hat{y}_j)^2$ by the method of **least squares**.

Considering only two independent variables, the multiple regression equation can be solved algebraically as follows:

$y = a + b_1x_1 + b_2x_2$; since 'a' is in the same plane as y and it can be derived by difference, we consider $y = b_1x_1 + b_2x_2$ for developing "**Normal equations**"; the normal equations (not related to normal distribution) are derived by considering coefficients of the constants in the equation, one at a time to multiply the entire equation followed by taking summation. In the equation under consideration, there are two constants, b_1 and b_2; coefficient of b_1 is x_1 and that of b_2 is x_2. Hence, for first normal equation, we multiply the whole equation by x_1, and for the second by x_2, and take summation. Hence, the normal equations are (1) $\Sigma x_1 y = \Sigma b_1 x_1^2 + \Sigma b_2 x_1 x_2$ (2) $\Sigma x_2 y = \Sigma b_1 x_1 x_2 + \Sigma b_2 x_2^2$; by taking constants out of Σ, and rearranging, we get the Normal equations (1) $b_1 \Sigma x_1^2 + b_2 \Sigma x_1 x_2 = \Sigma x_1 y$ (2) $b_1 \Sigma x_1 x_2 + b_2 \Sigma x_2^2 = \Sigma x_2 y$. These two equations can be solved as **simultaneous equations** which most Animal Science workers will be aware of.

Matrix algebra can simplify the procedure, especially when m is > 3 because solving for 3 unknowns by simultaneous equations itself is time–consuming. The method described below can be extended to any value of m.

On the left hand side (LHS) of the equations, if the constants are ignored, we get a (2 × 2) symmetric matrix with a right hand side (RHS) of (2 × 1) column vector. By inverting the LHS we get (2 × 2) inverse matrix which when multiplied the column vector of the RHS, we get (2 × 1) column vector giving the values of b_1 and b_2 as its elements. The same process is true for cases with more number of independent variables but becomes more and more complicated for manual calculation.

In the present case LHS = $\begin{bmatrix} \Sigma x_1^2 & \Sigma x_1 x_2 \\ \Sigma x_1 x_2 & \Sigma x_2^2 \end{bmatrix}$ whose inverse is given by

$$\begin{bmatrix} \dfrac{\Sigma x_2^2}{(\Sigma x_1^2)(\Sigma x_2^2)-(\Sigma x_1 x_2)^2} & \dfrac{-\Sigma x_1 x_2}{(\Sigma x_1^2)(\Sigma x_2^2)-(\Sigma x_1 x_2)^2} \\ \dfrac{-\Sigma x_1 x_2}{(\Sigma x_1^2)(\Sigma x_2^2)-(\Sigma x_1 x_2)^2} & \dfrac{\Sigma x_1^2}{(\Sigma x_1^2)(\Sigma x_2^2)-(\Sigma x_1 x_2)^2} \end{bmatrix}$$; alternatively, the determi-

nant $(\Sigma x_1^2)(\Sigma x_2^2)-(\Sigma x_1 x_2)^2$ can be designated as "D" and inverse of LHS will be

$$\begin{bmatrix} \dfrac{\Sigma x_2^2}{D} & \dfrac{-\Sigma x_1 x_2}{D} \\ \dfrac{-\Sigma x_1 x_2}{D} & \dfrac{\Sigma x_1^2}{D} \end{bmatrix}.$$

Now the inverse matrix is multiplied by the column vector of the RHS;

$$\begin{bmatrix} \dfrac{\Sigma x_2^2}{D} & \dfrac{-\Sigma x_1 x_2}{D} \\ \dfrac{-\Sigma x_1 x_2}{D} & \dfrac{\Sigma x_1^2}{D} \end{bmatrix} \begin{bmatrix} \Sigma x_1 y \\ \Sigma x_2 y \end{bmatrix} = \begin{bmatrix} \dfrac{(\Sigma x_2^2)(\Sigma x_1 y)-(\Sigma x_1 x_2)(\Sigma x_2 y)}{D} \\ \dfrac{(\Sigma x_1^2)(\Sigma x_2 y)-(\Sigma x_1 x_2)(\Sigma x_1 y)}{D} \end{bmatrix}$$. Therefore, if D =

$\left(\sum x_1^2\right)\left(\sum x_2^2\right) - \left(\sum x_1 x_2\right)^2$, the computational formulae are:

$$b_1 = \frac{\left(\sum x_2^2\right)\left(\sum x_1 y\right) - \left(\sum x_1 x_2\right)\left(\sum x_2 y\right)}{D} \text{ and } b_2 = \frac{\left(\sum x_1^2\right)\left(\sum x_2 y\right) - \left(\sum x_1 x_2\right)\left(\sum x_1 y\right)}{D}.$$

Finally, the intercept is calculated as, $a = \bar{y} - b_1 \bar{x}_1 - b_2 \bar{x}_2$.

Note: Each of the b_i's is referred to as **Partial regression coefficient.**

1.1.2.1. Example

To demonstrate various steps, an example with only two independent variables is considered; as already indicated, computers are generally used for computation of multiple linear regression equation and testing hypothesis.

The following hypothetical data refers to a study on influence of protein (%,) and energy (MJ/g,) in diet on 6th week body weight of broilers:

Protein, %, x_1	21.0	21.0	22.0	22.0	23.0	23.0	24.0	24.0	25.0	25.0
Energy, MJ/kg, x_2	10.2	10.4	10.6	10.8	11.0	11.2	11.4	11.6	11.8	12.0
Body weight, kg, y	1.20	1.30	1.40	1.50	1.60	1.70	1.85	2.00	2.05	2.08

$\sum x_1 = 230.0$, $\sum x_1^2 = 5310.00$, $\sum y = 16.68$, $\sum y^2 = 28.7414$, $\sum x_1 y = 387.85$, $\sum x_2 = 111.0$, $\sum x_2^2 = 1235.4$, $\sum x_2 y = 186.88$, $\sum x_1 x_2 = 2561$; therefore, $SS(x_1) = 20.00$, $SS(x_2) = 3.30$, $SS(y) = 0.9192$, $SCP(x_1 x_2) = 8.00$, $SCP(x_1 y) = 4.21$, $SCP(x_2 y) = 1.732$, m (number of independent variables) $= 2$ and $n = 10$. These values yield SS/SCP matrix as $\begin{bmatrix} 20.00 & 8.00 \\ 8.00 & 3.30 \end{bmatrix}$, $D = 2.0$,

an inverse of SS/SCP matrix as $\begin{bmatrix} 1.65 & -4.00 \\ -4.00 & 10.00 \end{bmatrix}$, which when multiplied by the RHS

$\begin{bmatrix} 4.210 \\ 1.732 \end{bmatrix}$ gives $b_1 = 0.0185$ and $b_2 = 0.48$; $a = -4.0855$; the multiple linear regression equation will be $y = -4.0855 + 0.0185 x_1 + 0.48 x_2$.

H_0: $\beta_1 = \beta_2 = 0$ ($\beta_i = 0$ for all i's); for testing the hypothesis, ANOVA has to be performed as shown below:

Source	v	SS	MSS = SS ÷ v	F
Total	$n - 1 = 9$	SSy = 0.9192		
Regression	$m = 2$	$\sum_{i=1}^{m} b_i SCP(x_i y) = 0.9092$	0.4546	324.714
Deviation	$n - m - 1 = 7$	0.0100	0.0014	

Coefficient of determination, $R^2 = 0.9092 \div 0.9192 = 0.9891$ or 98.91%; Multiple correlation coefficient $= \left(\sqrt{R^2}\right) = R = 0.9945$; Standard error (Multiple regression equation) = (Deviation MSS)$^{1/2}$ = 0.0374

Calculated value of F is > 4.74, the table value of $F_{0.05,\,2,7}$; hence, H_0 can be rejected.

Note:

1. R^2 can also be calculated as $\dfrac{F}{F + \dfrac{\upsilon \text{ for Deviations}}{\upsilon \text{ for Regression}}}$

2. F can be also be calculated as $\left(\dfrac{R^2}{1-R^2}\right)\left(\dfrac{\upsilon \text{ for Deviations}}{\upsilon \text{ for Regression}}\right)$

SS due to regression ($\upsilon = 2$) can be further split into components with $\upsilon = 1$; i.e. suppose first x_1 operates followed by x_2 and *vice versa* (Often called as "Stepwise regression"). Revisiting, Chapter "**Association between variables I**", we know that SS(regression) $= b \times \mathrm{SCP}_{xy} = (\mathrm{SCP}_{xy})^2 \div \mathrm{SSx}$; hence, the ANOVA can be modified as follows:

Source	υ	SS	MSS = SS ÷ υ	F
Total	$n - 1 = 9$	SSy = 0.9192		
Regression				
$x_1 + x_2$	$m = 2$	0.9092	0.4546	
x_1 alone	1	$(\mathrm{SCP}x_1 y)^2 \div \mathrm{SS}x_1 = 0.8862$	0.8862	633.00*
x_2 after x_1	1	$0.9092 - 0.8862 = 0.0230$	0.0230	16.42*
Deviation	$n - m - 1 = 7$	0.0100	0.0014	
x_2 alone	1	$(\mathrm{SCP}x_2 y)^2 \div \mathrm{SS}x_2 = 0.9090$	0.9090	649.29*
x_1 after x_2	1	$0.9092 - 0.9090 = 0.0002$	0.0002	0.14NS
Deviation	$n - m - 1 = 7$	0.0100	0.0014	

Table value of $F_{0.05,\,1,7} = 5.59$ NS < table value, Not significant   * > table value, Significant

It is interesting to note that even after the effect of protein levels, energy levels had a significant influence on body weight whereas *Vice versa* was not true which indicates the importance of energy levels for growth.

The method can be extended to any number of independent variables. The advantage of the stepwise regression is to eliminate unnecessary independent variables so that not only computation becomes easier but also reduces cost of experimentation, time involved in collection and recording of data, etc.

1.1.2.2 Testing partial regression coefficients

To test a two-tailed H_0: $\beta_i = 0$, se(b_i) is calculated as $\sqrt{\text{Deviation } MSS \times C_{ii}}$ where C_{ii} refers to the diagonal element of the inverse matrix of SS/SCP. In the above example, se(b_1) = 0.0481, and se(b_2) = 0.1183. With the availability of se values, statistic t can be calculated as the ratio of b_i to se(b_i) on υ of the deviation MSS (i.e. $n - m - 1$); Calculated values of t on $\upsilon = 7$ are 0.3846 and 4.057, respectively indicating that H_0 was acceptable for the partial regression of weights on protein but not on energy levels. It should be noted that it is not uncommon to record significant F test but not t test; if the t test is significant and F is not, it indicates high degree of correlation among the independent variables.

1.1.2.3 Standardized partial regression coefficients (β coefficient)

These indicate the relative importance of the independent variables and is calculated

by the formula $b_i^* = b_i \sqrt{\dfrac{SS(x_i)}{SS_y}}$; in the example above $b_1^* = 0.0863$ and $b_2^* = 0.9095$;

these do not have units unlike partial regression coefficients and they indicate the relative importance of the independent variable; in this case, energy levels appear to be more important than protein levels which was also indicated by t tests. However, this is not commonly calculated in Animal Science experiments.

1.1.2.4 Predicting y values

If the multiple regression equation is significant, it is worth using to predict y values for different values of x_i's provided that they are within the reasonable range employed for developing the equation. Procedures for computation of se (predicted y) are available both when none of the x_i's is 0 and when one or more x_i is zero; but they are not generally employed by Animal Science workers. Similarly, testing of difference between partial regression coefficients is also not in general practice. Nonetheless, if one is interested in such procedure, other publications may be referred to (as for instance Zar, 2003).

1.1.2.5 Multiple regression through origin

Situations in Animal Science data wherein a multiple regression equation through origin may have to be fit are rare; software for such procedure is available.

2. PARTIAL CORRELATION

Considering **Example 1.1.2.1**, $R = 0.9945$ which reflects the overall association between y, x_1 and x_2; hence, it is called **multiple correlation**. Calculation of product–moment correlation between any pair of variables is possible because all the values required are already calculated while processing for multiple regression equation. But, the major setback for such r is that it does not include the interactions among the variables. This aspect is taken care of while computing partial correlation coefficients. It is very important to note that y is no more a dependent variable because only when no variable is 'dependent', correlation/multiple correlation comes into picture. Hence, in the above example, y will be considered as variable x_3.

   With 3 variables designated d, e and f, utilizing the values calculated already, we get product–moment correlations $r_{de} = 0.9847$, $r_{df} = 0.9818$ and $r_{ef} = 0.9945$. By these

values, partial correlation coefficients can be calculated as $r_{def} = \dfrac{r_{de} - r_{df} \times r_{ef}}{\sqrt{\left(1 - r_{df}^2\right)\left(1 - r_{ef}^2\right)}}$.

Therefore, $r_{12.3} = 0.4173$, $r_{13.2} = 0.1378$ and $r_{23.1} = 0.8376$. When m is large, off-diagonals of the correlation matrix given under **Section 1.1(8)** directly gives the partial

correlations. To test H_0: $\rho_{de...} = 0$, se($r_{de...}$) is calculated as $\sqrt{\dfrac{1 - r_{de...}^2}{n - m}}$ where n is the

number of observations and m, number of variables. This is followed by calculation of statistic t on $\upsilon = (n - m)$ as the ratio of correlation to its se.

In the above example, $(n - m) = 7$, and $se(r_{12.3}) = 0.3435$, $se(r_{13.2}) = 0.3744$ and $se(r_{23.1}) = 0.2065$ and $t(r_{12.3}) = 1.215$, $t(r_{13.2}) = 0.368$ and $t(r_{23.1}) = 4.056$; of these calculated t values, only $t(r_{23.1})$ is > 2.365, the table value of $t_{0.05, 7}$; hence, H_0 concerning $r_{23.1}$ may not be accepted and those on $r_{23.1}$ and $r_{12.3}$ may be accepted. Again, partial correlation coefficient between energy and growth being significant supporting the conclusion drawn based on partial regression coefficient.

Partial correlation coefficients along with stepwise regression can help decide the number of independent variables to be considered.

11

Association Between Variables III
(Non-Linear Regression)

Association between variables discussed in Chapters "**Association between variables I and II**" is linear. However, such association can as well be non-linear, especially in biological variables; for instance, growth Vs age, multiplication of bacteria Vs time, etc. Several non-linear models are described, exponential growth, exponential decay, asymptotic regression, logistic growth etc. On some occasions, it is possible to convert non-linear model to linear models by appropriate transformations; but, it may be necessary that such transformation is not possible and a non-linear model has to be fit. It is for this reason, a brief description of non-linear models is given in this Chapter. Non-liner regression is also referred to as "**Curvilinear regression**" because when x and y values are plotted, a parabola results. Such data require to consider x^2 (2nd degree values of independent variable) as an independent variable; that means, the same independent variable is considered in two forms, x and x^2; extending the same logic, x^3, x^4, etc. can also be considered depending on the type of curve being involved. Hence, the independent variable is considered with different degrees (names) and such equations are often called **polynomials**; depending on the power of x employed, they are called variously as second degree/third degree, etc. polynomials. Symbolically, $y_i = \alpha + \beta_1 x_1 + \beta_2 x^2 + \beta_3 x^3 + \ldots + \beta_m x^m$. Hence, non-linear regression includes polynomial regression as well.

Hence, a general form of non-linear regression can be written as

$$y_i = a + \sum_{j=1}^{m} b_j x_i^j$$

where m is the highest degree to which x is considered; obviously, if $m = 1$, the equation is simple linear regression (*see* Chapter "**Association between variables I**" for details). Depending on value of m, they are called quadratic (2nd degree), cubic (3rd degree), quartic (4th degree), quintic (5th degree) …. regression (polynomial) models. Second degree polynomial ($m = 2$), exponential and logistic growth curves, exponential decay and asymptotic regression are often used in Animal Science.

Common non-linear functions (curves) an Animal Scientist may have to deal with are diagrammatically shown below.

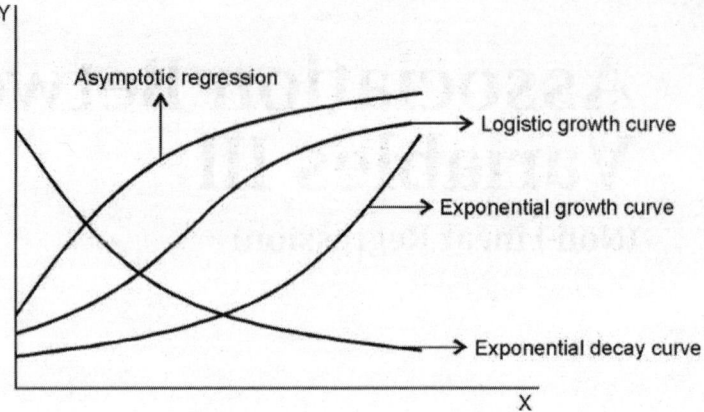

Fig. 11.1: Common non-linear curves

1. EQUATION (FUNCTION) CONVERTIBLE INTO A LINEAR FUNCTION

This category includes those equations which are already linear in nature but of higher degree; i.e. x has to be considered in the form of x^j where j takes the values 1, 2, 3 ... m. When $j = 1$, the equation is same as simple linear regression. Such functions where x is considered in various powers are often referred to as **Polynomial equations (functions)**. A polynomial equation, though more elaborate than that for linear function, can be fit manually with a little knowledge of matrix algebra or by using orthogonal polynomials (matrix method has been already outlined in Chapter **"Association between variables II"**) and hence, method of orthogonal polynomials is given in this Chapter.

1.1 Fitting a Polynomial Equation

1.2 Setting Power (*m*) of the Polynomial

At the beginning it is necessary to know up to what value of m ($m < n - 1$) the equation continues to be significant. This necessitates testing of b_i's when m is increased by 1 at a time; called **stepwise polynomial regression**. This procedure begins with $m = 1$ (linear regression) with H_0: $b = 0$; if H_0 is rejected, 2nd degree equation is fit with H_0: $b_2 = 0$; if H_0 is rejected again, 3rd degree equation is fit with H_0: $b_3 = 0$ and so on. It should be noted that partial regression coefficient, b_j corresponding to the degree of the polynomial is tested by Student's t test each time (as per the procedure given under **Section 1.1.2.2** Chapter "**Association between variables II**") but not the others because they have been already tested prior to the equation in question. The equation with the largest m in which H_0 is not acceptable is considered the best fit model for the data. Alternatively, F-test can also be used on $\upsilon = 1$ and υ of MSS corresponding to the equation with larger m by calculating F as the ratio of difference in SS due to regression for higher and lower degree models to deviation MSS for the higher degree model.

1.2.1 Computation

Calculations are basically on the same lines as those for multiple-regression, where instead of different x_i's, different powers of x are used. Accordingly, the elements of matrix will change from SCP to sum of different powers of x_i depending on m. Other than this, all the steps are essentially the same regarding construction and inversion of matrix, calculation of constants, ANOVA, etc.

But, it is evident that the procedure is tedious and most often than not requires computer. Notwithstanding this, one will be interested to fit the lowest degree equation whose R^2 will be the highest and in the process would like to know, if possible in the beginning itself, the value of m that gives the highest R^2. Unfortunately, there is no way to find out the best-fit polynomial. Therefore, we have to resort to stepwise polynomial regression as shown in **Example 1.2.1.1** taken from Zar (2003) to show the highlights of the stepwise polynomial regression:

1.2.1.1 Example (*Adapted from* **Zar, 2003**)

x, kg	y, hr	m	a	b_1	b_2	b_3	b_4	b_5	b_6
1.22	40.9	1	37.389	3.1269					
1.34	41.8		$t_{0.05, 17}$	20.709	H_0	Rejected			
1.51	42.4	2	40.302	0.6666	0.4540				
1.66	43.0		$t_{0.05, 16}$	2.720	H_0	Rejected			
1.72	43.4	3	32.767	10.4110	–3.3868	0.4701			
1.93	43.9		$t_{0.05, 15}$	2.549	H_0	Rejected			
2.14	44.3	4	6.9265	55.835	–31.487	7.7625	–0.6751		
2.39	44.7		$t_{0.05, 14}$	3.735	H_0	Rejected			
2.51	45.0	5	36.239	–9.1615	23.387	–14.346	3.5936	–0.3174	
2.78	45.1		$t_{0.05, 13}$	1.353	H_0	Accepted			
2.97	45.4	6	157.88	–330.98	364.04	–199.36	58.113	–8.6070	0.5096
3.17	46.2		$t_{0.05, 12}$	1.724	H_0	Accepted			
3.32	47.0				Conclusion				
3.50	48.6			Quartic ($m = 4$) regression is the best fit					
3.53	49.0								
3.85	49.7								
3.95	50.0								
4.11	50.8								
4.18	51.1								

1.3 Concept of Orthogonal Polynomials

The discussion regarding fitting a polynomial regression equation outlined above clearly indicates that the procedure is requires knowledge of matrices and elaborate calculation. To simplify these matters the concept of orthogonal polynomials has been introduced. Further, in animal science, the values of x_i are, on most occasions, equally spaced (for instance age in case of age *Vs* body weight) which facilitates manual fitting of **Orthogonal polynomials** by use of standard tables. Computer programs are available which create polynomials that are **mutually orthogonal**, i.e. minimized possibility of high correlation between different powers of x_i.

In the polynomial $y = b_0 + b_1 x^1 + b_2 x^2 + b_3 x^3 + \ldots$, x^i ($i = 1, 2, 3 \ldots$) is substituted by a polynomial of degree i in x, designated x_i. The coefficients are chosen in such a way that, over n values of the sample, $\Sigma \xi_i = 0$ and $\Sigma \xi_i \xi_j = 0$ ($i \# j$). Hence, the polynomial simplifies to $y = B_0 + B_1 \xi_1 + B_2 \xi_2 + B_3 \xi_3 + \ldots$. Owing to the orthogonal nature of different

polynomials, $B_0 = \bar{y}$ and minimizing of deviations from regression, we get $B_1 = \dfrac{\sum\limits_{i=1}^{n} \xi_1 y_i}{\sum \xi_1^2}$,

$B_2 = \dfrac{\sum\limits_{i=1}^{n} \xi_2 y_i}{\sum \xi_2^2}$, $B_3 = \dfrac{\sum\limits_{i=1}^{n} \xi_3 y_i}{\sum \xi_3^2}$ and so on. The values of $\sum \xi_i^2$ are given in standard tables

(see Appendix 9). While using Appendix 9, the following have to be observed:

1. The x_i's should be equally spaced i.e. difference between consecutive x_i's (d's) should be constant.
2. Usually, table of linear orthogonal contrasts contain only the upper half values of x; however, Appendix 9 gives all values suitable up to 5th degree equations.
3. For the terms whose power is an odd number (i.e. m is odd or subscript i of the polynomial is odd), signs are changed in the lower half and
4. For the terms whose power is an even number (i.e. m is even or subscript i of the polynomial is even), signs remain unchanged.
5. The values are for x_i's equally spaced with $d = 1$; hence, if $d \neq 1$, it is included during the retransformation of the equation to original scale.

1.3.1 Example

Body weights of broilers (kg) vs age (weeks) is given below for finding a best fit model by the method of orthogonal polynomials:

Age (wks), x_i	BW (kg), y_i	ξ_1 *	ξ_2 *	ξ_3 *	ξ_4 *	ξ_5 *
1	0.125	−5	15	−30	6	−3
2	0.350	−4	6	6	−6	6
3	0.750	−3	−1	22	−6	1
4	1.000	−2	−6	23	−1	−4
5	1.450	−1	−9	14	4	−4
6	2.000	0	−10	0	6	0
7	2.600	1	−9	−14	4	4
8	3.000	2	−6	−23	−1	4
9	3.500	4	−1	−22	−6	−1
10	3.750	3	6	−6	−6	−6
11	4.000	5	15	30	6	3
$\Sigma \xi_i^2$		110	858	4290	286	156
λ_i		1	1	5/6	1/12	1/40
$\Sigma \xi_i y$	$\Sigma y = 22.525$	46.125	1.775	−26.75	−1.15	1.075

(Contd.)

(Contd.)

Age (wks), x_i	BW (kg), y_i	ξ_1^*	ξ_2^*	ξ_3^*	ξ_4^*	ξ_5^*
B_i **	$\bar{y}$ = 2.047727	0.419318	0.002069	– 0.006235	– 0.004021	0.00689
Regression SS***		19.341051	0.003672	0.166798	0.004624	0.00741
B_i' ****		0.419318	0.002069	– 0.005196	– 0.000335	0.00017

* From Appendix 9, for $n = 11$

** Calculated as $\Sigma \xi_i y \div \Sigma \xi_i^2$

*** Calculated as $(\Sigma \xi_i y)^2 \div \Sigma \xi_i^2$ on $v = 1$

**** Calculated as a product of λ_i and B_i

$SS_y = (65.875625 - 22.525^2 \div 11) = 19.750568$ kg^2. With these values we can set up ANOVA table to test reductions in SS due to successive terms:

Source	v	SS	MSS = SS $\div v$	F
Total	$(n - 1) = 9$	SSy = 19.750568		
Reduction to Linear	1	19.341051	19.341051	377.83
Deviation	8	0.409517	0.051190	
Reduction to Quadratic	1	0.003672	0.003672	< 1
Deviation	8	19.746896	2.468362	
Reduction to Cubic	1	0.166798	0.116798	< 1
Deviation	8	19.583770	2.447971	
Reduction to Quartic	1	0.004624	0.004624	< 1
Deviation	8	19.745944	2.468243	
Reduction to Quintic	1	0.007410	0.007410	< 1
Deviation	8	19.743158	2.467895	

Table value of $F_{0.05, 1, 8} = 5.32$

It is clear from the above that only linear regression between body weight and age of broilers is significant. In fact, at one F value of quadratic component is found not significant, the analysis can be stopped; generally, it is advisable to test at least two higher degrees above the degree last detected to be significant. In any case, it is very obvious that the use orthogonal polynomials greatly reduces the calculation part; for instance, in the above example, it was necessary to construct, inverse and manipulate further at least 4 matrices of size 2×2 to 4×4 to get the same result as obtained above.

1.3.1.1 Conversion of B_i's to b_i's

The following steps have to be followed to obtain regression coefficients in the original scale:

1. Each of the B_i is multiplied by λ_i to get corresponding B_i' values and now the polynomial obtained contains b_i's and x_i's in the form of

   $$y = \bar{y} + B_1' \xi_1 + B_2' \xi_2 + B_3' \xi_3 + B_4' \xi_4 + B_5' \xi_5$$

2. Each of the B_i''s is the coefficient of ξ_i where n is the sample size, d is the difference between the successive values of x; which in the present example is unity and

a. $\xi_1 = (x - \bar{x}) \div d$

b. $\xi_2 = \xi_1^2 - (n^2 - 1) \div 12$

c. $\xi_3 = \xi_1^3 - (3n^2 - 7) \xi_1 \div 20$

d. $\xi_4 = [\xi_1^4 - (3n^2 - 1) \xi_1^2 \div 14] + [3(n^2 - 1)(n^2 - 9) \div 560]$

e. $\xi_5 = [\xi_1^5 - 5(n^2 - 7) \xi_1^3 \div 18] + [(15n^4 - 230n^2 + 407) \xi_1 \div 1008]$

A general formula for computation of $\xi_{(j+1)} = \xi_1 \xi_j - \dfrac{j^2 (n^2 - j^2)}{4(4j^2 - 1)} \xi_{(j-1)}$ where $j = 1, 2, 3$

... $(m - 1)$ facilitates calculations.

In the present example, only linear regression was found to be significant; hence, retransformation up to quadratic equation is given below:

1. $y = \bar{y} + B_1' \xi_1 + B_2' \xi_2$ where $\bar{y} = 2.047727$, $B_1' = 0.419318$, $B_2' = 0.002069$, $\xi_1 = (x - 6)$, $\xi_2 = (x - 6)^2 - 10$.

2. Therefore, $y = 2.047727 + 0.419318 \times (x - 6) + 0.002069 \times (x^2 - 12x + 26)$.

3. Finally, $y = -0.4144 + 0.3945x + 0.0021x^2$

Note:

1. It is relatively simple to retransform linear equation which will be as follows: $y = \bar{y} + B_1' \xi_1$ where $= 2.047727$, $B_1' = 0.419318$ and $\xi_1 = (x - 6)$. Hence, $y = 2.047727 + 0.419318 \times (x - 6)$ or $y = -0.4682 + 0.4193x$.

2. In addition, retransformation of equations requires algebraic rearrangement which becomes more and more complicated as m increases. In any case, computers greatly reduce this process.

1.3.2 Use of Orthogonal Polynomials when x_i's are Unequally Spaced

One of the conditions for using Appendix 9 is that difference between consecutive x_i's $(d_i's)$ should be constant. However, it is possible to develop orthogonal polynomials when $(d_i's)$ are not constant. This is demonstrated in the example below (the procedure can be extended to any n):

1.3.2.1 Example

Number of eggs of a parasite as a function of environmental temperature is as follows:

Temperature, °C, (x)	4	5	8	14	21	25	28
No. of parasite eggs, (y)	4	12	25	43	38	29	17

It is required to fit a quadratic equation by use of orthogonal polynomials, test significance of the equation and estimate the values of x and y in which the function attains the maximum value.

Since the d_i's are not constant, Appendix 9 can not be used; hence, the orthogonal polynomials have to be computed as follows:

x_i	$\xi_1 = x_i - \bar{x}$	x_i^2	$x_i\xi_1$	$x_i^2\xi_1$	$b_1\xi_1$	$x_i^2 - \dfrac{\sum_{i=1}^{n} x_i^2}{n}$	ξ'_2	ξ_2
4	−11	16	−44	−176	11011 ÷ 32	−2039 ÷ 7	11829 ÷ 224	11829
5	−10	25	−50	−250	10010 ÷ 32	−1976 ÷ 7	6838 ÷ 224	6838
8	−7	64	−56	−448	7007 ÷ 32	−1703 ÷ 7	−5447 ÷ 224	−5447
14	−1	196	−14	−196	1001 ÷ 32	−779 ÷ 7	−17921÷224	−17921
21	6	441	126	2646	−6006 ÷ 32	936 ÷ 7	−12090 ÷ 224	−12090
25	10	625	250	6250	−10010 ÷32	2224 ÷ 7	1098 ÷ 224	1098
28	13	784	364	10192	−13013 ÷32	3337 ÷ 7	15693 ÷ 224	15693
105	0	2151	576	18018	0	0	0	0

$n = 7$, $\bar{x} = 15$, $\lambda_1 = 1$, $b_1 = -(x_i^2\xi_1 \div x_i\xi_1) = -(1001 \div 32)$, $\xi'_2 = b_1\xi_1 + \xi_2 = \xi'_2 \times \lambda_2$ where $\lambda_2 = 224$ in this case.

With ξ_1 and ξ_2 values computed, the further calculations are similar to the **Example 1.3.1** discussed above.

Temperature, °C, (x)	4	5	8	14	21	25	28
No. of parasite eggs, (y)	4	12	25	43	38	29	17
ξ_1		−11	−10	−7	−1	6	10	13
ξ_2		11829	6838	−5447	−17921	−12090	1098	15693
$d_i's$			1	3	6	7	4	3

$$\sum_{i=1}^{n}y_i = 168, \ \sum_{i=1}^{n}y_i^2 = 5208, \ SS_y = 1176, \ d = \sum_{i=1}^{n}d_i - \frac{\sum_{i=1}^{n}d_i^2}{n} = 4 \ (n = 6 \text{ here})$$

Accordingly, $B_0 = \bar{y}$, $B_1 = \dfrac{\sum_{i=1}^{n}\xi_1 y_i}{\sum\xi_1^2}$ and $B_2 = \dfrac{\sum_{i=1}^{n}\xi_2 y_i}{\sum\xi_2^2}$. Hence, $B_0 = 24$, $B_1 = (357 \div 576)$

$= 0.619792$, $B_2 = (-938203 \div 931159488) = -0.001008$. This follows that $B_1' = B_1{}^*\lambda_1$ and $B_2' = B_2{}^*\lambda_2$ and $y = 24.0000 + 0.619792\xi_1 - 0.225792\xi_2$ which has to be retransformed to original scale as described in **Example 1.3.1** by replacing ξ_1 with $(x - \bar{x}) \div d$ and ξ_2 with $\xi_1^2 - \{(n^2 - 1) \div 12\}$. Therefore, the final equation on original scale will be $y = 24 + 0.619792 \{(x - 15) \div d\} - 0.225792 [\{(x - 15) \div d\}^2 - 4]$ or $y = 19.403748 + 0.578308x - 0.014112x^2$.or $y = 19.4037 + 0.5783x - 0.0141x^2$. The parabola has a maximum value at $x = 20.49$ (*see* **Section 1.4.1** below for explanation) when y will be 25.33.

(**Note:** Since d_i's are not constant, an average d is calculated as shown in the table above).

Further, $SS_{reg}(\text{Linear}) = (\Sigma\xi_1 y)^2 \div \Sigma\xi_1^2$; and $SS_{reg}(\text{Quadratic}) = (\Sigma\xi_2 y)^2 \div \Sigma\xi_2^2$; both on $\upsilon = 1$. As in the **Example 1.3.1**, deviation SS is given by $SS_y - SS_{reg}(\text{Linear})$ or $SS_{reg}(\text{quadratic})$ as the case may be on $\upsilon = (n - 2)$.

The ANOVA in this example will be as follows.

Source	υ	SS	MSS = SS ÷ υ	F
Total	$(n-1) = 6$	SSy = 1176		
Reduction to Linear	1	221.2656	221.2656	1.159
Deviation	5	954.7344	190.9469	
Reduction to Quadratic	1	945.2998	945.2998	20.488
Deviation	5	230.7002	46.1400	

Table value of $F_{0.05, 1, 5} = 6.61$; R^2(Linear) = 0.1882; R^2(Quadratic) = 0.8038

Both F values and R values clearly indicate that linear equation is not a good fit whereas, the quadratic model is a good fit for the given data.

1.4 Quadratic (2nd degree) Equation

As indicated already, this is by far the most commonly used polynomial in Animal Science and this equation is also popularly represented as $y = a + bx + cx^2$ by replacing b_0, b_1 and b_2 with a, b and c, respectively. Essentially same steps can be used as described under **Section 1.1.2.2**, Chapter "**Association between variables II**" for fitting the equation. However, orthogonal polynomials greatly reduce the computational work as shown below:

1.4.1 Maximum and Minimum Values

When b_2 or c is < 0, the parabola has a theoretical maximum and *vice versa*; in either case, the value of x for which the equation assumes the theoretical maximum/minimum (as the case may be) is given by the ratio of $(-b_1)$ or $(-b)$ to $(2b_2)$ or $(2c)$.

1.4.2 Example

The same data given in **Example 1.3.2.1** is considered with equal spacing between consecutive x_i values.

Temperature, °C, (x)	4	8	12	16	20	24	28	$\sum \xi_i^2$	λ
No. of parasite eggs, (y)	4	12	25	43	38	29	17		
ξ_1	-3	-2	-1	0	1	2	3	28	1
ξ_2	5	0	-3	-4	-3	0	5	84	1

$\xi_1 y = 86$, $\xi_2 y = -256$, $B_1 = (86 \div 28) = 3.017429$, $B_2 = (-256 \div 84) = -3.047619$, $\bar{y} = 24$; $B'_1 = B_1 * \lambda_1$ and $B'_2 = B_2 * \lambda_2$

Hence, $y = 24 + 3.017429\xi_1 - 3.047619\xi_2$; which has to be retransformed to original scale by substituting ξ_1 with $(x - \bar{x}) \div d$ and ξ_2 with $\xi_1^2 - \{(n^2 - 1) \div 12\}$. Therefore, the final equation on original scale will be $y = 24 + 3.017429\{(x - 16) \div 4\} - 3.047619[\{(x - 16) \div 4\}^2 - 4\}$ or $y = -24.641144 + 6.849595x - 0.190476x^2$; $y = -24.64 + 6.85x - 0.19x^2$ (Vs equation by matrix method $y = -24.86 + 6.86x - 0.19x^2$).

1.4.2.1 Maximum value

Since c is < 0, the parabola has a theoretical maximum at $x = -6.849595 \div (2 * -0.190476)$ = 17.98 when y will be 39.44. The quadratic equation for the same data by matrix method is $y = -24.857143 + 6.863095x - 0.190476x^2$ attaining a theoretical maximum value of 36.96 at $x = 18.01$.

Note: ξ_1 and ξ_2 values can be taken from Appendix 9; however, it is relatively easy to calculate orthogonal polynomials up to 2 levels for data with equal d; the same for the above example is shown below:

x_i	$\xi_1' = x_i - \bar{x}$	$\xi_1 = \xi_1' \div d$	$\xi_2' = \xi_1'^2 - c'$	$\xi_2 = \xi_2' \div d^2$
4	−12	−3	80	5
8	−8	−2	0	0
12	−4	−1	−48	−3
16	0	0	−64	−4
20	4	1	−48	−3
24	8	2	0	0
28	12	3	80	5
Σ 112	0	0	0	0
	$\Sigma\xi_1'^2 = 448$	$\Sigma\xi_1^2 = 28$		
	$\lambda_1 = 1$		$\lambda_2 = 1$	

1. $c' = \Sigma\xi_1'^2 \div n = 64$

2. ξ_2 can be calculated directly as $\xi_1^2 - c$ where $c = \Sigma\xi_1^2 \div n = 4$; to demonstrate the values of λ's, the circuitous method is shown above; since ξ_1 and ξ_2 are already integers, λ_1 and λ_2 are both unity; however, they are reduced to a smaller value by dividing with d and d^2, respectively. This part is undone during retransformation

3. It can be easily verified that $\xi_1' \times \xi_2' = 0$, $\xi_1' \times \xi_2 = 0$, $\xi_1 \times \xi_2' = 0$ and $\xi_1 \times \xi_2 = 0$; the primary prerequisite for orthogonality.

4. Lower half values of ξ_1 and ξ_2 are given in Appendix 9.

1.5 Multiple y_i Values for Each x_i

In Animal Science research, several values of dependent variable for each x is not unusual, especially in cases like Age vs body weight/milk production/egg production, etc., temperature vs egg production etc. The situation increases the accuracy of testing the fitted equation. The data is analyzed similar to one-way classification (*see* Chapter "**Analysis of variance**") and sum of squares between classes (x_i's in this case) is partitioned into sum of squares due to regression (linear, quadratic..., etc. as the case may be each with $v = 1$ and deviation) and sum of squares within classes.

1.5.1 Example

Let us take-up the same **Example 1.3.2.1** with multiple y_i's:

Temperature, °C	No of parasite eggs					$y_i.$	$\bar{Y}$
4	4	3	6	4	6	23	4.6
8	12	14	15	10	12	63	12.6
12	25	23	20	25	24	117	23.4
16	43	40	48	42	48	221	44.2
20	38	40	50	35	36	199	39.8
24	29	30	25	28	24	136	27.2
28	17	15	20	18	12	82	16.4
$x. = 112$; $y._j \rightarrow$	168	165	184	162	162	841	24.03
$\Sigma y._j^2$	5208	5059	6490	4838	5076	26671	

$y.. = 841$, $\Sigma\Sigma y..^2 = 26671$, $SS_y = 6462.971429$, $n_i. = 5$, $n._j = 7$, $n.. = 35$ (N)

To calculate sum of squares due to regression (only linear and quadratic are considered because they are commonly used in Animal Science), orthogonal polynomials already shown earlier but with $\bar{Y}$ values in place of y_i will be employed:

Temperature, °C, (x)	4	8	12	16	20	24	28	$\Sigma\xi_i^2$	λ
No. of parasite eggs,	4.6	12.6	23.4	44.2	39.8	27.2	16.4		
ξ_1	-3	-2	-1	0	1	2	3	28	1
ξ_2	5	0	-3	-4	-3	0	5	84	1

$\xi_1 y = 81$, $\xi_2 y = -261$, $B_1 = (81 \div 28) = 2.892857$, $B_2 = (-261 \div 84) = -3.111905$,
$= 24.03$; $B'_1 = B_1{}^* \lambda_1$ and $B'_2 = B_2{}^* \lambda_2$

Further, SS_{reg}(Linear) $= (\xi_1 y)^2 \div \Sigma\xi_1^2 = 234.321429$, SS_{reg}(Quadratic) $= (\xi_2 y)^2 \div \Sigma\xi_2^2 =$

810.964286; $SS_{temp} = \dfrac{\sum\limits_{i=1}^{7}(y_i.)^2}{n_i.} - \dfrac{y..^2}{n..} = (131849 \div 5) - (841^2 \div 35) = 6161.771429$. Now, the

ANOVA table can be laid as follows:

Source	υ	SS	MSS = SS ÷ υ	F
Total	$(N-1) = 34$	$SS_y = 6462.9714$		
Between temperatures	$(k-1) = 6$	6161.7714	1026.9619	95.468
Linear regression on x	1	234.3214	234.3214	21.783
Quadratic regression on x	1	810.9643	810.9643	75.389
Deviation from quadratic	$(k-3) = 4$	5116.4857	1279.1214	118.910
Within temperatures	$(N-k) = 28$	301.2000	10.7571	

Table value of $F_{0.05, 1, 28} = 4.20$; $F_{0.05, 4, 28} = 2.71$; $k =$ No of temperature classes

Note:

1. Both linear and quadratic regressions were significant; in addition, there is scope to test higher degree polynomials (up to quintic degree since 4 degrees of freedom are still available for deviations from regression).

2. Linear and quadratic equations can be developed as explained under **Section 1.4.2**.

3. Regarding subscripts used for x and y above, as well as analysis with unequal n_i. *see* Chapter "**One-factor analysis of variance**", "**Two-factor analysis of variance**" and "**Analysis of variance of more than two factors**" for explanation.

1.6 The Exponential Growth/Decay Curves

This is represented by the equation $y = a(b^x)$; since growth is generally involved, it is

also represented by $w = a(b^x)$. The equation is similar to compound interest formula if $b = 1 + r$, where r is the rate of interest (%) and $x = t$, the time (years). If $b < 1$, it is referred to as exponential decay curve; this is of particular interest in bioassays involving radioactive material.

Exponential growth curve is fit when rate of growth at any point of time is proportional to the growth attained till that time say as in case of log phase of growth of bacteria, growth of embryos etc.

1.6.1 Fitting Exponential Curve Models

Let us consider the growth equation: $y = a(b^x)$; taking logarithms on both sides, we

get log y = log a + x log b which is analogous to simple linear regression equation $y = a + bx$ (see Chapter "**Association between variables I**"). Therefore, solution to this equation is simply a modified version of that employed for simple linear regression i.e. log y is the dependent variable (instead of y) and the rest are the same. Hence, the computation is also the same excepting that log values of y are used in place of y. On the same lines in case of $y = a(e^{bx})$, taking $\log_e$ on both sides, $\log_e y = \log_e a + bx$; y in terms of $\log_e$ is considered as dependent variable. Fitting of these models in comparison to linear model is shown through an example below:

1.6.1.1 Example

Weight of chicken embryos during incubation as % of egg weight during 4th to 19th day of incubation is given below (Sreenivasaiah, *et al.*, 1984). It is necessary to fit an exponential growth curve to the data and check whether it is better than a simple linear model.

Age, d (x)	Weight, % of egg weight (y)	$\text{Log}_{10}\, y$	$\text{Log}_e\, y$
4	0.06	−1.2218	−2.8134
5	0.32	−0.4949	1.1394
6	0.65	−0.1871	0.4308
7	1.24	0.0934	0.2151
8	2.06	0.3139	0.7227

(Contd.)

(Contd.)

Age, d (x)	Weight, % of egg weight (y)	$\text{Log}_{10}\ y$	$\text{Log}_e\ y$
9	3.32	0.5211	1.2000
10	4.86	0.6866	1.5810
11	6.70	0.8261	1.9021
12	10.64	1.0269	2.3646
13	11.81	1.0723	2.4689
15	23.77	1.3760	3.1684
16	28.47	1.4544	3.3489
17	35.69	1.5525	3.5749
18	41.41	1.6171	3.7235
19	48.84	1.6888	3.8886

Computations

Linear model,
$y = a + bx$

$\sum_{i=4}^{19} x_i = 170$, $\sum_{i=4}^{19} x_i^2 = 2260$, $\sum_{i=4}^{19} y_i = 219.84$, $\sum_{i=4}^{19} y_i^2 = 7087.9910$, $\sum_{i=4}^{19} x_i y_i = 3556.43$,

$b_{yx} = 3.1947$, $a = -21.5509$, Regression equation: $y = -21.5509 + 3.1947x$; SS_y = 3866.0160, SS/MSS$_{reg}$ = 3402.0680, SS_e = 463.9480, MSS_e = 35.6883, F = 95.327 which is > 4.54, table value of $F_{0.05,\ 1,15}$; hence H_0: $\beta = 0$ rejected. Coefficient of determination, $R^2 = 0.88$ or $r = 0.9381$.

Exponential model

$\sum_{i=4}^{19} x_i = 170$, $\sum_{i=4}^{19} x_i^2 = 2260$, $\sum_{i=4}^{19} y_i = 10.3253$, $\sum_{i=4}^{19} y_i^2 = 17.395711$, $\sum_{i=4}^{19} x_i y_i = 173.0843$,

$b_{yx} = 0.1682$, $a = -1.2178$, Regression equation: $\log y = -1.2178 + 0.1682x$; in original scale, $y = 0.0606(1.4730^x)$; $SS_y = 10.2883$, SS/MSS$_{reg}$ = 9.4296, SS_e = 0.8587, $MSS_e = 0.0661$, F = 142.657 which is > 4.54, table value of $F_{0.05,\ 1,15}$; hence H_0: $\beta = 0$ rejected. Coefficient of determination, $R^2 = 0.9165$ or $r = 0.9573$.

Exponential model,

$\sum_{i=4}^{19} x_i = 170$, $\sum_{i=4}^{19} x_i^2 = 2260$, $\sum_{i=4}^{19} y_i = 26.9155$, $\sum_{i=4}^{19} y_i^2 = 93.2314$, $\sum_{i=4}^{19} x_i y_i = 415.1076$,

$b_{yx} = 0.3302$, $a = -1.9479$, Regression equation: $\log y = -1.9479 + 0.3302x$; in original scale, $y = 0.1426(e^{0.3302x})$; $SS_y = 44.9351$, SS/MSS$_{reg}$ = 36.3431, SS_e = 8.5920, $MSS_e = 0.6609$, F = 54.988 which is > 4.54, table value of $F_{0.05,\ 1,15}$; hence H_0: $\beta = 0$ rejected. Coefficient of determination, $R^2 = 0.8088$ or $r = 0.8993$.

Inference

All models satisfactory since R^2 is > 0.8 although the exponential model $y = a(b^x)$ explains more proportion of variability in embryo weights than the other two moels.

Note: Same method is used to fit exponential decay model, $y = a(b^{-x})$ or $y = a(e^{-bx})$.

2. EQUATION NOT CONVERTIBLE INTO A LINEAR FUNCTION

Equations under this category require knowledge of partial differentiation for manual computations. A general method of fitting such non-linear equations is given below which is followed by an example for fitting an asymptotic regression function:

2.1 Taylor's Theorem and Fitting Non-linear Regression

Following steps illustrate the general method of fitting non-linear regression:

1. Obtain initial values of a', b' and c' as estimates of a, b and c, respectively. This can be performed either by graphical methods or by other methods.
2. Taylor's theorem which states that if $f(a, b, c, x')$ is continuous in $a, b, c,$ and if $(a - a')$, $(b - b')$ and $(c - c')$ are small, then $f(a, b, c, x') \approx f(a', b', c', x') + f_a(a - a') + f_b(b - b') + f_c(c - c')$; '$\approx$' denoting 'approximately equal to' and f's are partial derivatives if f with respect to a, b and c, respectively evaluated at the point a', b' and c'.
3. In asymptotic curve $f(a, b, c, x') = y = a - b(c^x), f_a = 1, f_b = -(c')^x, f_c = -b'x(c')^{x-1}$.
4. By using the known values of a', b' and c', f, f_a, f_b and f_c can be calculated.
5. Therefore, the equation $y_i = f(a, b, c, x') + e_i \approx f + f_a(a - a') + f_b(b - b') + f_c(c - c') + e_i$.
6. Residual of y, y_{res}, is calculated as $y - f$ from the (multiple) linear regression equation obtained by replacing f_a by x_1, f_b by x_2 and f_c by x_3
7. The regression coefficients are only approximate and hence, second approximations, a'', b'' and c'' are used and the calculations are repeated (iteration process) till the reduction in y_{res} reduces steadily and becomes negligible.

Notwithstanding the method outlined above, on most occasions an Animal Scientist had better resort to computers to fit the non-linear equation to ensure accuracy ant save time.

2.2 Logistic and Gompertz Growth Curves

Logistic curve, $y = \dfrac{a}{(1 + bc^x)}$ is popular for studying growth in large populations (human beings, in particular). This follows that the model is suitable for studying dynamics of growth in animal populations as well. Gompertz curve, $y = a^{-b^{-cx}}$ is also used as an alternative to Logistic curve. In both equations, a, b and c are the constants. It is apparent that manual calculation to fit the above equations is not feasible and computer aid is compulsory. Both logistic and Gompertz curves have the typical sigmoid shape of a growth curve.

2.3 Asymptotic Regression

Asymptotic regression is represented as $y = a - b(c^x)$ or $y = a - b(e^{-cx})$; if the value of b or c is known, the function condenses into a simple linear model $y = a - x'$, where $x' = c^x$ and b^x, respectively. It is generally cumbersome to fit the equation manually and hence, computer programs available for the purpose can be made use of.

2.4   Dose–Response Relationship

This is very important consideration in Pharmacodynamics. It is suffice to mention that the dose (independent variable, x) is in log units and the response (dependent variable) is in proportion (%). This relationship is useful to find out the value of x when $y = 0.5$ or 50%; popularly referred to as **median effective dose or Median lethal dose** depending on the type of study. See Chapter "**Statistics in Specific Veterinary fields**" for details.

2.5   Others

Many other types of prediction equations is in vogue in Animal Science; for instance, egg production in Poultry, growth curves of different category of animals, disease incidence curves, milk production in dairy cattle etc. It is generally not possible to exhaust all the models because newer models are being proposed especially due to change in the production pattern of animals following changes in genetic make – up as well as environment provided in the form of management and healthcare. In any case, some of them are discussed in Chapter "Statistics in Specific Veterinary fields".

Important note: It is generally true that fitting Logistic, Gompertz and Assymptotic equations is highly cumbersome manually. Further, ready–made computer programs are available to get quick results. However, *it is not impossible to fit such equations with a Scientific Calculator*. Method of three points and Partial sums are two simple methods for the purpose. But, some derivations have to be done which require knowledge of basic Algebra. The procedure is shown in Appendices 13, 14 and 15. All the three equations are also fit by one of these methods (*see* Chapter "Analysis of Time Series" for details).

12

Transformations

For performing Analysis of Variance (ANOVA), certain assumptions are made (the details will be dealt in Chapter "**One-factor analysis of variance**"). It is essential to know that deviations from those assumptions can lead to erroneous conclusions. The transformations help bring the data closer to near Normality.

Failure to meet the assumptions for ANOVA is referred to as **error** which is classified into:

1. Gross error
2. Lack of independence error or association error
3. Unequal error variance due to nature of treatments
4. Non-additivity of effects and
5. Non-normality of errors

1. GROSS ERROR

If an observation is recorded, transcribed or read wrongly and/or a treatment is applied wrongly the treatment mean and variance are distorted. Consequent on this, conclusion(s) is(are) bound to be erroneous. Such errors constitute gross errors.

This can be corrected by deleting the observation(s) and using **missed-plot technique** to replace the value(s) for further analysis as discussed in Chapter "**Two-factor analysis of variance**". It is equally important to check all the observations and try locate the actual value and also to ensure that the same source of error has not affected other value(s).

In case of Two-way classification or Latin-square design (LSD), it is indeed difficult to detect gross errors because, the expected value depends on row, column and treatment effects. Under such circumstance, residual of the observations from their respective values can throw some light. In a Two-way classification, residual $D_{ij} = x_{ij} - \bar{X}_{i.} - \bar{X}_{.j} + \bar{X}_{..}$ and with Latin Square Design, residual $D_{ijk} = x_{ijk} - \bar{X}_{i..} - \bar{X}_{.j.} - \bar{X}_{..k} + 2\bar{X}_{...}$. If D_{ij} or D_{ijk} is extreme and the same is not explicable, the observation is rejected and calculated by missed-plot technique.

2. LACK OF INDEPENDENCE (ASSOCIATION) ERROR

Of the assumptions for ANOVA, that the error is independently and normally distributed with mean $= 0$ and same variance, σ^2 is extremely important. If a correlation exists among the errors for different replicates of the same treatment, ANOVA becomes erroneous. Hence, it is necessary that the same experimenter is involved in the entire experiment.

. Correlation between replicates of the same treatment is estimated by **Intra-class correlation (r_I)** as follows (n = number of replicates):

Source	Mean squares (MS)	Expected MS
Between classes	MS_b	$\sigma^2\{1 + (n-1)r_I\}$
Within classes	MS_w	$\sigma^2(1 - r_I)$

Therefore, $r_I = \dfrac{(MS_b - MS_w)}{\{MS_b + MS_w(n-1)\}}$ and $F = \dfrac{MS_b}{MS_w} = \dfrac{1+(n-1)r_I}{(1-r_I)}$. It is clear that if

$r_I = 0$, $F = 1$ and even if $r_I = +0.2$, when $n = 6$, the $F = 2.5$. Therefore, positive correlation among errors within a treatment seriously offset the accuracy of ANOVA by yielding false significant effects. This is applicable to t-test also.

Analysis of data having correlation among errors within a treatment is possible only when r_I is known. In any case skillful randomization obviates r_I and ensures validity of ANOVA.

3. UNEQUAL ERROR VARIANCE DUE TO NATURE OF TREATMENTS

It is possible that $\geq$ treatment(s) having variance different from that of the rest; this will result in increased F ratio and consequent significance detected when it actually does not exist. This effect is particularly evident when number of replicates per treatment is not uniform over all treatments.

If few treatments are involved, it is advisable to omit such treatment(s) from the main analysis. Conclusions can be tentatively given on the omitted treatment(s) by inspection of data itself. However, in case of LSD, special methods for this purpose have to be employed.

4. NON-ADDITIVITY OF EFFECTS

Analysis of variance also requires that the effects of factor(s) considered are additive. If the effects of rows and columns (two-way classification) are proportional (multiplicative), the error variance gets inflated severely curtailing the precision of the test; the severity directly proportional to the magnitude of non-additivity.

Tukey's test for additivity detects such situations and also helps select a suitable transformation; transformation is of the form of $y = x^p$ where x is the original scale and the power of x i.e. p should be such that the effects are additive. Therefore, if $p = \frac{1}{2}$, square root transformation, if $p = -1$, reciprocal transformation and when $p = 0$, logarithmic transformation are indicated because, x^p behaves like $\log x$ when p is small (*see* Chapter "**Two-factor analysis of variance**" for details).

5. NON-NORMALITY OF ERROR VARIANCE

For ANOVA, normal distribution is assumed; but, if the actual underlying distribution is skewed, again too many significant results are obtained.

If the magnitude of fixed effects (*see* Chapter **"One-factor analysis of variance"** for details) is moderate, effect of non-Normality is reasonably ignorable; lest, must be corrected by a suitable **variance–stabilizing transformation**. However, in distributions other than Normal distribution, variance is related to mean as in case of binomial and poisson distributions thereby making the variances unequal when treatment effects are large.

Let the transformation be $y = f(x)$ and $f'(x)$ be the derivative of $f(x)$ with respect to x. By Taylor expansion, $y = f(\mu) + f'(\mu) \times (x - \mu)$ where $E(y) = f(\mu)$ since $E(x - \mu) = 0$.

Similarly, $E\{y - f(\mu)^2\} = \{f'(\mu)\}^2 \times E(x - \mu)^2 = \{f'(\mu)\}^2 \sigma^2_x = \{f'(\mu)\}^2 \Phi(\mu)$. Therefore, to make σ^2_y independent of μ, $f(\mu)$ should be such that $\Phi(\mu)$ is constant. In other words, $f(\mu)$ is an indefinite integral of $\delta\mu\sqrt{\Phi(\mu)}$.

For Poisson distribution, $f(\mu) = \sqrt{\mu}$; i.e. $y = \sqrt{x}$ or **square-root transformation**. For Binomial distribution, $f(\mu) = \arcsin\sqrt{p}$; i.e. y is the angle whose sine is $\sqrt{p}$.

Variance on the transformed scale is obtained by calculating $\{f'(\mu)\}^2 \Phi(\mu)$. For Poisson distribution, since $\Phi(\mu) = \mu$ and $f(\mu) = \sqrt{\mu}$, $f'(\mu) = \frac{1}{2}\sqrt{\mu}$ and $\{f'(\mu)\}^2 \Phi(\mu) = \frac{1}{4}$. Hence, variance on the transformed scale is ¼.

5.1 Variance Stabilizing Transformations

5.1.1 Square-Root Transformation

Variance of counts of rare events or counts tend to be proportional to its mean; i.e. $s^2 = k\overline{X}$. Under such circumstances, square root transformation is effective. For instance, in Poisson events (*see* Chapter **"Probability distributions"**) wherein $k = 1$. Generally, the transformation employed is $\sqrt{x}$; but, if the counts are small (≤ 2), $\sqrt{x+1}$ or $\sqrt{x} + \sqrt{x+1}$ is preferable to $\sqrt{x}$ in order to stabilize the variance. Some authors also prefer $\sqrt{x+0.5}$ (for very small data and when some values are zero) or $\sqrt{(x+\frac{3}{8})}$. However, $\sqrt{x}$ or $\sqrt{x+0.5}$ is most commonly employed.

Means are converted to original scale by squaring. Since mean of a set of square root is < square root of the original mean, error mean square is added to each of the reconverted means as a rough correction.

This transformation affects both shape of the distribution as well as additivity; however, the transformation itself is too mild to cause severe changes in either of them unless effects of treatments and blocks are too large.

5.1.2 Arcsin or Angular Transformation for Proportions

Many traits in biological experiments are recorded as percentage values; the following are some of the examples:

1. Binomial (all or none) traits like fertility, hatchability, survivability (mortality)
2. Proportions like albumen, yolk and shell as a percentage of egg weight, cut-up parts as a percentage of live-weight and the like
3. Certain values as a percentage of the control treatment like weight gain in a particular treatment group as a percentage of control

These percentage values do not follow normal distribution which is a prerequisite for applying routine statistical procedures like ANOVA, Tests of significance etc., (the details are dealt in separate chapters), especially if the values are below 30% or above 70%.

Such data are recommended for an *arcsin* transformation as follows:

Let x be the percentage value and y be its arcsin value; then

$$y = \sin^{-1}\left(\sqrt{\frac{x}{100}}\right)$$

The statistical analyses will be performed replacing each of the values with its corresponding value calculated as above. In fact, ready-reference tables are available for obtaining *arcsin* values.

After the statistical analyses, arcsin Mean ($\bar{y}$) and *arcsin* Standard deviation (SD_{arc}) values are calculated and tests of significance performed for significant effects, if any.

Finally, when the results are tabulated, $\bar{y}$ is retransformed to the original scale as follows:

Let $\bar{x}$ be the mean on the original scale; then, $\bar{x} = 100\left(\sin^2 \bar{y}\right)$ and

$s = 50\left(\sin 2\bar{y}\right)\left(\sin 2s_{arc}\right)$

That means, standard deviation in percentage scale is equal to 50 times the product of the sine of twice the *arcsin* mean and sine of twice the *arcsin* standard deviation (Sreenivasaiah, 1985).

This short-cut method is accurate, simple and time-saving.

A Sample data pertaining to hen-housed egg production (%) over a period of 20 days is shown below to demonstrate the use of the short-cut method for retransformation of mean and standard deviation on *arcsin* scale back to the percentage scale.

% Hen-day egg prodn	Arcsin value	% Hen-day egg prodn	Arcsin value
8	16.43	45	42.13
10	18.43	40	39.23
10	18.43	42	40.40
18	25.10	39	38.65
12	20.27	40	39.23
16	23.58	48	43.85
25	30.00	56	48.45
20	26.57	35	36.27
30	33.21	40	39.23
38	38.06	36	36.87

	The result of calculations		
	% scale	*Arcsin* **scale**	**Retransformed (%)**
Sum	608	654.39	NA
Sum of squares	22428	23173.6395	NA
Mean	30.40	32.72	29.22
Standard deviation	14.41	9.61	14.97

However, this transformation is ineffective in removing heterogeneity in variance due to differences in n's which warrants a weighted analysis on *arcsin* scale. When $n < 50$, 0% should be equated to reciprocal of 4 times n; that is $[1 \div (4n)]$ and 100% equated to $[(n - ¼ n) \div n]$ before transforming to *arcsin* value. For binomial data, error variance (see Chapter **"One-factor analysis of variance"**) will be about $821 \div n$. Hence, in the angular scale, proportions near 0 and 1 are spaced out to increase their variance.

Other suggested *arcsin* transformations are as follows although they are not commonly used in Veterinary and Animal science fields:

$$\text{arcsin} = \sqrt{\dfrac{x + \dfrac{3}{8}}{n + \dfrac{3}{4}}}; \quad \text{arcsin} = \dfrac{1}{2}\left[\text{arcsin}\sqrt{\dfrac{x}{n+1}} + \text{arcsin}\sqrt{\dfrac{x+1}{n+1}}\right]$$

5.1.3 *Logarithmic Transformation*

When, in the original scale, the s varies directly as the $\overline{X}$; in other words, ratio of s to $\overline{X}$ (i.e. CV) is constant, this transformation is generally advised. If no zero value is encountered in the set of data, $\log x$ is used; else, $\log (x + 1)$ is employed. Logarithm of any base can be used; but base 10 is most commonly employed.

Retransformation of $\overline{X}$, is simply antilog $(\log \overline{X})$ and for s, the procedure is as follows:

Let $\overline{x}$ and s be the mean and standard deviation in log scale. Then, s in the original scale is obtained by the formula $s = \left[\dfrac{antilog(\overline{X}+s) - antilog(\overline{X}-s)}{2}\right]$

It is worth noting that the mean so obtained is nothing but the geometric mean of the observations (*see* Chapter **"Central tendency"**).

5.1.4 *Others*

5.1.4.1 Reciprocal transformation

Used when standard deviations of groups of data are proportional to the square of their means; the transformed value is the reciprocal of the original value; reciprocal of $(x + 1)$ is used when counts are involved.

5.1.4.2 Square transformation

This is virtually the opposite of square root transformation used when standard deviations of group means decrease as the magnitude of means increase; as the name indicates, the transformed value is simply the square of the original value.

5.1.4.3 Logit (Logistic) transformation

This transformation is used when predicted probability is < 0 or > 1; the transformation is done as follows: If In is the natural logarithm and P is the predicted probability,

$$\text{logit}(p) = In\left(\frac{p}{1-p}\right)$$

5.1.5 Analysis and interpretation of transformed data

All statistical analyses will be performed utilizing the transformed values which include hypotheses testing/ANOVA/Association between variables/Comparison of means, etc. However, when the final results are presented, the mean values are converted to original scale and along with superscripts, if any. Transformation of standard deviation to original scale can be done for logarithmic and *arcsin* transformations as described above.

13

One-Factor Analysis of Variance

Generally analysis of variance, designated ANOVA, is employed when (a) > 2 treatments are involved while studying a single variable and/or (b) ≥ 2 variables are involved. Let us consider a situation that $T_1, T_2 \ldots T_i$ are 'k' treatments (classes). In T_1 there are many observations; say $x_{11}, x_{12}, x_{13} \ldots x_{1j}$ observations and so on. Hence, each of the observation can be designated x_{ij} indicating jth observation of the ith treatment.

Obviously, these x_{ij}'s are variables and hence will have an overall mean $(\overline{X})$ and variance (s^2).

Further, it is also logical to state that each of the values would have been the same as overall mean, designated $\overline{x}_{..}$ (meaning of this notation is explained under "**Computations**") **if and only if**

1. There is no effect of ith treatment and
2. All the individuals (animals) allotted to each of the treatments are identical.
3. There is no other error whatsoever in any of the x_{ij}'s

In simple terms, it can be stated that $x_{ij} = \overline{x}_{..} \pm T_i \pm e_{ij}$ where T_i indicates effect of ith treatment (assignable cause of variation) and e_{ij} indicates differences between observations (animals, referred to as **error** or chance variation). In other words, ANOVA partitions the total variation in the given set of data into assignable and non-assignable (Chance) variation.

1. ASSUMPTIONS IN ANOVA

In the equation $X_{ij} = \overline{x}_{..} \pm T_i \pm e_{ij}$ the following important considerations/assumptions are worth noting:

1. All observations are independent of one another
2. **All effects (of Treatment T_i and Error e_{ij}) are additive.** In fact, ideally, data has to be subjected to Tukey's test of non-additivity before further analysis (*see* Chapter "**Two-factor analysis of variance**"). However, on most occasions, additivity is assumed.
3. The error associated with each of the observations, X_{ij}, is such that in some it is +ve, some others −ve and in some 0; in any case, the total of all error values is 0. That is,

error has a mean 0 but will have a variance (because the −ve values also become +ve due to squaring) σ^2. Hence, the second important assumption is that **error is Normally and independently distributed with mean 0 and variance σ^2**.

4. One more assumption that is made is that **variances of treatments are homogeneous;** this can be tested by Bartlett's test or Levene's test for homogeneity of variances (χ^2 distribution; see **Section 5**). It is not uncommon that homogeneity of variances is assumed as well. This hardly can cause severe damage to the conclusions especially if the n_i's are (nearly) equal because; the Bartlett's test itself is not immune to deviations from Normality!

2. DESIGN OF EXPERIMENTS

2.1. Basic Considerations

An experiment has to be "designed" (planned) so that the "treatments" (factor or group of factors) are properly allotted to the "experimental units" (subjects of experimentation be it an animal, product and the like).

2.1.1 Aims of Design of Experiments

1. To detect certain specified difference(s) or "effects" as "significant" with a known "confidence"
2. To get maximum information from the available resources
3. To select a proper "design" to ensure that the information obtained is worth the expense involved
4. The "design" should have a well-defined analytical procedure with all planned comparison of "treatments" possible independently on a scientific basis without loss of information; if unavoidable, only higher–order interactions may have to be ignored.

2.1.2 Basic Principles

1. Object of the experiment, variability in the experimental units, precision required of the estimates and that of comparisons must be well-defined
2. Should be least complicated to achieve the object of the experiment
3. When new treatment(s) is (are) being investigated, a tested treatment should be used as "Control"
4. Randomization of the experimental units to different treatments must conform to the requirements of tests of hypotheses
5. Possible methods of increasing precision like knowledge of previous experimentation may be utilized to decide:
   a. number of replications in each treatment
   b. type of grouping (blocking)—local control
   c. usefulness of including ancillary variable to obtain additional information

2.1.2.1 Randomization

This is a process employed to avoid bias in allotment of treatments to experimental units. Although it is ideal to have identical experimental units, it is practically impossible to obtain such units in any experiment for that matter, in general, and biological experiments, in particular. However, if the experimental units are allotted at random, there is sufficient ground to believe that the inherent variation between the experimental units would be equated among all the treatments; or there is no correlation among inherent variation of experimental units. Randomization process ensures equal "chance" to all the experimental units to be included in any particular treatment. Wherever possible, it is better to use random numbers while allotting experimental units. To sum up, **randomization makes errors of the individual observations independent with mean 0 variance σ^2**.

2.1.2.2 Replication

The number of times the effect of treatments is measured is referred to as replication. Repeated measurements (replications) are extremely important on following reasons:

1. To obtain proper estimate of error. If only one observation is made per treatment, it represents the effect of treatment + effect of the unit + error which is not distinguishable. Hence, all effects are mixed-up which is referred to as **confounded** and hence, none can be separated from one another. Therefore, at least 2 observations per treatment are mandatory.

2. To minimize standard error (se). For instance, se of difference between two means is $\sqrt{s^2\left(\dfrac{1}{n_1}+\dfrac{1}{n_2}\right)}$ with usual meanings for notations. Hence, if n_i's increase, se decreases; since se is the denominator of all tests of hypotheses (*see* Chapter "**Tests of hypotheses**"), it will facilitate elicit of smaller differences between treatments.

3. If s^2 is the variance due to error based on $\upsilon = n$, the **amount of information** from the data is defined as $\dfrac{1}{s^2}\left(\dfrac{n+1}{n+3}\right)$. It is interesting that the ratio $\left(\dfrac{n+1}{n+3}\right)$ increases rapidly as n increases from 1 to 10; thereafter, the increments are not that rapid. It is for this reason that **it is advisable to design an experiment so that υ for variance due to error is at least 10**.

4. The value of n depends on:
   a. amount of difference which is desired to be detectable by the experiment and
   b. the confidence level the experimenter desires

5. Without going to derivations, if it is desired to detect a difference of "d" between sample mean and μ, at $\alpha = 0.05$, then $n > \left(\dfrac{1.96\sigma}{d}\right)^2$

6. If it is desired to detect a difference of "d" between two sample means $\alpha = 0.05$, then $n > \left(\dfrac{2.228s}{d}\right)^2$ where s is the pooled standard deviation and 2.228 is the table value of $t_{0.05,\,10}$.

7. If sample of size n is drawn from a population of size N, and if $n_0 > \left(\dfrac{1.96\sigma}{d}\right)^2$, then

$$n = \dfrac{n_0}{1+\dfrac{n_0}{N}}$$

8. If it is desired to detect a difference of "d" between sample and population proportion (P), at $\alpha = 0.05$, then $n > \dfrac{1.96^2 PQ}{d^2}$

9. When estimate of σ^2/s^2 is not known, preliminary study, popularly referred to as **Pilot study** or **Uniformity trial** or **Benchmark survey** has to be conducted before the actual study.

2.1.2.3 Local control (blocking)

The term **blocking** originates, like many in "experimental designs", from agricultural experiments wherein fertility gradient of the soil is unavoidable. To remove (nullify, neutralize) the effect of fertility gradient, each of the treatments is **replicated (duplicated)** in each of the fertility levels so that the differences due to fertility is removed. Therefore, **a replicate is the one in which all treatments are repeated**. In case of Animal Science experiments, it may be necessary to logically group the experimental units into more homogenous groups so that variability among the experimental units is minimized; for instance, grouping as per sex, as per initial body weight, as per age, as per lactation number, etc. Ultimate aim is to ensure that animals within a group (block) have a comparably same effect on the variable under investigation.

2.1.2.4 Use of ancillary variable

If a variable under study is likely to be influenced by another factor which is not affected by treatments under investigation (hence not considered as a main factor for the study proper), inclusion of such factor(s) referred to as **Ancillary variable(s)** will help increase precision of the main investigation. The effect of ancillary variable is eliminated by analysis of covariance (ANACOV) so that true effects of the main factors can be detected. Examples in this category include day old chick weight as an ancillary variable for study of subsequent growth, assessment of sires (in large animal breeding experiments) through its daughters making use of dam values as ancillary variable.

2.2 Models of Experimental Design

It is in the fitness of things to recapitulate from **Section 2** of Chapter "**Association between variables I**" on models of experimental design. Conditions generally considered for classifying effects into **fixed** or **random** can be tabulated thus:

Criterion	Fixed effect (Model I)	Random effect (Model II)
Number of treatment groups	Small or finite	Large or even infinite
Number of underlying populations	Each treatment from a distinct population with its own mean	All drawn from the same population and the treatment mean is a random variable with a probability
Variability between groups	Not explainable by a distribution because each group has a distinct distribution	Since a common distribution is available, it can be explained by the distribution

2.2.1 Fixed–Effect Model (Model I)

Suppose a scientist is conducting an experiment to test the effect of four different floor–space allowances on growth rate of broilers. Since levels are specifically chosen, it is referred to as fixed–effect model. In this model:

1. H_0 will specify the means while stating equality as in this example, $H_0: \mu_1 = \mu_2 = \mu_3 = \mu_4$.

2. In addition, the equation for this model is generally represented as $x_{ij} = \mu + \alpha_i + \varepsilon_{ij}$ with α_i being the fixed effect where $\Sigma\alpha_i = 0$ and ε_{ij}, the error associated with the x_{ij}'s being normally distributed with mean 0 and variance σ^2; designated $\varepsilon_{ij} \sim N(0, \sigma^2)$.

3. F test is valid to test $\alpha_i = 0$.

4. When is H_0 false, MSS_T (mean sum of squares between treatments (classes) is an

$$\text{unbiased estimate of } \sigma^2 + \frac{n\sum_{i=1}^{k}\alpha_i^2}{(k-1)} \text{ ; this is referred to as \textbf{Expectation of Mean Square}}$$

(EMS). Usefulness of EMS will be enumerated under **Sections 4.2** and **5** of Chapter "**ANOVA for more than two factors**"

5. When repeated samples are drawn, they are from the same set of treatments (classes) and with the same α_i; therefore, when H_0 is false, the F distribution is referred to as **non-central F distribution**; however, Fisher's F distribution values only are employed.

2.2.2 Random–Effect Model (Model II)

Consider an experiment to find the effect of diurnal variation on certain hormone levels in layers; in this case, the diurnal variation is not controlled by the experimenter but comes as random variable; hence, this model is the random–effect model. In random model:

1. H_0 will be: there is no effect of diurnal variation on the hormone levels in layers.

2. In addition, the equation for this model is generally represented as $x_{ij} = \mu + A_i + \varepsilon_{ij}$ with A_i being the random effect where A_i is $\sim N(0, \sigma_A^2)$ which also means that $\Sigma A_i = 0$ and ε_{ij}, the error associated with the x_{ij}'s being Normally distributed with mean 0 and variance σ^2; designated $\varepsilon_{ij} \sim N(0, \sigma^2)$.

3. Consequent on the above factors, F test is valid in Model II also to test $\sigma_A = 0$.

4. When is H_0 false, MSS_T (mean sum of squares between treatments (classes) is an unbiased estimate (**Expectation of mean square, EMS**) of $\sigma^2 + n\sigma_A^2$; and MSS_E is EMS of σ^2.

5. Every time a new random sample is drawn and hence Fisher's F distribution is applicable.

6. Since each of the animals is assumed to be independent of each other animal, this design is often referred to as **completely randomized design (CRD)**.

2.2.3 Mixed Model (Model III)

If an experiment has both fixed and random effects, it is referred to as mixed model; For instance known sires are mated to random group of dams and the progeny values are considered as the criterion for analysis. Similarly, a Factorial experiment or a Randomized Block design (will be dealt in Chapters "**Two-factor analysis of variance**", "**Analysis of variance for more than two factors**" and "**Factorial experiments**") may include both random and fixed effects. In this model > 1 factors are involved and obviously, there is no question of one-factor ANOVA for mixed models.

Let us take the example of known sires each mated to dams at random and each dam produces progenies. The model can be represented as $x_{ijk} = \mu + \alpha_i + B_{ij} + \varepsilon_{ijk}$ where, the fixed effect, $\Sigma \alpha_i = 0$, whereas B_{ij} and ε_{ijk} are random variables representing dams and progenies, respectively. The MSS_{sires} estimates $\sigma^2 + n\sigma_B^2 + nb\dfrac{\sum_{i=1}^{k}\alpha_i^2}{(k-1)}$, $MSS_{dams/sire}$ estimates , $MSS_{progenies/dams/sire}$ estimates σ^2. Further, $MSS_{dams/sire}$ is a relevant MSS for testing MSS_{sires} by F ratio and if F value is < table value, sire effects are generally considered non-existent.

Note:

1. In a mixed model. If the dams are also fixed, then MSS_{sires} estimates $\sigma^2 + n\sigma_B^2 + nb\sigma_A^2$.

2. Generally, basic procedure of ANOVA does not differ between the models; but, further testing and interpretation do.

3. Since EMS is generally useful in Animal Breeding, it is dealt in Chapter "**Statistics in specific veterinary fields**".

3. COMPUTATIONS (MODELS I AND II)

The layout of the data can be represented as follows with indication of the notations generally used:

It is necessary to note the meaning of '.' used as subscript in Chapters on ANOVA. A subscript '.' indicates summation over the variable which is reduced as a '.' subscript; for instance, the x_{ij} values indicate that there are k treatments ($i = 1, 2, 3, ..., k$) each having j observations ($j = 1, 2, 3, ..., n_i$) observations to indicate summation of ith treatment, the usual notation will be $\sum_{j=1}^{n_i} x_{ij}$. But to make it simple, it is denoted x_i. To mean that summation is effected on j or all j or n_i observations within the ith treatment. This notation is simple and equally easy to understand in comparison to the usual notation. Similarly, $x_{i.}^2$ stands for sum of squares of j values in a particular ith treatment (class) and $x..$ indicates addition of all x_{ij} values (grand total), x^2 denotes total crude sum of squares or $\sum_{i=1}^{k}\sum_{j=1}^{n_i} x_{ij}^2$ {hence, **not same as** $(x..)^2$} and $\bar{x}_{..}$ indicates overall mean. As the classification level increases, this format of denoting sum and sum of squares facilitates understanding of the formulae.

Treatments →	T_1	T_2	T_3	....	T_i	Totals
Observations	x_{11}	x_{21}	x_{31}	....	x_{i1}	
	x_{12}	x_{22}	x_{32}	....	x_{i2}	
	.	.	.	....	.	
	.	.	.	....	.	
	x_{1j}	x_{2j}	x_{3j}	....	x_{ij}	
Totals, x_i.	x_1.	x_2.	x_3.	....	x_i.	x..
Sum of squares, x_i^2.	x_1^2.	x_2^2.	x_3^2.	....	x_i^2.	x^2..
No of observations, n_i	n_1	n_2	n_3	....	n_i	n.
Means	$\bar{x}_1$.	$\bar{x}_2$.	$\bar{x}_3$.		$\bar{x}_i$.	$\bar{x}$..

'.' indicates the subscript over which summation is effected

The table clearly suggests that there is only one known source of assignable variation (error being the unknown or non-assignable or chance variation) which is the sum of squares due to treatments (hence, such classification is referred to as **One-factor ANOVA** or **One-way classification** or **One-way ANOVA**). The procedure of ANOVA consists of calculating the following and then, by laying the ANOVA table:

1. Total sum of squares, TSS $= x_{..}^2 - \dfrac{(x_{..})^2}{n.}$ on $\upsilon = (n. - 1)$; $\dfrac{(x_{..})^2}{n.}$ is referred to as **Correction factor (C)**.

2. Treatment Sum of squares, $SS_T = \sum\limits_{i=1}^{k} \dfrac{(x_{i.})^2}{n_i} - C$ on $\upsilon = (k-1)$, where k is the number

of treatments (classes) and n_i's are different for treatments; if n_i's are same for all

treatments, it will be simplified into $\dfrac{\sum\limits_{i=1}^{k}(x_{i.})^2}{n_i} - C$.

3. Error sum of squares, $SS_E = TSS - SS_T$ on $\upsilon = (n. - k)$; in other words, SS_E

$= x_{..}^2 - \sum\limits_{i=1}^{k} \dfrac{(x_{i.})^2}{n_i}$ or, when n_i's are same for all treatments, $x_{..}^2 - \dfrac{\sum\limits_{i=1}^{k}(x_{i.})^2}{n_i}$.

4. When n_i's are different for treatments, weighted n_i per treatment can be calculated

as $n_i' = \dfrac{n. - \dfrac{\sum\limits_{i=1}^{k} n_i^2}{n.}}{k-1}$.

With the above calculations, the ANOVA table can be laid out as follows: $H_0: \mu_1 = \mu_2 = \mu_3 = \mu_4 ...,$ depending on number of treatments.

Source	υ	SS	MSS	F
Total	$(n.-1)$	TSS		
Treatments	$(k-1)$	SS_T	MSS_T	$(MSS_T \div MSS_E)^@$
Error	$(n.-k)$	SS_E	MSS_E	

MSS = Mean sum of squares = $(SS \div \upsilon)$; $^@$ on $\upsilon = (k-1)$ and $(n.-t)$ at set α

In ANOVA, means are tested depending on the variances (mean sum of squares) contributed by various treatments (MSS_T) against that due to error component (MSS_E). It is understandable that if the ratio of the former to the latter (F ratio) is ≤ 1, the observed difference could as well be due to error itself. Hence, F ratio must be > 1 for any effects to be significant. Standard tables of F are available (Appendix 5) to test the significance depending on degrees of freedom of both at set α.

If the calculated F value is $>$ Table value, H_0 is liable to be rejected and the treatments are significantly different.

Note: Calculation of sums of squares for treatments and error can be performed by Least–Squares technique which requires knowledge of matrix algebra.

3.1 Comparison of Treatment Means

If a control group is employed with which all other treatment(s) is (are) compared, it is advisable that the control group has more observations than the treatment groups; optimal size for control group can be calculated as $\sqrt{(k-1)}$ times the number of observations for treatment groups. The procedure for comparison of treatments is essentially same.

3.1.1 LSD Test (Student's t-Distribution)

3.1.1.1 Case of 2 treatments

In this case, Student's t test will yield the same result as that of ANOVA; the value of F obtained will be equal to t^2 value and MSS_E will be same as pooled variance in t test. In any case, since only two treatments are involved, there is no question of multiple comparisons.

3.1.1.2 Case of > 2 treatments

3.1.1.2.1 When n_i's are unequal

Standard error of the difference between two means is given by

$$se\left(\bar{X}_i - \bar{X}_j\right) = \sqrt{MSS_E\left(\frac{1}{n_i} + \frac{1}{n_j}\right)}$$

where n_i and n_j represent the number of observations for calculating $\bar{X}_i$ and $\bar{X}_j$, respectively. With the se of the difference being available, Student's t test can be performed as the ratio of difference to se of difference on $\upsilon = (n_i + n_j - 2)$ and set α. If the calculated value is $>$ table value (Appendix 3), the treatments are statistically different.

3.1.1.2.2 *When n_i's are equal*

Standard error of the difference between two means is given by $se\left(\overline{X}_i - \overline{X}_j\right) = \sqrt{\dfrac{2MSS_E}{n_i}}$

where n_i represent the number of observations per treatment. With the se of the difference being available, Student's t test can be performed as the ratio of difference to se of difference on $\upsilon = 2 \times (n_i - 1)$ and set α. If the calculated value is > table value (Appendix 3), the treatments are statistically different. Even with unequal number of observations per treatment, if the differences are not wide, weighted n can be used in place of n_i and comparisons made.

3.1.1.3 Least significant (critical) difference

Regardless whether n_i's are equal or unequal, $t = \dfrac{\left(\overline{X}_i - \overline{X}_j\right)}{\sqrt{MSS_E\left(\dfrac{1}{n_i} + \dfrac{1}{n_j}\right)}}$; therefore, if

$\left(\overline{X}_i - \overline{X}_j\right) > t\left(\sqrt{MSS_E\left(\dfrac{1}{n_i} + \dfrac{1}{n_j}\right)}\right)$, the difference will be significant. Hence, $t_{\upsilon, \alpha} \times$ se

(difference) is popularly referred to as **least significant (critical) difference (LSD)**. It is a general practice to calculate LSD and compare different combination of mean–pairs for significance in their difference.

3.1.2 Tukey's Test (q-Distribution)

This test is also a popular test used for multiple comparisons; it is same as LSD test except that the in place of Student's t values, q-distribution values are used and standard

error of difference is $se\left(\overline{X}_i - \overline{X}_j\right) = \sqrt{\dfrac{MSS_E}{2}\left(\dfrac{1}{n_i} + \dfrac{1}{n_j}\right)}$; where the MSS_E is divided by 2

(*cf*: LSD test). Since Student's t-distribution values are provided in Appendix 3, LSD test is used for comparisons and q-distribution values are not provided in this publication; however, the same can be accessed from several publications like Zar (2003) and others.

3.1.3 Scheffe's Test (S Test) for Multiple Contrasts

This test is primarily based on H_0: $\mu_A - \mu_B = 0$; however, this test is likely to detect more differences as significant than LSD or Tukey's test; i.e. increase the risk of Type II error and hence, generally not used in Animal Science. In any case, a general procedure is outlined below:

Suppose $\mu_1, \mu_2, \mu_3, ..., \mu_k$ are k sample means and H_0: $\{(\mu_1 + \mu_2 + \mu_3, ... + \mu_{k-1}) \div (k-1)\} - \mu_k = 0$, the S test comprises of allotting coefficient $\{1 \div (k-1)\}$ to each of the μ_{k-1}'s and (–) 1 to μ_k so that sum of all the coefficients = 0. The coefficients are designated c_i's

$(i = 1, 2, 3, ..., k)$. Then, the S statistic $= \dfrac{\left| \sum\limits_{i=1}^{k} c_i \overline{X_i} \right|}{se}$ where se, the standard error =

$\sqrt{MSS_E \left(\sum\limits_{i=1}^{k} \dfrac{c_i^2}{n_i} \right)}$. It is apparent that even combination of > I means can be compared with another combination of means and there is requisite of involving all the means while making a H_0; however, c_i's must be suitably allotted such that $\sum c_i = 0$. Critical value of S at set α for each contrast is $\sqrt{(k-1)F_{\alpha, k-1, n.-k}}$.

Confidence intervals for difference between two means can be calculated by $\left(\overline{X}_B - \overline{X}_A \right) \pm S_\alpha \sqrt{MSS_E \left(\dfrac{1}{n_A} + \dfrac{1}{n_B} \right)}$ and confidence interval for a contrast is given by $\sum\limits_{i=1}^{k} c_i \overline{X}_i \pm S_\alpha se$ where se is the standard error of contrast.

3.1.4 Range Tests

It can be noticed that in case of LSD test, the value of LSD is unaffected by the number of means in a range or group. Thus, it is generally agreed that LSD is less conservative when number of means increases. Hence, Range tests have been proposed; for instance by Newman and Keul, Dunnett, Duncan and others which are known to reduce Type–II error (*see* Chapter "**Tests of hypotheses**").

3.1.4.1 The Duncan's multiple range (DMR) test

Among multiple comparison tests, the **Duncan's multiple range (DMR) test** is probably most commonly used. Appendix 10 gives DMR values for $\alpha = 0.05$ and 0.01.

The procedure to locate the table value is as follows:
1. Arrange the mean values in an ascending or descending order.
2. Find out number of mean values between the means under test and add 2 to it (to include the means under comparison).
3. The number obtained @2 has to be located as column in Appendix 10 and the row is identified by the υ for MSS_E.
4. The DMR value is used in place of Student's t value for calculation of LSD.

3.1.4.2 The Student-Newman-Keuls' (SNK) test

The standard error of difference and the test statistic q are calculated similar to Tukey's test; but the table values for comparison are located for number of means in the range +2 (similar to DMR test). Table values of q-distribution is not provided in this publication.

3.1.4.3 Others

Scheffe has suggested a conservative test which is suitable for both equal and unequal observations per treatment. The critical difference, $s_L = \sqrt{(k-1)F_{0.05, (t-1), (n.-t)}}$ where k is the number of samples (treatments); however, LSD and DMR are commonly employed.

3.1.4.4 Confidence intervals after multiple comparisons

When a particular mean ($\bar{X}_i$) is found to be significantly different from others, confidence intervals at set α is given by $\bar{X}_i \pm t_{\alpha,\upsilon}\sqrt{\dfrac{MSS_E}{n_i}}$. On the contrary, if the means were found to be from the same population (H_0 being acceptable), a pooled mean is calculated as $\bar{X}_P = \dfrac{\sum\limits_{i=1}^{k} n_i \bar{x}_i}{\sum\limits_{i=1}^{k} n_i}$ whose confidence intervals at set α is given by

$\bar{X}_P \pm t_{\alpha,\upsilon}\sqrt{\dfrac{MSS_E}{\sum\limits_{i=1}^{k} n_i}}$. For Tukey's procedure, if a difference is found to be significant,

$(1-\alpha)$ confidence intervals are given by $\left(\bar{X}_B - \bar{X}_A\right) \pm q_{\alpha,\upsilon,k}se$ where se is the standard error of difference.

3.1.5 Indication of Significant Difference

When many means are involved, it becomes difficult to make statements on all possible significant differences. To resolve this, superscripts are placed on the mean values with a note "**Means bearing at least one common superscript are not significantly different (P ≤ α)**" when > 1 superscripts are given on any or many of the means or "**Means bearing different superscripts are significantly different (P ≤ α)**". The steps for this purpose are shown with the assumption that the mean values are 48, 58, 61, 62, 68, 71 and 72 with an LSD value of 10.1.

Step 1: Since superscript 'a' is generally put for the largest value, we had better arrange the means in a descending order.

Step 2: Subtract the LSD value from the largest value and locate the value obtained (or immediately greater vale among the group of means) among the means and draw a line embracing the means covered within the range; designate it as 'a'

72   71   68   62   61   58   48
a ────────────────

Step 3: Repeat Step 2 with second largest value and draw a line below the earlier one embracing the means covered within the range; designate it as 'b'

72   71   68   62   61   58   48
a ────────────────
     b ────────────────

Step 4: Repeat Step 2 with third largest value and draw a line below the earlier ones embracing the means covered within the range; designate it as 'c'

72   71   68   62   61   58   48
a ────────────────
     b ────────────────
         c ──────────────── and continue until the lowest value is either covered by a line or the difference between the penultimate and the last one is $\geq$ LSD

Step 5: After obtaining, place all the superscripts the particular value is underscored.

72   71   68   62   61   58   48

a ————————————

   b ——————————

      c ——————————

         ——————————

            d ——————————; hence, the means will have the
superscripts as 72^a, 71^{ab}, 68^{abc}, 62^{abc}, 61^{bc}, 58^{cd} and 48^d.

Note:
1. If any line to be drawn is only a superimposition of the previous one, it is ignored and the next value is considered; as for instance for the values 68, 62, 61 and 58 above.
2. If more than one set of values have to be compared within a table, different set of superscripts (a,b,c,d or m,n,o,p or x,y,z etc) can be employed. Different ways of presenting the significance of differences can be developed limited only by the imagination of the investigator!
3. When DMR is used, LSD differs for different comparisons.
4. The means can as well be arranged in an ascending order and the lines named accordingly, in a reverse sequence.

4.   MODEL EXAMPLES

4.1   Model I

Table below gives the gain in weights (kg) of pigs on three treatments for a period of 1 week. Test H_0: Means of weight gains is same among all treatments.

Treatments →	T_1	T_2	T_3	Totals
Observations	3	5	7	
	5	6	6	
	6	2	4	
	2	7	3	
		8	6	
		3	4	
		9		
		8		
Totals, $x_i.$ (kg)	16	48	30	$x.. = 94$
Sum of squares, $x^2_i.$	74	332	162	$x^2.. = 568$
No of observations, n_i	4	8	6	$n. = 18$
Means, kg	4.00	6.00	5.00	$\bar{x}.. = 5.22$

1. Total Sum of Squares, TSS $= 568 - (94^2 \div 18) = 77.1111$ on $v = 17$ and $(94^2 \div 18) = 490.8889$ is the CF.

2. Treatment sum of squares, $SS_T = (16^2 \div 4) + (48^2 \div 8) + (30^2 \div 6) - CF = 11.1111$ on $\upsilon = 2$,
3. Error sum of squares, $SS_E = TSS - SS_T = 77.1111 - 11.1111 = 66.0000$ on $\upsilon = 15$.
   With the above calculations, the ANOVA table can be laid out as follows:
   $H_0: \mu_1 = \mu_2 = \mu_3$

Source	υ	SS	MSS	F
Total	17	77.1111		
Treatments	2	11.1111	5.5556	1.262[NS]
Error	15	66.0000	4.4000	

Table value of $F_{0.05, 2, 15} = 3.68$; [NS] Not significant

The calculated F value is < Table value; therefore, H_0 may be accepted.

Note: Since H_0 is accepted, comparison of treatment means doesn't arise; the pigs gained 5.22 kg per week ($\bar{x}_{..}$) regardless of treatment.

4.2 Model II

The same procedure of ANOVA is applicable to Model II as well. The EMS can be utilized under relevant circumstances for further considerations like increased precision, reducing cost of experimentation, etc. These aspects are outlined through the following example:

From a large layer farm, 6 eggs from 5 layers were chosen at random and cholesterol content (g/g dry weight of yolk) estimated. It is necessary to know how precise the estimate of cholesterol has been and can the number of eggs considered per bird be reduced without affecting accuracy or not. Understandably, ANOVA is undertaken on H_0: There is no difference in cholesterol content of eggs.

Sl No	Cholesterol g/g dry weight of yolk						$x_{i.}$	$x^2_{i.}$
1	2.00	2.10	2.20	2.15	2.05	2.10	12.60	26.485
2	1.80	1.75	1.90	1.80	1.85	1.80	10.90	19.815
3	2.30	2.35	2.25	2.25	2.30	2.25	13.70	31.290
4	1.90	1.95	1.90	1.85	1.95	1.95	11.50	22.050
5	1.70	1.70	1.75	1.70	1.75	1.70	10.30	17.685
							$x_{..} = 59$	$x^2_{..} = 117.325$

Total SS = 1.2917; $SS_T = 1.2333$; $SS_{Deviations} = 0.0584$

Source	υ	SS	MSS	F	EMS
Total	29	1.2917			
Hens	4	1.2333	0.3083	134.043	$\sigma^2 + 66_A{}^2$
Error	25	0.0584	0.0023		σ^2

Table value of $F_{0.05, 4, 25} = 2.76$

Since calculated value of F > Table value, H_0 is liable to be rejected. Further, EMS showing the **components of variance** is useful in calculating $\sigma_A{}^2$, **component of**

variance for hens which in this example is 0.051. Variance of $\bar{x}_{..}$ as an estimate of μ is given by $\text{MSS}_T \div (n_i^* k) = \text{MSS}_T \div n_{..}$ where MSS_T is the mean sum of squares due to treatment (class; hens in this example), n_i is the number of observations (determinations, in this example) per treatment (class; hens in this example) and k is the number of treatments (class; hens in this example) and $n_{..}$ is the total number of observations. Hence, variance of $\bar{x}_{..} = 0.0103$. This includes both the effect of hens as well as error components.

4.2.1 Unequal n_i's for Treatments (Classes)

The procedure of ANOVA is same as described for equal observations wherein corresponding number of observations are used as denominator while calculating SS_T. But, for calculating variance component, σ_A^2, weighted n_i designated n_w can be

calculated as $\dfrac{1}{(k-1)}\left(n_{..} - \dfrac{\sum\limits_{i=1}^{k} n_i^2}{n_{..}}\right).$

4.2.2 Intra-Class Correlation (r_I)

This correlation is described under **Section 5.5** in Chapter "**Association between variables I**". However, it is in the fitness of things to mention that when $\sigma_A^2 > 0$, it is indicative that the members under the same treatment (class) are tending to behave alike. Under such circumstances, in Model II, it can be assumed that x_{ij}'s are distributed around the same mean and same variance σ_I^2 along with a correlation among members under same treatment (class), referred to as **Intra-class correlation, ρ_I**; it can be estimated as the ratio of σ_A^2 to $(\sigma_A^2 + \sigma^2)$.

From ANOVA, $\text{MSS}_E = \sigma_I^{2*}(1 - \sigma_I^2)$ and $\text{MSS}_T = \sigma_I^2 \times \{1 + (n-1) \times \rho_I\} = \sigma^2 + n\sigma_A^2$;

$\text{MSS}_E = \sigma_I^2 \times (1 - \rho_I)$; hence, $\text{MSS}_T - \text{MSS}_E$ estimates $n\rho_I\sigma_I^2$ and $r_I = \dfrac{\text{MSS}_T - \text{MSS}_E}{[\text{MSS}_T + (n-1)\text{MSS}_E]}$.

In **Example 4.2**, $r_I = (0.051 - 0.0023) \div \{0.051 + (24 \times 0.0023)\} = 0.4586$.

4.2.3 Cost of Experimentation

Suppose the experiment has to be redone with n_i' observations per k' treatment (hen),

variance of $\bar{x}_{..} = \dfrac{\sigma_A^2}{k'} + \dfrac{\sigma^2}{n_i'k'} \approx \dfrac{0.051}{k'} + \dfrac{0.0023}{n_i'k'}$. Since σ_A^2 is larger, it is reasonable that k'

has to be increased and n_i' reduced to minimize variance of $\bar{x}_{..}$. Assuming that the cost of determining cholesterol (Rs 75 per determination) is 50 times that of egg, data from 15 hens with one egg per hen costs Rs ($15 \times 75 + 15 \times 1\frac{1}{2}$) = Rs 1147.5 *Vis-à-vis* Rs ($30 \times 75 + 30 \times 1.5$) = Rs 2295.00 for the set of data in **Example 4.2**. However, the new estimate of variance of $\bar{x}_{..} = (0.051 \div 15) + (0.0023 \div 15) = 0.0036$ which is not only far lesser than 0.0103 in the original experiment and also half as costly as the original experiment.

In general, cost (C) of making n_i' determination on each of the k' units selected at random from the population @ Rs c per determination is given by $C = c_k k' + ck'n_i'$ where c_k is cost of selecting a unit (say Rs 0.10); and n_i' required to minimize the

variance of $\bar{x}_{..} = \sqrt{\dfrac{c_k \sigma^2}{c\sigma_A^2}}$ which, in the above example works out to be $\sqrt{\dfrac{0.1 \times 0.0023}{75 \times 0.051}} =$

0.008; since n_i' can't be a fraction, the minimum of single determination per hen is required to ensure minimum value of variance of $\bar{x}_{..}$. It also emphasizes the fact that the number of hens had better be increased rather than number of eggs per hen in order to increase precision and reduce costs.

5. TEST FOR HOMOGENEITY OF VARIANCES

5.1 Bartlett's Test

Testing of homogeneity of two variances by F test is described in Chapter "**Tests of hypotheses**". But when > 2 variances have to be tested for homogeneity, Bartlett's test is resorted to.

The statistic B is calculated as $B = \left(In\ s_P^2 \right) \left(\displaystyle\sum_{i=1}^{k} v_i \right) - \displaystyle\sum_{i=1}^{k} v_i In\ s_i^2$ where k is the number

of samples and $s_P^2 = \dfrac{\displaystyle\sum_{i=1}^{k} SS_i}{\displaystyle\sum_{i=1}^{k} v_i}$ where SS_i is the sum of squares (i.e. $s_i^2 \times v_i$). the distribution

of B's is approximately χ^2 on $v = (k-1)$ and more accurately so when it is divided by

a correction factor C which is calculated as $C = 1 + \dfrac{1}{3(k+1)} \left(\displaystyle\sum_{i=1}^{k} \dfrac{1}{v_i} - \dfrac{1}{\displaystyle\sum_{i=1}^{k} v_i} \right)$. To facilitate

computation, natural log is replaced by $2.3026 \times \log 10$ while calculating B statistic.

Hence, $B = 2.3026 \left[\left(\log_{10} s_P^2 \right) \left(\displaystyle\sum_{i=1}^{k} v_i \right) - \displaystyle\sum_{i=1}^{k} v_i \log_{10} s_i^2 \right]$ and $B_C = \dfrac{B}{C}$ which follows χ^2

distribution on $v = (k-1)$

5.2 Example

In a feeding trial on pigs, five protein levels were under investigation. The treatments had unequal number of animals and the variance and v of each treatment is tabulated. Before proceeding for ANOVA, it was thought necessary to run a test for homogeneity of variances. Hence, it is required to test H_0: Variances of all the treatments are homogenous.

s_i^2	υ_i	$s_i^2 \times \upsilon_i$	$\text{Log}_{10}\, s_i^2$	$\text{Log}_{10}\, s_i^2 \times \upsilon$
4.50	10	45	0.6532	6.532
10.50	10	105	1.0212	10.120
21.50	20	430	1.3324	26.648
4.00	30	120	0.6021	18.063
1.00	30	30	0.00	0
Totals	100	$\sum_{i=1}^{k} SS_i = 730$	3.6089	60.463

$$s_p^2 = (730 \div 100) = 7.30,\ \log_{10} s_p^2 = -0.1367,\ \sum_{i=1}^{k} \frac{1}{\upsilon_i} = 0.3166,\ C = 1.0256$$

Therefore, $B = 2.3026 \times \{(0.8633 \times 100) - 60.463\} = 59.561$; and $B_C = 58.074$ which is $>$ 9.49, the table value of $\chi^2_{0.05,\,4}$. Hence, H_0 is rejected.

5.2.1 Multiple Comparison of Variances

In **Example 5.1**, the variances were not homogenous. Hence, it becomes necessary to compare the variances as it was done for means. Analogous to Tukey's test (*see* **Section 2.1.2** above), $q = \dfrac{\left| In\ s_A^2 - In\ s_B^2 \right|}{se\left(In\ s_A^2 - In\ s_B^2 \right)}$ where the denominator is given by $\sqrt{\dfrac{1}{\upsilon_A} + \dfrac{1}{\upsilon_B}}$ when $\upsilon_A \neq \upsilon_B$ and when $\upsilon_A = \upsilon_B$; the numerator can be multiplied by 2.3026 to use $\log_{10}$ values. The calculated q value is compared with critical values of Tukey's q distribution on $\upsilon = \infty$, 5 and set α. The procedure to place superscripts on the variances depending on the results of comparisons is same as described under **Section 2.1.3** above.

In the example under consideration, the comparisons are shown below:

Sl No	s_i^2	υ_i	$\text{Log}_{10}\, s_i^2$	Comparisons	
1	4.50	10	0.6532	1 Vs 2: $q = 1.895$	2 Vs 4: $q = 2.643$
2	10.50	10	1.0212	1 Vs 3: $q = 4.038$	2 Vs 5: $q = 6.440$
3	21.50	20	1.3324	1 Vs 4: $q = 0.322$	3 Vs 4: $q = 5.825$
4	4.00	30	0.6021	1 Vs 5: $q = 4.120$	3 Vs 5: $q = 10.628$
5	1.00	30	0.00	2 Vs 3: $q = 1.850$	4 Vs 5: $q = 5.369$

Table value of $q_{0.05,\,\infty,\,5} = 3.858$

The multiple comparisons can be indicated by the following superscripts: 4.50^b, 10.50^{ab}, 21.50^a, 4.00^b, 1.00^c; the values bearing at least one common letter superscript are not significantly different ($P \leq 0.05$).

Note: Table values of Tukey's q distribution are not provided in this publication.

5.3 Levene's Test

This test is simpler than the Bartlett's test because it uses the average of absolute deviations instead of variance. The absolute deviations are used in place of individual observations and one-factor ANOVA is performed as described above. Then, if F value between treatments (classes) is < table value at set α and the relevant $\upsilon - s$, then, the variances are considered homogenous. This test is not commonly employed and if at all homogeneity is tested, Bartlett's test is used in Animal Science.

6. KRUSKAL–WALLIS TEST (ANOVA BY RANKS) (NON-PARAMETRIC ANOVA)

This can be used when one-way ANOVA is not applicable and it is $\approx 95\%$ ($3 \div \pi$) as powerful as ANOVA. When the samples are not from Normal population and/or population variances are not homogenous, if number of groups, $k = 2$, Kruskal–Wallis test $\equiv$ Mann–Whitney test (*see* Chapter "**Tests of hypotheses**").

6.1 Example

A hypothetical example is given below regarding infestation of an intestinal parasite from a large-scale abattoir. It is required to test H_0: The parasite is equally abundant at all sections of the intestine at $\alpha = 0.05$. The numbers were allotted ranks without giving weightage to classification; i.e. combined ranks (*see* Chapter "**Tests of hypotheses**"):

Upper intestine		Middle intestine		Lower intestine	
Number	Rank*	Number	Rank*	Number	Rank*
3	10	18	4	9	7
6	9	22	1	11	6
2	11	19	3	12	5
1	12	20	2	8	8
Totals, R_i	42		10		26

* Combined rank; $n_1 = 4$, $n. = 16$

The Kruskal–Wallis statistic, $H = \dfrac{12}{n.(n.+1)} \sum_{i=1}^{k} \dfrac{R_i^2}{n_i} - 3(n.+1)$. In the above example,

$H = 45.846$ which is > 5.692, the table value of $H_{0.05,\,4,4,4}$ (Appendix 11). If $k > 5$, $H \approx \chi^2$ on $\upsilon = (k-1)$. Hence, H_0 is liable to be rejected.

6.2 Multiple Comparisons

When H_0 is rejected, multiple comparisons become a necessity. However, comparisons are done among sum of ranks of each group instead of means by calculating

$se = \sqrt{\dfrac{n_i(n_ik)(n_ik+1)}{12}}$. In the present example, rank for sum of the ranks is 1 for middle intestine, 2 for lower intestine and 3 for upper intestine with sum of the ranks as 10, 26 and 42 respectively. The se calculated by the above formula ($n_i = 4$, $k = 3$) is 7.211. The difference in sum of ranks is divided by the se to obtain calculated value of statistic q. The table value of $q_{\alpha,\,\infty,\,k}$ is compared to draw conclusions. The table value of q in the present case is 3.314 at $\alpha = 0.05$ and hence, minimum difference to be significant is $7.211 \times 3.314 = 23.9$. If the rank totals are allotted superscripts as described under **Section 2.1.3** above, it will be 42^b, 26^b, 10^a; indicating that number of parasites in middle intestine was significantly different from the other two regions (Note that the '^{a}' is used on the lower value because they are rank totals).

Note:

1. H can also be calculated as the ratio of SS_T to total MSS by applying the procedure for ANOVA on the combined Ranks as described under **Section 6.1** above.

2. Sum of all the Ranks, ΣR_i or R. should be $\{n. \times (n. + 1)\} \div 2$

3. Since the test is not commonly used in Animal Science, table values of q distribution are not provided in this publication. They can be accessed from other publications like Zar, 2003 and

4. For the same reason, unequal observations are also not discussed; but,

5. If there is (are) tied ranks, a correction factor, $C = 1 - \dfrac{\displaystyle\sum_{i=1}^{m}\left(t_i^3 - t_i\right)}{n.^3 - n.}$ is calculated followed by corrected

H, $H_c = H \div C$ where t_i is the number of ties in the ith group and m is the number of groups with tied ranks.

7. TEST FOR DIFFERENCE AMONG SEVERAL MEDIANS

This test, applicable when $n \geq 20$, is similar to χ^2 test for $2 \times k$ contingency table (*see* Chapter "**Tests of hypotheses**"). The data will consist of frequencies above median (forming f_{1k} values) and frequencies not above median (forming f_{2k} values) from k samples. It is rare that a median test with multiple samples is encountered in animal science.

8. HOMOGENEITY OF MULTIPLE CVs

Comparison of CVs from two samples has been outlined in Chapter "**Tests of hypotheses**"; the same can be extended to compare multiple CVs as follows: when

number of samples, $k > 3$, $\chi^2 = \dfrac{\displaystyle\sum_{i=1}^{k} \upsilon_i V_i^2 - \dfrac{\left[\displaystyle\sum_{i=1}^{k} \upsilon_i V_i\right]^2}{\displaystyle\sum_{i=1}^{k} \upsilon_i}}{V_P^2\left(0.5 + V_P^2\right)}$ on $\upsilon = (k-1)$ at set α; where Pooled

CV, $V_P = \dfrac{\displaystyle\sum_{i=1}^{k} \upsilon_i V_i}{\displaystyle\sum_{i=1}^{k} \upsilon_i}$.

8.1 Example

The following are the hypothetical values of CV in respect of 5 groups of pigs referred to in the **Example 6.1** above: H_0: All CVs are homogenous

Sl No	V_i	v_i	$v_i V_i$	$v_i V_i^2$
1	0.0550	10	0.550	0.030250
2	0.0925	10	0.925	0.085563
3	0.0330	20	0.660	0.017800
4	0.0155	30	0.465	0.007208
5	0.0110	30	0.330	0.003630
Totals	0.207	100	2.930	0.144451

$$V_P = \left(\sum_{i=1}^{k} v_i V_i \div \sum_{i=1}^{k} v_i \right) = (2.93 \div 100) = 0.0293$$

$\chi^2 = 3.779$ which is < 9.49, the table value of $\chi^2_{0.05,\,4}$. Hence, H_0 may be accepted.

9. WEIGHTED LINEAR REGRESSION

In case of one-factor ANOVA, if the treatments (classes) have unequal frequencies and the treatments consist of an independent variable having graded effect on the variable in question is used at different levels, then, weighted linear regression can be fit for such data. In simpler terms, this is a case of multiple (but unequal) y_i's for each x_i.

The ANOVA is first performed as described above to ascertain that the treatments are significant as a prerequisite. Then the linear regression of $\bar{y}_{i.}$ against x_i. is fit; or the regression equation is $\hat{\bar{y}}_{i.} = a + b\bar{x}$ and the constants are calculated as: $a = \bar{y}_{..} - b\bar{x}$

where $\bar{y}_{..}$ and $\bar{x}$ are weighted means and $b = \dfrac{\sum_{i=1}^{k} n_i x_i \bar{y}_{i.}}{\sum_{i=1}^{k} n_i x_i^2}$; the weighted means are

calculated (see Chapter "**Central tendency**") as $\bar{y}_{..} = \dfrac{\sum_{i=1}^{k} n_i \bar{y}_{i.}}{\sum_{i=1}^{k} n_i} = \dfrac{\sum_{i=1}^{k} y_{i.}}{\sum_{i=1}^{k} n_i} = \dfrac{\sum_{i=1}^{k} y_{..}}{\sum_{i=1}^{k} n_i}$ and

$\bar{x} = \dfrac{\sum_{i=1}^{k} n_i x_i}{\sum_{i=1}^{k} n_i}$. Further, SCP or $\left(\sum_{i=1}^{k} n_i x_i \bar{y}_{i.} \right) = \sum_{i=1}^{k} x_i y_{i.} - \dfrac{\left(\sum_{i=1}^{k} n_i x_i \right)(y_{..})}{\sum_{i=1}^{k} n_i}$

and SS_x or $\sum_{i=1}^{k} n_i x_i^2 = \sum_{i=1}^{k} n_i x_i^2 - \dfrac{\left(\sum_{i=1}^{k} n_i x_i \right)^2}{\sum_{i=1}^{k} n_i}$ (analogous to simple linear regression

calculation; see Chapter "**Association between variables I**")

9.1 Example

The following table gives a hypothetical data on effect of different protein levels on weight gain (kg) in broilers by 6 weeks of age. Let us use the method of weighted regression to study the data. H_0: Growth rate is same with all protein levels

Sl No	Protein levels, %					
	16	18	20	22	24	
1	0.5	0.8	1.3	1.6	1.8	
2	0.6	0.8	1.2	1.5	1.9	
3	0.4	0.9	1.3	1.7	2.1	
4	0.5	0.7	1.1	1.5	1.7	
5		0.7	1.0		1.6	
6			1.1			
7			1.0			Totals
$y_i.$	2.0	3.9	8.0	6.3	9.1	29.3
n_i	4	5	7	4	5	25
$\bar{y}_i.$	0.50	0.78	1.14	1.575	1.82	
$\sum_{j=1}^{n_i} y_{ij}^2$	1.02	3.07	9.24	9.95	16.71	39.99

One-factor ANOVA performed as described above yielded the following:

Source	υ	SS	MSS	F
Total	24	5.6504		
Between protein levels	4	5.3298	1.3325	83.281
Error	20	0.3206	0.0160	

Table value of $F_{0.05, 4, 20} = 2.87$

The calculated value of F > table value and hence, there is a scope for weighted regression analysis. The same is as follows:

$$\sum_{i=1}^{k} x_i y_i. = 16 \times 2 + 18 \times 3.9 + 20 \times 8 + 22 \times 6.3 + 24 \times 9.1 = 619.2; \sum_{i=1}^{k} n_i x_i = 4 \times 16 + 5$$

$$\times 18 + 7 \times 20 + 4 \times 22 + 5 \times 24 = 502; y.. = 29.3, \sum_{i=1}^{k} n_i x_i^2 = 4 \times 16^2 + 5 \times 18^2 + 7 \times 20^2 + 4$$

$$\times 22^2 + 5 \times 24^2 = 10260 \text{ and } \sum_{i=1}^{k} n_i = 25; \text{ therefore, } SCP = 30.8560, SS_x = 179.84, b_{yx} =$$

0.1716, $SS_{regression} = b_{yx} \times SCP = 5.2949$ on $\upsilon = 1$. Introducing this value in the ANOVA table, we get the following result (H_0: There is no linear association between protein levels and weight gain):

Source	υ	SS	MSS	F
Total	24	5.6504		
Linear regression	1	5.2949	5.2949	16.516
Deviation from regression (Between protein levels)	3	0.0349	0.0116	< 1
Error	20	0.3206	0.0160	

Table value of $F_{0.05, 3, 20} = 3.10$ and $F_{0.05, 1, 20} = 4.35$

It is obvious that H_0 is not tenable.

10. NOMINAL SCALE DATA

Multiple sample analysis of nominal scale data is similar to $2 \times c$ or $r \times c$ contingency table may be set up and analyzed by χ^2 test as described in Chapter "**Tests of hypotheses**".

14

Two-Factor Analysis of Variance

In this Chapter, two factors will be considered operating and their effects on the population mean will be investigated. An experiment with two factors saves on time, effort and cost to conduct separate experiments with one factor at a time. Analysis of effect of > 1 factor on μ is also referred to as **factorial analysis of variance**. It is important to note that non-parametric tests with > 1 factors are not generally powerful and accurate to prescribe for routine use to derive conclusions.

With two or more factors under consideration, there appears a scope for testing whether a factor has a similar effect at all levels of another factor or not; this is referred to as **interaction effect** which was non-existent with one-factor ANOVA. In simple terms, interaction is the dependence of effect of one variable on the level of other variable.

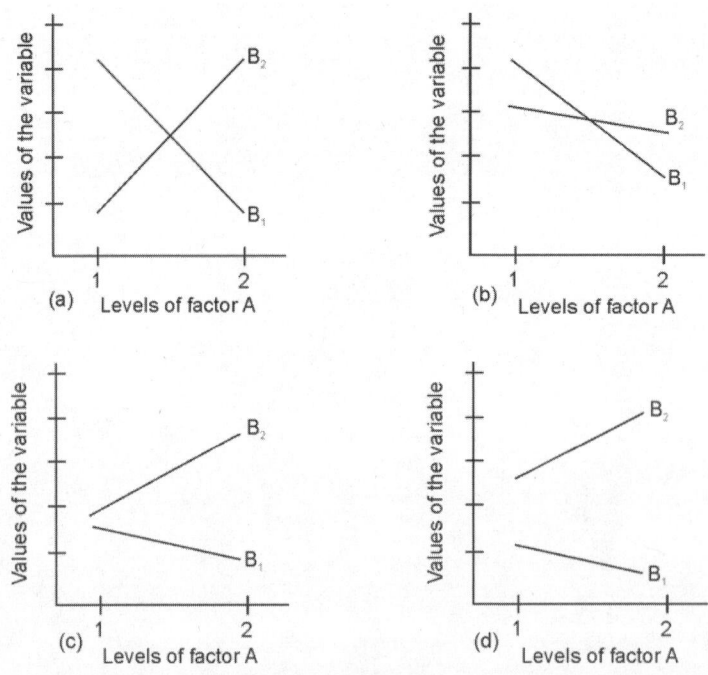

Fig. 14.1: Effects of factors and interaction (*Adapted from* Zar, 2003)

The meaning of the above diagram is summarized in the table below:

Figure	Effect of A	Effect of B	Interaction effect
(a)	Nil	Nil	Large
(b)	Large	Nil	Slight
(c)	Nil	Large	Large
(d)	Large	Large	Large

Another aspect that is worth considering is the concept of **replication**. This is basically from the Agricultural studies wherein fertility gradient of the soil is unavoidable. To remove (nullify, neutralize) the effect of fertility gradient, each of the treatments is **replicated (duplicated)** in each of the fertility levels so that the differences due to fertility is removed as sum of squares due to replicates; which, obviously, must be significant. Therefore, the following aspects are noteworthy:

1. A replicate is the one in which all treatments are repeated and
2. **(Mean) sum of squares between replicates is assumed to be significant**; else, it is waste of time, money and effort. If the replicate effect is not significant, the same result(s) can be obtained without replicating the treatments.
3. Replication itself can be one of the factors; it is generally called a **block** and the experimental design as **randomized block design (RBD)**.
4. In Animal Science experiments, blocking can be done on criteria like location, age groups, body weights, temperature, etc.
5. Factor A and B combine (cross) each other in the cells of the table; hence, this classification is also referred to as **crossed classification**.
6. The mathematical model, with interaction, can be written as follows: $x_{ijk} = \mu + \alpha_i + \beta_j + \eta_{ij} + e_{ijk}$ where η_{ij} is the interaction effect which can be estimated only when > 1 determinations per cell are available.

1. BLOCKING IN ANIMAL EXPERIMENTS

If animals from the same parents are allotted to different treatments or body weight of animals for experiment is arranged in an ascending/descending order and they are allotted, one at a time, at random, to each of the treatments in a sequence, the body weight of the animals forms a **block;** similarly, sex of the animals can act as block (equal number allotted to each of the treatments); sometimes both body weight and sex are used when it is called **double blocking;** say when equal number of chicks of either sex from the same breeding flock with comparable weights allotted to different treatments.

The term "**Block**" is actually an extension of the term "**Pair**" and hence, RBD ANOVA is an extension of paired t–test. When animals are reared in cages, all treatments are allotted at random to cages in each tier (if there are tiers) so that it will reasonably assure that all animals in each of the treatments have the same environment. Therefore, in an RBD, blocks represent the random effects and the other factor the fixed effects. Random numbers can be used to allot either treatment or animal. An example of an RBD is shown overleaf:

Block	Treatments (Diets)			
I	3	4	1	2
II	1	3	2	4
III	3	2	4	1
IV	4	2	1	3
V	1	4	3	2

While analyzing such data they are re-tabulated stratifying as per treatment and block to apply the ANOVA procedure.

2. DATA STRUCTURE

(m observations, x_{ijk}, per treatment combination)

		Factor A ($i = 1, 2, 3 \ldots a$)					Factor B Totals, $x_{.j.}$'s	Factor B Sum of squares, $x^2_{.j.}$'s	Factor B $n_{.j}$'s = $m*a$
		1	2	3	...	a			
Factor B ($j = 1, 2, 3 \ldots b$)	1	x_{111} x_{112} $x_{113\ldots}$ x_{11k} Total $= x_{11.}$	x_{211} x_{212} $x_{213\ldots}$ x_{21k} Total $= x_{21.}$	x_{311} x_{312} $x_{313\ldots}$ x_{31k} Total $= x_{31.}$	...	x_{a11} x_{a12} $x_{a13\ldots}$ x_{a1k} Total $= x_{a1.}$	$x_{.1.}$	$x^2_{.1.}$	$n_{.1}$
	2	x_{121} x_{122} $x_{123\ldots}$ x_{12k} Total $= x_{12.}$	x_{221} x_{222} $x_{223\ldots}$ x_{22k} Total $= x_{22.}$	x_{321} x_{322} $x_{323\ldots}$ x_{32k} Total $= x_{32.}$	...	x_{a21} x_{a22} $x_{a23\ldots}$ x_{a2k} Total $= x_{a2.}$	$x_{.2.}$	$x^2_{.2.}$	$n_{.2}$
	3	x_{131} x_{132} $x_{133\ldots}$ x_{13k} Total $= x_{13.}$	x_{231} x_{232} $x_{233\ldots}$ x_{23k} Total $= x_{23}$	x_{331} x_{332} $x_{333\ldots}$ x_{33k} Total $= x_{33}$	...	x_{a31} x_{a32} $x_{a33\ldots}$ x_{a3k} Total $= x_{a3}$	$x_{.3.}$	$x^2_{.3.}$	$n_{.3}$
		. . .	. . .	. . .	.	. . .			

(Contd.)

(Contd.)

	Factor A ($i = 1, 2, 3 \ldots a$)					Factor B Totals, $x_{\cdot j \cdot}$'s	Factor B Sum of squares, $x^2_{\cdot j \cdot}$'s	Factor B $n_{\cdot j}$'s = $m*a$
	1	2	3	...	a			
b	x_{1b1}	x_{2b1}	x_{3b1}		x_{ab1}			
	x_{1b2}	x_{2b2}	x_{3b2}		x_{ab2}			
	$x_{1b3\ldots}$	$x_{2b3\ldots}$	$x_{3b3\ldots}$		$x_{ab3\ldots}$	$x_{\cdot b \cdot}$	$x^2_{\cdot b \cdot}$	$n_{\cdot b}$
	x_{1bk}	x_{2bk}	x_{3bk}		x_{abk}			
	Total $= x_{1b \cdot}$	Total $= x_{2b \cdot}$	Total $= x_{3b \cdot}$		Total $= x_{ab \cdot}$			
Factor A Totals $x_{i \cdot \cdot}$'s	$x_{1 \cdot \cdot}$	$x_{2 \cdot \cdot}$	$x_{3 \cdot \cdot}$		$x_{a \cdot \cdot}$	Grand total = $x \ldots$		
Factor A Sum of squares, $x^2_{i \cdot \cdot}$'s	$x^2_{1 \cdot \cdot}$	$x^2_{2 \cdot \cdot}$	$x^2_{3 \cdot \cdot}$		$x^2_{a \cdot \cdot}$		TSS = $x^2 \ldots$	
Factor A $n_{i \cdot}$'s = $m*b$	$n_{1 \cdot}$	$n_{2 \cdot}$	$n_{3 \cdot}$		$n_{a \cdot}$			$n_{\cdot \cdot}$ = $m*a*b$

$$x_{\ldots} = \sum_{i=1}^{a}\sum_{j=1}^{b}\sum_{k=1}^{m} x_{ijk} \text{ and } x^2_{\ldots} = \sum_{i=1}^{a}\sum_{j=1}^{b}\sum_{k=1}^{m} x^2_{ijk} \text{ which is} \neq (x_{\ldots})^2$$

3. CALCULATIONS

Irrespective of the Model of experiment, the calculation is performed as follows; however, denominator for calculation of F values does differ between models which will be given after ANOVA table.

3.1 Sum of Squares

Total SS, $\text{TSS} = x^2_{\ldots} - \dfrac{(x_{\ldots})^2}{n_{\cdot\cdot}}$ on $\upsilon = (n_{\cdot\cdot} - 1)$

SS due to Factor A, $SS_A = \displaystyle\sum_{i=1}^{a} \dfrac{(x_{i\cdot\cdot})^2}{n_{i\cdot}} - \dfrac{(x_{\ldots})^2}{n_{\cdot\cdot}}$ on $\upsilon = (a - 1)$

SS due to Factor B, $SS_B = \displaystyle\sum_{j=1}^{b} \dfrac{(x_{\cdot j\cdot})^2}{n_{\cdot j}} - \dfrac{(x_{\ldots})^2}{n_{\cdot\cdot}}$ on $\upsilon = (b - 1)$

SS due to cells, $SS_C = \displaystyle\sum_{j=1}^{b} \dfrac{(x_{ij\cdot})^2}{n_{ij}} - \dfrac{(x_{\ldots})^2}{n_{\cdot\cdot}}$ on $\upsilon = (ab - 1)$

SS due to Interaction AB, $SS_{AB} = SS_C - SS_A - SS_B$ on $\upsilon = (ab - 1) - (a - 1) - (b - 1) = (a - 1)(b - 1)$

SS due to error, SS_E = Total SS $- SS_C$ on $\upsilon = (n.. - 1) - (ab - 1) = (n.. - ab)$

3.1.1 Unequal Observation for Treatment Combinations

1. When m is same for all treatment combinations, $n_{ij} = m$, $n_{i\cdot} = m \times b$ and $n_{\cdot j} = m \times a$ and $n.. = m \times a \times b$
2. Hence, to make the formulae relevant even when m's are unequal, the denominators are given in terms of n's.
3. When m is not same, υ for SSE will be υ for TSS $- \upsilon$ for SS_C
4. Unequal frequencies are more common than not in quantitative genetics; further, for computing variance components, weighted n's are required; these are separately dealt in Chapter "**Statistics in Specific Veterinary fields**".

3.2 ANOVA

H_0's: 1.There is no effect of Factor A 2. There is no effect of Factor B and 3. There is no effect of Interaction between Factors A and B in the population sampled.

Source	υ	SS	MSS	F@
Total	$(n.. - 1)$	TSS		
Cells	$(ab - 1)$	SS_C		
Factor A	$(a - 1)$	SS_A	MSS_A	$(MSS_A \div MSS_E)$
Factor B	$(b - 1)$	SS_B	MSS_B	$(MSS_B \div MSS_E)$
Interaction AB	$(a - 1)(b - 1)$	SS_{AB}	MSS_{AB}	$(MSS_{AB} \div MSS_E)$
Error	$(n.. - ab)$	SS_E	MSS_E	

MSS = Mean Sum of squares = $(SS \div \upsilon)$; @ Refers to Model I

Calculated values of F are compared with tabulated values at set α with corresponding υ of MSS of numerator and denominator to test each of the above Null hypotheses.

3.2.1 Calculation of F in Models I, II and III

MSS that has to be used as denominator for calculation of F statistic under different Models of experimental design is tabulated below: Obviously, numerator will be the respective MSS for the factor/interaction.

Effect	MSS to be used as denominator		
	Model I	Model II	Model III
Factor A		MSS_{AB}	
Factor B	MSS_E	MSS_{AB}	MSS_E
Interaction AB		MSS_E	

3.2.2 Pooling of MSS$_{AB}$ when not Statistically Significant

When MSS_{AB} is not statistically significant, SS_{AB} and SS_E can be pooled with pooling of corresponding υ's i.e. $(a - 1)(b - 1) + (n.. - ab) = n.. - (a + b - 1)$ from which a pooled

MSS_E can be obtained; this MSS_E is preferred to test the effects of Factors A and B. However, some reservations regarding such a practice have also been indicated since such a pooling is likely to reduce the confidence levels in stating probability of Type I error although it does reduce probability of Type II error. In this publication, pooling is not resorted to even when MSS_{AB} is not significant to ensure that the Type I error does not exceed the stated α.

3.2.3 Multiple Comparisons

Comparison of differences between means, if found significant, and construction of confidence intervals is similar to procedures given in Chapter "**One-factor analysis of variance**" by utilizing MSS_E and corresponding υ. Usually, LSD test is employed in Animal Science.

3.3 Example

3.3.1 More than One Observation per Treatment Combination

The following hypothetical data are about weight gain of broilers reared sexes separate to test the effect of a commercial supplementation (unequal $m's$):

Variable: Weight gain (kg) by 6 weeks		Factor A (Supplementation)	
		Yes	No
Factor B (Sex)	Male	2.0,1.8,2.1,2.3,1.9,2.2	1.8,1.2,1.5,2.1
	Female	1.8,1.7,1.8,1.6,1.7	1.6,1.7,1.6,1.5,1.8

The cell totals and sum of squares with n_{ij}'s is as follows:

Variable: Weight gain (kg) by 6 weeks, n_{ij}, x_{ij}, x^2_{ij}		Factor A (Supplementation)		$n_{.j}$	$x_{.j}$	$x^2_{.j}$
		Yes	No			
Factor B (Sex)	Male	6, 12.3, 25.39	4, 6.6, 11.34	10	18.9	36.73
	Female	5, 8.6, 14.82	5, 8.2, 13.50	10	16.8	28.32
$n_{i.}$		11	9		$n.. = 20$	
$x_{i..}$		20.9	14.8		$x... = 35.7$	
$x^2_{i..}$		40.21	24.84		$x^2... = 65.05$	

Total   SS $= 65.05 - (35.7^2 \div 20) = 1.3255$
$SS_A = (20.9^2 \div 11) + (14.8^2 \div 9) - (35.7^2 \div 20) = 0.3233$
$SS_B = (18.9^2 \div 10) + (16.8^2 \div 10) - (35.7^2 \div 20) = 0.2205$
$SS_C = (12.3^2 \div 6) + (6.6^2 \div 4) + (8.6^2 \div 5) + (8.2^2 \div 5) - (35.7^2 \div 20) = 0.6205$ and
$SS_{AB} = (0.6205 - 0.3233 - 0.2205) = 0.0767$

The ANOVA table will be as follows (Model I):
H_0's: 1. There is no effect of supplementation on weight gain 2. There is no difference between sexes in weight gain and 3. There is no effect of Interaction between supplementation and sexes in the population sampled.

Source	v	SS	MSS	F
Total	$(n.. - 1) = 19$	1.3255		
Cells	$(ab - 1) = 3$	0.6205		
Factor A	$(a - 1) = 1$	0.3233	0.3233	7.331
Factor B	$(b - 1) = 1$	0.2205	0.2205	5.000
Interaction AB	$(a - 1)(b - 1) = 1$	0.0767	0.0767	1.739
Error	$(n.. - ab) = 16$	0.7050	0.0441	

Table values of $F_{0.05, 1, 16} = 4.49$

H_0's 1 and 2 are not acceptable whereas No.3 is acceptable.

The means of various factors can be presented as a $(a + 2) \times (b + 2)$ contingency table:

	Supplemented	Not supplemented	Pooled
Males	2.05	1.65	1.89[a]
Females	1.72	1.64	1.68[b]
Pooled	1.90[p]	1.64[q]	

Value bearing different superscripts within the last column (a, b) or last row (p, q) are significantly different ($P \leq 0.05$)

Note: Since only two means are available for sex and supplementation, LSD test is not required to compare them and superscripts have been put directly.

3.3.2 One Observation per Treatment Combination

In this case, the cell totals are not available and hence, SS_C, consequent on which SS_{AB} can not be calculated. Rest of the calculations is analogous to that discussed in the **Example 2.3.1** above.

The following data of number of bacterial colonies in 3 petri dishes (PD 1, 2 and 3) over 3 periods of time (T 1, 2 and 3) is considered as an example. We would like to test H_0: 1.There is no difference in number of bacterial colonies between Petri dishes and 2. There is no difference in number of bacterial colonies between different periods. ($a = 3$ and $b = 3$)

	PD 1	PD 2	PD 3	$x_i.$	n_i	$\bar{x}_i.$	$x^2_i.$
T 1	50	39	46	135	3	45	6137
T 2	135	102	150	387	3	129	51129
T 3	286	150	227	663	3	221	155825
$x._j$	471	291	423	$x.. = 1185$			
n_j	3	3	3	$n. = 9$			
$\bar{x}._j$	157	97	141			$\bar{x}.. = 131.67$	
$x^2._j$	102521	34425	76145				$x^2.. = 213091$

$$\text{Total SS} = x_{..}^2 - \frac{(x_{..})^2}{n_{.}} = 57066, \quad SS_T = \sum_{i=1}^{a} \frac{(x_{i\cdot})^2}{n_i} \text{ or } \frac{\sum_{i=1}^{a}(x_{i\cdot})^2}{n_i} = 46496 \text{ as } n_i \text{ is same on}$$

$$\upsilon = (a - 1) = 2; \text{ similarly, as } n_j \text{ is same, } SS_{PD} = \sum_{j=1}^{b} \frac{(x_{\cdot j})^2}{n_j} \text{ or } \frac{\sum_{j=1}^{b}(x_{\cdot j})^2}{n_j} = 5792 \text{ on } \upsilon = (b - 1)$$

$= 2$; finally, SS_E (residuals) $= \text{Total SS} - SS_T - SSP_{PD} = 4778$ on $\upsilon = (a - 1)(b - 1) = 2$

Source	υ	SS	MSS	F
Total	8			
Periods	2	46496	23248.0	19.463
Petri dishes	2	5792	2896.0	2.424
Error or residuals	4	4778	1194.5	

Table value of $F_{0.05, 2, 4} = 6.94$ and $F_{0.05, 1, 3} = 10.13$

Therefore, H_0 No. 1 is not acceptable whereas No. 2 is acceptable.

Note: For SS_E, $\upsilon = (a - 1)(b - 1)$ which is same as that of SS_{AB} when > 1 observations are available for treatment combinations.

4. TUKEY'S TEST OF NON-ADDITIVITY

It was mentioned in the Chapter "**One-factor analysis of variance**" that test for additivity (non-additivity) of effects is available. Since the test simulates two-factor ANOVA, the same is presented below:

A general procedure is described below considering i rows and j columns with observations designated x_{ij} with other usual notations as described above: H_0: Row and column effects are additive

	Col 1	Col 2	Col 3	$x_{i\cdot}$	$\bar{x}_{i\cdot}$	$d_i = \bar{x}_{i\cdot} - \bar{x}_{..}$	$w_i = \Sigma x_{ij} d_j$	$w_i d_i$
Row 1	x_{11}	x_{12}	x_{13}	x_{1j}	$\bar{x}_{1\cdot}$			
Row 2	x_{21}	x_{22}	x_{23}	x_{2j}	$\bar{x}_{2\cdot}$			
Row 3	x_{31}	x_{32}	x_{33}	x_{3j}	$\bar{x}_{3\cdot}$			
$x_{\cdot j}$	$x_{\cdot 1}$	$x_{\cdot 2}$	$x_{\cdot 3}$	$x_{..}$				
$\bar{x}_{j\cdot}$	$\bar{x}_{1\cdot}$	$\bar{x}_{2\cdot}$	$\bar{x}_{3\cdot}$	$\bar{x}_{4\cdot}$				

$d_j = \bar{x}_{j\cdot} - \bar{x}_{..}$

Check: $\Sigma d_i = 0$ and $\Sigma d_j = 0$; $N = \Sigma\Sigma x_{ij} d_i d_j$ or $\Sigma w_i d_i$; $D = (\Sigma d_i^2) \times (\Sigma d_j^2)$

Then, $B = N \div D$ and SS for non-additivity $= B \times N$ or $N^2 \div D$ on $\upsilon = 1$. The value of B is useful in identification of transformation required if H_0 is not acceptable. Let us check with an example.

4.1 Example

Example 2.3.2 already discussed above is considered again to test H_0: Row and column effects are additive.

	PD 1	PD 2	PD 3	$x_{i \cdot}$	$\bar{x}_{i \cdot}$	$d_i = \bar{x}_{i \cdot} - \bar{x}_{\cdot \cdot}$	$w_i = \Sigma x_{ij} d_j$	$w_i d_i$
T 1	50	39	46	135	45	−86.67	343.55	−29775.4785
T 2	135	102	150	387	129	−2.67	1282.71	−3424.8357
T 3	286	150	227	663	221	89.33	4161.79	371772.7007
$x_{\cdot j}$	471	291	423	1185				
$\bar{x}_{j \cdot}$	157	97	141		131.67			
$d_j = \bar{x}_{j \cdot} - \bar{x}_{\cdot \cdot}$	25.33	−34.67	9.33			0		

$N = \Sigma\Sigma x_{ij} d_i d_j$ or $\Sigma w_i d_i$; $D = (\Sigma d_i^2) \times (\Sigma d_j^2) = 15498.6667 \times 1930.6667 = 29922759.69$

$N = 338572.3865$; SS due to non-additivity $= 3830.9054$; $B = 0.011315$

ANOVA for the above data is already computed into which the above values are introduced as follows:

Source	υ	SS	MSS	F
Periods	2	46496.0000	23248.0000	19.463
Petri dishes	2	5792.0000	2896.0000	2.424
Residuals	4	4778.0000	1194.5000	
Non-additivity	1	3830.9054	3830.9054	12.135
Remainder	3	947.0946	315.6982	

Table value of $F_{0.05, 2, 4} = 6.94$ and $F_{0.05, 1, 3} = 10.13$

Therefore, H_0 is not acceptable. To know the type of transformation that may be required, calculate $p = (1 - B^* \bar{x}_{\cdot \cdot})$ and investigate power p of x_{ij} in original scale such that effects are additive in the scale $y = x^p$. If $p = \frac{1}{2}$, square-root transformation, if $p = -1$, reciprocal or inverse transformation, if $p \rightarrow 0$, log (natural logarithm) transformation and so on. In the present example, since $p = -0.4898$ i.e. $\rightarrow (-\frac{1}{2})$ and hence,

transformation of x_{ij}'s as $x_{ij}^{-\frac{1}{2}}$ or $\dfrac{1}{\sqrt{x_{ij}}}$ appears to be appropriate. The transformation

may be put to effect and checked as follows:

	PD 1	PD 2	PD 3	$x_{i\cdot}$	$\bar{x}_{i\cdot}$	$d_i = \bar{x}_{i\cdot} - \bar{x}_{\cdot\cdot}$	$w_i = \Sigma x_{ij} d_j$	$w_i d_i$
T 1	0.1414	0.1601	0.1474	0.4489	0.1496	0.0471	0.000198	0.000009
T 2	0.0861	0.0990	0.0817	0.2668	0.0889	−0.0136	0.000169	−0.000002
T 3	0.0591	0.0817	0.0664	0.2072	0.0691	−0.0334	0.000228	−0.000008
$x_{\cdot j}$	0.2866	0.3408	0.2955	0.9229				
$\bar{x}_{\cdot j}$	0.0955	0.1136	0.0985		0.1025			
$d_j = \bar{x}_{\cdot j} - \bar{x}_{\cdot\cdot}$	−0.0070	0.0111	−0.0040			0		

$N = \Sigma\Sigma x_{ij} d_i d_j$ or $\Sigma w_i d_i$; $D = (\Sigma d_i^2) \times (\Sigma d_j^2) = 0.000188 \times 0.003519 = 0.000001$

$N = -0.000001$; SS due to non-additivity $= 0.000002$; $B = -1$ and $p = 1.10$ (i.e. $\to 1$) indicating that the transformation was effective. This can be further verified by ANOVA on the transformed scale:

Source	υ	SS	MSS	F
Periods	2	0.010570	0.005285	440.417
Petri dishes	2	0.000563	0.000282	23.500
Residuals	4	0.000047	0.000012	
Non–additivity	1	0.000002	0.000002	< 1
Remainder	3	0.000045	0.000015	

Table value of $F_{0.05, 2, 4} = 6.94$ and $F_{0.05, 1, 3} = 10.13$

The ANOVA is in confirmation that the transformation was effective not only in making the effects additive but also larger F values demonstrated the effects of both periods and Petri dishes; the latter failed to be significant on original scale. Further, mere inspection of the data also indicates that the variances are also made homogenous (the range of values in each classification by row and column is reduced) by the transformation.

5. MISSED-PLOT TECHNIQUE

5.1 One Missing Observation

The terminology is again from the field of Agriculture which actually refers to missing observation(s) in RBD. Missing observation(s) is expectable in animal experiments like for instance, eggs of the experiment being broken, blood sample destroyed, etc. Under such conditions, missed observation of the ith group and jth block can be estimated as $\hat{x}_{ij} = \dfrac{ax_{i\cdot} + bx_{\cdot j} - x_{\cdot\cdot}}{(a-1)(b-1)}$ where the totals refer to those with the available data.

Obviously, the estimated value is used for further analysis; but, bias is unavoidable due to estimated value. The bias in the SS_T (groups SS) can be corrected by subtracting

the correction factor $\dfrac{\left[x_{\cdot j} - (a-1)\hat{x}_{ij}\right]^2}{a(a-1)}$; further, since the estimate is calculated, υ for Total SS is reduced by 1.

5.1.1 *Example*

The following data pertains to 36 rats (6 litter mates from 6 litters). Rats each from each of the litters are subjected to 6 treatments (a rat per treatment) to increase bone ash content. Bone ash % after treatment is given below; however, datum pertaining to rat from 5th litter allotted to treatment 2 was lost. It is now required to predict the missed value and conduct ANOVA.

Litter No.	Treatment No.						$x_{\cdot j}$	$x^2_{\cdot j}$
	1	2	3	4	5	6		
I	21	38	36	25	35	43	198	6880
II	25	30	41	32	36	46	210	7642
III	24	33	42	34	36	47	216	8090
IV	23	33	43	31	38	46	214	7988
V	25	x_{25}	42	24	36	49	209*	7751*
VI	23	32	41	34	38	44	212	7770
$x_{i\cdot}$	141	199*	245	180	219	275	$x_{\cdot\cdot} = 1259*$	$x^2_{\cdot\cdot} = 46121*$

Estimated integer value for x_{25} = 33; * includes estimated x_{25} value of 33

$$\hat{x}_{25} = \frac{6\times166 + 6\times176 - 1226}{5\times5} = 33.04 \approx 33;$$ hence, x_{25} is considered as 33 and ANOVA performed as described under **Section 3.3.2** to obtain the following SS: $SS_{Litter} = 33.4722$,

$SS_T = 1885.4722$, Correction factor for $SS_T = \dfrac{[176-5\times33]^2}{6\times5} = 4.0333$; Corrected $SS_T = 1881.4389$, $SS_E = 176.0611$ on $\upsilon = 24$ (instead of 25). The ANOVA table is given below: H_0: There is no effect of treatment on bone ash content

Source	υ	SS	MSS	F
Litter	5	33.4722	6.6944	< 1
Treatments	5	1881.4389	376.2878	51.294
Error	24@	176.0611	7.3359	

@1 degrees of freedom lost due to estimation; Table value of $F_{0.05\ 5,\ 24} = 3.90$

Calculated value is > table value and hence, H_0 is not acceptable.

Note: Standard error of difference between T2 and others is given by $\sqrt{MSS_E\left[\dfrac{2}{b} + \dfrac{a}{b(a-1)(b-1)}\right]}$

which is used in place of $\sqrt{\dfrac{2MSS_E}{b}}$; the latter is used as se of difference between any two means other than the one which had the missed observation.

5.2 > 1 Missing Observation

Number of missing observations should be $< 10\%$ of $n_{..}$ and $< (a-1)$; then, one of the the following procedures can be used:

5.2.1 One-by-One Replacement

1. All but one missing observations can be replaced either with $\bar{x}_{i.}$ or $\bar{x}_{..}$.
2. The last missed observation is estimated as described under **Section 5.1**
3. This is followed by discounting one of the values replaced (other than that is estimated in Step 2 above) and calculation by the procedure at **Section 5.1**
4. The procedure is repeated till all the missing values were estimated by the formula given in **Section 5.1**
5. For each block having one missed observation, the bias is corrected as given in **Section 5.1**
6. For each block with > 1 missed observation, bias is calculated as $\sum\limits^{m'} x_{ij}^2$

$$+\frac{x_{.j}^2}{a-m'}-\frac{\left(x_{.j}+\sum\limits^{m'}\hat{x}_{ij}\right)^2}{a}$$ where m' is the number of missed observations in block j

and bias is pooled over all missing data in a particular block. The sum of all bias calculated is subtracted from the SST (groups SS) and υ for Total SS is reduced by m'.

5.2.2 Simultaneous Equations

5.2.2.1 Values of different treatments and blocks

Suppose two values, x and y belonging to different treatments as well as different blocks are missing (say treatment 1 block 1 and treatment 2 block 2); then, they are estimated separately as one missing value assuming that the other is available; i.e. x

$$=\frac{ax_{1.}+bx_{.1}-(x_{..}+y)}{(a-1)(b-1)}\text{ and }y=\frac{ax_{2.}+bx_{.2}-(x_{..}+x)}{(a-1)(b-1)}.$$ Two equations are obtained and

they can be easily solved as simultaneous equations (by direct method or Doolittle method or Matrix method).

5.2.2.2 Values belonging to same block

Suppose two values, x and y belonging to same block are missing (say treatment 1 block 1 and treatment 2 block 1); then, they are estimated separately as one missing value assuming that the other is available; i.e. $x =\dfrac{ax_{1.}+b(x_{.1}+y)-(x_{..}+y)}{(a-1)(b-1)}$ and $y =$

$$\frac{a(x_{1.}+x)+bx_{.2}-(x_{..}+x)}{(a-1)(b-1)}.$$ Two equations are obtained and they can be easily solved

as simultaneous equations (by direct method or Doolittle method or Matrix method).

5.2.2.3 Values belonging to same treatment

Suppose two values, x and y belonging to same treatment are missing (say treatment 1 block 1 and treatment 1 block 2); then, they are estimated separately as one missing value assuming that the other is available; i.e. $x = \dfrac{ax_{1.} + bx_{.1} + y(a-1) - x_{..}}{(a-1)(b-1)}$ and

$y = \dfrac{ax_{1.} + bx_{.2} + x(a-1) - x_{..}}{(a-1)(b-1)}$. Two equations are obtained and they can be easily solved as simultaneous equations (by direct method or Doolittle method or Matrix method).

Note: Even when > 2 observations are missing, simultaneous equations can be developed as above and solved either by Matrix method or by the method of Least–squares. Further, variance between two means is more complicated when > 1 observations are missing; it is briefly outlined below:

Standard error of difference between two treatment means is where effective number of counts for the two treatments in question, say $A(T_1)$ and $B(T_2)$. In each of the rows, each of the treatments is allotted counts as follows:

Features in the block (row)	Count	
	r_1	r_2
Both treatments A and B occur	1	1
A occurs, B missing	½	0
A missing	0	0

Let us assume that in **Example 5.2.2** two observations, x_{11} and x_{66} are missing. Then, for comparing treatments T_1 and T_2, The counts for 6 blocks will be; 0,0; 1,1; 1,1; 1,1; 1,1 and 1,1, respectively; $r_1 = r_2 = 5$; similarly between T_1 and T_6, the counts will be; 0,0; 1,1; 1,1; 1,1; 1,1;1,½, respectively; and $r_1 = 5$ and $r_2 = 4½$.

Standard error of difference multiplied by the table value of t on υ for MSS_E at set α gives LSD value for the comparison.

6. NON-PARAMETRIC TWO-FACTOR ANOVA (FRIEDMAN'S ANOVA BY RANKS)

When the data does not meet the requirements of ANOVA with respect to Normality and equality of variances (homoscedasticity), then this test is an alternative. Suppose, the data given in **Example 6.1** is subjected to this test, the following will be the result:

H_0: Egg cholesterol levels are same for all drugs

Hens	Drug 1	Drug 2	Drug 3	Drug 4	$R_{.j}$	$R^2_{.j}$
1	220 (8)	235 (3)	180 (19)	200 (16)	46	690
2	225 (6)	230 (4)	175 (20)	205 (14)	44	648
3	223 (7)	234 (2)	190 (18)	215 (10)	37	477
4	210 (12)	238 (1)	200 (16)	200 (16)	45	657
5	218 (9)	228 (5)	210 (12)	210 (12)	38	394
$R_{i.}$	42	15	85	68	$R_{..} = 210$	$R^2_{..} = 2866$

Value in the parentheses indicates rank; $a = 4$, $b = 5$; R's refer to Rank sums

$$\chi_c^2 = \frac{12}{ab(a+1)} \sum_{i=1}^{a} R_{i.}^2 - 3b(a+1) = 1376.3 \text{ with 2 ties with 3 ranks tied in each. Therefore,}$$

$\Sigma t = 2 \times (3^3 - 3) = 48$ and correction factor, $C = 1 - \dfrac{\Sigma t}{b(a^3 - a)} = 0.84$. The corrected $\chi_c^2 =$

$\chi_c^2 \div C = 1638.452$ which is > 7.8, the table value of χ_c^2 for $a = 4, b = 5$ (see Appendix 8); hence, H_0 is not acceptable.

If a two-factor ANOVA is computed on ranks, the result will be:

H_0: Egg cholesterol levels are same for all drugs

Source	υ	SS	MSS	F
Total	19	661.0		
Hens	4	17.5	4.3750	< 1
Drugs	3	562.6	187.5333	27.817
Residual	12	80.9	6.7417	

Table value of $F_{0.05, 3, 12} = 3.49$

Calculated value of F is > table value and hence, H_0 is not acceptable.

Note:

1. Calculation of is similar to Kruskal-Wallis statistic, H (see **Section 6** Chapter "**One-factor analysis of variance**")

2. If $a = 2$, Wilcoxon paired – sample test and if $b = 2$, Spearman's Rank correlation have to be employed (see **Section 3.2.1.2**, Chapter "**Tests of hypotheses**")

3. If $a > 6$ and $b > 10$, $\chi_c^2 \approx \chi^2$ distribution

6.1   Friedman's Test with Multiple Observations per Cell

When m observations per cell (m being same for all cells) are available, the

statistic $\chi_c^2 = \dfrac{12}{abm^2(ma+1)} \sum_{i=1}^{a} R_{i.}^2 - 3b(ma+1)$ can be calculated as those of one obser-

vation per cell. With unequal values of m, the procedure is complicated and beyond the scope of this publication.

6.2   Multiple Comparisons

On the same lined of LSD test, for Friedman's non-parametric test, standard error of

difference between **rank sums** $(R_A - R_B) = \sqrt{\dfrac{ab(a+1)}{12}}$ and when various groups are

compared with a "Control" group, the standard error is calculated as $\sqrt{\dfrac{ab(a+1)}{6}}$; if

mean of the ranks is used, the denominator in the above formulae for standard error will be $12b$ and $6b$, respectively.

In the above example, se = 5.92 and critical value of Student's $t_{0.05, 19}$ = 2.179 and LSD = 12.9. With the LSD value, multiple comparisons among the Rank sums give the following: (as per the procedure described in **Section 3.1.5**, Chapter **"One-factor analysis of variance"**)

	Drug 1	Drug 2	Drug 3	Drug 4
Rank sum	42^b	15^a	85^d	68^c

Means bearing different superscripts are significantly different (P ≤ 0.05)

Note: Since lower rank indicates higher value for the variable, superscripts are allotted by arranging rank sums in an ascending order.

7. DICHOTOMOUS NOMINAL–SCALE DATA (COCHRAN'S Q TEST)

Data under this category are rare in animal science; in any case, a hypothetical data on occurrence of Avian Influenza stratified by type of rearing and different farms is considered for explaining the method. Since the occurrence or non-occurrence of the disease is an attribute, only 0 (non-occurrence) and 1 (occurrence) are recorded.

Note: If any block (Farm) has only 1 or 0 for all treatments (rearing systems), it is deleted from analysis.

Farms	Rearing system				
	Intensive-floor	Intensive-cages	Semi-intensive	Extensive	$x_{.j}$
1	1	0	1	1	3
2	0	0	1	1	2
3	0	0	1	1	2
4	1	0	0	1	2
5	0	0	1	1	2
6	0	0	1	1	2
$x_{i.}$	2	0	5	6	$x_{..} = 13$
Means	0.333	0.000	0.833	1.000	

$a = 4, b = 6$

H_0: Occurrence of Avian Influenza is not related to rearing system

Test statistic $Q = \dfrac{(a-1)\left[\sum\limits_{i=1}^{a} x_{i.}^2 - \dfrac{(x_{..})^2}{a}\right]}{x_{..} - \dfrac{\sum\limits_{j=1}^{b} x_{.j}^2}{a}} = (68.25 \div 5.75) = 11.87$ on $\upsilon = (a-1)$. Cochran's

Q is distributed $\approx \chi^2$ especially when a is at least 4 and $a*b$ is at least 24. The calculated value in the present example is > 7.81, the table value of $\chi^2_{0.05, 3}$; hence, H_0 is not acceptable indicating that occurrence of Avian Influenza is indeed influenced by rearing systems.

Note: When $a = 2$, Cochran's test is same as McNemar's test (*see* **Section 3.2.1.3** Chapter **"Tests of hypotheses"**)

7.1   Multiple Comparisons

For pair-wise comparisons, the test statistic is S which is the ratio of difference between means to the standard error (se) of the difference; the latter is given by the

formula $se = \sqrt{2 \left(\dfrac{ax.. - \sum\limits_{j=1}^{b} x_{.j}^2}{ab^2 (a-1)} \right)}$ and the critical value of S at set $\alpha = \sqrt{\chi_{\alpha,\, (a-1)}^2}$. In the

present example, se = 0.326 and critical value of S at α = 0.05 is 2.795; hence, minimum difference between the means to be significant is $S*se$ = 0.911. Now the means can be allotted superscripts by the procedure described in **Section 3.1.5** Chapter "**One-factor analysis of variance**" as follows:

	Intensive-floor	Intensive-cages	Semi-intensive	Extensive
Means	0.333[ab]	0.000[b]	0.833[ab]	1.000[a]

Means bearing at least one common superscript are not significantly different (P $\leq$ 0.05)

It is clear that the birds reared outdoor (Extensive system or range system) have the maximum risk of the disease whereas those in cages have the least risk.

8.   POOLING SEVERAL ANOVA RESULTS

It is necessary that, in any field of specialization, an experiment is repeated several times in space and time before arriving at a final recommendation. That means, several ANOVA are available pertaining to, say different locations, years or methods, etc. based on varying number of replications on a particular trait or treatment. It may be necessary to **consolidate** all these results to arrive at a more general and acceptable conclusion which can be **recommended**. Therefore, the consolidated analysis aims at checking whether there is any interaction between results and different sets of conditions from where the results have originated. The procedure for consolidated analysis of data from several two-factor ANOVAs is briefly given below; the method can be extended to higher order ANOVA results as well with suitable modifications in calculation of pooled error variance depending on the significance of Bartlett's test of homogeneity of variances and interaction effects in consolidated ANOVA.

8.1   The Data

From each of the sources, data on treatment totals, number of replications, and MSS_E along with its υ are obtained.

8.2   Bartlett's Test of Homogeneity of Variances

Since the above data has a wide base, this test is mandatory prerequisite; the procedure is described in **Section 5.1** Chapter "**One-factor Analysis of Variance**". If the MSS_E's

are found heterogeneous, **weighted MSS$_E$** is calculated as $MSS_E^W = \dfrac{\sum\limits_{i=1}^{k} r_i MSS_{E(i)}}{\sum\limits_{i=1}^{k} r_i}$ where

r_i is the number of replicates for $MSS_{E(i)}$. On the contrary, if the MSS_E's are found homogeneous, a pooled MSS_E is calculated as $MSS_E^P = \dfrac{\sum\limits_{i=1}^{k} v_i MSS_{E(i)}}{\sum\limits_{i=1}^{k} v_i}$ where v_i is the v

for $MSS_{E(i)}$.

8.3 Analysis of the Data

The various sources of ANOVA are considered as columns and treatment totals as rows to develop a consolidated ANOVA as per the procedure given for RBD with > 1 observations in **Sections 3 and 4** above. It is worth noting that the treatment totals directly give the respective row x column total (with number of replication being the number of observations for the total for calculation of interaction). MSS_E^P calculated in

the Bartlett's test (on $v = \sum\limits_{i=1}^{k} v_i$) is used as the MSS_E for this ANOVA if the variances

are homogeneous; otherwise, MSS_E^W will be used as MSS_E.

Further analysis depends on significance of interaction effects:

1. If the interaction effects are not significant, the MSS_T is divided by MSS_E^P for F test. If MSS_T is significant, treatment means are tabulated with **standard error of**

    mean as $\sqrt{\dfrac{MSS_E^P}{k}}$

2. If the interactions are significant, the totals obtained are converted to respective means by dividing them with corresponding number of replications so that replications can be ignored. Now analysis again proceeds like that for RBD with one observation per cell with the following exception: MSS_E calculated for table of means will be the SS for interactions and pooled MSS_E for calculation of F

    values is computed as $\dfrac{1}{k}\left(\sum\limits_{i=1}^{k} \dfrac{MSS_{E(i)}}{r_i} \right)$; the MSS_T is divided by $MSS_{Interaction}$ for F

    test. If MSS_T is significant, treatment means are tabulated with **standard error of**

    mean as $\sqrt{\dfrac{MSS_{Interaction}}{k}}$ and LSD calculated on $MSS_{Interaction}$.

8.4 Example

In feeding trials on pigs at five different research centers, five protein levels were under investigation on their effect on weekly weight gain (kg). The extract of the results comprising of totals for each treatment along with number of replications, MSS_E and its v from each of the centers is tabulated below for developing a consolidated ANOVA:

Treatment (i= 1 to k); k = 5	Research center (j = 1 to 5)					Treatment totals, $x_{i.}$
	1	2	3	4	5	
1	24	27	29	20	22	122
2	35	38	32	42	45	192
3	48	50	40	40	42	220
4	40	38	43	39	40	200
5	50	60	52	55	60	277
Location totals, $x_{.j}$	197	213	196	196	209	
r_i or n_{ij}	6	6	4	8	10	$\sum_{i=1}^{k} r_i = 34$
Total observations[#], $n_{.j}$	30	30	20	40	50	$n.. = 170$
$MSS_{E(i)}$	4.50	10.50	21.50	4.00	1.00	$\sum_{i=1}^{k} MSS_{E(i)} = 41.50$
v for $MSS_{E(i)}$	20	20	12	32	36	$\sum_{i=1}^{k} v_i = 120$

[#] $k * r_i$ or $k * n_{ij}$

Before proceeding for consolidated ANOVA, it is necessary to run a test for homogeneity of variances on H_0: Variances of all the locations are homogenous.

s_i^2	v_i	$s_i^2 * v_i$	$Log_{10} s_i^2$	$Log_{10} s_i^{2*}v$
4.50	20	90	0.6532	13.0640
10.50	20	210	1.0212	20.4240
21.50	12	258	1.3324	15.9888
4.00	32	128	0.6021	19.2672
1.00	36	36	0.00	0.0000
Totals	120	$\sum_{i=1}^{k} SS_i = 722$	3.6089	68.7440

$s_P^2 = (722 \div 120) = 6.0167$, $\log_{10} s_P^2 = 0.7794$, $\sum_{i=1}^{k} \frac{1}{v_i} = 0.2424$, C = 1.0195

Therefore, B = 2.3026 × {(0.7794 × 120) − 68.7440} = 57.0676; and B_C = 55.9759 which is > 9.49, the table value of $\chi^2_{0.05, 4}$. Hence, H_0 is rejected.

$$MSS_E^P = s_P^2 = 6.0167; \quad MSS_E^W = \frac{\sum_{i=1}^{k} r_i MSS_{E(i)}}{\sum_{i=1}^{k} r_i} = (218 \div 34) = 6.4118$$

Now, consolidated ANOVA can proceed similar to that of RBD with > 1 observations per cell (number of replications representing the number of observations per cell). The various SS will be: {C = $(x..)^2 \div n..$} = 6012.4765

SS due to treatments, $SS_T = \dfrac{\sum\limits_{i=1}^{k}\left(x_{i.}\right)^2}{\sum\limits_{i=1}^{k} r_i} - C = 366.2588$; SS due to locations, SS_L

$= \sum\limits_{i=1}^{k}\dfrac{\left(x_{.j}\right)^2}{n_{i.}} - C = 548.2768$; SS due to interactions, $SS_{TxL} = \sum\limits_{i=1}^{k}\dfrac{\left(x_{ij}\right)^2}{r_i} - C - SS_T - SS_L =$

50.5379. The consolidated ANOVA table is as follows:

H_0's:

1. There is no effect of treatments on weekly weight gain of piglets
2. There is no effect of interactions on weekly weight gain of piglets

Source	υ	SS	MSS	F
Locations	4	548.2768		
Treatments	4	366.2588	91.5647	14.281
Treatment × Location interaction	16	50.5379	3.1586	< 1
MSS_E^W	120		6.4118	

@ Variances heterogeneous; Table value of $F_{0.05,\,4,\,120} = 3.92$; Standard Error of Mean $(se) = \sqrt{MSS_E^W}$ = 2.532 kg

Based on the calculated F values, H_0 No. 2 can be accepted whereas H_0 No. 1 is not acceptable.

Since interaction effects are not significant; pooled treatment means can be compared by the LSD test (*see* Chapter "**One-factor analysis of variance**") as follows:

Treatments	1	2	3	4	5	se, kg	LSD, kg
Means, kg	3.588[c]	5.647[b]	6.471[b]	5.882[b]	8.147[a]	2.532	1.216

Values bearing common letter superscripts are not significantly different (P < 0.05)

To enumerate the further analysis it is assumed that the interaction effects were significant. In such a case, the following procedure has to be adopted:

8.4.1 ANOVA of (Weighted) Means

Each of the treatment totals obtained in the original data is divided by respective number of replications to obtain a table of mean values; obviously, this table gives the mean values stratified by treatment and locations and all values have number of replications as unity. In other words, effect of unequal replications is ignored.

Analysis of the table so formed will proceed similar to RBD with one observation per cell and the MSS_E calculated will be considered as $MSS_{Interaction}$; MSS_E for calculation

of F values will be $\dfrac{1}{k}\left(\sum\limits_{i=1}^{k}\dfrac{MSS_{E(i)}}{r_i}\right) = 1.695$. The table of means and ANOVA are shown

below.

Treatment	Research center					Treatment totals, x_i.
	1	2	3	4	5	
1	4.000	4.500	7.250	2.500	2.200	20.450
2	5.833	6.333	8.000	5.250	4.500	29.910
3	8.000	8.333	10.000	5.000	4.200	35.533
4	6.667	6.333	10.750	4.875	4.000	32.625
5	8.667	10.000	13.000	6.875	6.000	44.542
Location totals, $x_{.j}$	33.167	35.499	49.000	24.500	20.900	$x_{..} = 163.06$
$MSS_{E(i)}$	4.50	10.50	21.50	4.00	1.00	
r_i	6	6	4	8	10	

$x^2_{..} = 1229.1911; C = \{(x_{..})^2 \div_{ij}\} = 1063.5425$

Total SS = 165.6486; SS_L = 96.1153; SS_T = 61.2145; SS_{LxT} = 8.3188. Now, ANOVA table can be set-up as follows:

H_0's:
1. There is no effect of treatments on weekly weight gain of piglets
2. There is no effect of interactions on weekly weight gain of piglets

Source	v	SS	MSS	F
Locations	4	96.1153		
Treatments	4	61.2145	15.3036	9.029
Treatment × Location interaction	16	8.3188	0.5199	< 1
Error	120		1.695	

Table value of $F_{0.05, 4, 120}$ = 3.92; Standard Error of Mean $(se) = \sqrt{MSS_E}$ = 1.302 kg; LSD = 0.625 kg

Based on the calculated F values, H_0 No. 2 can be accepted whereas H_0 No. 1 is not acceptable. Further, Pooled treatment means can be compared as described above:

Treatments	1	2	3	4	5	se, kg	LSD, kg
Means, kg	4.090[c]	5.982[b]	7.107[b]	6.525[b]	8.908[a]	1.302	0.625

Values bearing common letter superscripts are not significantly different (P < 0.05)

Note: Results obtained are the same because the interaction effects were not significant in the first place itself.

8.5   Limitations of Consolidated ANOVA

1. Unless the variances are homogeneous, replications are same and interaction effects are not significant, the procedure is not very precise.
2. If the interaction is not significant, $SS_{Interaction}$ may be pooled with that of pooled Error to obtain a better estimate of MSS_E (see **Section 3.2.2** above on this aspect). If the MSS_E's are heterogeneous, in spite of all weightages, the result can not be considered highly reliable.

15

ANOVA for More than Two Factors

It is not uncommon that an experiment is designed with > 2 factors affecting a variable. In general, the analytical procedures are extensions of those discussed in one- and two-factor ANOVA with modifications in H_0, number of interactions, and testing under Models I, II and III. Understandably, with at least one more factor appearing in the classification, the notations used also change; albeit on the same logic. Since > 3 factors being considered is a rare case, only three-factor ANOVA is discussed and the reader is referred to other publications for information concerning multi–factor ANOVA.

Presently, it is not common that ANOVA itself is performed manually with an electronic calculator; and much less a multi-factor (multivariate) ANOVA. In any case, procedure is outlined below for a three-factor ANOVA which can be extended with careful modifications for a multivariate ANOVA. However, description of multivariate analysis is beyond the scope of this publication.

1. DATA STRUCTURE

Let us assume three factors a, b and c at p, q and r levels, respectively; i.e. a_i's ($i = 1, 2,$ ... p), b_j's ($j = 1, 2,$ ... q), and c_k's ($k = 1, 2,$ ... r); Therefore, each cell is designated ijk. If each cell ijk has only one observation, then each observation can be designated x_{ijk}. On the other hand, if each cell ijk has m values ($m = 1, 2$ ... l), then each observation can be designated x_{ijkl}.

By extending the logic on notations in two-way ANOVA with one and m observations per cell, the following will be the notations for totals, crude sum of squares and number of observations:

	m observations/cell			One observation/cell		
	Total	Crude SS	n	Total	Crude SS	n
Factor A	$x_{i...}$	$x^2_{i...}$	$n_{i..}$	$x_{i..}$	$x^2_{i..}$	$n_{i.}$
Factor B	$x_{.j..}$	$x^2_{.j..}$	$n_{.j.}$	$x_{.j.}$	$x^2_{.j.}$	$n_{.j}$
Factor C	$x_{..k.}$	$x^2_{..k.}$	$n_{..k}$	$x_{..k}$	$x^2_{..k}$	$n_{.k}$
Interaction AB	$x_{ij..}$	$x^2_{ij..}$	$n_{ij.}$	$x_{ij.}$	$x^2_{ij.}$	n_{ij}
Interaction AC	$x_{i.k.}$	$x^2_{i.k.}$	$n_{i.k}$	$x_{i.k}$	$x^2_{i.k}$	n_{ik}

(Contd.)

194

	m observations/cell			One observation/cell		
	Total	Crude SS	n	Total	Crude SS	n
Interaction BC	$x_{\cdot jk\cdot}$	$x^2_{\cdot jk\cdot}$	$n_{\cdot jk}$	$x_{\cdot jk}$	$x^2_{\cdot jk}$	n_{jk}
Interaction ABC	$x_{ijk\cdot}$	$x^2_{ijk\cdot}$	n_{ijk}	*	*	*
Overall	$x_{\cdots\cdot}$	$x^2_{\cdots\cdot}$	$n_{\cdots}$	$x_{\cdots}$	$x^2_{\cdots}$	$n_{\cdot\cdot}$

* Not feasible because $m = 1$; $\quad x^2_{\cdots\cdot} = \sum\limits_{i=1}^{p}\sum\limits_{j=1}^{q}\sum\limits_{k=1}^{r}\sum\limits_{l=1}^{m} x^2_{ijkl}$ and $x^2_{\cdots} = \sum\limits_{i=1}^{p}\sum\limits_{j=1}^{q}\sum\limits_{k=1}^{r} x^2_{ijk}$

As indicated in earlier Chapters on ANOVA, $x^2_{\cdots\cdot} \neq \left(x_{\cdots\cdot}\right)^2$ and $x^2_{\cdots} \neq \left(x_{\cdots}\right)^2$. Formulae for calculation of various SS are shown in the following table where, correction factor $C = (x_{\cdots\cdot})^2 \div n_{\cdots}$ or $(x_{\cdots})^2 \div n_{\cdot\cdot}$ for $m > 1$ and $m = 1$, respectively; they are applicable even for unequal m's:

Source	m observations/cell	One observation/cell
Total SS	$x^2_{\cdots\cdot} - C$	$x^2_{\cdots} - C$
Factor A(SS_A)	$\sum\limits_{i=1}^{p} \dfrac{\left(x_{i\cdots}\right)^2}{n_{i\cdots}} - C$	$\sum\limits_{i=1}^{p} \dfrac{\left(x_{i\cdots}\right)^2}{n_{i\cdot}} - C$
Factor B(SS_B)	$\sum\limits_{j=1}^{q} \dfrac{\left(x_{\cdot j\cdots}\right)^2}{n_{\cdot j\cdot}} - C$	$\sum\limits_{j=1}^{q} \dfrac{\left(x_{\cdot j\cdot}\right)^2}{n_{\cdot j}} - C$
Factor C(SS_C)	$\sum\limits_{k=1}^{r} \dfrac{\left(x_{\cdot\cdot k\cdot}\right)^2}{n_{\cdot\cdot k}} - C$	$\sum\limits_{k=1}^{r} \dfrac{\left(x_{\cdot\cdot k}\right)^2}{n_{\cdot k}} - C$
Factor AB(SS_{AB})	$\sum\limits_{i=1}^{p}\sum\limits_{j=1}^{q} \dfrac{\left(x_{ij\cdots}\right)^2}{n_{ij\cdot}} - C - SS_A - SS_B$	$\sum\limits_{i=1}^{p}\sum\limits_{j=1}^{q} \dfrac{\left(x_{ij\cdot}\right)^2}{n_{ij}} - C - SS_A - SS_B$
Factor AC(SS_{AC})	$\sum\limits_{i=1}^{p}\sum\limits_{k=1}^{r} \dfrac{\left(x_{i\cdot k\cdot}\right)^2}{n_{i\cdot k}} - C - SS_A - SS_C$	$\sum\limits_{i=1}^{p}\sum\limits_{k=1}^{r} \dfrac{\left(x_{i\cdot k}\right)^2}{n_{ik}} - C - SS_A - SS_C$
Factor BC (SS_{BC})	$\sum\limits_{j=1}^{q}\sum\limits_{k=1}^{r} \dfrac{\left(x_{\cdot jk\cdot}\right)^2}{n_{\cdot jk}} - C - SS_B - SS_C$	$\sum\limits_{j=1}^{q}\sum\limits_{k=1}^{r} \dfrac{\left(x_{\cdot jk}\right)^2}{n_{jk}} - C - SS_B - SS_C$
Factor ABC (SS_{ABC})	$\sum\limits_{i=1}^{p}\sum\limits_{j=1}^{q}\sum\limits_{k=1}^{r} \dfrac{\left(x_{ijk\cdot}\right)^2}{n_{ijk}} - C - SS_A - SS_B - SS_C$ $- SS_{AB} - SS_{AC} - SS_{BC}$	*
Error(SS_E)	Total SS $- SS_A - SS_B - SS_C -$ $SS_{AB} - SS_{AC} - SS_{BC} - SS_{ABC}$	Total SS $- SS_A - SS_B - SS_C -$ $SS_{AB} - SS_{AC} - SS_{BC}$

* Not feasible because $m = 1$

The ANOVA table with υ for respective SS is given below:

Mathematical model: $x_{ijk} = \bar{x} + \alpha_i + \beta_j + \gamma_k + \alpha\beta_{ij} + \alpha\gamma_{ik} + \beta\gamma_{jk} + \alpha\beta\gamma_{ijk} + e_{ijk}$ ($\alpha\beta\gamma_{ijk}$ included only when m > 1).

Source	υ (m > 1)	υ (m = 1)	MSS	F[@]
Total	$n... - 1$	$n.. - 1$		
Factor A(SS$_A$)	$p - 1$	$p - 1$	MSS$_A$	
Factor B(SS$_B$)	$q - 1$	$q - 1$	MSS$_B$	
Factor C(SS$_C$)	$r - 1$	$r - 1$	MSS$_C$	
Factor AB(SS$_{AB}$)	$(p-1)(q-1)$	$(p-1)(q-1)$	MSS$_{AB}$	
Factor AC(SS$_{AC}$)	$(p-1)(r-1)$	$(p-1)(r-1)$	MSS$_{AC}$	
Factor BC(SS$_{BC}$)	$(q-1)(r-1)$	$(q-1)(r-1)$	MSS$_{BC}$	
Factor ABC(SS$_{ABC}$)	$\upsilon_A \times \upsilon_B \times \upsilon_C$	[#]	MSS$_{ABC}$[##]	
Error (SS$_E$)	$pqr(m-1)$[###]	$\upsilon_A \times \upsilon_B \times \upsilon_C$	MSS$_E$	

[#] Not feasible because $m = 1$; [##] Only if $m > 1$; [###] When m's are same; otherwise, calculated by difference between υ of Total SS and total υ of other sources; [@] Ratio of respective MSS to MSS$_E$.

1.1 Example

Three strains of broilers ($p = 3$) were fed on three levels of calorie–protein (CP) ratio ($q = 3$) to find the effects as per sex of broilers ($r = 2$). Five birds of each sex were allotted ($m = 5$) to each of the treatment combinations. The data on six–week body weight (kg) of 90 broilers (*abcm* or $n...$) is presented below as per strain of broilers. The following H$_0$'s have to be tested:

1. Body weight of all strains of broilers is same ($\alpha_i = 0$)
2. Body weight at all levels of CP ratio is same ($\beta_j = 0$)
3. Body weight of sexes is same ($\gamma_k = 0$)
4. Body weight of broilers is independent of CP ratio ($\alpha\beta_{ij} = 0$)
5. Body weight of broilers is independent of sex ($\alpha\gamma_{ik} = 0$)
6. Effect of CP ratio is independent of sex ($\beta\gamma_{jk} = 0$)
7. Body weight of broilers is independent of CP ratio and sex ($\alpha\beta\gamma_{ijk} = 0$)

Note: If $m = 1$, H$_0$ on $\alpha\beta\gamma_{ijk}$ is not possible.

Body weight, kg	Strain 1		Strain 2		Strain 3	
	♂	♀	♂	♀	♂	♀
CP 120 ratio	1.0, 1.1, 1.2, 1.2, 1.1	0.8, 0.8, 0.9, 0.9, 1.0	0.9, 0.8, 0.9, 0.8, 1.0	0.7, 0.8, 0.7, 0.9, 0.8	1.2, 1.0, 1.3, 1.0, 1.1	1.0, 1.0, 0.9, 1.1, 1.0
130	1.3, 1.2, 1.4, 1.2, 1.3	1.0, 1.1, 1.0, 1.0, 1.2	1.1, 1.2, 1.1, 1.1, 1.0	0.9, 0.9, 1.0, 0.8, 0.9	1.4, 1.5, 1.4, 1.3, 1.2	1.1, 1.2, 1.2, 1.1, 1.2
140	1.7, 1.8, 1.6, 1.6, 1.5	1.5, 1.4, 1.4, 1.3, 1.3	1.3, 1.4, 1.3, 1.5, 1.3	1.1, 1.0, 1.2, 1.0, 1.1	2.0, 2.1, 1.8, 1.9, 1.9	1.5, 1.6, 1.6, 1.5, 1.5

The cell totals and crude SS ($x_{ijk\cdot}$ and $x^2_{ijk\cdot}$) and other marginal and interaction totals of above table are summarized below:

	Strain 1 ♂		Strain 1 ♀		Strain 2 ♂		Strain 2 ♀		Strain 3 ♂		Strain 3 ♀	
$n_{ijk}=5$	$x_{ijk\cdot}$	$x^2_{ijk\cdot}$	$x_{ijk\cdot}$	$x^2_{ijk\cdot}$	$x_{ijk\cdot}$	$x^2_{ijk\cdot}$	$x_{ijk\cdot}$	$x^2_{ijk\cdot}$	$x_{ijk\cdot}$	$x^2_{ijk\cdot}$	$x_{ijk\cdot}$	$x^2_{ijk\cdot}$
CP 120	5.6	6.30	4.4	3.90	4.4	3.90	3.9	3.07	5.6	6.34	5.0	5.02
ratio 130	6.4	8.22	5.3	5.65	5.5	6.07	4.5	4.07	6.8	9.30	5.8	6.74
140	8.2	13.50	6.9	9.55	6.8	9.28	5.4	5.86	9.7	18.87	7.7	11.87
$x_{i\cdot k\cdot}$		20.2		16.6		16.7		13.8		22.1		18.5
$x^2_{i\cdot k\cdot}$		28.02		19.10		19.25		13.00		34.51		23.63

$x_{ij\cdot\cdot}$	Str1	Str2	Str3	$x_{i\cdot k\cdot}$	Str1	Str2	Str3	$x_{\cdot jk\cdot}$	CP1	CP2	CP3	$x_{\cdot\cdot k\cdot}$
CP1	10.0	8.3	10.6	♂	20.2	16.7	22.1	♂	15.6	18.7	24.7	59.0
CP2	11.7	10.0	12.6	♀	16.6	13.8	18.5	♀	13.3	15.6	20.0	48.9
CP3	15.1	12.2	17.4	$x_{i\cdot\cdot}$	36.8	30.5	40.6	$x_{\cdot j\cdot}$	28.9	34.3	44.7	
ni.. = 30				n.j. = 30				n..k = 45	n... = 90	$x^2_{\cdot\cdot\cdot\cdot}$ 137.51	$x_{\cdot\cdot\cdot\cdot}$ 107.9	

With the totals of main factors and interactions ready, SS can be easily computed by applying the formulae tabulated earlier. They are as follows:

Source	υ	SS	MSS	F
Total SS	89	8.1499		
Strains (SS$_A$)	2	1.7349	0.8675	109.96
CP levels (SS$_B$)	2	4.2996	2.1498	272.51
Sex (SS$_C$)	1	1.1334	1.1334	143.68
Strain x CP levels (SS$_{AB}$)	4	0.2560	0.0640	8.13
Strain x Sex (SS$_{AC}$)	2	0.0109	0.0055	<1
CP levels x Sex (SS$_{BC}$)	2	0.0992	0.0500	6.31
Strain x CP levels x sex (SS$_{ABC}$)	4	0.0471	0.0118	1.49
Error (SS$_E$)	72	0.5680	0.0079	

Table values: $F_{0.05,\,1,\,72} = 3.98$, $F_{0.05,\,2,\,72} = 3.13$ and $F_{0.05,\,4,\,72} = 2.50$

Therefore, all the main factors appeared to have significant effect on body weight of broilers whereas, both two- and three-factor interactions were not statistically perceptible as significant. Hence, H$_0$'s 1, 2 and 3 are not acceptable whereas, Nos 4, 5, 6 and 7 are acceptable. The means can be compared by the method of LSD (see Chapter "**One-factor analysis of variance**"); the same is shown below:

All values in kg	Strains	CP levels	Sex
LSD	0.046	0.046	Not required
1	1.227[b]	0.963[c]	1.311[a]
2	1.017[c]	1.143[b]	1.087[b]
3	1.353[a]	1.490[a]	

Means bearing different superscript within a column are significantly different (P < 0.05)

Note:

1. If any of the two-factor interactions is significant, corresponding means are tabulated, LSD values calculated on the respective number of observations for the interaction (mr for AB and mq for AC and mp for BC;) and superscripts allotted. For instance, two-factor interaction tables in the above example will be:

Strain × Sex interaction	Strain 1	Strain 2	Strain 3	Means for sexes
♂	1.347	1.113	1.473	1.311^A
♀	1.107	0.920	1.233	1.087^B
Means for Strains	1.227^Y	1.017^Z	1.353^X	

and

CP levels × Sex interaction	CP ratio 1	CP ratio 2	CP ratio 3	Means for sexes
♂	1.040^d	1.247^c	1.647^a	1.311^A
♀	0.886^e	1.040^d	1.333^b	1.087^B
Means for CP levels	0.963^Z	1.143^Y	1.490^X	$LSD_{CP \times Sex} = 0.065$

2. If ABC interaction is significant, a $3 \times 3 \times 2$ table of means has to be developed and means compared by LSD with suitable change in number of observations (m) while calculating LSD (5 in the present example).

3. If $m = 1$, there is no question of ABC interaction because that itself is the estimate of SS_E.

4. If m is unequal among cells, the analytical procedure is as described above with careful use of number of observations for the corresponding totals while calculating SS. However, while calculating LSD, number of observations does require some clarification. If two means are compared at a time, separate LSD values can be easily computed and comparisons made. Similarly, in a random–effects model, number of observations is essential for calculating variance components. In either case, if a common value for number of observations has to be made, for instance with

respect to factor A in this example, it can be calculated as $\dfrac{1}{p-1}\left[n_{...} - \dfrac{\sum\limits_{i=1}^{p} n_{i..}^{2}}{n_{...}} \right]$. The logic can be

extended to other factors as well. Such computations are mostly resorted to by Animal Geneticist while estimating heritability and correlations (see Chapter "**Statistics in Specific Veterinary fields**"). In addition, the same formula with suitable modification in subscripts is suitable in one– and two-factor ANOVA also.

2. LATIN SQUARE DESIGN

In RBD, the blocking is restricted to rows in such a way that variation within blocks is assumed to be entirely due to fixed effect forming the columns. However, it is possible two-way blocking in such a way all treatments occur in all the rows and columns with a condition that each of the treatments appears once and only once in any row or column. For instance, with three treatments (A, B and C) the arrangements can be as follows:

A	B	C
B	C	A
C	A	B

Obviously, in this design, number of treatments = number of rows = number of columns and the smallest Latin square possible is the one shown above. Pens and barns can be allotted by this method although it is not very common because positional variation is not reckoned as an important source of variation in animal science unlike Agricultural trials. However, several combinations of Latin squares are possible; for instance, 12 alternatives of a 3 × 3, 576 of a 4 × 4, 161280 of 5 × 5, etc. are possible indicating its suitability for Switch-over and Switch-back trials if each column is designated for a particular (large) animal and the entire trial is replicated with a different configuration of the Latin square.

Note: Latin squares in which a treatment occurs only once in each row and column are referred to as **Graeco–Latin Squares**.

2.1 Analytical Procedure

Let us assume p treatments ($i = 1, 2, 3 \dots p$) were used in a trial based on Latin – square design. Obviously, there will be p rows ($j = 1, 2, 3 \dots p$) and p columns ($k = 1, 2, 3 \dots p$). Hence, x_{ijk} represents value of ith treatment in the jth row and kth column. With the notations as described in **Section 1** above, the procedure is summarized in the table below where, correction factor $C = (x...)^2 \div p^2$. In addition, rows and columns may represent factors like period, age, a specific animal (as in case of large animal), animal pens, barns, sheds, etc.

Source	v	SS	MSS	F@
Total	$p^2 - 1$	$x^2... - C$		
Treatments (SS$_T$)	$p - 1$	$\dfrac{\sum_{i=1}^{p}(x_{i..})^2}{p} - C$	MSS$_A$	
Rows (SS$_R$)	$q - 1$	$\dfrac{\sum_{j=1}^{q}(x_{.j.})^2}{q} - C$	MSS$_B$	
Columns (SS$_C$)	$r - 1$	$\dfrac{\sum_{k=1}^{r}(x_{..k})^2}{r} - C$	MSS$_C$	
Error (SS$_E$)	$(p-1)(p-2)$	Total SS $-$ SS$_T$ $-$ SS$_R$ $-$ SS$_C$	MSS$_E$	

Since $p = q = r$, they can replace each other in all the formulae
@ F values are calculated for each MSS with MSS$_E$ as denominator

Note:

1. The entire Latin-square can be replicated; in the latter case, replicate sum of squares as well as interactions will be calculated analogous to three-factor ANOVA for $m > 1$ detailed above. Such experiments are not common in animal science.

2. Latin-squares are replicated to balance the residual effects in case of switch–over trials which will be discussed in the next section.

2.1.1 *Example*

The following example for Latin square design without replication is considered. Suppose, four treatments ($p = 4$) were tried on four cows ($q = 4$; rows) over four 30 days' periods ($r = 4$; columns) to study the effect on milk yield (kg) and the data obtained were as follows:

	Period 1	Period 2	Period 3	Period 4	$x._{.j.}$
Cow 1	C24	B36	D35	A32	127
Cow 2	A32	D40	C23	B35	130
Cow 3	B40	C26	A30	D38	134
Cow 4	D45	A35	B30	C25	135
$x.._{.k}$	141	137	118	130	$x... = 526$

$x_i...$ values for treatments A, B, C and D are 129, 141, 98 and 158, respectively; $x^2... = 17894$ and $C = 17292.25$

The ANOVA table can be set-up as follows:

H_0's: 1. There is no effect of treatments on monthly milk yield
2. There is no effect of Cows on monthly milk yield
3. There is no effect of Periods on monthly milk yield

Source	v	SS	MSS	F
Total	15	601.75		
Treatments(SS_T)	3	480.25	160.0833	27.443
Cows(SS_R)	3	10.25	3.4167	< 1
Periods(SS_C)	3	76.25	25.4167	4.357
Error(SS_E)	6	35.00	5.8333	

Table value of $F_{0.05, 3, 6} = 4.76$

Depending on the calculated value, it is reasonable to reject H_0 No.1 and accept H_0 Nos 2 and 3.

Note: Residual effects, if any, of the treatment(s) previously exposed to get confounded with treatment effects in this design. To obviate this, switch-over and switch-back trials can be used (*see* **Section 3** below).

2.1.2 *Missed-plot technique*

3.1.2.1 One observation missing

Suppose value pertaining to treatment 1 (A), Cow 2 and period I is missing in the above example; the data will be as follows:

	Period 1	Period 2	Period 3	Period 4	$x._{.j.}$
Cow 1	C24	B36	D35	A32	127
Cow 2	A—(19)	D40	C23	B35	98 (117)
Cow 3	B40	C26	A30	D38	134
Cow 4	D45	A35	B30	C25	135
$x.._{.k}$ 109 (128)	137	118	130	$x... = 494$ (513)	

$x_i...$ values for treatments A, B, C and D are **129 (116)**, 141, 98 and 158, respectively; $x^2... = $ (17231) and $C = $ (16448.0625)

Note: Value in the parentheses indicates those after the estimated value is included for calculation of sums and sums of squares; the highlighted values correspond to before the estimate of missed value being comsidered.

Least square estimate of missing value is $\dfrac{p\left(x_{i..} + x_{.j.} + x_{..k}\right) - 2x_{...}}{(p-1)(p-2)}$; all values required

for the above equation are calculated above (due to missed value) and highlighted.

Hence, the missed value $= \dfrac{4(97+98+109) - 2\times494}{(4-1)(4-2)} = 19$. This value is replaced for x_{112}

and ANOVA is performed.

A correction for SST for upward bias calculated as $\left[\dfrac{\left(x_{...} - (p-1)x_{i..} - x_{.j.} - x_{..k}\right)}{(p-1)(p-2)}\right]^2$ (all

totals inclusive of the estimated value; those in parentheses in the table above) and standard error of difference between treatment mean which had missed observation

and others is given by $\sqrt{\dfrac{2}{p} + \dfrac{1}{(p-1)(p-2)}}$ and between those with no observation

missing by $\sqrt{\dfrac{2MSS_E}{p}}$. Consequent on this procedure õ of total SS and SS_E are reduced

by 1.

2.1.2.2 > 1 observations missing

Analogous to RBD, missed observation(s) can be estimated by simultaneous equation method in Latin square design also utilizing the same computational formulae with a reduction in υ of total SS (consequently for SS_E) by 1 for each of the estimated value. However, in case of Latin square design, the counts are allotted as follows as a prerequisite for calculation of variance of difference between two means (*see* **Section 5.2.2** of Chapter "**Two-factor analysis of variance**" for details):

Cell	Features in the cell (unit) to which A is allotted		Count	
	Same row	Same column	r_1	r_2
A occurs	B occurs	B occurs	1	1
A occurs	B does not occur in one of these		$\frac{2}{3}$	0
A occurs	B not available in both		$\frac{1}{3}$	0
A missing	Regardless		0	0

For enumerating the allotment of counts, let us consider the following lay-out of Latin square design with missed observations indicated by*:

			Columns		
Rows	1	2	3	4	5
1	D	E	C	B	A
2	C	D	A	E	B*
3	E	A*	B*	D	C
4	B	C	E	A	D
5	A	B	D	C	E

The allotment of counts, with respect to treatments A and B, is given below:

Row number		Features		Count	
	Cell	Same row	Same column	r_1	r_2
1	A occurs	B occurs	B does not occur	$\frac{2}{3}$	0
2	A occurs	B does not occur	B does not occur	$\frac{1}{3}$	0
3	A does not occur	B does not occur	B occurs	0	0
4	A occurs	B occurs	B occurs	1	1
5	A occurs	B occurs	B occurs	1	1
Total	3	2			

After getting r_1 and r_2 values, standard error of difference between two means and LSD are calculated as in case of RBD.

3. SWITCH (CROSS)-OVER AND SWITCH-BACK EXPERIMENT

3.1 Switch-over design

In large-animal experimentation, particularly in Nutrition experiments, two main constraints, beside others, are:

1. Number of animals for trials is always limited due to both cost constraints and availability of the statistically calculated number of animals and
2. Variation within animals is large because unlike small animals like poultry, obtaining large animals of minimum within animal variation is difficult.

Therefore, the same experimental subjects are used for different treatments, but at different times, one after another. For instance, if a particular drug/supplement is being tested for its growth-stimulating ability, the randomly allotted animals can be fed for a known period of time on each of the diets and growth measured; this can be followed by feeding the next feed and so on. There are some constraints in such an arrangement:

1. The residual effect(s) of the treatment(s) the animals have already undergone before a particular treatment is given; in simple terms, will there be any difference if the order of application of treatments altered?
2. That the previous treatment has no influence on the response of the animals to the next treatment(s) in line can't be guaranteed every time.
3. Growth potency of the animal species/breed is assumed to be constant over the entire experimental period; that means, broilers grow fastest during the initial

periods and tend to grow slower later on; if a treatment is applied during the period when growth is likely to be at peak the response for the treatment gets confounded and hence, biased in favor of the treatment applied. This is the reason that switch-over experiments are not advisable for fast growing animals.

In spite of the above limitations, if data is available, it is a case of repeated measures on the same experimental unit and ANOVA for such data is shown through an example below:

3.1.1 *Example*

Data on egg cholesterol (mg%) on 5 birds subjected to 4 different drugs is given below:
Test H_0: The egg cholesterol content was same in eggs under all drugs

Hens	Drug 1	Drug 2	Drug 3	Drug 4	$x_{.j}$	$x^2_{.j}$
1	220	235	180	200	835	176025
2	225	230	175	205	835	176125
3	223	234	190	215	862	186810
4	210	238	200	200	848	180744
5	218	228	210	210	866	187708
$x_{i.}$	1096	1165	955	1030	$x.. = 4246$	$x^2.. = 907412$

$$\text{Total SS} = x^2_{..} - \frac{(x_{..})^2}{n_.} = 5986.2 \text{ on } \upsilon = (n. - 1) = 19, \text{SS}_{\text{Hens}} = \frac{\sum_{j=1}^{b}(x_{.j})^2}{a} - \frac{(x_{..})^2}{n_.} = 212.7 \text{ on}$$

$\upsilon = (b - 1) = 4$ where a = number of treatments = 4, $n.$ = total number of observations = $a \times b = 20$, b = number of hens = 5; $\text{SS}_{\text{Within hens}}$ = Total SS – SS_{Hens} = 5773.5 on $\upsilon = (n. - b)$ or

$$b \times (a - 1) = 15; \text{SS}_{\text{Drugs}} \text{ i.e. } \text{SS}_T = \frac{\sum_{i=1}^{a}(x_{i.})^2}{b} - \frac{(x_{..})^2}{n_.} = 4847.4 \text{ on } \upsilon = (a - 1) = 3 \text{ ans SS}_{\text{Residual}}$$

$= \text{SS}_{\text{Within hens}} - \text{SS}_{\text{Drugs}} = 926.1$ on $\upsilon = (a - 1)(b - 1) = 12$. Finally, the ANOVA table is as follows:

Source	υ	SS	MSS	F
Total	19	5986.2		
Hens	4	212.7		
Within hens	15	5773.5		
Drugs	3	4847.4	1615.800	20.937
Residual	12	926.1	77.175	

Table value of $F_{0.05, 3, 12} = 3.49$

Calculated value of F > table value and hence, H_0 is liable for rejection. $\text{LSD}_{0.05}$

$$= 2.179 \times \sqrt{\frac{2 \times 77.175}{5}} = 12.107. \text{ The mean values for various drugs can be allotted}$$

superscripts as per the procedure described in **Section 3.1.5** Chapter "**One-factor analysis of variance**":

	Drug 1	Drug 2	Drug 3	Drug 4
Mean	219.2[b]	233.0[a]	191.0[d]	206.0[c]

Means bearing different superscripts are significantly different (P d" 0.05)

It may be concluded that cholesterol levels in eggs reduced due to the drugs with drugs 1, 4 and 3 causing significant progressive reductions from that of drug 1. It can be noted that the above example is similar to two-factor ANOVA with slight modification.

A switch-over design by using Latin square models, can be a candidate for three-factor ANOVA.

3.1.2 *Latin squares for estimating residual effects*

Under the assumption that the correlation between residual effect and treatment effect is 0 and the residual effect itself wanes off after one succeeding period, if treatments can be "**Balanced**" in such a way that every treatment is applied in every order possible, computation of both treatment (Main) effects and residual effects will be easier. It is easy to visualize that Latin squares can be very handy for this purpose.

3.1.2.1 Balancing treatment sequences

Three (A B and C) treatments will be considered to discuss the balancing of treatment and residual effects by Latin squares. Two squares of power t (t = number of treatments; 3 in this example) can be written simultaneously by alternating the sequence of columns as is shown below: (sequence of writing the columns is indicated as sequence number)

	Latin – square I			Latin – square II		
Sequence of writing columns →	1	3	5	2	4	6
	A	C	B	B	C	A
	B	A	C	C	A	B
	C	B	A	A	B	C

It can be seen that the squares are mirror images of one another. This procedure is also called "**Slicing**"; with odd-numbered squares, if the sliced squares are superimposed, we get a square containing letters (treatments) appearing only once in combination with itself and other treatments; such squares are referred to as "**Orthogonal Latin squares**". In the above case, the orthogonal square will be:

AB	BC	CA
CC	AA	BB
BA	CB	AC

(t – 1) Number of such squares are possible for Latin square of power t (such that t is a prime number of or $t = m^n$ where m and n are prime numbers). Same logic holds for different values of t. Sets of mutually orthogonal squares are also available, albeit not provided in this publication.

3.1.2.2 Application of treatments

Treatment sequence (as indicated by the columns of the squares) is allotted at random to animals. If the sets of squares are repeated, animals can be allotted in groups (blocks) and allotted at random to the columns. If the experiment is repeated over a period(s) of time, each time, animals (blocks) are allotted at random separately for each square.

3.1.2.3 Example

The data is presented below are on the effect of three diets (A, B and C, $j = 1, 2, \ldots q$) on monthly milk yield (kg/30 d) of cows over 3 periods ($k = 1, 2, \ldots r$) over four Latin squares ($i = 1, 2, \ldots p$); 3 sequences in each, $l = 1, 2, 3, \ldots s$). The data collected will be analyzed under the assumptions already indicated earlier. In the example, $p = 4, q = r = 3, s = 12$

Period	Square I Sequence 1	2	3	Within square period total, $x_{ij \cdot 1}$	Square II Sequence 4	5	6	Within square period total, $x_{ij \cdot 1}$
1	A150	B170	C100	420	A135	B150	C80	365
2	B175	C90	A140	405	C90	A140	B160	390
3	C90	A140	B160	390	B180	C75	A125	380
Sequence total $x_{ijk \cdot}$	415	400	400	Square total, $x_{\cdot jkl} = 1215$	405	365	365	Square total, $x_{\cdot jkl} = 1135$

Period	Square I Sequence 1	2	3	Within square period total, $x_{ij \cdot 1}$	Square II Sequence 4	5	6	Within square period total, $x_{ij \cdot 1}$
1	A160	B180	C90	430	A125	B160	C90	375
2	B165	C100	A130	395	C100	A120	B180	400
3	C80	A150	B170	400	B170	C95	A115	380
Sequence total, $x_{ijk \cdot}$	405	430	390	Square total, $x_{\cdot jkl} = 1225$	395	375	385	Square total, $x_{\cdot jkl} = 1155$

Treatment totals, $x_{\cdot j \cdot \cdot} = 1630, 2020$ and 1080 for treatment A, B and C, respectively, Period totals, $x_{\cdot \cdot k \cdot} = 1590, 1590$ and 1550 for Period 1, 2 and 3, respectively, $x_{\cdot \cdot \cdot \cdot} = 4730$ and $x^2_{\cdot \cdot \cdot \cdot} = 662400$.

$$\text{Total SS} = x^2_{\cdot \cdot \cdot \cdot} - \frac{(x_{\cdot \cdot \cdot \cdot})^2}{pqr} = 40930.5556; \quad SS_T \text{ (SS due to treatments)} = \frac{\sum_{j=1}^{p}(x_{\cdot j \cdot \cdot})^2}{pr} - \frac{(x_{\cdot \cdot \cdot \cdot})^2}{pqr}$$

$= 37172.2222$ on $\upsilon = (q - 1) = 2$; $SS_{P/S}$ (SS due to Periods within square)

$$= \frac{\sum\limits_{k=1}^{r}\left(x_{ij \cdot l}\right)^{2}}{q} - \frac{\sum\limits_{i=1}^{p}\left(x_{\cdot jkl}\right)^{2}}{qr} = 611.1111, \text{ on } \upsilon = p^{*}(q-1) = 8 \text{ and } SS_{S} \text{ (SS due to sequences)} =$$

$$\frac{\sum\limits_{l=1}^{s}\left(x_{ijk \cdot}\right)^{2}}{k} - \frac{\left(x_{\cdots}\right)^{2}}{ijk} = 1397.2222 \text{ on } \upsilon = (s-1) = 11 \text{ and finally, } SS_{E} \text{ (SS due to Error)} =$$

Total $SS - SS_{T} - SS_{P} - SS_{S} = 1750.0001$. Now, ANOVA table ignoring residual effects can be set–up as follows:

H_{0}: 1) There is no effect of treatments on monthly milk yield 2) There is no effect of periods on monthly milk yield and 3) There is no effect of sequence of applying treatments on monthly milk yield

Source	υ	SS	MSS	F
Total	35	40930.5556		
Treatments	2	37172.2222	18586.1111	148.689
Periods	8	611.1111	76.389	< 1
Sequences	11	1397.2222	127.0202	1.016
Error	14	1750.0001	125.0000@	

Table value $F_{0.05, 2, 14} = 3.74$ and $F_{0.05, 11, 14} = 2.56$ @Ignoring residual effects

Since F calculated for Treatments is > table value, H_{0} No. 1 is liable to be rejected whereas, Nos. 2 and 3 are acceptable. Comparison of treatment means can be done as described earlier in Chapter "**One-factor analysis of variance**"; standard error of treatment difference is $\sqrt{\dfrac{2MSS_{E}}{pr}}$ and standard error of each treatment mean = $\sqrt{\dfrac{MSS_{E}}{pr}}$; The treatment means (kg) along with superscripts are: 135.833[b], 168.333[a], 90.000[c]. (LSD = 9.791 kg).

Note:

1. Since $q = r$, qr can be replaced by q^{2} or r^{2}
2. Periods are considered subset of the Latin square; such type of "nesting" is common in genetic studies; more on this is discussed in Chapter "**Statistics in specific veterinary fields**".

3.1.2.4 Estimation of direct (main) and residual effects

This is in continuation of Total SS, SS_{T}, SS_{P} and SS_{S} shown above. The additional sums of squares to be calculated are sum of squares due to direct effects adjusted for residual effects and sum of squares due to residual effects adjusted for direct effects and error.

3.1.2.4.1 Calculation of direct and residual effects adjusted for each other

First, total of observations which represent those after a particular treatment is applied are added; for instance, let us consider treatment A; in square I column 1, after treatment A, two values 165 and 80 kg are available; in column 2, there is no value after Treatment A and in column 3, 170 is the value after the treatment A. Same way, the values are located in squares II, III and IV; obviously, totally 8 values available for each of the treatments because in every square, Treatment A occurs as the last treatment once leaving only two more columns for residual effects. Further, it is assumed that the residual effects last for only one succeeding period and therefore, the value soon after the application of new treatment succeeding treatment A represents residual effect, if any, along with the effect of the new treatment applied. In the above example, totals are:

Treatment A: 175 + 160 + 90 + 75 + 165 + 170 +100 + 95 = 1030 kg (R_A)

Treatment B: 90 + 90 + 140 + 125 + 80 + 100 + 120 + 115 = 860 kg (R_B)

Treatment C: 140 + 140 + 180 + 160 + 150 + 130 + 170 +180=1250 kg (R_C).

Check: Sum of residual totals for treatments A, B and C = $x... - x._{.1}.$; i.e. grand total − total of period 1 (over all squares); in this case, it was indeed found that (1030 + 860 + 1250) = (4730 − 1590).

Next stage is to calculate totals of all sequences in which a particular treatment occurred last; obviously, in every square, only once a treatment appears last and hence, there will be that many number of sequences of this type as are squares. In the above example, the values are:

Treatment A: 400 + 365 + 430 + 385 = 1580 kg (S_A)

Treatment B: 400 + 405 + 390 + 395 = 1590 kg (S_B)

Treatment C: 415 + 365 + 405 + 375 = 1560 kg (S_C).

Two more quantities have to be estimated as follows:

$L = x._{.1}. - q \times x.... = (1590 - 3 \times 4730) = -12600$ and

$M = q \times x._{.1}. - (q + 2) \times x.... = (3 \times 1590 - 5 \times 4730) = -18880$

3.1.2.4.1.1 Direct effects adjusted for residual effects

Direct effect adjusted for residual effects for q^{th} treatment, DR_j for each of the treatments

is given by $pq \times (q^2 - q - 2) \times \delta_j = (q^2 - q - 1) \times x._{.j}. + q \times R_j + S_j + L$; Check: $\sum_{j=1}^{q} DR_j = 0$. In

the example; $DR_A = 220$, $DR_B = 1670$ and $DR_C = -2230$; $\delta_A = 4.583$, $\delta_B = 34.792$ and $\delta_C = -39.375$

3.1.2.4.1.2 Residual effects adjusted for direct effects

Residual effect adjusted for direct effects for q^{th} treatment, RS_j for each of the treatments

is given by $pq \times (q^2 - q - 2) \times \rho_j = q \times x._{.j}. + q^2 \times R_j + q \times S_j + M$; Check: $\sum_{j=1}^{q} RS_j = 0$; in the

present case, $RS_A = 20$, $RS_B = -310$ and $RS_C = 290$; $\rho_A = 0.417$, $\rho_B = -6.458$ and $\rho_C = 6.042$. The same are tabulated below:

	$x._{.j}..$	R_j	S_j	DR_j	δ_j	$\bar{x}_{.+} + \delta_j$	RS_j	ρ_j
A	1630	1030	1580	220	4.583	135.972	20	0.417
B	2020	860	1590	1670	34.792	166.181	−310	−6.458
C	1080	1250	1560	−1890	−39.375	92.014	290	6.042
Total	4730*	3140**	4730*	0	0	394.167***	0	0

* $= x....$; ** $= x.... - x._{.1}.$; $\bar{x}_{....} = (x_{....} \div pqr) = (4730 \div 36) = 131.389$; *** $= 3\,\bar{x}_{....}$

3.1.2.5 Calculation of sum of squares and ANOVA

SS due to direct effects (adjusted), $SS_{DR} = \dfrac{\sum\limits_{j=1}^{q} DR_j^2}{pq\left(q^2-q-1\right)\left(q^2-q-2\right)} = 26705.8333$; SS due

to residual effects (adjusted), $SS_{RS} = \dfrac{\sum\limits_{j=1}^{q} RS_j^2}{pq^2\left(q^2-q-2\right)} = 1254.1667$; both on $\upsilon = (q-1) = 2$.

Finally, the ANOVA table including adjusted effects is as follows:

Source	υ	SS	MSS	F
Total	35	40930.5556		
Periods	8	611.1111	76.389	1.849
Sequences	11	1397.2222	127.0202	3.074
Treatments, unadjusted		37172.2222		
Direct effects, adjusted	2	26705.8333	13352.9167	323.163
Residual effects, adjusted	2	3762.5000	1881.2500	45.529
Error	12	495.8334@	41.3195	

Table value of $F_{0.05,\,8,\,12} = 2.85$, $F_{0.05,\,11,\,12} = 2.72$ and $F_{0.05,\,2,\,12} = 3.88$@ Including residual effects = Total SS $-$ SS$_{T(Unadjusted)} -$ SS$_P -$ SS$_S -$ SS$_{RS}$

Note: If the same experiment is continued for next period, mean values after cumulative effect is given by $\bar{x}._{j..} + \delta_j + \rho_j$

3.1.2.5.1 Comparison of adjusted means

Standard error of difference between two adjusted means of direct effects is given by

the formula $\sqrt{\dfrac{2MSS_E}{pq}\left(\dfrac{q^2-q-1}{q^2-q-2}\right)}$ and those adjusted of residual effects by

$\sqrt{\dfrac{2MSS_E}{pq}\left(\dfrac{q^2}{q^2-q-2}\right)}$; in both, MSS$_E$ including residual effects has to be employed.

These values multiplied by students t value on υ for error and set α give the corresponding LSD values which can be used to compare and allot superscripts as described in Chapter "**One-factor analysis of variance**". In this example, LSD for direct effects at $\alpha = 0.05$ is $2.179 \times 8.608 = 6.393$ kg; hence the superscripts for the means are: 135.972^b, 166.181^a, 92.014^c; similarly for adjusted residuals, LSD $= 8.577$ kg and superscripts on means adjusted for residual effects are 131.806^b, 124.93^c, 137.431^a. Standard error of difference between two cumulative effects (direct + residual) is

$\sqrt{\dfrac{2MSS_E}{pq}\left[\dfrac{(q+1)(2q-1)}{q^2-q-2}\right]}$; however, in this case, MSS$_E$ ignoring residual effects has to be employed.

The covariance between direct and residual effects is estimated by $\left[\dfrac{MSS_E}{p}\left(\dfrac{1}{q^2-q-2}\right)\right]$

= 2.5825 kg²; the correlation coefficient being the ratio of covariance to geometric mean of variances (13352.9167 and 1881.2500), it is apparent that they are not correlated (r = 0.005).

3.1.2.6 Extra period to ensure balanced design

In the above model, it was evident that direct effects are more accurately estimated because, the ratio of variance of difference between two residual effects to that of

difference between two direct effects is $\dfrac{q^2}{\left(q^2-q-1\right)}$ which goes on decreasing as number

of treatments (q) increases; for instance, in the example above, for q = 3, it is 1.8, for q = 4, it will be 1.45, for q = 5, it will be 1.32 and so on. But, to make the ratio unity, the'/ number of treatments required will be so large (> 30) that neither it is feasible economically nor will that many large animals will be normally available for experimentation.

Hence, if an extra period is added and repeat the last treatment in each sequence in the period number (r + 1), it means that every treatment is preceded by itself and same number of times as each other treatment. Hence, the design becomes not only completely balanced as far as residual effect is concerned but also makes direct and residual effects orthogonal.

For q = 3, the design would be

A	B	C		A	B	C
B	C	A		C	A	B
C	A	B		B	C	A
C	A	B		B	C	A

With the same notations as described under **Section 3.1.2.5** above, the following

can be estimated: $DR_j = (q+1)x_{.j..} - S_j - x_{....}$ and $\delta_j = \dfrac{DR_j}{pq(q+2)}$; $SS_{DR} = \dfrac{\displaystyle\sum_{j=1}^{q} DR_j^2}{pq(q+1)(q+2)}$

regardless whether residual effects are included or not included. Similarly,

$RS_j = qR_j + x_{..1.} - x_{....}$ and $\rho_j = \dfrac{RS_j}{pq^2}$; $SS_{RS} = \dfrac{\displaystyle\sum_{j=1}^{q} RS_j^2}{pq^2}$. Standard error of difference between

two direct effect means and that of two residual effects is $\sqrt{\dfrac{2MSS_E(q+1)}{pq(q+2)}}$ and

$\sqrt{\dfrac{2MSS_E}{pq}}$, respectively. Obviously, ratio of the variances has reduced to $\dfrac{(q+2)}{(q+1)}$ which

will be 1.25 when q = 3, 1.20 when q = 4 and so on. Further, variance of difference

between two cumulative effects (unadjusted MSS_E to be used) is $\dfrac{2MSS_E}{pq}\left[\dfrac{(2q+3)}{(q+2)}\right]$

3.2 Switch-Back Design

In Switch-over design there was a possibility of residual effect which could not be accounted for and statistical procedure shown is likely to be complicated for an Animal Science worker. Further, there was no guarantee that if the order of treatments is altered, the same result would be obtained; it is true that use of Latin squares does take care of the order of treatments but, needs more animals and/or time. In addition, subjects may require some adjustment period before a correct response can be measured; therefore, the values recorded at the beginning can be unreliable, though not biased. Hence, if an animal is given treatment A followed by treatment B (switch-over) and again reverted back to treatment A (switch-back) it ensures that treatment responses are devoid of residual effects especially if another animal is on B – A – B regime simultaneously. Hence, this design is also referred to as "**Counterbalanced**" design.

Suppose two animals (E and F) are used in this design with two treatments A (Control) and B, the following table shows the plan of experiment:

Period	Animal E	Animal F
I	Treatment A_1	Treatment B_1
II	Treatment B_2	Treatment A_2
III	Treatment A_3	Treatment B_3

In animal E, effect of treatment B is given by $\{B_2 - \frac{1}{2}(A_1 + A_3)\}$ and in animal F, by $\{\frac{1}{2}(B_1 + B_3) - A_2\}$ removing the residual (linear) effect over periods in each of the animals. The assumption made in this case is that expected performance of each of the animals in Period II can be estimated by linear interpolation between Periods I and III (by use of orthogonal polynomials).

More treatments can be compared by this method provided a pair of animals is available for each pair of treatment comparisons; for instance, for 4 treatments, 6 comparisons are possible taking 2 treatments at a time (*see* Chapter "**Probability**" for calculation of combinations) and 6 pairs of animals are required. Thus the design is powerful enough to give accurate results even with relatively smaller number of animals because each animal acts as its own control also.

Let us take-up the same aspect in statistical terms; suppose two treatments A and B were tested for two periods (I and II) on two sets (E and F) of n animals each, the set E animals were given Treatment A in period I and B in period II; *vice versa* in case of set F; the lay-out will be:

	Sets of r animals each	
Periods	**E**	**F**
I	A	B
II	B	A

Ignoring residual effects, the treatment difference is obviously the values of treatment A in periods I and II as a deviation of values of treatment B in periods I and II; i.e. $(P_IA + P_{II}A) - (P_IB + P_{II}B)$ which, by rearrangement is $(P_I - P_{II}) \times (A - B)$ or interaction between treatment and periods (PT). In other words, treatment difference is

confounded with PT effect and hence, testing treatment difference becomes less accurate.

Suppose, one more period (III) is added to repeat the same treatments as in period I, the lay-out will be as follows:

| Periods | Sets of r animals each | |
	E	F
I	A	B
II	B	A
III	A	B

Now, PT has υ of 2 which can be divided into its orthogonal components (linear, PT_L and quadratic, PT_Q) on $\upsilon = 1$ each where $PT_L = (P_{III} - P_I) \times (A - B)$ and $PT_Q = (P_I - 2 \times P_{II} + P_{III}) \times (A - B)$; of these, the former can not give any information about treatment differences and only the latter can.

Alternatively, if one more period (IV) is added to repeat the same treatments as in period II, the lay-out will be as follows:

| Periods | Sets of r animals each | |
	E	F
I	A	B
II	B	A
III	A	B
IV	B	A

Now, PT has υ of 3 which can be divided into its orthogonal components (linear, PT_L, quadratic, PT_Q and cubic, PT_C) on $\upsilon = 1$ each where $PT_L = (-3P_I - P_{II} + P_{III} + 3P_{IV}) \times (A - B)$, $PT_Q = (P_I - P_{II} - P_{III} + P_{IV}) \times (A - B)$ and $PT_C = (3 \times P_{II} - P_I - 3 \times P_{III} + P_{IV}) \times (A - B)$. In this case, the quadratic component can not give any information about treatment differences whereas, the other two components provide. Since higher order interactions often tend to be not significant, it is advisable to prefer higher order interactions. But, calculations become more and more complex as the degree of the equation advances. In any case, in animal experiments, cubic component itself is less likely and hence, treatment difference can be estimated on the cubic effect contrast $(3 \times P_{II} - P_I - 3 \times P_{III} + P_{IV}) \times (A - B)$.

Note: Orthogonal contrasts are given in Appendix 9; accordingly, for $n = 3$ (3 periods), linear contrasts are –1, 0 and 1; quadratic are 1, –2 and 1; therefore, $PT_L = (-P_I + 0 \times P_{II} + P_{III}) \times (A - B)$ or $PT_L = (P_{III} - P_I) \times (A - B)$. Similarly, $PT_Q = (P_I - 2 \times P_{II} + P_{III}) \times (A - B)$. On the same lines, linear, quadratic and cubic equations are derived for $n = 4$ (4 periods) with contrasts being –3, –1, 1, 3 (linear), 1, –1, –1, 1 (quadratic) and –1, 3, –3, 1 (cubic).

Extending the above discussion, for k periods, PT will have $\upsilon = (k - 1)$ and if the treatments are switched back and forth as shown above, the highest $(k - 1)$th degree component of PT interaction provides the estimate of treatment effect with least chance of confounding with PT. Further, if a_i's are binomial coefficients (calculated as $^{k-1}C_i$; see Chapter "**Probability**" for details), the $(k - 1)$th degree component of PT interaction is given by the formula: $\{P_k - a_1 P_{k-1} + a_2 P_{k-2} - a_3 P_{k-3} + \ldots + (-1)^{k-1} P_I)\} \times (A - B)$.

3.2.1 Estimation of Treatment Effects

Each animal in this design will yield data for all the k periods albeit on different treatments. Each of these observations can be converted into $(k-1)$th degree component of PT interaction is given by the formula given above: $\{P_k - a_1 P_{k-1} + a_2 P_{k-2} - a_3 P_{k-3} + \ldots + (-1)^{k-1} P_1)\}$ and designated x_{ij} meaning value of jth animal of ith set ($i = 1, 2$ and $j = 1, 2, \ldots r$). If there are 2 sets of animals, there will be $2r$ values.

3.2.1.1 Without blocking

If $2r$ animals are allotted at random to the two sets (without forming into blocks), the ANOVA will be as follows:

$$\text{Total SS} = x_{..}^2 - \frac{(x_{..})^2}{2r}$$

$$\text{SS due to treatments } SS_T = \frac{\left(\sum_{j=1}^{r} x_{1j} - \sum_{j=1}^{r} x_{2j}\right)^2}{2r} \text{ on } \upsilon = 1 \text{ and}$$

SS due to error, SSE = Total SS $- SS_T$ on $\upsilon = 2 \times (r-1)$

3.2.1.2 With blocking

If animals were paired on a criterion and members of each pair allotted at random to the two sets, the ANOVA will be as follows:

$$\text{Total SS} = x_{..}^2 - \frac{(x_{..})^2}{2r}, \quad \text{SS due to treatments } SS_T = \frac{\left(\sum_{j=1}^{r} x_{1j} - \sum_{j=1}^{r} x_{2j}\right)^2}{2r} \text{ on } \upsilon = 1, \text{ SS}$$

$$\text{between pairs, } SS_P = \frac{\sum_{j=1}^{r}\left(x_{1j} + x_{2j}\right)^2}{2} - \frac{(x_{..})^2}{2r} \text{ on } \upsilon = 1 \text{ SS due to error, SSE = Total SS} -$$

$SS_T - SS_P$ on $\upsilon = (r-1)$.

3.2.1.3 Example (with blocking)

An experiment with 10 pairs of piglets ($r = 10$; number of sets = 2) was designed to test two diets of varying Calorie–Protein (CP) ratio *viz.* 120 and 140 on weight gain (kg) over 3 periods of 15 days each. One of each pair was allotted at random to the treatments in each of the periods; set 1 was given treatments A, B and A whereas, set 2 was given B, A and B during period 1, 2 and 3, respectively forming a switch-back trial. The data collected were as follows (each one of the pair receiving treatments A, B and A, and B, A and B during periods 1, 2 and 3, respectively):

Pairs	Period I		Period II		Period III	
	A	B	B	A	A	B
1	4.00	6.25	6.00	4.00	4.25	5.75
2	3.50	6.25	5.75	3.75	3.75	6.00
3	4.50	7.00	7.00	4.75	4.50	7.00
4	3.25	6.50	6.50	3.75	3.75	6.75
5	3.75	6.50	6.00	4.00	4.00	6.25
6	3.50	6.25	5.50	3.50	3.75	6.00
7	4.00	7.25	7.00	4.25	4.00	7.00
8	2.75	6.25	6.00	3.00	3.25	6.25
9	3.75	7.00	6.75	3.75	4.00	7.00
10	4.00	6.50	6.50	4.25	4.00	6.50

The above data needs re-tabulation to facilitate application of orthogonal polynomials:

1st member of pair ↓	Set 1			2nd member of pair ↓	Set 2		
	Period I	Period II	Period III		Period I	Period II	Period III
	A	B	A		B	A	B
1	4.00	6.00	4.25	1	6.25	4.00	5.75
2	3.50	5.75	3.75	2	6.25	3.75	6.00
3	4.50	7.00	4.50	3	7.00	4.75	7.00
4	3.25	6.50	3.75	4	6.50	3.75	6.75
5	3.75	6.00	4.00	5	6.50	4.00	6.25
6	3.50	5.50	3.75	6	6.25	3.50	6.00
7	4.00	7.00	4.00	7	7.25	4.25	7.00
8	2.75	6.00	3.25	8	6.25	3.00	6.25
9	3.75	6.75	4.00	9	7.00	3.75	7.00
10	4.00	6.50	4.00	10	6.50	4.25	6.50

As discussed in **Section 3.2** above, linear contrast do not separate treatment effects and therefore, contrasts pertaining to quadratic degree are applied for each piglet value within each set i.e. $(P_I - 2 \times P_{II} + P_{III})$; for instance, the values corresponding to periods I, II and III of 1st member of the pair 1 (x_{11}) (4.00, 6.00, 4.25) will be converted to $(4.00 - 2 \times 6.00 + 4.25) = -3.75$; for x_{12}, it will be $(3.50 - 2 \times 5.75 + 3.75) = -4.25$ and so on; these values are tabulated below:

Pair	1	2	3	4	5	6	7	8	9	10	Total
1st member	-3.75	-4.25	-5.00	-6.00	-4.25	-3.75	-6.00	-6.00	-5.75	-5.00	-49.75
2nd member	4.00	4.75	4.50	5.75	4.75	5.25	5.75	6.50	6.50	4.50	52.25

$x.. = 52.25 - 49.75 = 2.50; x^2.. = 535.1250; \sum\limits_{j=1}^{10} x_{1j} = -49.75$ and $\sum\limits_{j=1}^{10} x_{2j} = 52.25$; Total SS

$= 535.1250 - (2.5)^2 \div 20 = 534.8125$; SST $= (-49.75 - 52.25)^2 \div 20 = 260.2563$; SSP $= (-3.75 + 4.00)^2 + (-4.25 + 4.75)^2 + \dots + (-5.00 + 4.50)^2 \div 2 = 2.8750$ and SSE $= 271.9937$. With these, ANOVA table can be set–up as follows:

H_0: Treatments have no significant effect on weight gain in piglets

Source	v	SS	MSS	F
Total	19	535.1250		
Pairs	9	2.8750	0.3194	< 1
Treatments	1	260.2563	260.2563	8.612
Error	9	271.9937	30.2215	

Table value of $F_{0.05, 1, 9} = 5.12$

Calculated value of F is > table value and hence, H_0 is liable to be rejected.

3.3 General

Both switch-over and switch-back designs are not suitable to measure long-term and cumulative effects and when a strong residual effect is suspected. On the same lines, if a treatment affects animal adversely, the designs are unsuitable as in the case of extremely low plane of nutrition rendering the animal permanently affected making the residual and main effects non–additive. There is another limitation in that number of treatments can not exceed number of periods in both designs; under such circumstance, incomplete block design, balanced carefully to residual effects, can be used. But for these, both designs are very efficient in obtaining accurate information with smaller number of animals. Incomplete block designs are not commonly employed in animal science; in any case, only a brief account of it is given in **Section 5.3** later in this Chapter.

4. HIERARCHICAL OR NESTED CLASSIFICATION (MODEL III)

The discussions on three-factor ANOVA including Latin-squares, Switch-over and Switch-back trials are primarily fixed models (Model I). In these designs of collecting data, all combination of factors (in rows and columns) is considered; hence, such designs are also referred to as **crossed** designs. But, it is possible all such combinations may not be possible and/or relevant and one factor may occur in combination of a second factor whereas another level of the same factor may appear in combination with different levels or forms of the second factor (usually the 2nd factor being at random). This is particularly true in Population Genetics for estimation of heritability, breeding value, etc. In such cases, typically there will be a super-classification containing a sub-group which, in turn, will have another sub-group. Selected (known, fixed) sires are mated at random to dams to obtain progenies on which measurement(s) is (are) made. Since groups within groups are encountered, such classification is also referred to as **Nested** or **Hierarchical** classification. Examples on this type of data are given in section on **Animal genetics** in Chapter "**Statistics in specific veterinary fields**". However, such data can also be available in other fields of study as well; for instance, nutrition, animal management, etc. hence, a brief account of the design is as follows:

4.1 One Level Nesting

4.1.1 Data Structure

Let us assume there are p factors ($i = 1, 2 \ldots p$) each of them in combination with q levels ($j = 1, 2 \ldots q$, distinct for each p) of another factor and each combination has r observations ($k = 1, 2 \ldots r$). The data structure ($p = 4$ and $q = 4$) with usual notations for sums and sums of squares will be as follows:

Factor A		1				2				3				4		
Factor B	1	2	3	4	5	6	7	8	9	10	11	12	13	14	15	16
	x_{111}	x_{121}	x_{141}													x_{1161}
						x_{272}										
									x_{393}							
		x_{124}														
$x_{ij\cdot}$ (Factor B totals)	$x_{11\cdot}$	$x_{12\cdot}$	$x_{13\cdot}$							$x_{110\cdot}$						$x_{116\cdot}$
n_{ij}	n_{11}	n_{12}	n_{13}	n_{14}	n_{21}	n_{22}	n_{23}	n_{24}	n_{31}	n_{32}	n_{33}	n_{34}	n_{41}	n_{42}	n_{43}	n_{44}
$x_{i\cdot\cdot}$ (Factor A totals)		$x_{1\cdot\cdot}$				$x_{2\cdot\cdot}$				$x_{3\cdot\cdot}$				$x_{4\cdot\cdot}$		
$n_{i\cdot}$		$n_{1\cdot}$				$n_{2\cdot}$				$n_{3\cdot}$				$n_{4\cdot}$		
Grand total						$x\ldots$ on total observations of $n_{\cdot\cdot}$										

Sum of squares of all observations, regardless of factors A and B, is designated $x^2\ldots$

which is otherwise, $\sum\limits_{i=1}^{p}\sum\limits_{j=1}^{q}\sum\limits_{k=1}^{r} x_{ijk}^2$; on the same lines, it is easy to visualize that $x_{ij\cdot}$, $x_{i\cdot\cdot}$,

$x\ldots$, $n_{i\cdot}$ and $n_{\cdot\cdot}$ represent $\sum\limits_{k=1}^{r} x_{ijk}$, $\sum\limits_{j=1}^{q}\sum\limits_{k=1}^{r} x_{ijk}$, $\sum\limits_{i=1}^{p}\sum\limits_{j=1}^{q}\sum\limits_{k=1}^{r} x_{ijk}$, $\sum\limits_{j=1}^{q} n_{ij}$ and $\sum\limits_{i=1}^{p}\sum\limits_{j=1}^{q} n_{ij}$, respectively. It is important to note that $x^2\ldots \neq (x\ldots)^2$. The formulae given below are valid even for unequal number of observations.

4.1.2 Analysis of Data

Correction factor, $C = (x\ldots)^2 \div n_{\cdot\cdot}$
Total SS $= x^2\ldots - C$ on $v = (pqr - 1)$

SS due to factor A, $SS_A = \sum\limits_{i=1}^{p} \dfrac{(x_{i\cdot\cdot})^2}{n_{i\cdot}} - C$ on $v = (p - 1)$

SS due to factor B, $SS_B = \sum\limits_{i=1}^{p}\sum\limits_{j=1}^{q} \dfrac{(x_{ij\cdot})^2}{n_{ij}} - C$ on $v = (q - 1)$

SS due to factor B within factor A, $SS_{B/A} = (SS_B - SS_A)$ or $\sum_{i=1}^{p}\sum_{j=1}^{q}\frac{\left(x_{ij\cdot}\right)^2}{n_{ij}} - \sum_{i=1}^{p}\frac{\left(x_{i\cdot\cdot}\right)^2}{n_{i\cdot}}$ on $\upsilon = p(q-1)$.

SS due to error, SS_E = Total SS $- SS_A - SS_{B/A}$; or Total SS $- SS_B$ on $\upsilon = pq(r-1)$.

H_0's:
1. There is no difference between levels or forms of factor A and
2. There is no difference between levels or forms of factor B within factor A

Source	υ	SS	MSS	F
Total	$pqr - 1$			
Factor A	$p - 1$	SS_A	MSS_A	$MSS_A \div MSS_{A/B}$
Factor B	$pq - 1$	SS_B		
Factor B/A	$p(q - 1)$	$SS_{A/B}$	$MSS_{A/B}$	$MSS_{A/B} \div MSS_E$
Error	$pq(r - 1)$	SS_E	MSS_E	

Note: Denominator for calculation of F value to test effect of Factor A is $MSS_{A/B}$ but not MSS_E.

Note:
1. In genetic studies, Factor A will be usually sires and Factor B dams; each sire (fixed effect) mated to different dams (random effect) to get progenies on whom the measurements (x_{ijk}) are made; obviously, all sires can't be mated to all dams. Value of q need not be same under all p's and value of k's (n_{ij}'s) need not be same in all pq's; weightages are given to unequal number of observations, if any. The expectation mean squares are equated to the MSS to calculate components of variance for further computations like heritability, correlations, etc.

2. In addition, it is not always possible to obtain data on sires and dams of the progenies (full–sib data), especially in large animal breeding. Data on either sire or dam, usually the latter, only will be available (half-sib data). With such data, components of variance due to error and dam (or sire) will be calculated for further computations.

3. For more, *see* Section **Animal Genetics** in Chapter "**Statistics in specific veterinary fields**".

4.1.3 Example

The following example on effect of different drugs hemoglobin levels (g%) in dogs is considered. Let us assume there are 3 drugs ($i = 1, 2, 3$) each of them in obtained from three different sources ($j = 1, 2, 3$, distinct for each drug) and each of the drugs was tried on 6 dogs ($k = 1, 2, \ldots 6$). The results on hemoglobin levels (g %) was as follows: ($n_{ij} = 6$, $n_{i\cdot} = 16$ and $n.. = 54$)

Drugs	A				B			C	
Sources	1	2	3	4	5	6	7	8	9
x_{ijk}'s	8.00	8.25	8.00	10.00	12.00	11.75	9.00	9.50	10.00
	8.25	8.50	9.00	12.00	11.00	11.50	9.25	9.50	9.50
	8.00	8.25	8.50	10.75	11.25	11.00	9.75	9.75	10.00
	7.75	8.50	8.00	10.25	11.00	11.25	9.00	9.25	9.00
	8.00	8.00	8.25	11.00	10.75	10.75	9.25	9.50	9.25

(Contd.)

(Contd.)

Drugs		A			B			C	
Sources	1	2	3	4	5	6	7	8	9
	8.00	8.00	8.00	11.25	11.00	11.00	9.50	9.75	9.75
x_{ij}	48.00	49.50	49.75	65.25	67.00	67.25	56.50	57.25	57.50
$x_{i..}$		147.25			199.50			171.25	
$x...$			518.00; $C = (518^2 \div 54) = 4968.9630$						
$x^2...$			5052.5; Total SS $= (5052.5 - C) = 83.5370$						

SS due to drugs, $SS_D = \{(147.25^2 + 199.50^2 + 171.25^2) \div 18\} - C = 76.0023$
SS due to sources, $SS_S = \{(48^2 + 49.50^2 + ... + 57.5^2) \div 6\} - C = 76.7870$
SS due to sources within drugs, $SS_{S/D} = SS_S - SSD = 0.7847$
SS due to error, $SS_E = $ Total SS $- SS_S = 6.7500$
The ANOVA table is as follows:
H_0's:
1. There is no difference between drugs on hemoglobin levels and
2. There is no difference between sources of each of the drugs

Source	v	SS	MSS	F
Total	53			
Drugs	2	76.0023	38.0012	253.341
Sources	8	76.7870		
Sources within drugs	6	0.7847	0.1308	< 1
Error	45	6.7500	0.1500	

Table value of $F_{0.05, 2, 45} = 2.81$

Based on the calculated value of F, it can be concluded that effect of drugs on hemoglobin levels was significant and sources of drugs were not significantly different.

5. OTHER DESIGNS

5.1 Split-Plot Design

This is yet another design more popular in agricultural experiments used when one of the factors requires more experiment material than others. Owing to its limited use, one numerical example is given below:

5.1.1 *Example*

The following data corresponds to a large dairy farm maintained on pasture, each having four separate areas (split plots). Treatments were applied on pastures ($i = 4$) with additional mineral supplements to split plots ($k = 2$). The experiment was conducted on three replications (blocks; $j = 3$; $l = 3$). The data on inter-calving period (yrs) is tabulated below:

Plot	Block	Pasture	Mineral	ICP	Plot	Block	Pasture	Mineral	ICP
1	2	1	1	2.00	7	3	1	1	1.50
1	2	1	2	3.00	7	3	1	2	1.50
2	2	3	2	1.50	8	3	4	2	1.50
2	2	3	1	1.75	8	3	4	1	1.50
3	2	2	1	3.50	9	1	1	2	2.50
3	2	2	2	3.25	9	1	1	1	2.75
4	2	4	1	1.25	10	1	2	1	3.75
4	2	4	2	1.50	10	1	2	2	3.25
5	3	2	2	3.75	11	1	3	1	2.75
5	3	2	1	3.00	11	1	3	2	2.25
6	3	3	2	1.75	12	1	4	2	1.25
6	3	3	1	2.00	12	1	4	1	1.50

Uncorrected sum of squares of all the 24 observations = 138.9375 (x^2....); Total SS = 16.3099. The above data can be rearranged into 2×2 tables as follows to facilitate further calculations:

Totals, $n_{ij\cdot} = 2$	Block 1	Block 2	Block 3	Factor A totals, $x_i\ldots$, $n_i\cdot\cdot = 6$
Pasture 1	5.25	5.00	3.00	13.25
Pasture 2	7.00	6.75	6.75	20.50
Pasture 3	5.00	3.25	3.75	12.00
Pasture 4	2.75	2.75	3.00	8.50
Block totals, $x_{\cdot j\cdot}$, $n_{\cdot j} = 8$	20.00	17.75	16.50	$x\ldots = 54.25$, $n\ldots = 24$

Note: Totals in cells represent $x_{ij}\cdot$.

This table subjected to ANOVA as per RBD with 2 observations per cell yielded the following results (see Chapter "**Two-factor analysis of variance**" for details of procedure):

SS due to blocks, $SS_B = 0.7865$; SS due to pasture treatment, $SS_P = 12.7161$ and SS due to interaction, $SS_{B \times P} = 1.5885$ (it is otherwise SS due to error for this table)

Similarly, another 2×2 table can be formed thus:

Totals, $n_{i\cdot k} = 3$	Mineral 1	Mineral 2	Factor A totals, $x_i\ldots$, $n_i\cdot\cdot = 6$
Pasture 1	6.25	7.00	13.25
Pasture 2	10.25	10.25	20.50
Pasture 3	6.50	5.50	12.00
Pasture 4	4.25	4.25	8.50
Factor B totals, $x_{\cdot\cdot k}$, $n_{\cdot\cdot k} = 12$	27.25	27.00	$x\ldots = 54.25$, $n\ldots = 24$

Note: Totals in the cells represent $x_{i\cdot k}\cdot$.

This table subjected to ANOVA as per RBD with 3 observations per cell yielded the following results (*see* Chapter "**Two-factor analysis of variance**" for details of procedure):

SS due to mineral supplements, $SS_M = 0.0026$, SS due to interaction, $SS_{P \times M} = 0.2579$ and SS due to error, $SS_E =$ Total SS $- SS_B - SS_P - SS_{B \times P} - SS_M - SS_{P \times M} = 0.9583$ (it is otherwise SS due to error for this table). With these, ANOVA table can be set-up:

H_0's:

1. There is no effect of pasture treatment on inter-calving period
2. There is no effect of mineral supplements on inter-calving period
3. There is no effect of pasture x mineral supplement interaction on inter-calving period

Source	v	SS	MSS	F
Total	23	16.3099		
Blocks	2	0.7865	0.3933	
Pasture treatment (A)	3	12.7161	4.2387	16.013
Main-plot error, $SS_{B \times P}$	6	1.5885	0.2647	
Mineral supplement (B)	1	0.0026	0.0026	< 1
Pasture x Mineral supplement (A × B)	3	0.2579	0.0860	< 1
Split–plot Error, SS_E	8	0.9583	0.1198	

Table value of $F_{0.05,3,6} = 4.76$

Based on the calculated value of F, H_0 No. 1 can be rejected. Comparison of means is by LSD procedure is done for effects of factors A, B and A × B interactions, whichever statistically significant. The procedure is described in Chapter "**One-factor analysis of variance**"; value used as the denominator for calculating F value is considered as MSS_E for calculating LSD for the effect concerned. In this example, only effects of Factor A (Pasture treatments) has been found to be significant for which $MSS_{B \times P}$ will be used as SS_E. The comparison of means ($\alpha = 0.05$) is shown below:

Pasture treatment	1	2	3	4	LSD, yrs
Means, yrs	2.208[b]	3.417[c]	2.000[ab]	1.417[a]	0.727

Since lower ICP is desirable, superscripts are allotted from lower value onwards. Values bearing common letter superscript are not significantly different (P < 0.05)

5.2   Double–Blocking

For instance, if "Breeds" form the main block and each of them is used for testing some diets during each of their lactations, "Lactation" forms the second blocking which is nested within the breed. Such situations are referred to as "Double-blocking". Data structure with b breeds (main blocks) with l lactations in each breed (nested within breed) and t treatment within each lactation, utilizing blt number of animals is shown below considering $b = 2$ ($i = 2$), $l = 3$ ($j = 3$) and $t = 3$ ($k = 3$) requiring 18 animals (305 d milk yields in '000 kg are given):

Breeds		A				B			
		Lactations		$x_{i \cdot k}$		Lactations		$x_{i \cdot k}$	$x_{\cdot \cdot k}$
Treatments	I	I	II		I	II	III		
1	4.1	6.8	7.0	17.9	5.8	8.3	8.4	22.5	40.4
2	4.9	8.6	8.7	22.2	7.9	10.8	11.0	29.7	51.9
3	6.9	11.3	11.0	29.2	11.6	12.0	11.9	35.5	64.7
$x_{ij \cdot}$	15.9	26.7	26.7		25.3	31.1	31.3	$x...$	157.0
$x_{i \cdot \cdot}$		69.3				87.7		$x^2...$	1475.32

Number of observations: Breeds = 9 ($n_{i \cdot \cdot}$), Lactations within breed = 3 ($n_{ij \cdot}$), Treatments = 6 ($n_{\cdot \cdot k}$), Treatment × Breed interaction = 3 ($n_{i \cdot k}$), Total ($n...$) = 18

Since both nesting of blocks and treatments in blocks are involved, ANOVA has to be performed involving both as follows:

H_0's:
1. There is no effect of breeds on 305 d lactation milk yield
2. There is no effect of lactations within breeds on 305 d lactation milk yield
3. There is no effect of treatments on 305 d lactation milk yield
4. There is no effect of breed × treatment interactions on 305 d lactation milk yield

The sums of squares are calculated as follows:

Correction factor, $C = (x...)^2 \div n... = 1368.3889$

Total SS $= x^2... - C = 106.9311$

SS due to breeds, $SS_B = \sum_{i=1}^{b} \dfrac{(x_{i \cdot \cdot})^2}{n_{i \cdot \cdot}} - C = 18.8089$ on $\upsilon = (b-1) = 1$

SS due to lactations within breeds, $SS_{L/B} = \sum_{i=1}^{b} \sum_{j=1}^{l} \dfrac{(x_{ij \cdot})^2}{n_{ij \cdot}} - \sum_{i=1}^{b} \dfrac{(x_{i \cdot \cdot})^2}{n_{i \cdot \cdot}} = 33.6622$ on $\upsilon = b(l-1) = 4$

SS due to treatments, $SS_T = \sum_{k=1}^{t} \dfrac{(x_{\cdot \cdot k})^2}{n_{\cdot \cdot k}} - C = 49.2544$ on $\upsilon = (t-1) = 2$

SS due to breed × treatment interaction, $SS_{B \times T} = \sum_{i=1}^{b} \sum_{k=1}^{t} \dfrac{(x_{i \cdot k})^2}{n_{i \cdot k}} - C - SS_B - SS_T = 0.7078$ on $\upsilon = (b-1)(t-1) = 2$ and finally, SS due to error, SSE = Total SS $- SS_B - SS_{L/B} - SS_T - SS_{B \times T} = 4.4978$ on $\upsilon = b(l-1)(t-1) = 8$. The ANOVA table will be as follows:

Source	υ	SS	MSS	F
Total	17	16.3099		
Breeds	1	18.8089	18.8089	33.454
Lactation within breeds	4	33.6622	8.4156	14.968
Treatment	2	49.2544	24.6272	43.803
Breed × Treatment	2	0.7078	0.3539	< 1
Error	8	4.4978	0.5622	

Table values of $F_{0.05,1,8} = 5.32$, $F_{0.05,4,8} = 3.84$, $F_{0.05,2,8} = 4.46$

Based on the calculated values of F, except H_0 No. 4, the others are liable to be rejected.

Note: Several types of blocking can be considered; like body weights within sex, breeds within lactation, egg production within season of hatch, etc. In each case, ANOVA can be developed depending on H_0's.

5.3 Balanced Incomplete Block Design

This design used in agricultural experiments has limited use in Animal Science. As the name indicates, instead of each block containing all treatments, it will have lesser number of treatments; hence, it is an incomplete block. It is qualified as **balanced** because the treatments are so allotted that each treatment pair occurs for the same number of times in each block. Suppose seven treatments have to be allotted to seven blocks, in an RBD, the minimum number of animals required will be 49 (one observation per cell). In simple terms, each treatment has seven determinations (replications, r). If we can allot the treatments in such a way that only 3 blocks (columns) are allotted in each row of (treatment); only 21 animals would suffice. In this case, number of blocks, $b = 7$, number of treatments, $t = 7$ and number of replications, $r = 3$. One such arrangement can be:

				Blocks			
Treatments	1	2	3	4	5	6	7
1	T_1	T_1	T_1				
2		T_2	T_2	T_2			
3	T_3			T_3		T_3	
4			T_4			T_4	T_4
5	T_5				T_5		T_5
6		T_6			T_6	T_6	
7		T_7		T7			T_7

It the above table, each block (column) has 3 treatments, each row (treatment) has 3 blocks allotted to it (3 replications, $r = 3$) and the next very important aspect, in any two rows or columns, only once a par of treatments appear one below the other (rows) or side by side (columns). To put it in other words, if, in the above table, 1 is allotted for presence of each treatment and 0 for no treatment being allotted, the sum of products over any two rows or columns will be 1. This number of appearance of a pair of treatments is designated λ whose value is 1 in the above arrangement.

Unlike agricultural plots, animals are not static; hence, the above table can be rewritten as:

Replications				Blocks			
	1	2	3	4	5	6	7
1	T_1	T_1	T_1	T_2	T_2	T_3	T_4
2	T_3	T_6	T_2	T_3	T_5	T_4	T_5
3	T_5	T_7	T_4	T_7	T_6	T_6	T_7

Another example of arrangement of 7 treatments in 4 replications is given below:

Replications	Blocks						
	1	2	3	4	5	6	7
1	T_1	T_3	T_7	T_1	T_2	T_5	T_2
2	T_4	T_6	T_1	T_2	T_7	T_3	T_4
3	T_7	T_5	T_2	T_3	T_3	T_4	T_5
4	T_6	T_7	T_5	T_6	T_4	T_1	T_6

It is evident in the above table that none of the blocks is complete but has only 4 treatments and every pair of treatments occurs only twice in any block pair; in 1st and 2nd blocks, treatments 6 and 7, in 2nd and 3rd blocks, treatments 7 and 5 and so on. Blocks can represent litters (in pigs, mice, rabbits, etc.) and replications, the animals in each block.

Let us consider a numerical example for the above set of incomplete blocks where $t = 7$, $r = 4$, $k = 4$ (Block size) and $\lambda = 1$:

5.3.1 Example

The following data pertains to weekly weight gain (g) of full-sibs (hens) from 7 genetic groups subjected to 7 different diets.

Hens	Genetic groups (Blocks)						
	1	2	3	4	5	6	7
1	$86.3T_1$	$105.0T_3$	$229.0T_7$	$86.5T_1$	$99.2T_2$	$98.5T_5$	$99.5T_2$
2	$123.5T_4$	$182.9T_6$	$87.2T_1$	$90.0T_2$	$217.3T_7$	$115.0T_3$	$132.0T_4$
3	$209.8T_7$	$97.5T_5$	$98.1T_2$	$103.0T_3$	$105.4T_3$	$141.7T_4$	$96.8T_5$
4	$173.8T_6$	$209.8T_7$	$90.0T_5$	$195.5T_6$	$150.0T_4$	$86.0T_1$	$185.3T_6$
Totals	593.4	595.2	504.3	475.0	571.9	441.2	513.6

Grand Total = 3694.6, Crude Total SS = 549203.88

	Totals			
Treatments (T_i)	All blocks containing the treatment*	Blocks (B_j)	$(2) \div r$	$Q_i = (3) - (4)$
(1)	(2)	(3)	(4)	(5)
346.0	2013.9	593.4	503.475	89.925
386.8	2064.8	595.2	516.200	79.000
428.4	2083.3	504.3	520.825	−16.525
547.2	2120.1	475.0	530.025	−55.025
382.8	2054.3	571.9	513.575	58.325
737.5	2177.2	441.2	544.300	−103.100
865.9	2264.8	513.6	566.200	−52.600
3694.6	14778.4 (Check = 3694.6 × 4)	3694.6	3694.600	

* Totals of blocks 1, 3, 4 and 6 for T_1, blocks 3, 4, 5 and 7 for T_2 .. Blocks 1, 2, 3 and 5 for T_7.

$$\sum_{i=1}^{7} T_i^2 = 2192509.54, \quad \sum_{j=1}^{7} B_j^2 = 1971842.10, \quad \sum_{i=1}^{7} Q_i^2 = 34426.5075 \quad C = 3694.6^2 \div 28 =$$

108078.8629.

Total SS = Crude SS – C = 61701.41

SS due to genetic groups (unadjusted), $SS_G' = \sum_{j=1}^{7} \dfrac{B_j^2}{r} - C = 5458.0550$

SS due to treatments (adjusted), $SS_T = \dfrac{k}{\lambda t} \sum_{i=1}^{7} Q_i^2$ where k = block size (4 in this

example). Hence, $SS_T = \dfrac{4}{7} \sum_{i=1}^{7} Q_i^2 = 19672.2900$ and finally, Intra-block error, SSE = Total

SS – SS_G' – SS_T = 405.6806

The ANOVA table will be:

H_0: There is no difference in body weight gain due to treatments

Source	υ	SS	MSS	F
Total	27	61701.4100		
Blocks (unadjusted)	6	5458.0550	909.6758	< 1
Treatments (adjusted)	6	19672.2900	3278.7150	1.345
Error	15	36571.0650	2438.0710	

Table values of $F_{0.05, 6, 15} = 2.79$

Since calculated value of F is < table value, H_0 appears to be acceptable.

Note:

1. Unadjusted SS due to genetic groups, SS_G', if found significant, can be adjusted as follows:

Unadjusted SS due to Treatments, $SS_T' = \sum_{i=1}^{7} \dfrac{k}{\lambda t} Q_i$ and adjusted SS due to genetic groups, $SS_G =$

$SS_G' + SS_T - SS_T'$ on $\upsilon = (t-1) = 7$ to calculate MSS_G. It can be tested against MSS_E (2438.0710 in this example)

2. If SS_T is significant, standard error of difference between two treatments can be calculated as

$\sqrt{\dfrac{2kMSS_E}{\lambda t}}$ and LSD calculated as per the procedure described in Chapter "**One–factor analysis**

of variance". Adjusted treatment means are given by Overall Mean + $\dfrac{k}{\lambda t} Q_i$ where Overall

Mean = Grand Total ÷ (rt); in this example, overall mean = (3694.6 ÷ 28) = 131.95. Likewise, adjusted treatment means (g) are:

Treatments	1	2	3	4	5	6	7
Means, g	183.34	177.09	122.51	100.51	165.28	73.04	101.89

Obviously, a difference of nearly 110 g is not detected significant; but, the difference is definitely of practical importance. Hence, although H_0 appears acceptable, it needs to be verified again. An experiment with complete RBD is preferable because it is more efficient than incomplete block design. However, LSD in the above example was 121.94 g which proves that the treatments were indeed statistically homogeneous.

6. EMS IN DIFFERENT MODELS

Calculation of expectation mean square (EMS) and, consequently, the components of variance depend on the model of experimental design; the same is outlined below: (Regardless of the Model, if number of observations are unequal among the cells, suitable weighted number of observations have to be computed; for details *see* Section "**Animal genetics**" in Chapter "**Statistics in specific veterinary fields**")

6.1 RBD

In an RBD, the EMS is defined as follows:

	Model I (Fixed-effect)	**Model II (Random-effect)**
Treatments	$\sigma_e^2 + k\left(\dfrac{\sum_{i=1}^{t} t_i^2}{(t-1)}\right)$	$\sigma_e^2 + k_t^2$
Error	σ_e^2	σ_e^2

k = number of replications (blocks); t = number of treatments

6.2 Two-Factor ANOVA

Two factors, A and B, at levels a and b, respectively in r replications per treatment combination is considered. EMS of an effect contains:

1. Its component of variance times the number of observations used to estimate the factor and
2. Variance component of its interaction with **random effects**, if any, times the number of observations for the interaction.

	Model I (Fixed)	**Model III (A fixed, B random)**
Factor A	$\sigma_e^2 + rb\left(\dfrac{\sum_{i=1}^{a}\alpha_i^2}{(a-1)}\right)$	$\sigma_e^2 + r\sigma_{AB}^2 + rb\left(\dfrac{\sum_{i=1}^{a}\alpha_i^2}{(a-1)}\right)$
Factor B	$\sigma_e^2 + ra\left(\dfrac{\sum_{j=1}^{b}\beta_j^2}{(b-1)}\right)$	$\sigma_e^2 + ra\sigma_B^2$

(Contd.)

(Contd.)

	Model I (Fixed)	**Model III (A fixed, B random)**
Interaction AB	$\sigma_e^2 + r\left(\dfrac{\displaystyle\sum_{i=1}^{a}\sum_{j=1}^{b}(\alpha\beta)_{ij}^2}{(a-1)(b-1)}\right)$	$\sigma_e^2 + r\sigma_{AB}^2$
Error	σ_e^2	σ_e^2

6.3 Mixed model

If the fixed effect, $E^F = \dfrac{\displaystyle\sum_{i=1}^{a}\alpha_i^2}{(a-1)}$, random effect, $E^R = \sigma_e^2$, and k^E is the ratio of total number of observations to that employed to estimate the effect, i.e. $(N \div n^E)$, then EMS of effect E, EMS^E will be the summation of the following:

1. σ_e^2, the MSS_E
2. All effects in a hierarchical order contained within the effect (i.e. lower than the effect concerned) times the number of observations for each of the effects (except for MSS_E)
3. All interactions of the factor concerned with other **random** effects times the number of observations for each of the interactions (except for MSS_E)

Let us develop EMS for a hypothetical design of an experiment. Suppose, in a poultry breeding farm, a nutrition experiment of feeding breeder ration (at p levels of linoleic acid on egg weight; fixed effect) was conducted with s sires each mated to d dams and the crossbred pullets were allotted at w pullets per treatment at random (s, d and w are random effects). The EMS will be as follows:

Source	υ	MSS	EMS
Treatment, P	$p-1$	P	$\sigma_e^2 + w\sigma_{PD}^2 + wd\sigma_{PS}^2 + sdw\left(\dfrac{\displaystyle\sum_{t=1}^{p}\alpha_t^2}{(p-1)}\right)$
Sires, S	$s-1$	S	$\sigma_e^2 + pw\sigma_D^2 + pdw\sigma_S^2$
Dams within sires, D	$s(d-1)$	D	$\sigma_e^2 + pw\sigma_D^2$

(Contd.)

(Contd.)

Source	υ	MSS	EMS
P x S interaction	$(p-1)(s-1)$	PS	$\sigma_e^2 + w\sigma_{PD}^2 + wd\sigma_{PS}^2$
P x D interaction	$s(p-1)(d-1)$	PD	$\sigma_e^2 + w\sigma_{PD}^2$
Error	$sdp(w-1)$	E	σ_e^2

Note: The EMS also help identify the proper MSS to be used as denominator while calculating F for testing significance; for instance, to test P, PS has to be used; similarly, D for S, E for D and PD, and PD for PS so that, if F is > 1, it is due to the effect under test of significance.

16

Factorial Experiments

At the outset, it is very important to note that the ANOVA dealt in Chapters 13, 14 and 15 are also **factorial** to the extent that effect of each of the factors was elucidated. That means, each of the factors was studied in separate experiments; for example, effect of protein levels on growth rate, effect of calcium on egg shell strength, etc. The main constraint was that one of the factors was fixed to study the other factor. If, say two factors A and B each at two **levels** a_1 and a_2 and b_1 and b_2, respectively have to be evaluated in all combinations, the earlier designs or methods become less suitable. In **Factorial experiments** the treatments are the combination of **levels** of different factors involved; hence the terminology. It is important to note that the treatments (all combinations of levels of all factors) so formed can be applied under CRD, RBD or Latin square design. In the example given above, the four treatments possible will be a_1b_1, a_1b_2, a_2b_1 and a_2b_2; each set of observations (replication) gives:

Simple effects	Effect	Estimate	Main effects (Mean of simple effects)
AB_H	Effect of A when B is held at higher level	$a_2b_2 - a_1b_2$	$A = \frac{1}{2}(AB_H + AB_L)$
AB_L	Effect of A when B is held at lower level	$a_2b_1 - a_1b_1$	
A_HB	Effect of B when A is held at higher level	$a_2b_2 - a_2b_1$	$B = \frac{1}{2}(A_HB + A_LB)$
A_LB	Effect of B when A is held at lower level	$a_1b_2 - a_1b_1$	

Without going to the proof involved, it is interesting to note that in a factorial experiment with 2 factors each at 2 levels forming 4 treatments, 2 replications (totally 8 observations) are suffice to result in variance of either of the Main effects to be $\frac{1}{2}(\sigma^2)$; in other words, if r replications are available, variance of the main effects will be $(\sigma^2 \div r)$. In comparison to single-factor designs, factorial experiments need $\frac{1}{2}$ the number of observations.

Notwithstanding the above, it is also possible to test whether factor A has the same effect at two levels of factor B or not and *vice versa*; this is referred to as **two-factor interaction** which is estimated by $\frac{1}{2}[(a_2b_2 - a_1b_2) - (a_2b_1 - a_1b_1)]$ for factor A and $\frac{1}{2}[(a_2b_2 - a_2b_1) - (a_1b_2 - a_1b_1)]$ for factor B. It is obvious that both of them are one and the same; and is referred to as **AB Interaction** (Multiplication by $\frac{1}{2}$ in case of interaction is conventional after Yates who introduced it).

1. TWO-FACTOR EXPERIMENTS

A factorial experiment with two factors each at two levels is a 2×2 or 2^2 Factorial experiment. Similarly, three factors with 2 levels in each will be $2 \times 2 \times 2$ or a 2^3 experiment (totally 8 treatments), two factors with 3 levels in each will be 3×3 or 3^2 experiment (totally 9 treatments) and so on. That means, the base indicates levels and the power, the number of factors. Some times, there could be two factors one at 3 and the other at 2 levels, making a 3×2 factorial experiment with 6 treatments or 3 factors at 2, 3 and 4 levels resulting in $2 \times 3 \times 4$ factorial experiment with 24 treatments. Various such combinations are possible.

1.1 2^2 Factorial Experiment

1.1.1 Notations

Generally practiced notation for main effects and interactions are as follows for a two factor, each at two levels, experiment which can be extended to other combinations of factors and levels:

2^2 Experiment		Factor A (denoted A)		
		Higher level	**Lower level**	**Total**
Factor B	Higher level	ab	b	$b + ab$
(denoted B)	Lower level	a	(1)	$(1) + a$
Total		$a + ab$	$(1) + b$	

Note: Half the difference between column totals is the main effect A; Half the difference between row totals is the Main effect B; Half the difference between diagonals = $\frac{1}{2}[(1) + ab - (a + b)]$ = Interaction effect (denoted AB)

1.1.2 Sum and Sum of Squares

Let us consider Main effect A; its average effect is $\frac{1}{2}[(a_2b_2 - a_1b_2) + (a_2b_1 - a_1b_1)]$ which on expansion will be $\frac{1}{2}(a_2b_2) + \frac{1}{2}(a_2b_1) - \frac{1}{2}(a_1b_2) - \frac{1}{2}(a_1b_1)$; same way, Main effect B = $\frac{1}{2}[(a_2b_2) + (a_1b_2) - (a_2b_1) - (a_1b_1)]$ which on expansion will be $\frac{1}{2}(a_2b_2) + \frac{1}{2}(a_1b_2) - \frac{1}{2}(a_2b_1) - \frac{1}{2}(a_1b_1)$ and Interaction AB is given by $\frac{1}{2}[(a_2b_2 - a_1b_2) - (a_2b_1 - a_1b_1)]$. If the experiment has r replications, $\frac{1}{2}$ will be replaced by $(1 \div 2r)$. Hence, 2 or $2r$ will be the divisor to obtain average (mean) effect A, B and AB. Extending the logic, the multiplier for sum of squares will be $(\frac{1}{2})^2$ or $\frac{1}{4}$ and with r replications, $(1 \div 4r)$ or the divisor for sum of squares will be $4r$.

In generalized terms, if an experiment with n factors each at 2 levels (2^n experiment) is conducted with r replications; divisor for different effects/calculations are tabulated below:

2^n Experiment	Main effect	
n = No. of factors; r = No. of replications	Mean	SS
Divisor	$2^{(n-1)}r$	$2^n r$

Therefore, the multipliers for treatment totals (orthogonal contrasts) and divisors for calculating mean and SS are:

Main effects	Treatment totals (1)	a	b	ab	Sum*	Sum of squares (SS)**	Divisor for Mean	SS
A	-1	1	-1	1	[A]	$[A]^2$	2r	4r
B	-1	-1	1	1	[B]	$[B]^2$		
AB	1	-1	-1	1	[AB]	$[AB]^2$		

* Sum of treatment totals weighted with corresponding multipliers; i.e. [A] = $a + ab - b - (1)$; [B] = $b + ab - a - (1)$ and [AB] = $(1) + ab - a - b$** on $\sigma = 1$

Note: Multiplier for main effect (row) is the product of the multipliers for the other two. For instance, multiplier for (1) of AB is the product of those of A and B with respect to (1); i.e. $(-1) \times (-1)$. It can also be noted that multipliers of any Main effect as well as sum of the products of the multipliers of any two main effects add to zero (analogous to orthogonal polynomials). Hence these are the **orthogonal** (factorial) **Contrasts** used in estimating, sums, means and sum of squares of factorial effects. Such orthogonal contrasts are available for all factorial experiments facilitating computations.

Sum of squares due to treatment, replications, if any, and error are calculated similar to the one showed in Chapter "**Two-factor analysis of variance**" or Chapter "**ANOVA for more than two factors**" in all the factorial experiments. But, the factorial experiment is unique in that the υ available for treatments is partitioned (factorized) into main and interaction effects with υ of 1 each.

1.1.2.1. Yates' algorithm for a 2^2 experiment

Factorial effects can also be calculated by Yates' method of sums and differences which is shown below:

Treatments	Treatment totals*	Cycle 1	Cycle 2	Effect
(1)	(1)	$(1) + a$	$(1) + a + b + ab$	Grand total
a	a	$b + ab$	$a - (1) + ab - b$	A
b	b	$a - (1)$	$ab - a + b - (1)$	B
ab	ab	$ab - b$	$ab - b - a + (1)$	AB

* Total over r replications

The procedure is to add two consecutive values of the previous column starting from the top till all values are covered; this gives values for top half the column being filled. It is followed by subtracting first from the second from two consecutive values of the previous column again from the top of the column till all values are covered; this gives the values for the bottom half of the column being filled. When a column is filled completely, it completes one **cycle**. The procedure is continued till the first value in the column represents grand total or for **n cycles**.

The advantages of this method are quite obvious: one need not know the contrasts which are difficult to find out as the factors increase and **this method is applicable to any 2^n factorial experiment**. The computations are simply mechanical addition and subtraction cycles; **the number of cycles in a 2^n factorial experiment will be** n; even otherwise, end of cycles can be easily visualized when all treatment totals appear into the first cell of the column.

1.1.2.2 Example

The following data refers to a study on the effect of floor space (Factor A, 2 levels, 700 and 900 cm²/bird) and protein content in diet (Factor B, 2 levels, 18 and 22%), totally 4 treatments ($t = 4$), on 6 weeks' weight gain (kg) in broilers over 5 replications ($r = 5$). The results are as follows:

Factor A, cm²/bird	700	900	700	900	
Factor B, %	18	18	22	22	Total (replication)
Treatment notation	(1)	a	b	ab	
1	0.85	1.12	1.28	1.90	5.15
2	0.78	1.21	1.35	1.78	5.12
3	0.82	1.18	1.29	1.89	5.18
4	0.80	1.06	1.40	1.93	5.19
5	0.75	1.10	1.25	1.79	4.89
Treatment total	4.00	5.67	6.57	9.29	Overall = 25.53
Treatment Means	0.800	1.134	1.314	1.858	

Total crude SS = 35.5773, $C = 25.53^2 \div 20 = 32.5890$

Total SS = Total Crude SS − C = 2.9883 on $\upsilon = (rt - 1) = 19$

SS due to replications, $SS_R = \dfrac{5.15^2 + 5.12^2 + 5.18^2 + 5.19^2 + 4.89^2}{t} - C = 0.0154$ on $\upsilon = (r - 1) = 4$

SS due to treatments, $SS_T = \dfrac{4.00^2 + 5.67^2 + 6.57^2 + 9.29^2}{r} - C = 2.9346$ on $\upsilon = (t - 1) = 3$

and SS due to error, SS_E = Total SS − SS_R − SS_T = 0.0383 on $\upsilon = (r - 1) \times (t - 1) = 12$.

SS_T can be partitioned into A, B and AB each on $\upsilon = 1$ by employing the **contrasts** as follows:

Treatments	(1)	a	b	ab	Main effect			
Totals	4.00	5.67	6.57	9.29	Total	SS*	Mean**	sem***
A	−1	1	−1	1	4.39	0.9636	0.439	0.0253
B	−1	−1	1	1	6.19	1.9158	0.619	
AB	1	−1	−1	1	1.05	0.0551	0.105	
						2.9345		

* Divisor $2^n r = 20$, ** Divisor $2^{(n-1)} r = 10$; *** Standard Error of factorial effect Mean = $\sqrt{\dfrac{MSS_E}{r}}$

1.1.2.2.1 *Main effect totals by Yates' algorithm*

Application of Yates' method for the above example is as follows:

Treatments	Treatment totals*	Cycle 1	Cycle 2	Effect
(1)	4.00	9.67	25.53	Grand total
a	5.67	15.86	4.39	A
b	6.57	1.67	6.19	B
ab	9.29	2.72	1.05	AB

* Total over 5 replications

It can be seen that the same values are obtained by this method also.

The final ANOVA table is shown below:

H_0s:

1. There is no effect of floor space on weight gain of broilers
2. There is no effect of protein levels in diet on weight gain of broilers
3. There is no effect of interaction between floor space and protein levels in the diet on weight gain of broilers

Source	v	SS	MSS	F
Total	19	2.9883		
Replications	4	0.0154		
Treatments	(3)	(2.9346)		
A	1	0.9636	0.9636	301.125
B	1	1.9158	1.9158	598.688
AB	1	0.0551	0.0551	17.219
Error	12	0.0383	0.0032	

Table value of $F_{0.05,1,12} = 4.75$

The calculated values of F are > tabulated values and hence all the H_0s are liable for rejection.

Note:

1. Although interaction effects are significant, they were not as profound as the effects of A and B; hence, it is suffice if the conclusions are based on the H_0s already drawn.
2. If one is interested to compare the means of the 4 treatments, it can be done by calculating standard error of difference between two means as $\sqrt{\dfrac{2MSS_E}{r}}$ (= 0.036 kg) and follow with the LSD test explained in Chapter "**One-factor analysis of variance**". The comparison of treatment means is shown below:

Treatments	(1)	*a*	*b*	*ab*	*sem*	LSD, kg
Mean, kg	0.800[d]	1.134[c]	1.314[b]	1.858[a]	0.0253	0.078

Means bearing different superscripts are significantly different (P < 0.05)

1.1.3 *Procedure when AB is Significant*

If interaction AB is significant, as in the above example, a further study of the treatment means is made as follows:

2^2 Experiment weight gain, kg		Floor space, cm²/bird		Difference
		700	900	
Protein, %	18	(1) 0.800[d]	(a) 1.134[c]	– 0.334
	22	(b) 1.314[b]	(ab) 1.858[a]	– 0.544
	Difference	– 0.514	– 0.724	

Standard error of difference = 0.0358 kg; LSD = 0.078 kg

With the fact that *ab* is ideal for broiler growth, it is apparent that when protein level in the diet was not ideal, increasing the floor space allowance to optimum level did compensate although, such an effect was more evident with ideal protein levels in the feed. On the other hand, even with unfavorable floor space, restoring protein levels to ideal value, resulted in an overwhelming compensation in terms of weight gain; albeit, such an effect was the best with *ab*. Hence, protein content in the diet appears to have more influence on weight gain of broilers than floor space allowance.

1.2 Two-Factor Experiment: General

Suppose two factors with *a* and *b* levels, respectively forming totally *ab* treatments are employed in an experiment which may be laid-out as per CRD, RBD or any other design. Hence, υ for different sources of variation will be: Total $(ab - 1)$, Factor A $(a - 1)$, Factor B $(b - 1)$, Interaction AB $(a - 1) \times (b - 1)$. In a 2^2 experiment, AB has υ of only 1 and hence, no further analysis is possible. However, when *a* and/or *b* is (are) > 2, υ of AB interaction will be > 1 and can be further investigated by partitioning AB into as many parts as are υ. The following are generally agreed principles as far as interactions are concerned:

1. When F value for interaction effect is > 1, even if it is not significant, it had better be looked into carefully by comparing the mean values involved.
2. Larger the main effect, larger will be the interactions too.

1.2.1 *Example*

An example on weight gain of broilers on two Calorie–Protein (CP) ratio regimen (Factor A; 140 and 160) with 3 feeding methods (Factor B; Pellets, Mash and Cafeteria) is given below (replications, $r = 6$); obviously, there will be 6 treatments ($t = 6$) and υ for treatments will be 5 which will be split into 1 for Main effect A, 2 for Main effect B and 2 for interaction AB.

Factor A	140			160			
Factor B	Pellets	Mash	Cafeteria	Pellets	Mash	Cafeteria	Total
1	2.01	1.89	1.65	1.87	1.53	1.63	10.58
2	1.94	1.79	1.48	1.74	1.59	1.58	10.12
3	1.86	1.93	1.76	1.82	1.40	1.67	10.44
4	2.05	1.88	1.59	1.61	1.63	1.49	10.25

(Contd.)

(*Contd.*)

Factor A		140			160			
Factor B	Pellets	Mash	Cafeteria	Pellets	Mash	Cafeteria	Total
5	2.00	1.75	1.43	1.73	1.49	1.73	10.13
6	1.91	1.83	1.80	1.82	1.50	1.77	10.63
Total	11.77	11.07	9.71	10.59	9.14	9.87	62.15

Factor A totals: 32.55 and 29.60; Factor B totals: 22.36, 20.21 and 19.58

Total crude SS = 108.3627; $C = (62.15^2 \div 36) = 107.2951$
Total SS = $(108.3627 - 62.15^2 \div 36) = 1.0676$

SS due to replications, $SS_R = 0.0417$; SS due to treatments, $SS_T = 0.7827$ and SS due to error, SS_E = Total SS $- SS_R - SS_T = 0.2432$; υ for SS_R, SS_T and SS_E are 5, 5 and 25, respectively. The υ for SS_T can be partitioned into main effects and interactions by regular ANOVA method as:

$$\text{Main effect A} = \frac{32.55^2 + 29.60^2}{18} - C = 0.2417 \text{ on } \upsilon = 1$$

$$\text{Main effect B} = \frac{22.36^2 + 20.21^2 + 19.58^2}{12} - C = 0.3541 \text{ on } \upsilon = 2$$

Interaction AB = SS_T – Main effect A – Main effect B = 0.1869 on $\upsilon = 2$

Note: Total SS and SS due to replications, treatments and error are calculated by the procedures given in Chapters 13–15.

Now, the ANOVA table can be laid-out as follows:

H_0s:
1. There is no effect of CP ratio on weight gain of broilers
2. There is no effect of feeding regimen on weight gain of broilers
3. There is no effect of interaction between CP ratio and feeding regimen on weight gain of broilers

Source	υ	SS	MSS	F
Total	35	1.0676		
Replications	5	0.0417		
Treatments	(5)	0.7827		
A	1	0.2417	0.2417	24.918
B	2	0.3541	0.1771	18.253
AB	2	0.1869	0.0935	9.634
Error	25	0.2432	0.0097	

Table value of $F_{0.05,1,25} = 4.24$; $F_{0.05,2,25} = 3.38$

The calculated values of F are > tabulated values and hence all the H_0s can be rejected.

It can be noticed that υ for Factor B and Interaction AB are > 1; hence, it may be necessary partition υ for treatments (5) into υ of 1 each so that more accurate conclusions can be drawn. If the treatments have r replications, they can be listed as along with orthogonal contrasts and divisors for SS as:

| Factor A | | 140 | | | 160 | | Divisor |
| Factor B | Pellets | Mash | Cafeteria | Pellets | Mash | Cafeteria | for SS |
Comparison			Ortho- gonal	contrasts			
CP ratio	1	1	1	−1	−1	−1	tr
Mash Vs others*	1	−2	1	1	−2	1	$2tr$**
Interaction of Mash Vs others with CP ratio	1	−2	1	−1	2	−1	$2tr$**
Pellet Vs cafeteria	1	0	−1	1	0	−1	$r(t-2)$ ***
Interaction with CP ratio	1	0	−1	−1	0	1	$r(t-2)$ ***

* Mash commonly used feeding regimen ** Mash included twice *** Mash excluded

Note: Procedure for development of the above orthogonal contrasts is beyond the scope of this publication.

Sum of squares for the above comparisons ($\upsilon = 1$) are calculated below:

Comparison	Totals*	Divisor for SS	SS	F[@]
CP ratio	2.95	36	0.2417	24.918
Mash Vs others*	1.52	72	0.0321	3.309[NS]
Interaction of Mash Vs others with CP ratio	−2.84	72	0.1120	11.546
Pellet Vs cafeteria	2.78	24	0.3220	33.196
Interaction with CP ratio	1.34	24	0.0748	7.711

* By using contrasts given above SS due to treatments, SS_T 0.7826
[@] MSS_E of 0.0097 calculated above used as denominator NS not significant

Excepting comparison of mash with others, all other comparisons, including interactions, were significant ($P < 0.05$).

Of all the comparisons, Pellet vs Cafeteria was most overwhelming followed by the effect of CP ratio. The mean values of these are shown along with standard error of

difference between means calculated by $\sqrt{MSS_E \left(\dfrac{1}{n_1} + \dfrac{1}{n_2} \right)}$ where n_1 and n_2 represent

the number of observations used for computation of the means in question.

kg	Factor A		Difference	se of difference
Factor B	140	160	Difference	se of difference
Pellet	1.962	1.765	0.197	0.057 kg
Cafeteria	1.618	1.645	−0.027	
Difference	0.344	0.120		Note: $(n_1 = n_2 = 6)$
se of difference	0.057 kg			

The above result clearly demonstrates that increasing CP ratio from 140 to 160 in pellets caused significant loss in weight gain whereas, it had no significant effect in Cafeteria system (the birds able to adjust energy/CP intake themselves). Similarly, increasing CP ratio alone could cause severe growth depression regardless of the feeding regimen.

2. EXPERIMENTS WITH MORE THAN 2 FACTORS

2.1 2^3 and 2^n Factorial Experiments

When each of the factors in a three–factor experiment is at two levels, we have $2 \times 2 \times 2 = 2^3 = 8$ treatments; hence, referred to as 2^3 **factorial experiment**. The calculations and setting up of ANOVA are simply the extension of 2^2 factorial experiment discussed in **Section 1.1** above. A numerical example given below will demonstrate the procedure:

2.1.1 Example

Two lysine levels (Factor A, 0.2 and 0.6%) were considered through two Protein levels (Factor B, 12 and 14%) on either sex (Factor C, male and female) daily weight gain (kg) of piglets; all the 8 treatment combinations in 8 replications ($r = 8$). The data stratified as per factors and replications is given below for statistical analyses:

Lysine, %	0.2	0.6	0.2	0.6	0.2	0.6	0.2	0.6	
Protein, %	12	14	12	14					
Sex	Female				Male				
Treatments	(1)	a	b	ab	c	ac	bc	abc	Total
1	1.03	0.87	1.48	1.09	1.11	1.22	1.52	1.38	9.70
2	0.99	1.16	1.53	1.47	1.09	1.34	1.27	1.40	10.25
3	0.97	1.00	1.22	1.09	0.97	1.13	1.45	1.08	8.91
4	1.21	1.14	1.57	1.17	1.21	1.19	1.24	1.39	10.12
5	1.19	1.36	1.13	1.01	1.29	1.25	1.34	1.17	9.74
6	0.99	1.00	1.16	1.24	0.85	1.34	1.67	1.46	9.71
7	1.24	1.32	1.43	1.13	0.96	1.32	1.32	1.21	9.93
8	0.99	1.29	1.19	1.43	0.99	1.41	1.22	1.21	9.73
Total	8.61	9.14	10.71	9.63	8.47	10.20	11.03	10.30	78.09

Total crude SS = 97.3211; $C = (78.09^2 \div 64) = 95.2820$; Total SS = 97.3211 – C = 2.0391

SS due to replications, SS_R = 0.1411; SS due to treatments, SS_T = 0.7986 ($\upsilon = 2^n – 1 = 7$) and sum of squares due to error, SS_E = Total SS – SS_R – SS_T = 1.0994; υ for SS_R, SS_T and SS_E are 7, 7 and 49, respectively. (**Note:** Total SS and SS due to replications, treatments and error are calculated by the procedures given in Chapters 13, 14 and 15).

The υ for SS_T will be partitioned into individual effects and interactions by using Yates' algorithms:

Treatments	Totals*	Cycle 1	Cycle 2	Cycle 3	Effect	SS**
(1)	8.61	17.75	38.09	78.09	Grand total	95.2820@
a	9.14	20.34	40.00	0.45	A	0.0032
b	10.71	18.67	–0.55	5.25	B	0.4307
ab	9.63	21.33	1.00	–4.07	AB	0.2588
c	8.47	0.53	2.59	1.91	C	0.0570
ac	10.20	–1.08	2.66	1.55	AC	0.0375
bc	11.03	1.73	–1.61	0.07	BC	0.0001
abc	10.30	–0.73	–2.46	–0.85	ABC	0.0113
				SS due to treatments, SS_T 0.7986		

* Total over 8 replications (r) ** $(Effect)^2 \div 2^n r$ where $n = 3$; @ = Correction factor

Now, all the SS values are available for the ANOVA table:

H_0s:
1. There is no effect of lysine on weight gain of piglets
2. There is no effect of protein levels on weight gain of piglets
3. There is no effect of sex of piglet on its weight gain
4. There is no effect of interaction (two- or three-way) between lysine, protein and sex of piglets on their weight gain.

Source	υ	SS	MSS	F
Total	63	2.0391		
Replications	7	0.1411		
Treatments	(7)	(0.7986)	(0.1141)	(5.094)
A	1	0.0032	0.0032	< 1
B	1	0.4307	0.4307	19.228
AB	1	0.2588	0.2588	11.554
C	1	0.0570	0.0570	2.545
AC	1	0.0375	0.0375	1.674
BC	1	0.0001	0.0001	< 1
ABC	1	0.0113	0.0113	< 1
Error	49	1.0994	0.0224	

Table value of $F_{0.05,1,49}$ = 4.03; ($F_{0.05,7,49}$ = 2.20)

Considering the calculated values of F *vs* table value, H_0 Nos 1 and 3 appear acceptable and others are not; in case of H_0 No 3, except interaction AB, none was significant. That means the effects of B and AB were the only significant effects. Their means can be compared by the methods already described in Chapter "**One–factor analysis of variance**".

Weight gain, kg	Lysine, %		Mean
Protein, %	0.2	0.6	
12	$(1) + c = 1.068^r$	$a + ac = 1.209^q$	1.138^b
14	$b + bc = 1.359^p$	$ab + abc = 1.246^q$	1.302^a
Mean	1.213	1.227	

LSD, kg for AB interaction = 0.106

Means bearing different superscripts (a, b) within the last column and (p, q, r) in the table are significantly different (P < 0.05)

Note: Calculation of LSD for comparison of various effects and interactions are based on the principles described in Chapter "**One-factor analysis of variance**". However, for sake of convenience, the formulae are listed below:

1. LSD for Main effect $= t_{\alpha,\upsilon_E}\sqrt{\dfrac{2MSS_E}{2^{(n-1)}r}}$ and

2. LSD for Interaction effects involving m factors $= t_{\alpha,\upsilon_E}\sqrt{\dfrac{2MSS_E}{2^{(n-m)}r}}$

In the above example, $n = 3$ and $r = 7$; therefore, LSD for Main effects can be calculated

as $t_{\alpha,\upsilon_E}\sqrt{\dfrac{2MSS_E}{4r}}$; LSD for 2 factor interactions (AB, AC and BC) by $t_{\alpha,\upsilon_E}\sqrt{\dfrac{2MSS_E}{2r}}$ and

LSD for 3 factor interaction (ABC) by $t_{\alpha,\upsilon_E}\sqrt{\dfrac{2MSS_E}{r}}$. Although treatment means (simple

effects) are not generally compared, if one wishes to do so, LSD can be calculated as

$t_{\alpha,\upsilon_E}\sqrt{\dfrac{2MSS_E}{r}}$. These general rues are applicable to all 2^n factorial experiments.

In this example also treatments effects were significant and hence, the comparison of treatment means is given below:

Treatments	(1)	a	b	ab	c	ac	bc	abc
Means, kg	1.076^d	1.143^{cd}	1.339^{ab}	1.204^{bcd}	1.059^d	1.275^{abc}	1.379^a	1.288^{abc}

Means bearing at least one common letter superscript are not significantly different (P < 0.05); LSD = 0.150 kg

Males on 14% protein diet performed the best followed by males on 14% protein + 0.6% lysine in the diet and males on 0.6% lysine in that order. The poorest performance was by the female piglets on 12% protein with 0.2% lysine.

2.2   A 2 × 3 × 4 Experiment

This is a case where all factors are not employed in same number of levels. For instance, marinating spent–hen carcasses in 0, 3 and 6% STPP solution (Factor A, 3 levels) for 3, 6 and 9 h (Factor B, 3 levels) to study its effect during storage for 0 (fresh), 4 and 8 d at 4°C (refrigerated) and for 30 and 60 d at −20°C (frozen) (Factor C, 5 levels) forms 3 × 3 × 5 Factorial experiment of 45 treatments as performed by Sreenivasaiah (1985), with 3 replications. Analysis of such data is by formation of suitable 2 × 2 tables and calculation of main effects (considering row and column totals) and interactions (by using the cell values).

A numerical example of a 2 × 3 × 4 (three–factor) experiment is analyzed below to demonstrate various steps:

2.2.1   Example

Let us consider an experiment involving 2 stocking densities (Factor A, 2 levels; 11 and 15 birds per m²) fed on 3 protein levels (Factor B, 3 levels; 17, 20 and 23%) each on 4 lysine levels (Factor C, 4 levels; 0.3, 0.6, 0.9 and 1.2%) in 5 replications on weight gain (kg) of broilers. This is a 2 × 3 × 4 experiment (24 treatments) with 5 replicates employing 120 broilers. The hypothetical data is given below:

Treatment combination			Replications					
Birds/m²	Protein, %	Lysine, %	1	2	3	4	5	Total, x_{ijk}
11	17	0.3	0.48	0.42	0.40	0.36	0.31	1.97
		0.6	0.55	0.48	0.60	0.47	0.42	2.52
		0.9	0.75	0.80	0.65	0.75	0.87	3.82
		1.2	1.10	1.20	0.90	0.97	1.00	5.17
	20	0.3	0.70	0.69	0.75	0.80	0.80	3.74
		0.6	0.65	0.88	0.93	1.00	0.97	4.43
		0.9	1.10	1.08	1.07	1.15	0.98	5.38
		1.2	1.45	1.36	1.58	1.25	1.31	6.95
	23	0.3	0.97	0.85	0.76	0.90	0.64	4.12
		0.6	1.20	1.47	1.54	1.42	1.53	7.16
		0.9	1.53	1.67	1.72	1.61	1.59	8.12
		1.2	2.04	2.00	1.97	2.10	1.84	9.95
15	17	0.3	0.40	0.38	0.32	0.25	0.27	1.62
		0.6	0.48	0.42	0.47	0.39	0.36	2.12
		0.9	0.65	0.60	0.58	0.45	0.57	2.85
		1.2	1.00	1.10	0.84	0.76	0.92	4.62
	20	0.3	0.53	0.49	0.51	0.49	0.60	2.62
		0.6	0.55	0.68	0.75	0.69	0.77	3.44
		0.9	0.92	0.84	0.80	0.91	0.78	4.25
		1.2	1.10	1.00	0.97	1.05	1.03	5.15

(Contd.)

(Contd.)

Treatment combination			Replications					
Birds/m²	Protein, %	Lysine, %	1	2	3	4	5	Total, $x_{ijk\cdot}$
23	0.3		0.77	0.75	0.64	0.70	0.59	3.45
	0.6		1.10	1.25	1.20	1.30	1.33	6.18
	0.9		1.35	1.45	1.49	1.57	1.38	7.24
	1.2		1.65	1.74	1.59	1.69	1.80	8.47
			23.02	23.60	23.03	23.03	22.66	115.34
			26.2144	27.9796	26.9763	27.3499	26.2084	

Total crude SS, $x^2\ldots = 134.7286$; $C = 110.8610$; Total SS $= 134.7286 - C = 23.8676$; SS

due to replications, $\text{SS}_R = \dfrac{\sum\limits_{l=1}^{r}\left(x_{\cdots l}\right)^2}{abc} - C = 0.0189$; SS due to treatments,

$$\text{SS}_T = \dfrac{\sum\limits_{i=1}^{a}\sum\limits_{j=1}^{b}\sum\limits_{k=1}^{c}\left(x_{ijk\cdot}\right)^2}{r} - C = 23.0812$$

For this example, the following subscripts and formulae for calculation of SS are used (analogous to those shown in Chapter "**Analysis of variance for more than two factors**"):

	Subscript	Levels	Totals Notation	n
Stocking density	i	2 (a)	$x_{i\cdots}$	bcr = 60
Protein levels	j	3 (b)	$x_{\cdot j\cdots}$	acr = 40
Lysine levels	k	4 (c)	$x_{\cdot\cdot k\cdot}$	abr = 30
Replications	l	5 (r)	$x_{\cdots l}$	abc = 24
ABC interaction			$x_{ijk\cdot}$	r = 5
Grand total			$x_{\cdots}$	abcr = 120

| Total crude SS | | Sum of squares $x^2_{\cdots}$ | |

SS due to	Calculation	Notation	v
Total	$x^2\ldots - C^*$		abcr − 1
Replication	$\dfrac{\sum\limits_{l=1}^{r}\left(x_{\cdots l}\right)^2}{abc} - C$	SS_R	r − 1
Factor A	$\dfrac{\sum\limits_{i=1}^{a}\left(x_{i\cdots}\right)^2}{bcr} - C$	SS_A	a − 1

(Contd.)

(Contd.)

Total crude SS		Sum of squares	
		x^2...	
SS due to	Calculation	Notation	v
Factor B	$\dfrac{\sum\limits_{j=1}^{b}\left(x_{.j..}\right)^2}{acr}-C$	SS_B	$b-1$
Factor C	$\dfrac{\sum\limits_{k=1}^{c}\left(x_{..k.}\right)^2}{abr}-C$	SS_C	$c-1$
Interaction AB	$\dfrac{\sum\limits_{i=1}^{a}\sum\limits_{j=1}^{b}\left(x_{ij..}\right)^2}{cr}-C-SS_A-SS_B$	SS_{AB}	$(a-1)(b-1)$
Interaction AC	$\dfrac{\sum\limits_{i=1}^{a}\sum\limits_{k=1}^{c}\left(x_{i.k.}\right)^2}{br}-C-SS_A-SS_C$	SS_{AC}	$(a-1)(c-1)$
Interaction BC	$\dfrac{\sum\limits_{j=1}^{b}\sum\limits_{k=1}^{c}\left(x_{.jk.}\right)^2}{ar}-C-SS_B-SS_C$	SS_{BC}	$(b-1)(c-1)$
Interaction ABC	$\dfrac{\sum\limits_{i=1}^{a}\sum\limits_{j=1}^{b}\sum\limits_{k=1}^{c}\left(x_{ijk.}\right)^2}{r}-C-@$	SS_{ABC}	$(a-1)(b-1)(c-1)$
Error	By difference	SS_E	$abc(r-1)$

$* \ C = (x....)^2 \div (abcr); \ @ \ (SS_A + SS_B + SS_C + SS_{AB} + SS_{AC} + SS_{BC})$

The 2 × 2 tables needed for the calculation of the above SS and the values thereon are given below:

$x_{ij...}$ values	Stocking density, birds/m^2		
Protein,%	11	15	Factor B totals, $x_{.j...}$
17	13.48	11.21	24.69
20	20.50	15.46	35.96
23	29.35	25.34	54.69
Factor A totals, $x_{i....}$	63.33	52.01	115.34

SS due to stocking density, $SS_S = 1.0679$

SS due to protein levels, $SS_P = 11.4819$

SS due to interaction, $SS_{SxP} = 0.0979$

| $x_{i \cdot k}$ values | Stocking density, birds/m² | | Factor C totals, $x_{\cdot \cdot k}$. |
Lysine,%	11	15	
0.3	9.83	7.69	17.52
0.6	14.11	11.74	25.85
0.9	17.32	14.34	31.66
1.2	22.07	18.24	40.31
Factor A totals, $x_{i \cdot \cdot}$	63.33	52.01	115.34

SS due to lysine levels, $SS_L = 9.2199$
SS due to interaction, $SS_{SxL} = 0.0569$

| $x_{\cdot jk}$ values | Protein levels, % | | | Factor C totals, $x_{\cdot \cdot k}$. |
Lysine,%	17	20	23	
0.3	3.59	6.36	7.57	17.52
0.6	4.64	7.87	13.34	25.85
0.9	6.67	9.63	15.36	31.66
1.2	9.79	12.10	18.42	40.31
Factor B totals, $x_{\cdot j \cdot}$	24.69	35.96	54.69	115.34

SS due to interaction, $SS_{PxL} = 1.1143$
SS due to interaction $SS_{SxPxL} = 0.0424$
SS due to error, $SS_E = \text{Total SS} - SS_R - SS_T = \text{Total SS} - SS_R - SS_S - SS_P - SS_L - SS_{SxP} - SS_{SxL} - SS_{SxL} - SS_{SxPxL} = 0.7675$
Now, the ANOVA table will be laid-out as follows:
H_0s:
1. There is no effect of stocking density (A) on weight gain of broilers
2. There is no effect of protein levels (B) on weight gain of broilers
3. There is no effect of lysine levels (C) on weight gain of broilers
4. There is no effect of interaction AB on weight gain of broilers
5. There is no effect of interaction AC on weight gain of broilers
6. There is no effect of interaction ABC on weight gain of broilers

Source	υ	SS	MSS	F
Total	119	23.8676		
Replications	4	0.0189		
Treatments	(23)	(23.0812)	(1.0035)	(125.438)
Stocking density, A	1	1.0679	1.0679	133.488
Protein levels, B	2	11.4819	5.7410	717.625
AB	2	0.0979	0.0490	6.125
Lysine levels, C	3	9.2199	3.0733	384.163
AC	3	0.0569	0.0190	2.375[NS]

(Contd.)

(Contd.)

Source	υ	SS	MSS	F
BC	6	1.1143	0.1857	23.213
ABC	6	0.0424	0.0071	< 1
Error	96	0.7675	0.0080	

Table value of $F_{0.05,1,96} = 3.96$; $F_{0.05,2,96} = 3.09$; $F_{0.05,3,96} = 2.70$; $F_{0.05,6,96} = 2.19$ ($F_{0.05,23,96} = 1.63$)

Comparison of calculated values of F with corresponding table values, it is evident that except interactions AC and ABC, all other effects were significant. Therefore, H_0 Nos 5 and 7 are acceptable and all others are fit for rejection.

Calculation of LSD for comparison of various effects and interactions are based on the principles described in Chapter "**One-factor Analysis of Variance**". However, the general formula for calculation of standard error of difference between two means

of each of the effect is: $\sqrt{\dfrac{2MSS_E}{w}}$ where value of w varies with the effect/interaction

considered for comparisons as follows:

Comparison	Treatments	A	B	C	AB	AC	BC	ABC
w	r	bcr	acr	abr	cr	br	ar	r
Example	5	60	40	30	20	15	10	5
$LSD_{0.05}$, kg	0.112	0.032	0.040	0.046	0.056	0.065	0.079	0.112

The standard error so calculated is multiplied by table value of t at set α and υ of MSS_E i.e. $\{abc(r-1)\}$ to get LSD value which can be used to allot superscripts. With the LSD values available, allotment of superscript has been described with several examples in this Chapter and also in Chapters 13–15; hence, not shown in this chapter again.

3. POLYNOMIAL RESPONSE CURVE AND RESPONSE SURFACE

When [3] 1 factor(s) is (are) quantitative, response curve or response surface can be fit to estimate levels of the factor(s) that is likely to maximize/minimize the value of the dependent variable in consideration. Both these aspects are dealt in a separate chapter.

4. CONFOUNDING

Under practical situations, two aspects have important influence on design of a factorial experiment:

1. Number of factors: as number of factors and/or levels increases arithmetically, the number of treatments increases geometrically; for instance, a 2^2 experiment has 4, 2^3 has 8, 2^4 has 16 and so on; similarly, a 2^2 experiment has 4, 3^2 has 9, 4^2 has 16 and so on. When number of treatments is very large, it will be difficult to have sufficient number of animals (especially large animals) for experimentation and, even if available, it is difficult to get sufficient number of homogenous groups to replicate all the treatments.

2. High-order interactions: again, as number of factors and/or levels increases, several higher order interactions, which of less practical significance, do come into picture; if these can be avoided, number of treatments can be reduced. Such reductions are possible only when such interaction effects are made indistinguishable from block (local control) effect to facilitate evaluation of more important comparisons more efficiently; this process is called **Confounding**.

4.1 Process of Confounding

For confounding, each replication is subdivided into ≥ 2 groups (blocks) over which equal number of treatments are distributed in such a way that those interaction(s) which are considered less important are confounded with the group (block) effects so that the other treatments are compared more effectively. Needless to state that treatment combinations are allotted to groups (blocks) at random.

4.1.1 Complete Confounding

The general procedure to confound any interaction/effect can be generalized as follows:
1. Obtain the estimate of the effect in terms of treatments; last cycle of Yates algorithm is the easiest way for it.
2. Group the treatments as per sign into those with positive sign and those with negative sign.
3. Assign the above groups to separate blocks allotting at treatments at random to a block.

For convenience, the last cycle of the Yates' table is given in full form in terms of treatments involved so that it would facilitate identifying of effect confounded as well as planning confounding in an experiment:

	(1)	*a*	*b*	*ab*	*c*	*ac*	*bc*	*abc*
Grand total	+	+	+	−	+	+	+	+
A	−	+	−	+	−	+	−	+
B	−	−	+	+	−	−	+	+
AB	+	−	−	+	+	−	−	+
C	−	−	−	−	+	+	+	+
AC	+	−	+	−	−	+	−	+
BC	+	+	−	−	−	−	+	+
ABC	−	+	+	−	+	−	−	+

Notes:
1. Grand total is the summation of all treatment totals; hence, all are +
2. For main effects (A, B and C), all treatments which contain the letter (*a*, *b* and *c*, respectively) are +; for instance, for main effect A, treatments *a*, *ab*, *ac* and *abc* are + and so on.
3. For any interaction, the signs are simply the product of the signs allotted to the treatments in respect of each of its constituent factors; for instance, in case of interaction AB, multiply rows pertaining main effect A and main effect B.

Note: The above is also useful in calculating adjusted value of treatment effects by following the column signs; for example, adjusted value for treatment c = Overall mean + Q where Q is the summation of treatment means weighted by respective contrasts; i.e. $(-A - B + AB + C - AC - BC + ABC)$ in case of treatment c.

4.1.1.1 Confounding in a 2^3 experiment

With three factors, A, B and C, the highest order of interaction is ABC which is estimated as $\frac{1}{4}\{abc - bc - ac + c - ab + b + a - (1)\}$; by rearranging these as per signs, $\frac{1}{4}\{abc + a + b + c - ac - ab - bc - (1)\}$ or, $\frac{1}{4}[\{abc + a + b + c\} - \{ac + ab + bc + (1)\}]$. In order to confound interaction ABC, the treatments with '+' sign $\{abc + a + b + c\}$ and those with '−'sign $\{ac + ab + bc + (1)\}$ are allotted in different blocks, at random. Hence, each replication will have 2 blocks containing treatments as above. Therefore, if there are r replications, there will be $2r$ blocks; thus providing υ of $(2r - 1)$ for blocks. Total SS will have a υ of $(8r - 1)$ and SS due to treatments will have a υ of 6 (one each for A, B, AB, C, AC and BC; ABC confounded); obviously, SS due to error will have υ of $6(r - 1)$.

4.1.1.2 Example

Example 2.1.1 is used to demonstrate complete confounding of interaction ABC. The treatments are given in 2 groups (blocks); one containing the treatments (1), ab, ac and bc and (1); the other containing, a, b, c, and abc.

| | **Treatments** | | | | | | | | |
| | **Group 1** | | | | **Group 2** | | | | |
Replications	**(1)**	**ab**	**ac**	**bc**	**a**	**b**	**c**	**abc**	**Total**
1	1.03	1.09	1.22	1.52	0.87	1.48	1.11	1.38	9.70
2	0.99	1.47	1.34	1.27	1.16	1.53	1.09	1.40	10.25
3	0.97	1.09	1.13	1.45	1.00˙	1.22	0.97	1.08	8.91
4	1.21	1.17	1.19	1.24	1.14	1.57	1.21	1.39	10.12
5	1.19	1.01	1.25	1.34	1.36	1.13	1.29	1.17	9.74
6	0.99	1.24	1.34	1.67	1.00	1.16	0.85	1.46	9.71
7	1.24	1.13	1.32	1.32	1.32	1.43	0.96	1.21	9.93
8	0.99	1.43	1.41	1.22	1.29	1.19	0.99	1.21	9.73
Total	8.61	9.63	10.20	11.03	9.14	10.71	8.47	10.30	78.09

For calculation of SS due to groups, Groups x replication table has to be developed by computing sums of each group within replication.

Replications	**1**	**2**	**3**	**4**	**5**	**6**	**7**	**8**	**Totals**
Group 1	4.86	5.07	4.64	4.81	4.79	5.24	5.01	5.05	39.47
Group 2	4.84	5.18	4.27	5.31	4.95	4.47	4.92	4.68	38.62

SS due to Groups = $\{(4.86^2 + 5.07^2 + \ldots 4.84^2 + 5.18^2 + \ldots + 4.68^2) \div 4\} - C = (382.2737 \div 4) - 95.2820 = 0.2864$

Note: Groups are **nested** within replications; therefore, SS due to groups on $\upsilon = (rg - 1)$ can be split into SS due to replications (on $\upsilon = r - 1$) + SS due to groups within replication {on $\upsilon = r(g - 1)$} where g = number of groups within a replication (*see* Chapter "**Analysis of variance for more than two factors**" for details).

SS due to other Main effects and interactions are computed similar to an experiment without confounding (as shown in **Example 2.1.1**); but, SS due to ABC is not calculated. Therefore, the ANOVA table can be laid as follows:

H_0s:

1. There is no effect of confounding (MSS due to groups is not significant)
2. There is no effect of lysine on weight gain of piglets
3. There is no effect of protein levels on weight gain of piglets
4. There is no effect of sex of piglet on its weight gain
5. There is no effect of interaction (two-way) between lysine, protein and sex of piglets on their weight gain.

Source	υ	SS	MSS	F
Total	63	2.0391		
Groups	15	0.2864	0.0191	< 1
Treatments	(6)	(0.7873)	(0.1312)	(5.704)
A	1	0.0032	0.0032	< 1
B	1	0.4307	0.4307	18.726
AB	1	0.2588	0.2588	11.252
C	1	0.0570	0.0570	2.478
AC	1	0.0375	0.0375	1.630
BC	1	0.0001	0.0001	< 1
ABC	Not calculated			
Error	42	0.9654	0.0230	

Table value of $F_{0.05,15,42} = 1.92$; $(F_{0.05,6,42} = 2.32)$; $F_{0.05,1,42} = 4.07$

That effect of grouping is not significant indicates that H_0 No.1 is acceptable and the confounding was not effective; therefore, there is no likelihood of any change in other conclusions as well; which indeed, is true.

Considering the calculated values of F *Vs* table value, H_0 Nos 2 and 4 appear acceptable and others are not; in case of H_0 No 3, except interaction AB, none was significant. That means the effects of B and AB were the only significant effects. Their means have been compared under **Example 2.1.1**; the same procedure can be followed by replacing the value of MSS_E by the one calculated above (0.0224 by 0.0230).

4.1.2 *Partial Confounding*

Unlike in complete confounding where a particular effect was confounded in all replications, in partial confounding the following two alternatives are possible:

1. Not all the replications need have confounding in the first place
2. Secondly, even in those replications where confounding of an effect is planned, different effects may be involved in different replications

Hence, many combinations of partial confounding are possible. An illustration of a 2^3 factorial experiment with 4 replications each with confounding of different effects is given below:

Replications	1		2		3		4	
Groups	1	2	3	4	5	6	7	8
	abc	ab	abc	ac	abc	ab	abc	ab
Treatments	a	ac	ab	bc	bc	ac	ac	bc
	b	bc	c	a	a	b	b	a
	c	(1)	(1)	b	(1)	c	(1)	c
Confounds	ABC		AB		BC		AC	

Such experiments in which the confounding of interaction effect is not uniform in all the replications are said to be **partially confounded**. It is understood that a main effect is not confounded because such an experiment will defeat its own aim.

4.1.2.1 Implications of partial confounding

1. Main effects A, B and C remain unaltered
2. In the above set of replications, ¾ of information about each of the interactions AB, AC, BC and ABC are available because in only one of the 4 replications confounding of an interaction is effected.
3. Consequent on (2) above, the denominator for calculating SS to the confounded interactions reduces according to the information (observations involved) obtained; in the current illustration, reduces from 4 to 3. Analysis of such an experiment is given with a numerical example.

4.1.2.2 Example (confounding in a 2^3 experiment)

The same **Example 2.1.1** will be considered, but with data of only 4 replications;

Replication 1 (ABC confounded)									Totals		
Group 1 (–ve)				Group 2 (+ve)							
(1)	ab	ac	bc	a	b	c	abc	Group 1	Group 2	Replication 1	
1.03	1.09	1.22	1.52	0.87	1.48	1.11	1.38	4.86	4.84	9.70	

Replication 2 (AB confounded)

Group 3 (+ve)Group 4 (–ve)

abc	(1)	ab	c	bc	a	b	ac	Group 3	Group 4	Replication 2
1.40	0.99	1.47	1.09	1.27	1.16	1.53	1.34	4.95	5.30	10.25

Replication 3 (BC confounded)

Group 5 (–ve)Group 6 (+ve)

b	ac	c	ab	abc	bc	(1)	a	Group 5	Group 6	Replication 3
1.22	1.13	0.97	1.09	1.08	1.45	0.97	1.00	4.41	4.50	8.91

Replication 4 (AC confounded)

Group 7 (+ve)Group 8 (–ve)

abc	ac	b	(1)	c	bc	ab	a	Group 7	Group 8	Replication 4
1.39	1.19	1.57	1.21	1.21	1.24	1.17	1.14	5.36	4.76	10.12

Treatment totals (over all groups) Total Crude SS48.5672

(1)	a	b	ab	c	ac	bc	abc	Grand total	38.98
4.20	4.17	5.80	4.82	4.38	4.88	5.48	5.25	38.98	

Number of observations: Total: 32 Replications: 8 Main effects: 4 Groups: 4

Treatment totals that are added in the respective interaction confounded are put in one group and those which are subtracted in the other; this is indicated in the parentheses against groups. All the main effect and group totals as well as number of observations for each of them are indicated in the above table.

Calculation of SS is as per a regular 2^3 experiment; but, the effects that are partially confounded will be corrected after obtaining values of SS.

4.1.2.2.1 Adjustment factors (AF) for confounded effects

The procedure for calculation of adjustment factor for an effect that is confounded is as follows: (ABC interaction is considered for illustration)

1. Identify the effect confounded in the replication; replication 1, ABC
2. Identify the group (block) that contains treatments that carry positive sign for calculation of the effect that is confounded had it not been confounded; replication 1, group 2
3. Subtract the total of the group (block) containing treatments that have negative sign from that of the group that has treatments having positive signs; the resultant value is the AF; replication 1, ABC, $(4.84 - 4.86) = -0.02$
4. The AF is applied after obtaining the effect totals in the nth cycle of the Yates' algorithm; in this case $n = 3$.

Hence, Yates' algorithm method, AF and corrected totals thereon are shown below:

Treatments	Totals*	Cycle 1	Cycle 2	Cycle 3	AF	Totals	Effect	SS**
(1)	4.20	8.37	18.99	38.98	–	38.98		C
a	4.17	10.62	19.99	–0.74	–	–0.74	A	0.0171
b	5.80	9.26	–1.01	2.72	–	2.72	B	0.2312
ab	4.82	10.73	0.27	–1.68	–0.35	–1.34	AB	0.0748
c	4.38	–0.03	1.25	1.00	–	1.00	C	0.0313
ac	4.88	–0.98	1.47	1.28	0.60	0.68	AC	0.0193
bc	5.48	0.50	–0.95	0.22	0.09	0.13	BC	0.0007
abc	5.25	–0.23	–0.73	0.22	–0.02	0.24	ABC	0.0024

** For effects not confounded $\dfrac{(\text{Total})^2}{2^n r}$; for confounded effects $\dfrac{(\text{Total})^2}{2^n (r-f)}$; where $n = 3$; $r = 4$ and f = number of replicates in which the effect is confounded (1 in this case)

Total SS = 1.0847

SS due to groups, $SS_G = 0.1982$, on $\upsilon = (rg - 1) = 7$

SS due to replications, $SS_R = 0.1369$, on $\upsilon = (r - 1) = 3$

SS due to groups within replication, $SS_{G/R} = (SS_G - SS_R) = 0.0613$, on $\upsilon = r(g - 1) = 4$

SS due to treatments, $SS_T = 0.6407$ on $\upsilon = 2^n - 1 = 7$

SS due to error, $SS_E = (\text{Total SS} - SS_R - SS_{G/R} - SS_T)$ or Total SS $-SS_G - SS_T) = 0.2458$

The ANOVA table is as follows:

H_0's:

1. Confounding is not effective
2. There is no effect of treatments on weight gain of piglets

3. There is no effect of lysine on weight gain of piglets
4. There is no effect of protein levels on weight gain of piglets
5. There is no effect of sex of piglet on its weight gain

Source	v	SS	MSS	F
Total	31	1.0847		
Groups	7	0.1982	0.0283	1.953
Replications	3	0.1369	0.0456	3.147
Groups within replications	4	0.0613	0.0153	1.057
Treatments	(7)	0.6407	0.0915	6.312
Lysine, A	1	0.0171	0.0171	1.179
Protein levels, B	1	0.2312	0.2312	15.945
AB	1	0.0748	0.0748	5.159
Sex of piglets, C	1	0.0313	0.0313	2.159
AC	1	0.0193	0.0193	1.331
BC	1	0.0007	0.0007	< 1
ABC	1	0.0024	0.0024	< 1
Error	17	0.2458	0.0145	

Table values $F_{0.05,1,17} = 4.45$; $F_{0.05,3,17} = 3.20$; $F_{0.05,4,17} = 2.96$; $(F_{0.05,7,17} = 2.63)$

Effect of grouping within a replicate to confound the interaction effects has not been effective because neither MSS between groups nor between replications is significant. Of the individual factors, only protein levels were found to have significant influence on growth of piglets. Hence, H_0's 1, 3 and 5 are acceptable and 2 and 4 are rejected. Comparison of means for protein levels by LSD is same as shown under **Example 2.1.1** above.

4.1.2.3 Confounding ≥ 2 effects in a replication

In the example above, in each of the replication only one effect was confounded. However, it is possible to confound more than one effect in the same replication as well. For instance let us consider signs for treatment with respect to BC and AC.

	(1)	a	b	ab	c	ac	bc	abc
AC	+	–	+	–	–	+	–	+
BC	+	+	–	–	–	–	+	+

Groups are formed within a replication in the following way:
1. One group will have treatments which have positive sign in both; i.e. Group 1 allotted (1) and abc
2. One group is allotted treatments which carry positive sign for AC and negative for BC; i.e. Group 2 is allotted b and ac
3. One group is allotted treatments which carry negative sign for AC and positive for BC; i.e. Group 3 is allotted a and bc
4. One group is allotted treatments which carry negative sign for both AC and BC; i.e. Group 4 is allotted ab and c

With the above allotment, the contrasts for the groups to confound BC, AC and consequently AB are as follows:

Effect confounded	Group 1	Group 2	Group 3	Group 4
BC	1	1	−1	−1
AC	1	−1	1	−1
AB	1	−1	−1	1

It can be noticed that if BC and AC are confounded, then AB also gets automatically confounded because AB is the generalized interaction between BC and AC. The generalized interaction between any two effects can be deduced by canceling–out common letters; like between BC and AC, C is canceled to get AB or A is the generalized interaction between BC and AC.

Note: This concept can be extended to any number of factors and levels. While designing such experiments, one needs to be very careful in allocation of treatments, randomization, collection and tabulation of data. Basis of analysis of such data is no different from what is already explained in various chapters including the current one; but, with suitable modifications in the denominator for calculation of Means and SS.

4.1.2.4 Confounding in a 3^2 experiment

Let us consider two factors A and B, each at 3 levels 0, 2 and 3. Obviously, the nine treatment combinations that are possible with designations are shown in a 2×2 table to calculate main effects A and B from marginal totals and interaction AB from the cell values:

		Levels of A			Totals for B
		0	**1**	**2**	
	0	a_0b_0, (00)	a_1b_0, (10)	a_2b_0, (20)	(00) + (10) + (20)
Levels of B	1	a_0b_1, (01)	a_1b_1, (11)	a_2b_1, (21)	(01) + (11) + (21)
	2	a_0b_2, (02)	a_1b_2, (12)	a_2b_2, (22)	(02) + (12) + (22)

Totals for A(00) + (01) + (02)(10) + (11) + (12)(20) + (21) + (22)

Therefore, totals for calculation of SS for various effects are:

Row section	Main effect A, $\upsilon = 2$	Main effect B, $\upsilon = 2$
	(00) + (01) + (02)	(00) + (10) + (20)
	(10) + (11) + (12)	(01) + (11) + (21)
	(20) + (21) + (22)	(02) + (12) + (22)
Diagonal sections	Interaction AB(I), $\upsilon = 2$	Interaction AB(J), $\upsilon = 2$
Interaction AB $\upsilon = 4$	(00) + (11) + (22)	(00) + (12) + (21)
	(01) + (12) + (20)	(01) + (10) + (22)
	(02) + (10) + (21)	(02) + (11) + (20)

With the above information, it is possible to form groups (blocks) within a replication to confound a desired effect; for instance, if 3 groups (blocks) are formed similar to the row totals used for computation of AB(I), the SS between groups becomes indistinguishable with that of AB(I); in other words, AB(I) gets confounded. The same logic is applicable for other effects as well.

4.1.2.4.1 Meaning of AB(I) and AB(J)

An alternative method of locating the diagonal sections is shown in Fig. 16.1.

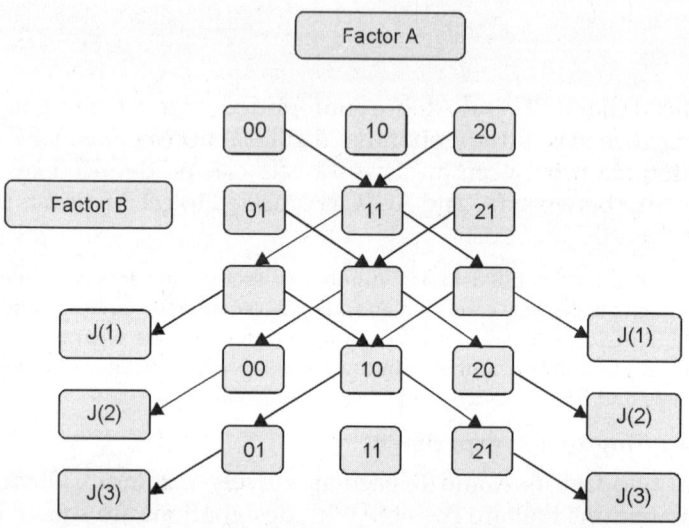

Fig 16.1: Diagonal sections in a 3^2 experiment

The procedure is to write the treatment with Factor A as columns and B as rows. The first two rows are repeated and arrows are drawn to identify the diagonal sections as indicated. If the treatments along the arrows are applied through separate groups in a replication, the corresponding diagonal section will be confounded; it can be checked that the same treatments are grouped in the example that follows.

Yet another way of finding the treatments in a group to confound AB(I) and AB(J) is to find the treatments that give the values 0, 1 and 2 for $x_1 + x_2$ [for AB(I)] and 0, 1 and 2 for $x_1 + 2x_2$ [for AB(J)] where x_1 refers to levels of Factor A and x_2 refers to Factor B. The rule is, if the total of levels of both factors add to 0 or the total when divided by the number of levels (3 in this case) leaves no remainder, then that treatment is considered as $x_1 + x_2 = 1$; treatments that fall into this category are 00, 12 and 21; hence they are the treatments to be in a group to confound I(1). Similarly, treatments 10, 01 and 22 do not add to zero and when divided by 3, leave a remainder of 1; hence they are the treatments to be in a group to confound I(2); and treatments 11, 20 and 02 leave a remainder of 2 on division by 3 and hence are the treatments to be grouped to confound I(3). Since coefficients of both x_1 and x_2 are unity, it is also designated $A_L B_L$.

On the same lines, we can find the treatment combinations which yield 0, 1 and 2 as remainder their levels are added as $x_1 + 2x_2$ and divided by 3. Treatments that fall into this category of giving no remainder are 00, 11 and 22; hence they are the treatments to be in a group to confound J(1). Similarly, treatments 10, 21 and 02 when divided by 3, leave a remainder of 1; hence they are the treatments to be in a group to confound J(2); and treatments 01, 12 and 20 leave a remainder of 2 on division by 3 and hence are the treatments to be grouped to confound J(3). Since coefficient of x_2 is 2, it is also referred to as designated $A_L B_Q$.

Both the methods explained above have a common advantage that they are applicable to any number of factors and levels.

Let us consider a numerical example to know the procedure for analyses of a 3^2 experiment:

4.1.2.5 Example (Confounding in a 3^2 experiment)

Data on respiratory rate per min from a 3^2 experiment involving 36 Golden Retrievers given vitamin C (Factor A) @ 0, 250 and 500 mg/d and subjected to three temperature regimen (Factor B) *viz.* 12, 24 and 36 °C are given below with usual notations for the treatments. Let us identify the interaction confounded, if any, and proceed developing an ANOVA:

Group	Replication 1			Total	Group	Replication 2			Total
1	36 (00)	40 (01)	70 (02)	146	4	32 (00)	31 (10)	29 (20)	92
2	32 (10)	38 (11)	65 (12)	135	5	43 (01)	36 (11)	31 (21)	110
3	30 (20)	32 (21)	45 (22)	107	6	75 (02)	69 (12)	50 (22)	194
Totals	Replication 1			388		Replication 2			396
Group	Replication 3			Total	Group	Replication 4			Total
7	36 (00)	35 (11)	48 (22)	119 (i_1)	10	33 (00)	70 (12)	35 (21)	138 (j_1)
8	45 (01)	70 (12)	31 (20)	146 (i_2)	11	41 (01)	32 (10)	54 (22)	127 (j_2)
9	78 (02)	35 (10)	34 (21)	147 (i_3)	12	72 (02)	40 (11)	30 (20)	142 (j_3)
Totals	Replication 3			412		Replication 4	407		
Treatments	(00)	(01)	(02)	(10)	(11)	(12)	(20)	(21)	(22)
Totals	137	169	295	130	149	274	120	132	197

Grand total: 1603; Total Crude SS = 79951; C = 71378.0278; Total SS = 8572.9722
Note: All totals are unadjusted

For calculation of SS due to vitamin C levels and temperature, a 2 × 2 table is necessary and the same is as follows:

Totals of respiratory rates (Unadjusted)		Vitamin C, mg/d			Total (Level)
		0	250	500	
Temperature, °C	12	137 (00)	130 (10)	120 (20)	387 (0)
	24	169 (01)	149 (11)	132 (21)	450 (1)
	36	295 (02)	274 (12)	197 (22)	766 (2)
Total (level)		601 (0)	553 (1)	449 (2)	1603

Before proceeding to the next stage, it is necessary to identify effect(s) confounded, if any; in this example, the following are confounded:

Replication	1	2	3	4
Confounded with	A	B	AB(I)	AB(J)

4.1.2.5.1 Adjustment factors (AF) for totals

Factor A is confounded in Replication 1; the totals of group 1 which is synonymous with total for 0 level of Factor A i.e. treatment (00); hence, its total, 146 is subtracted from total of Factor A, Level 0 (601) to get the adjusted total: (601 – 146) = 455 over (12 – 3) = 9 observations. The same procedure is followed for rest of the confounded effects. For AB(I) and AB(J), the corresponding treatment totals from 2 × 2 table of unadjusted totals are added and the total from the replicate confounding the effect is subtracted. For example, to calculate adjusted total of AB(i_1), unadjusted totals of (00), (11) and (22) are added from all replications (137 + 149 + 197) and total of i_1 from replication 3 in which it was confounded (119) is subtracted to get the adjusted total; and so on. Consequent on this, the adjusted totals for Factors A and B are shown below:

	Adjusted totals (number of observations)			
Levels	Factor A	Factor B	AB(I)	AB(J)
0	455 (9)	295 (9)	364 (9)	405 (9)
1	418 (9)	340 (9)	417 (9)	369 (9)
2	342 (9)	572 (9)	410 (9)	422 (9)
Totals	1215 (27)	1207 (27)	1191 (27)	1196 (27)

Note: Totals of AB(I) and AB(J) can also be obtained by forming a 3 x 3 table keeping the treatment structure as in Replication 3 and 4, respectively and obtaining information about each of the treatments from the replications where the effect is not confounded.

4.1.2.5.2 Calculation of various SS and ANOVA

Total SS = 8572.9722

SS due to groups (blocks), SS_G = 2492.9722 on $\upsilon = (rg - 1) = 11$

SS due to replications, SS_R = 38.9722 on $\upsilon = (r - 1) = 3$

SS due to groups (blocks) within replications, $SS_{B/R}$ = 2454.0000 on $\upsilon = r(g - 1) = 8$

SS due to treatments (Calculated from unadjusted totals and Grand Total by usual method), SS_T = 8413.2222

SS due to Factor A, $SS_{Vit} = \dfrac{\left(455^2 + 418^2 + 342^2\right)}{9} - \dfrac{1215^2}{27} = 737.5556$ on $\upsilon = 2$

SS due to Factor B, $SS_{Temp} = \dfrac{\left(295^2 + 340^2 + 572^2\right)}{9} - \dfrac{1207^2}{27} = 4910.2963$ on $\upsilon = 2$

SS due to interaction (calculated from unadjusted totals and grand total by usual method), $SS_{VitxTemp} = SS_T - SS_{Vit} - SS_{Temp} = 2765.3703$

$$\text{SS due to AB(!)} = \frac{\left(364^2 + 417^2 + 410^2\right)}{9} - \frac{1191^2}{27} = 184.2222 \text{ on } \upsilon = 2$$

$$\text{SS due to AB(J)} = \frac{\left(405^2 + 369^2 + 422^2\right)}{9} - \frac{1196^2}{27} = 162.7407 \text{ on } \upsilon = 2$$

SS due to error, $SS_E = \text{Total SS} - SS_R - SS_T = 120.7778$ on $\upsilon = 16$

All components calculated are laid into an ANOVA table:

H_0s:

1. There is no effect of confounding (MSS due to groups is not significant)
2. There is no effect of vitamin C on respiratory rate Golden retrievers
3. There is no effect of temperature on respiratory rate Golden retrievers
4. There is no effect of interaction (two-way) between vitamin C and temperature on respiratory rate Golden retrievers.

Source	υ	SS	MSS	F
Total	31	8572.9722		
Groups	11	2492.9722	226.6338	30.023
Replications	3	38.9722	12.9907	1.721[NS]
Groups within replications	8	2454.0000	306.7500	40.6367
Treatments (Unadjusted)	8	8413.2222	1051.6528	139.318
Vitamin C, A	2	737.5556	368.7778	48.8538
Temperature, B	2	4910.2963	2455.1482	325.245
Interaction Vit × Temp, AB	4	2765.3703	691.3426	91.586
AB(I)	2	184.2222	92.1111	12.202
AB(J)	2	162.7407	81.3704	10.780
Error	16	120.7778	7.5486	

Table values $F_{0.05}$: $(11,16) = 2.45$, $(3,16) = 3.24$, $(8,16) = 2.59$, $(2,16) = 3.63$ and $(4,16) = 3.01$; [NS] Not significant

MSS between groups is highly significant, confirming that confounding has been effective. Therefore, all H_0's are rejected.

4.1.2.5.3 *Retrieving inter-group information*

On most occasions, only higher order interactions are confounded; hence, information from replication(s) with confounding on the effect confounded is generally ignored. However, if any of the main effects is (are) confounded, as was the case in the above example, if inter-group information could be retrieved, it does serve purpose. This may be performed easily if all the effects are confounded in one of the replications uniformly as in the example above. Such design is also referred to as **balanced incomplete block design** (*see* Chapter "**ANOVA for more than two factors**" for details). The procedure is briefly as follows:

Step I: Calculation of total SS, SS due to replications and SS due to treatments is same by ignoring confounding (based on unadjusted totals). In the example under study, Total SS = 8572.9722, SS_R = 38.9722 and SS_T = 8413.2222. The treatment totals (Unadjusted) are utilized as:

Treatments	Unadjusted totals, t	B_t^*	W_t^{***}	Adjusted totals
(00)	137	495	34	
(01)	169	529	−6	
(02)	295	629	−28	
(10)	130	501	−11	m was negative;
(11)	149	506	26	hence ignored
(12)	274	613	−27	
(20)	120	487	15	
(21)	132	502	−9	
(22)	197	547	6	
	1603 = G	4809**	0	

* Total of all blocks in which the treatment is a constituent;

** Since each of the groups has 3 treatments ($k = 3$), it is included 3 times, hence, = 3G;

*** Calculated as $kt - (k+1)B_t + G$ and ΣW_t is always 0; $\Sigma W_t^2 = 3844$

Step II: $SS_{B/R}$ after adjusting for treatment effects = $\dfrac{\Sigma W_t^2}{k^3(k+1)}$ = (3844 ÷ 108) = 39.5926

on $\upsilon = 8$; hence, **inter-group** MSS due to error, $MSS_{E(a)}$ = (39.5926 ÷ 8) = 4.9491

Step III: Intra-group SS due to error, $SS_{E(b)}$ = Total SS − SS_R − $SS_{B/R}$(adj) − SS_T(Unadj) = 8572.9722 − 38.9722 − 4.9491 − 8413.2222 = 115.8287; hence, MSS due to error, $MSS_{E(b)}$ = (115.8287 ÷ 16) = 7.2393

Step IV: A weighting factor required for adjusting treatment totals can be calculated as: $m = \dfrac{MSS_{E(b)} - MSS_{E(a)}}{k^2 MSS_{E(b)}}$ = −0.0352. Since the value m is negative, it is ignored in the present case; otherwise, adjusted treatment totals are given by $t + mW_t$.

Step V: An **Effective MSS$_E$** is calculated as $MSS_{E(b)}(1 + km)$ = 6.9845; however, since m is negative, this is not applicable in the current case.

Step VI: A 2 × 2 table of adjusted treatment totals is made and SS due to main effects ad interaction are calculated and tested against **Effective MSS$_E$**

Step VII: All the subsequent procedures of calculation of means, standard errors and LSD are as per procedures already described in the previous Chapters 13–15.

5. EXPERIMENTS WITH REPEATED MEASURES

Quite often an animal gives > 1 measurements for the same trait; for example, milk yield in different lactations, litter size, wool yield etc. Such data requires slightly different analytical procedure mainly because lactation number is not a "treatment" and so are litter number and shearing yield. Let us consider a numerical example to know about the analysis of such data:

Data on milk yield (tons) of three breeds of milch animals during 3 periods of 100 d and over 4 lactations are given below.

Milk yield (tons)		Lactation				
Breed	100 d periods	I	II	III	IV	Period totals
Jersey	1	1.5	1.9	1.7	1.7	6.8
	2	1.8	2.5	2.1	2.2	8.6
	3	2.0	2.6	2.2	2.1	8.9
Lactation totals		5.3	7.0	6.0	6.0	24.3
HF	1	1.8	2.5	2.3	2.1	8.7
	2	2.6	3.5	3.0	2.9	12.0
	3	3.1	4.2	3.6	3.2	14.1
Lactation totals		7.5	10.2	8.9	8.2	34.8
Crosbreds	1	0.7	1.0	0.9	0.8	3.4
	2	1.0	1.5	1.1	0.9	4.5
	3	1.2	1.8	1.2	1.1	5.3
Lactation totals		2.9	4.3	3.2	2.8	13.2
Overall totals		15.7	21.5	18.1	17.0	72.3

By following usual method, we can calculate:

Total crude SS = 500.81 (Lactation totals used); C = 435.6075; Total SS = 65.2025

SS due to breeds, SS_B = 58.3350 on $v = 2$

SS due to lactations, SS_L = 6.1758 on $v = 3$

SS due to error, SS_E = 0.6917 on $v = 6$

H_0's:

1. There is no difference between breeds in milk yield
2. There is no difference between lactations

Source	v	SS	MSS	F
Total	11	65.2025		
Breeds	2	58.3350	29.1675	252.971
Lactations	3	6.1758	2.0586	17.854
Error	6	0.6917	0.1153	

Table values $F_{0.05,2,6}$ = 19.33

Since the calculated values of F were > table values, H_0's are rejected.

Note:

1. The lactation effect is significant; it can be split into linear, quadratic and cubic components by use of orthogonal polynomials as described in Chapter "**Association between variables III**".
2. For testing periods and other interactions, suitable 2 × 2 tables can be formed and analyzed as described in earlier Chapters. If periods are significant, linear and quadratic equations can be fit by use of orthogonal polynomials as described in earlier Chapter "**Association between variables III**".

6. EXPECTATION MEAN SQUARES (EMS)

The method of writing components of EMS for a calculated MSS has been described in **Section 6** of Chapter **"Analysis of variance for more than two factors"**. Therefore, EMS in a two- and three-factor experiment is tabulated below. It is generally true that in an experiment involving more than two factors, all factors will be neither fixed nor random; hence, only mixed effect model is considered for a three-factor experiment.

| | Two-factor Experiment (Factors A and B) | | |
MSS	Model I (Fixed)	Model II (Random)	Mixed (A fixed)
A	$\sigma^2 + nbk^2_A$	$\sigma^2 + n\sigma^2_{AB} + nb\sigma^2_A$	$\sigma^2 + n\sigma^2_{AB} + nbk^2_A$
B	$\sigma^2 + nak^2_B$	$\sigma^2 + n\sigma^2_{AB} + na\sigma^2_B$	$\sigma^2 + na\sigma^2_{AB}$
AB	$\sigma^2 + nk^2_{AB}$	$\sigma^2 + n\sigma^2_{AB}$	$\sigma^2 + n\sigma^2_{AB}$
Error	σ^2	σ^2	σ^2
	Three-factor Experiment (Factors A, B and C)		
	A fixed, B and C random		
A	$\sigma^2 + n\sigma^2_{ABC} + nc\sigma^2_{AB} + nb\sigma^2_{AC} + nbck^2_A$		
B	$\sigma^2 + na\sigma^2_{BC} + nac\sigma^2_B$		
AB	$\sigma^2 + n\sigma^2_{ABC} + nc\sigma^2_{AB}$		
C	$\sigma^2 + na\sigma^2_{BC} + nab\sigma^2_C$		
AC	$\sigma^2 + n\sigma^2_{ABC} + nb\sigma^2_{AC}$		
BC	$\sigma^2 + na\sigma^2_{BC}$		
ABC	$\sigma^2 + n\sigma^2_{ABC}$		
Error	σ^2		

k = number of observations; a, b and c are levels of A, B and C, respectively

17

Response Curve and Response Surface

In a factorial experiment, it is not necessary that all factors must be continuous or quantitative; in fact, in the **Example 2.1.1** in Chapter "**Factorial experiments**" one of the factors is sex of the piglets. However, it is not uncommon that one or more factors will be not only quantitative, but also the levels considered will be equally spaced, say as in case of Sreenivasaiah (1985) where STPP levels were 0, 3 and 6%, durations of marinating were 3, 6 and 9 h, set for refrigeration storage was 0, 4 and 8 d and set for frozen storage was 0, 30 and 60 d. It is under such situations, another dimension for factorial analysis appears; to investigate whether there is any association linear/ quadratic/cubic, etc. between levels of factor(s), the independent variable, and the criterion studied (dependent variable). This would help in the following aspects:

1. Quantify the relationship, if any
2. Predict the effect of level(s) of factor(s) not included in the study but within the range included
3. Whenever the association is parabolic (quadratic), predict maxima/minima value, as the case may be

Since **response** of the dependent variable is studied, it is referred to as **response curve/surface**.

1. POLYNOMIAL RESPONSE CURVE

Regression equations can be fit depending on the significance of SS obtained in the analysis of association that follows. If quadratic component were to be significant, a theoretical maximum/minimum value, as the case may be, (maximum in this example) can be calculated (as ratio of $-b$ to $2c$); hence, such a parabola is often referred to as **Response Curve**. The utility of such a derived value is when the experiment is repeated, the levels can be fixed on either side of the maximum/minimum value to ascertain the validity of prediction. Otherwise, equation(s) of the degree(s) that is (are) significant can be derived.

Response curve can be derived only when at least 3 levels are used for a factor that is quantitative; if it is equally spaced, it is convenient to use the orthogonal contrasts readily available (Appendix 9) or they have to be derived; otherwise, matrices/computer assistance becomes necessary.

1.1. Example

The following example pertains to egg production of a group of 5 hens allotted to each of the 12 treatments comprising of layer mash containing 3 levels of protein in combination with 4 levels of lysine in a 3 × 4 factorial experiment. Only total number of eggs produced by 5 birds is given along with total crude SS below:

Lysine, %, factor (L)	Protein, % (factor P)			Totals	Means
	15	18	21		
0.2	48	111	138	297	19.8
0.4	63	123	138	324	21.6
0.6	84	129	141	354	23.6
0.8	102	135	135	372	24.8
Totals	297	498	552	Grand total	Overall mean
Means	14.85	24.90	27.60	1347	$\bar{y} = 22.45$

Total crude SS = 32658 (SS of egg production of all 60 hens)
Step I: Computation of ANOVA by methods already described earlier.
Total sum of squares = 2417.85
Sum of squares due to protein levels, $SS_P = 1805.70$
Sum of squares due to lysine levels, $SS_L = 218.85$
Sum of squares due to interaction, $SS_{PxL} = 183.90$
Sum of squares due to error, $SS_E = 209.40$
Now, the ANOVA table will be:
H_0s:
1. There is no effect of protein levels on egg production
2. There is no effect of lysine levels on egg production
3. There is no effect of interaction between protein and lysine on egg production

Source	v	SS	MSS	F
Total	59	2417.85		
P	2	1805.70	902.9500	206.980
L	3	218.85	72.9500	16.722
PxL	6	183.90	30.6500	7.026
Error	48	209.40	4.3625	

Table value of $F_{0.05,2,48} = 3.19$; $F_{0.05,3,48} = 2.80$; $F_{0.05,6,48} = 2.30$

It is evident that treatment and interaction effects are significant and hence, all H_0s are rejected.
Step II: Since 3 levels are available for protein, linear and quadratic components can be fit by using **orthogonal contrasts** (Appendix 9) as shown below (*see* Chapter "**Association between variables III**" for details):

	Protein levels, % (r = 20)			Component Totals ($\xi_i y_i$)	SS[@]	F
Totals, (y_i) →	15	18	21			
	297	498	552			
	ξ_i's (Appendix 9)					
Linear	−1	0	1	255	1625.625	372.636
Quadratic	1	−2	1	−147	180.075	41.278
	SS_P = 1805.700			SS_P	1805.700	
			MSS_E; υ = 48		4.3625	

Table value of $F_{0.05,1,48}$ = 4.04; [@] Calculated as $\dfrac{\left(\sum \xi_i y_i\right)^2}{r\sum \xi_i^2}$

Step III: Partitioning SS_L into linear, quadratic and cubic components (since 4 levels are available) by using orthogonal contrasts.

	Lysine levels, % (r = 15)				Component Totals ($\xi_i y_i$)	SS[@]	F
Totals, (y_i's) !	0.2	0.4	0.6	0.8			
	297	324	354	372			
	ξ_i's (Appendix 9)						
Linear	−3	−1	1	3	255	216.75	49.685
Quadratic	1	−1	−1	1	−9	1.35	< 1
Cubic	−1	3	−3	1	−15	0.75	< 1
	SS_L = 218.85				SS_L	218.85	
				MSS_E; υ − 48		4.3625	

Table value of $F_{0.05,1,48}$ = 4.04; [@] calculated as $\dfrac{\left(\sum \xi_i y_i\right)^2}{r\sum \xi_i^2}$

It is clear that the effect of lysine levels was primarily linear.

Step IV: Both linear and quadratic components, especially the former in case of protein levels being overwhelming, were significant. Hence, linear and quadratic equations for protein levels can be computed as follows:

1. Linear equation: $y = \bar{y} + B_1' \xi_1$ where $B_1' = \lambda_1 B_1$; $B_1 = \dfrac{\sum \xi_i y_i}{\sum \xi_i^2} = 6.375$; $\lambda_1 = 1$ (Appendix 9);

   hence, B_1' = 6.375. $\xi_1 = (x - \bar{x}) \div d$; d = 3 (difference between successive levels of protein), = Average of protein levels = 18; $\bar{y}$ = 22.45; therefore,
   y = 22.45 + 6.375 {$(x - 18) \div 3$} = − 15.800 + 2.125x.

2. Quadratic equation: $y = \bar{y} + B_1' \xi_1 + B_2' \xi_2$ where $y = \bar{y} + B_1' \xi_1$ = −15.8 + 2.125x.
   $\xi_1 = (x - 18) \div 3$; = −1.225; $B_2' = \lambda_2 B_2$; λ_2 = 3 (Appendix 9); hence, B_2' = −3.675;
   $\xi_2 = \xi_1^2 - (n^2 - 1) \div 12$ where n number of levels = 3; therefore,

$$\xi_2 = \left(\frac{x-18}{3}\right)^2 - \frac{2}{3} = \frac{x^2 - 36x + 318}{9}.$$

Finally, quadratic equation will be

$$y = -15.8 + 2.215x - 3.675\left(\frac{x^2 - 36x + 318}{9}\right) = -145.6500 + 16.9150x - 0.4083x^2.$$

It can be noticed that the coefficient of x^2 is negative and hence, the equation has a theoretical maximum value at $x = 20.7139\%$ protein when y will be 29.538 eggs. The response curve is graphically shown below:

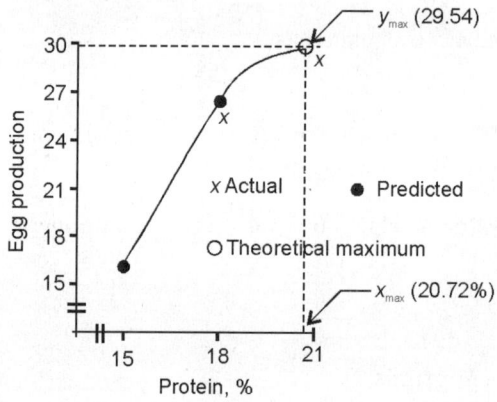

Fig. 17.1: Response curve

Hence, the experiment may be repeated say, with 19, 21 and 23% protein levels to confirm the result.

Note: If $x = (-b \div 2c)$ or $b + 2cx$ is equated to economic values, $(P_x \div P_y)$, where P_x and P_y are market prices of x and y, we get **economic response** and optimum dose at which maximum yield can be expected can be obtained by solving $b + 2cx = (P_x \div P_y)$; or by $x = \dfrac{P_x - bP_y}{2cP_y}$.

2. POLYNOMIAL RESPONSE SURFACE

When two factors are quantitative, and each of them is employed at least at 3 levels, preferably equally spaced, provides a possibility of computing an equation to help predict levels of the two factors to maximize y (dependent variable). This is like an extended response curve with two independent variables and similar to multiple regression but with quadratic and interaction components. Such equations are referred to as **Response surface** and are represented as $y = a + b_1x_1 + b_2x_1^2 + b_3x_2 + b_4x_1x_2$. Obviously, linear and quadratic components of one factor, linear component of the other and interaction between the two have to be significant to proceed to fit response surface. Orthogonal polynomials (Appendix 9) can be used to facilitate computations when the levels are equally spaced; else, designer contrasts have to be calculated as described in Chapter "**Association between variables III**". A numerical example follows to outline various steps involved in the process:

2.1 Example

Let us revisit **Example 1.1** in which linear and quadratic components were calculated.

Lysine, %, Factor (L)	Protein, % (Factor P)			Totals	Means
	15	18	21		
0.2	48	111	138	297	19.8
0.4	63	123	138	324	21.6
0.6	84	129	141	354	23.6
0.8	102	135	135	372	24.8
Totals	297	498	552	Grand total	Overall mean
Means	14.85	24.90	27.60	1347	$\bar{y} = 22.45$

Total crude SS = 32658 (SS of egg production of all 60 hens)

Step I: Computation of ANOVA already given above.

It was evident that protein, lysine and interaction effects were significant.

Step II: Now, let us compute linear, quadratic and cubic components of protein levels for each of the lysine levels:

Protein, %		Lysine % (Factor L): Totals (r = 15), y_i				
Linear contrasts, ξ_l		0.2	0.4	0.6	0.8	
15	−1	48	63	84	102	
18	0	111	123	129	135	
21	1	138	138	141	135	$\Sigma \xi_l y_i$
$\xi_l y_i$		90	75	57	33	255
Quadratic contrasts, ξ_q		0.2	0.4	0.6	0.8	
15	1	48	63	84	102	
18	−2	111	123	129	135	
21	1	138	138	141	135	$\Sigma \xi_q y_i$
$\xi_q y_i$		−36	−45	−33	−33	−147

Since totals are used, SS due to linear effects of protein levels,

$$P_L = \frac{\left(\sum \xi_l y_i\right)^2}{r \sum \xi_l^2} = 1625.625; \text{ similarly, quadratic effects, } P_Q = \frac{\left(\sum \xi_q y_i\right)^2}{r \sum \xi_q^2} = 180.075.$$

Note:

1. In each of these, r is taken as 20 because for each of the protein levels there were 20 observations.
2. $P_L + P_Q = SS_P = 1805.7$

It is now possible to test these on $\upsilon = 1$ on MSS_E already calculated on $\upsilon = 48$ as 4.3625; obviously, both components are highly significant.

Step III: To test interaction of linear and quadratic components of protein levels, $P_L L$, $P_Q L$, respectively, with lysine levels as follows:

SS due to P_LL on $\upsilon = 3$ is calculated as $\dfrac{90^2 + 75^2 + 57^2 + 33^2}{5\sum \xi_{i}^2} - \dfrac{225^2}{20 \sum \xi_{i}^2} = 180.675$ where

$\sum \xi_{1}^2 = 2$, the sum of squares of contrasts; hence, MSS due to $P_LL = 60.225$ yielding an F value of 13.805 against MSS_E of 4.3625. Similarly, SS due to P_QL on $\tilde{o} = 3$ is calculated

as $\dfrac{-(36)^2 + (-45)^2 + (-33)^2 + (-33)^2}{5 \sum \xi_{q}^2} - \dfrac{(-147)^2}{20 \sum \xi_{q}^2} = 3.225$ where $\sum \xi_{q}^2 = 6$, the sum of squares

of contrasts; hence, MSS due to $P_QL = 1.075$ yielding an F value of < 1 against MSS_E of 4.3625.

Note:

1. In each of these, r is taken as 5 for the first term because for each of the protein levels within a lysine level, there were 5 observations and as 20 for the other term because total number of observation for a protein level is 20.

2. $P_LL + P_QL = SS_{PxL} = 183.9$

Therefore, it is reasonable to expect that the interaction, response to protein levels with the lysine levels, is primarily linear.

Step IV: Confirm the findings in Step III that interaction is indeed linear by partitioning SS due to P_LL on $\upsilon = 3$ into linear, quadratic and cubic components P_LL_L, P_LL_Q and P_LL_C each on $\upsilon = 1$ as follows:

It is now ascertained that the interaction effects were mainly linear in nature. With the above partitioning of SS, a consolidated ANOVA can be laid:

Lysine, %	0.2	0.4	0.6	0.8			
$P_L = \xi_i y_i$	90	75	57	33			
	Contrasts, ξ_i's (Appendix 9)				Totals	SS@	F
P_LL_L	−3	−1	1	3	−189	178.605	40.941
P_LL_Q	1	−1	−1	1	−9	2.025	< 1
P_LL_C	−1	3	−3	1	−3	0.045	< 1
					SS due to P_LL	180.675	

Calculated as $\dfrac{(\text{Total})^2}{2r \sum \xi_i^2}$ where $r = 5$, the number of observations per treatment combination

Step V: That the effects of protein levels is quadratic and the weight gain increases linearly with increased lysine levels at each level of protein can be expressed as a

Source	υ	SS	MSS	F
Total	59	2417.850		
P	2	1805.700	902.9500	206.980
P Linear, P_L	1	1625.625	1625.6250	372.636
P Quadratic, P_Q	1	180.075	180.0750	41.278

(Contd.)

Source	v	SS	MSS	F
L	3	218.850	72.9500	16.722
L Linear, L_L	1	216.750	216.7500	49.685
L Quadratic, L_Q	1	1.350	1.3500	< 1
L Cubic, L_C	1	0.750	0.7500	< 1
Interaction, PxL	6	183.900	30.6500	7.026
$P_L L_L$	1	178.605	178.6050	40.941
$P_L L_Q$	1	2.025	2.0250	< 1
$P_L L_C$	1	0.045	0.0450	< 1
$P_Q L_L + P_Q L_Q + P_Q L_C$	3[@]	3.225	1.0750	< 1
Error	48	209.400	4.3625	

Table value of $F_{0.05,2,48} = 3.19$; $F_{0.05,3,48} = 2.80$; $F_{0.05,6,48} = 2.30$; $F_{0.05,1,48} = 4.04$; [@] Not partitioned because L_Q and L_C were not significant

Response surface: $y = \bar{y} + b_1 P_L + b_2 P_Q + b_3 L_L + b_4 P_L L_L$

Hence, the equation in the coded scale will be $y = 22.450 + 6.375 P_L - 1.225 P_Q + 0.850 L_L$

Factors (x_i's)		Total (y_i's)	Orthogonal contrasts (ξ_i's)			
Protein (P)%	Lysine (L)%	($r = 5$)	P_L	P_Q	L_L	$P_L L_L$*
			$\frac{1}{3}(P - 18)$	$(3P^2_L - 2)$	$10(L - 0.5)$	
15	0.2	48	−1	1	−3	3
	0.4	63	−1	1	−1	1
	0.6	84	−1	1	1	−1
	0.8	102	−1	1	3	−3
18	0.2	111	0	−2	−3	0
	0.4	123	0	−2	−1	0
	0.6	129	0	−2	1	0
	0.8	135	0	−2	3	0
21	0.2	138	1	1	−3	−3
	0.4	138	1	1	−1	−1
	0.6	141	1	1	1	1
	0.8	135	1	1	3	3
		$\Sigma \xi_i y_i$	255	−147	255	−189
		$\Sigma \xi_i^2$	8	24	60	40
6.375	−1.225	0.85	−0.945			

* by multiplying contrasts of P_L and L_L; $\bar{y} = 22.45$;

$-0.945 P_L L_L$. This equation can be decoded by undoing the calculations done to develop orthogonal contrasts; that means, by substituting $P_L = \frac{1}{3}(P - 18)$, $P_Q = (3P^2_L - 2)$, $L_L = 10(L - 0.5)$ and $P_L L_L = \{\frac{1}{3}(P - 18)\}\{10(L - 0.5)\}$. The equation in terms of protein, lysine and interaction on original scale to get **mean value** for any treatment combination of protein and lysine levels will be: $y = -178.25 + 14.40P - 0.41P^2 + 65.20L - 3.15PL$. The predicted ($y'$) and actual values of means are tabulated below:

The response surface so developed can be utilized to predict a response and also to

Lysine, %, Factor (L)	Protein, % (Factor P)			Means	
	15	18	21	Actual	Predicted, y'
0.2, actual	9.6	22.2	27.6	19.8	
0.2, predicted, y'	9.09	21.81	27.15		19.35
0.4, actual	12.6	24.6	27.6	21.6	
0.4, predicted, y'	12.68	23.51	26.96		21.05
0.6, actual	16.8	25.8	28.2	23.6	
0.6, predicted, y'	16.27	25.21	26.77		22.75
0.8, actual	20.4	27.0	27.0	24.8	
0.8, predicted, y'	19.86	26.91	26.58		24.45
Means, actual	14.85	24.90	27.60	Overall mean	
Means, predicted, y'	14.475	24.36	26.865	22.45	21.90

"$(y - y')^2 = 5.3688 = $ (SS due to interaction PxL – SS due to $P_L L_L$) which forms only 0.22 % of Total SS.

calculate a probable combination of the two factors to maximize y; both have high practical utility.

18

Analysis of Covariance

In the preceding chapters on ANOVA the observations were assumed to be independent of influence from any other factor other than the ones that were under consideration. For example, when we conduct a growth trial on broilers, it is definitely necessary to select chicks that are of uniform birth weight and preferably from the same genetic background as well. Otherwise, there is a possibility that the day-old chick weight may influence growth rates independent of the experimental factors and make the results less reliable. The same situation can be viewed the other way also; if effect(s) of such variable(s), referred to as **auxiliary or ancillary variable(s)**, is (are) removed before the actual comparisons are made to ensure both efficiency and reliability of the test; in other words, inclusion of such auxiliary variable(s) helps reduce MSS_E thereby add to the efficiency of the test. The procedure for adjusting for effect of auxiliary variable is referred to as **analysis of covariance or ANACOV**; covariance is the numerator for calculation of association between variables (*see* Chapters 9–11).

It is easy to visualize that such corrections need regression analysis which is followed by ANOVA; hence, in Animal Science terminology, ANACOV is the hybrid between regression analysis and ANOVA. Advantages of ANACOV include, apart from adding to precision and reliability of experiments, study of regressions in multiple classifications and also to know the nature of treatment effects.

Assumptions for ANACOV are the same as ANOVA; in addition, it is also assumed that correct form of regression line is fit, treatment and regression effects need not be additive and that the x's are not affected by the treatments. In addition, it also assumes that the slopes of the regression lines and the residual mean squares are homogenous.

The ANACOV is indeed a large area in statistics and hence, only a brief account is given through numerical examples; readers interested in further information must access books specially dedicated to ANACOV.

1. PRELIMINARIES FOR ANACOV

The data structure is as follows (k = number of treatments and each treatment has n pairs of observations):

			Treatments			
	T_1	T_2		T_i	T_k	
	y_{11}	$x_{11}\ y_{21}$	$x_{21}\ \cdots\ y_{i1}$		$x_{i1}\ y_{k1}$	x_{k1}
	y_{12}	$x_{12}\ y_{22}$	$x_{22}\ \cdots\ y_{i2}$		$x_{i2}\ y_{k2}$	x_{k2}
	$\vdots$	$\vdots\quad\vdots$	$\vdots\quad\vdots\quad\vdots$		$\vdots\quad\vdots$	$\vdots$
	y_{1j}	$x_{1j}\ y_{2j}$	$x_{2j}\ \cdots\ y_{ij}$		$x_{ij}\ y_{kj}$	x_{kj}
	y_{1n}	$x_{1n}\ y_{2n}$	$x_{2n}\ \cdots\ y_{in}$		$x_{in}\ y_{kn}$	x_{kn}
Totals	$y_{1\cdot}$	$x_{1\cdot}\ y_{2\cdot}$	$x_{2\cdot}\ \cdots\ y_{i\cdot}$		$x_{i\cdot}\ y_{k\cdot}$	$x_{k\cdot}$
Sum of squares	$y^2_{1\cdot}$	$x^2_{1\cdot}\ y^2_{2\cdot}$	$x^2_{2\cdot}\ \cdots\ y^2_{i\cdot}$		$x^2_{i\cdot}\ y^2_{k\cdot}$	$x^2_{k\cdot}$
Grand total and total crude SS			$x_{\cdot\cdot},\ y_{\cdot\cdot},\ x^2_{\cdot\cdot}$ and $y^2_{\cdot\cdot}$			
Cross products	$\displaystyle\sum_{j=1}^{n} x_{1j}y_{1j}$	$\displaystyle\sum_{j=1}^{n} x_{2j}y_{2j}$	$\displaystyle\sum_{j=1}^{n} x_{ij}y_{ij}$		$\displaystyle\sum_{j=1}^{n} x_{kj}y_{kj}$	
Total cross products			$\displaystyle\sum_{i=1}^{k}\sum_{j=1}^{n} x_{ij}y_{ij}$			

Step I: At the beginning, it is necessary to know whether the auxiliary variable under consideration has any effect or not. This can be tested by calculating SS due to regression (overall) and testing it as per methods enumerated in Chapter "**Association between variables I**"; total cross products is considered for the purpose. This step is based on the assumption of homogeneity of regression coefficients in each of the treatments. In short, it involves calculation of:

$$T_{yy} = y^2\!.. - \{(y..)^2 \div nk\};\ T_{xx} = x^2\!.. - \{(x..)^2 \div nk\};\ T_{xy} = \sum_{i=1}^{k}\sum_{j=1}^{n} x_{ij}y_{ij} - \{(\,x..\ y..) \div nk\};\ b_{yx} = T_{xy}$$

$\div T_{xx}$; SS due to regression $= b_{yx}T_{xy}$ on $\upsilon = 1$; SS due to error, $SS_E = T_{yy} -$ SS due to regression on $\upsilon = (n - 2)$ and $MSS_E = SS_E \div (nk - 2)$; F on $\upsilon = 1$ and $(nk - 2)$ must be significant to consider adjusting the effects of auxiliary variable.

Step II: If the overall regression is significant, the next stage is to assess whether it is really worthwhile proceeding with ANACOV or not. This Step is also essentially same as Step I, but each of the treatment groups are considered as separate entities. T_{yy}, T_{xx}, T_{xy} and b_{yx} are calculated using treatment-wise values and ANOVA to compute residual SS for each of the regression carried-out with suitable changes in n's. It is summarized below:

Source (1)	T_{yy} (2)	T_{xx} (3)	T_{xy} (4)	b_{yx} (5)	υ (6)	Regression SS (7)	Residual SS* (2 – 7)
T_1	T_{1yy}	T_{1xx}	T_{1xy}	b_{1yx}	1	$b_{1yx}T_{1xy}$	SS_{1E}
T_2	T_{2yy}	T_{2xx}	T_{2xy}	b_{2yx}	1	$b_{2yx}T_{2xy}$	SS_{2E}
$\vdots$	$\vdots$	$\vdots$	$\vdots$	$\vdots$	$\vdots$	$\vdots$	$\vdots$
T_k	T_{kyy}	T_{kxx}	T_{kxy}	b_{kyx}	1	$b_{kyx}T_{kxy}$	SS_{kE}

(Contd.)

Source (1)	T_{yy} (2)	T_{xx} (3)	T_{xy} (4)	b_{yx} (5)	υ (6)	Regression SS (7)	Residual SS* $(2-7)$
Pooled	$\sum\limits_{i=1}^{k} T_{iyy}$	$\sum\limits_{i=1}^{k} T_{ixx}$	$\sum\limits_{i=1}^{k} T_{ixy}$	$b_{pyx} = \dfrac{\sum\limits_{i=1}^{k} T_{ixy}}{\sum\limits_{i=1}^{k} T_{ixx}}$	k	$b_{pyx} \sum\limits_{i=1}^{k} T_{ixy}$	SS_{PE}**and $\sum\limits_{i=1}^{k} SS_{iE}$ ***

* Each on $\upsilon = (n-2)$; ** On $\upsilon = k\,(n-1) - 1^{@}$; *** Designated SS_{TE}; on $\upsilon = k\,(n-2)$; **Note:** @ One degree of freedom subtracted due to computation of b_{pyx}

Step III: Now, a different kind of ANOVA is laid to test whether deviation from regression is significant or not.

Source	υ	SS	MSS	F
Total	$k(n-1) - 1$	SS_{PE}		
Within treatments, Pooled	$k(n-2)$	SS_{TE}	MSS_E	
Deviation from regression	$(k-1)$	Difference	MSS_R	$MSS_R \div MSS_E$

ANACOV can be taken-up if and only if F ratio is not significant. However, generally Steps I, II and III are assumed to yield suitable result and ANACOV is performed. Therefore, a numerical example is not provided for the above steps.

2. ANACOV IN A CRD

Data from a CRD is analyzed as described in Chapter "**One-factor analysis of variance**". The algebraic model, with usual meaning for notations, is modified to include the regression term as: $y_{ij} = \alpha_i + \beta\left(x_{ij} - \bar{x}_{..}\right) + e_{ij}$ and therefore, mean of the dependent variable, $\bar{y}_{ij} = \alpha_i + \beta\left(\bar{x}_{ij} - \bar{x}_{..}\right) + \bar{e}_{ij} = \alpha_i + \beta\left(\bar{x}_{ij} - \bar{x}_{..}\right)$ (error has a mean 0 and variance $\acute{o}^2$). Hence, $\alpha_i = \bar{y}_{ij} - \beta\left(\bar{x}_{ij} - \bar{x}_{..}\right)$; the term $-\beta\left(\bar{x}_{ij} - \bar{x}_{..}\right)$ refers to the adjustment due to ANACOV. **The equation $\alpha_i = \bar{y}_{ij} - \beta\left(\bar{x}_{ij} - \bar{x}_{..}\right)$ clearly indicated that ANACOV involves the error or residual component but not the treatment component.**

2.1 Procedure of ANACOV

The data obtained from an experiment conducted on CRD will be the same as shown under **Section 1**. Hence, only totals, SS and cross products are shown below:

Step I: Computation of sums, SS and sum of cross products (SCP)

		Treatments			
	T_1	T_2		T_i	T_k
Totals	$y_1.$	$x_1.\ y_2.$	$x_2. \ \ \dots \ \ y_i.$	$x_i.\ y_k.$	$x_k.$
Sum of squares	$y^2_1.$	$x^2_1.\ y^2_2.$	$x^2_2. \ \ \dots \ \ y^2_i.$	$x^2_i.\ y^2_k.$	$x^2_k.$
Grand Total and Total Crude SS			$x..,\ y..,\ x^2..$ and $y^2..$		
Total cross products			$\displaystyle\sum_{i=1}^{k}\sum_{j=1}^{n} x_{ij}y_{ij}$		

With the availability of the above information, ANOVA with respect to both x and y, separately and **analysis of products** have to be developed; for the former two, the method is discussed in Chapter "**One-factor analysis of variance**"; the latter is outlined here:

Step II: Analysis of products is essentially similar to analysis of squares with the only change that instead of squaring each value/totals, the corresponding values/totals of x and y are multiplied. All the three are tabulated in notation form along with ANOVA and analysis of products for easy understanding:

	Variable x	Product xy	Variable y
Sum	$x..$	—	$y..$
Total SS	$SS_X =$	$SCP_{XY} =$	$SS_Y =$
$\upsilon = nk - 1$	$x^2.. - \dfrac{(x..)^2}{nk}$	$\displaystyle\sum_{i=1}^{k}\sum_{j=1}^{n} x_{ij}y_{ij} - \dfrac{(x..)(y..)}{nk}$	$y^2.. - \dfrac{(y..)^2}{nk}$
Between treatments	$SS_{T(X)} =$	$SCP_{T(XY)} =$	$SS_{T(Y)} =$
$\upsilon = k - 1$	$\displaystyle\sum_{i=1}^{k} \dfrac{(x_i.)^2}{n} - \dfrac{(x..)^2}{nk}$	$\dfrac{\sum_{i=1}^{k} x_i.y_i.}{n} - \dfrac{(x..)(y..)}{nk}$	$\displaystyle\sum_{i=1}^{k} \dfrac{(y_i.)^2}{n} - \dfrac{(y..)^2}{nk}$
Error*	$SS_{E(X)}$	$SCP_{E(XY)}$	$SS_{E(Y)}$
$\upsilon = k(n-1)$			

Reduction due to regression on $u = 1$ $SS_{R(Y)} =$

Note: Regression coefficient, $b = \dfrac{SCP_{E(xy)}}{SS_{E(x)}}$ $\dfrac{\left(SCP_{E(xy)}\right)^2}{SS_{E(x)}}$

Deviations from regression, on $\upsilon = k(n-1) - 1$ $SS_D = SS_{E(Y)} - SS_{R(Y)}$

* SS within treatments, by difference = (Total SS – Between treatments); Deviation Mean Sum of squares, $MSS_D = SS_D \div \{\, k(n-1) - 1\,\}$

Step III: Calculation of adjusted means: Means of each of the treatments can be adjusted by the formula: $\bar{y}_i. - b(\bar{x}_i. - \bar{x}..)$ which is derived at the beginning of this section.

Step IV: Tests of significance and confidence limits are all as described in relevant Chapters earlier; but MSS_D is used as the MSS_E for all purposes. The difference between

ith and jth treatment mean can be estimated as: $\bar{y}_{i.} - \bar{y}_{j.} - b(\bar{x}_{i.} - \bar{x}_{j.})$ and the variance

of this difference is given by: $MSS_D \left[\dfrac{2}{n} + \dfrac{(\bar{x}_{i.} - \bar{x}_{j.})^2}{SS_{E(X)}} \right]$.

Step V: Calculating efficiency of ANACOV as $\dfrac{MSS_{E(Y)}}{MSS_D \left(1 + \dfrac{MSS_{E(Y)}}{SS_{E(X)}} \right)}$, where $MSS_Y =$

$\dfrac{SS_{E(Y)}}{k(n-1)}$.

2.2 Example

The data below refers to a feeding trial on cows fed control (A), urea-supplemented (B), sorghum-supplemented (C) and corn-supplemented (D) diets. Milk yield per d over 40 d experimental period (y_i's) is compared with that per d before the experiment (x_i's). It is necessary to check whether ANACOV is worthwhile to increase precision of results.

2.2.1 Calculation of Sums, SS and Cross–Products

	Treatment A		Treatment B		Treatment C		Treatment D	
	x	y	x	y	x	y	x	y
	15.8	15.9	16.6	20.0	15.2	30.0	14.9	20.5
	15.4	16.0	15.6	20.5	14.8	27.3	14.9	19.3
	16.5	16.3	11.6	22.0	17.8	35.0	20.8	27.0
	15.5	15.3	13.4	25.5	17.1	33.3	19.4	22.5
	14.4	15.3	15.3	26.0	16.9	32.8	17.1	21.0
	20.3	21.8	18.0	27.5	18.2	35.0	17.6	22.5
	17.1	16.5	13.2	23.0	15.9	30.8	18.2	22.0
	11.0	10.8	15.3	25.3	15.2	30.5	14.0	15.5
Totals	126.0	127.9	119.0	189.8	131.1	254.7	136.9	170.3
SS	2032.16	2106.81	1799.46	4555.84	2160.03	8158.91	2382.43	3699.49
CP	2067.53	2832.19	4197.11	2963.62				

The above values are tabulated for easy location below:

	Treatments							
	A		B		C		D	
Totals	126.0	127.9	119.0	189.8	131.1	254.7	136.9	170.3
Grand total and total crude SS	$SSx.. = 513.0$, $y.. = 742.7$, $x^2.. = 8374.08$, $y^2.. = 18521.05$							
Total cross products	$\displaystyle\sum_{i=1}^{k}\sum_{j=1}^{n} x_{ij}y_{ij} = 12060.45$							

2.2.2 Developing ANOVA and ANACOV

Now, the ANOVA and ANACOV are in the following table:

	Variable x	Cross product xy	Variable y
Sum	$x.. = 513.0$	12060.45	$y.. = 742.7$
Total SS on $\upsilon = 31$	$SS_X = 150.0488$	$SCP_{XY} = 154.0406$	$SS_Y = 1283.4472$
Between treatments $\upsilon = 3$	$SS_{T(X)} = 21.6963$	$SCP_{T(XY)} = 19.4456$	$SS_{T(Y)} = 1044.4759$
Error* on $\upsilon = 28$	$SS_{E(X)} = 128.3525$	$SCP_{E(XY)} = 134.5950$	$SS_{E(Y)} = 238.9713$
	Reduction due to Regression on $\upsilon = 1$		$SS_{R(Y)} = 141.1411$
	Deviations from regression, on $\upsilon = 27$		$SS_D = 97.8302$

* SS within treatments, by difference = (Total SS – Between treatments); Deviation mean sum of squares, $MSS_D = SS_D \div 27 = 3.6233$; Regression Coefficient, $b = 1.0486$

That the unadjusted $MSS_{E(y)}$ was $238.9713 \div 28 = 8.5347$ was reduced to $MSS_D = 3.6233$ (more than halved), confirms the usefulness of the auxiliary variable.

2.2.3 Adjusted Means and Comparisons

The computation of adjusted means is tabulated below for easy reference:

Treatments	Means (unadjusted)		Adjustment factor $-b(\bar{x}_{i.} - \bar{x}_{..})$	Means (adjusted)
	x	y		
A	15.75	15.99	0.29	16.28
B	14.88	23.72	1.21	24.93
C	16.39	31.84	– 0.38	31.46
D	17.11	21.29	– 1.13	20.16

$\bar{x}_{..} = 16.03$; $b = 1.05$; Sum of adjustment factors = 0

Variance of difference between two adjusted means can be calculated by entering the means under comparison into $3.6233\left[\dfrac{2}{8} + \dfrac{(\bar{x}_{i.} - \bar{x}_{j.})^2}{128.3525}\right]$. The LSD is calculated as per procedure described in Chapter "**One-factor analysis of variance**"; in any case, the values are tabulated below:

Means		Variance	$sd = \sqrt{\text{Variance}}$	$LSD(t_{0.05,27} * sd)$
$\bar{x}_{i.}$	$\bar{x}_{j.}$			
	23.72	2.5926	1.61	3.30
15.99	31.84	7.9977	2.83	5.81
	21.29	1.6988	1.30	2.67

(Contd.)

Means		Variance	$sd = \sqrt{\text{Variance}}$	LSD($t_{0.05,27}$*sd)
$\bar{x}_{i.}$	$\bar{x}_{j.}$			
23.72	31.84	2.7671	1.66	3.41
	21.29	1.0725	1.04	2.13
31.84	21.29	4.0478	2.01	4.12

LSD values indicated that all the treatments were different from one another and hence the superscripts are 15.99[d] (A) 23.72[b] (B) 31.84[a] (C) 21.29[c] (D).

Efficiency of ANACOV in this case was 2.21 emphasizing that procedure was worthwhile undertaking.

2.2.4 The F Test for Adjusted Means

Analogous to multiple regression equations (*see* Chapter "**Association between variables II**"), a H_0: there is no difference between adjusted means can be made by the calculations already available to which "Treatment + Error" line is computed based on H_0 is added. The same is shown below (theoretical aspects of this part may be obtained from other publications):

	Variable x	Cross product xy	Variable y
Sum	x.. = 513.0	12060.45	y.. = 742.7
Total SS on υ = 31	SS_X = 150.0488	SCP_{XY} = 154.0406	SS_Y = 1283.4472
Between treatments υ = 3	$SS_{T(X)}$ = 21.6963	$SCP_{T(XY)}$ = 19.4456	$SS_{T(Y)}$ = 1044.4759
Error* on υ = 28	$SS_{E(X)}$ = 128.3525	$SCP_{E(XY)}$ = 134.5950	$SS_{E(Y)}$ = 238.9713
Treatment + Error, on υ = 31 (on H_0)	$SS_{H0E(X)}$ = 150.0488	$SCP_{H0E(XY)}$ = 153.6356	$SS_{H0E(Y)}$ = 1283.4472

Reduction due to regression on υ = 1, (on H_0) $SS_{H0R(Y)}$ = 157.3081

Deviations from regression$_{H0'}$ on υ = 29, (on H_0) SS_{H0D} = 1126.1391

Mean deviations from regression$_{H0'}$ on υ = 2, (on H_0) MSS_{H0D} = 563.0696

* SS within treatments, by difference = (Total SS – Between treatments); Deviation mean sum of squares, $MSS_D = SS_D \div 27 = 3.6233$; Regression coefficient, b = 1.0486

The ratio of variances **MSS$_{H0D}$** and **MSS$_D$** follows F distribution on υ = 2 and 26; the calculated value is (563.0696 ÷ 3.6233) = 155.402 which is > 3.37, the tabulated value of F at α = 0.05. Hence, H_0 is rejected.

3. ANACOV IN A RBD

Suppose in the **Example 2.2**, each of the 8 animals per treatment is considered as a block, the same data can be analyzed as RBD (*see* Chapter "**Two-factor analysis of variance**" for details).

H_0:

1. There is no effect on pre-treatment production on subsequent yield of dairy cows
2. There is no effect of treatments on milk yield of dairy cows

3.1 Calculation of Sums, SS and SCP

Cow no	Treatment A		Treatment B		Treatment C		Treatment D		Cow totals	
	x	y	x	y	x	y	x	y	x	y
1	15.8	15.9	16.6	20.0	15.2	30.0	14.9	20.5	62.5	86.4
2	15.4	16.0	15.6	20.5	14.8	27.3	14.9	19.3	60.7	83.1
3	16.5	16.3	11.6	22.0	17.8	35.0	20.8	27.0	66.7	100.3
4	15.5	15.3	13.4	25.5	17.1	33.3	19.4	22.5	65.4	96.6
5	14.4	15.3	15.3	26.0	16.9	32.8	17.1	21.0	63.7	95.1
6	20.3	21.8	18.0	27.5	18.2	35.0	17.6	22.5	74.1	106.8
7	17.1	16.5	13.2	23.0	15.9	30.8	18.2	22.0	64.4	92.3
8	11.0	10.8	15.3	25.3	15.2	30.5	14.0	15.5	55.5	82.1
Totals	126.0	127.9	119.0	189.8	131.1	254.7	136.9	170.3	513.0	742.7
CP	2067.53	2832.19	4197.11	2963.62	12060.45					

3.2 Developing ANOVA and ANACOV

Now, the ANOVA and ANACOV are in the following table:

Source	v	Variable x	Cross product xy	Variable y
Total	31	$SS_X =$ 150.0488	$SCP_{XY} =$ 154.0406	$SS_Y =$ 1283.4472
Between cows	7	$SS_{C(X)} =$ 49.1938	$SCP_{C(XY)} =$ 74.6506	$SS_{C(Y)} =$ 130.4397
Between treatments	3	$SS_{T(X)} =$ 21.6963	$SCP_{T(XY)} =$ 19.4456	$SS_{T(Y)} =$ 1044.4759
Error	21	$SS_{E(X)} =$ 79.1587	$SCP_{E(XY)} =$ 59.9444	$SS_{E(Y)} =$ 108.5316
Treatment + Error	24	100.8550	79.3900	1153.0075
Regression (Error)	1	$(SCP_{E(XY)})^2 \div SS_{E(X)}$	45.3940	
Regression (Treatment + Error)	1	$79.39^2 \div 100.855$	62.4934	
Error (Corrected)	20	$108.5316 - 45.3940$	63.1376	
Treatment + Error (Corrected)	23	$1153.0075 - 62.4934$	1090.5141	
Treatment (Corrected)	3	$1090.5141 - 63.1376$	1027.3765	

$b_{yx} = (59.9444 \div 79.1587) = 0.7573$ is used for computing adjusted treatment means

ANOVA table for testing SS due to regression and SS due to treatments (corrected) can now be laid as follows:

Source	υ	SS	MSS	F
Regression	1	45.3940	45.3940	14.379
Treatments (Corrected)	3	1027.3765	342.4588	108.479
Error (Corrected)	20	63.1376	3.1569	

Table value of $F_{0.05,1,20} = 4.35$; $F_{0.05,3,20} = 3.10$

3.3 Comparison of Treatment Means

Since calculated values of F were > table values, the H_0's are rejected.

Means		Variance*	$sd = \sqrt{\text{Variance}}$	LSD($t_{0.05, 20}$ *sd)
$\bar{x}_{i\cdot}$	$\bar{x}_{j\cdot}$			
	23.72	3.78	1.94	4.05
15.99	31.84	13.35	3.65	7.61
	21.29	2.19	1.48	3.09
23.72	31.84	4.09	2.02	4.21
	21.29	1.08	1.04	2.17
31.84	21.29	6.35	2.52	5.26

$$* \text{ Calculated as } 3.1569 \left[\frac{2}{8} + \frac{\left(\bar{x}_{i\cdot} - \bar{x}_{j\cdot}\right)^2}{63.1376} \right]$$

LSD values indicated that all the treatments were different from one another and hence the superscripts are 15.99[d] (A) 23.72[b] (B) 31.84[a] (C) 21.29[c] (D).

Efficiency of ANACOV in this case was 1.54 emphasizing that procedure was worthwhile undertaking.

Note:

1. Calculation of adjusted treatment means and their comparison is same as under ANACOV in a CRD

2. In spite of increase in LSD values, the overall result of treatment comparisons is the same

3. That the unadjusted $MSS_{E(y)}$ was 108.5316 ÷ 21 = 5.1682 was reduced to $MSS_D = 3.1569$ (approximately to 61%), confirms the usefulness of the auxiliary variable in spite of local control (blocking) in the form of cows.

4. POOLING OF REGRESSION LINES

When data on regression analysis for the same set of associated variables is available, it may be necessary to develop a pooled estimate. But, it is mandatory that the lines must be homogenous with respect to elevation (α), slope (β) and residual variances (σ^2) in order that they can be pooled. ANACOV assumes homogeneity of slopes and residual mean squares thereby making it inapplicable for this purpose.

4.1 Example

Let us consider the same **Example 2.1** with the assumption that the treatments are different sources of information on the association of the same variables x (say first month milk production, kg/d) and y (say 305 d milk production, kg/d) in order to discuss this aspect (only sums, SS and cross-products listed; data on control and Sorghum deleted):

Report	A		B	
	x	y	x	y
Totals	119.0	189.8	136.9	170.3
SS	1799.46	4555.84	2382.43	3699.49
Corrected SS	29.3350	52.8350	39.7288	74.2288
CP (Corrected CP)	2832.19 (8.9150)		2963.62 (49.3613)	

υ for regression = 1, for residual = 6 and for total = 7

The above data can be processed as follows:

Step I: Comparison of residual SS (H_0: Residual SS are homogenous among the different sources)

Source		υ	Σx^2	Σxy	Σy^2	b	υ	SS	MSS
								Residuals from b	
Residuals	A	7	29.3350	8.9150	52.8350	0.3039	6	50.1257	8.3543
	B	7	39.7288	49.3613	74.2288	1.2425	6	12.8995	2.1499
							12	63.0252	5.2521
Slopes	Pooled	14	69.0638	58.2763	127.0638	0.8438	13	77.8900	5.9915
	Difference between slopes (by subtracting υ and SS from previous line; MSS calculated separately)						1	14.8648	14.8648
ElevationsBetween**	1		20.0256	–21.8157	23.7656				
(A + B)*	15		89.0894	36.4606	150.8294		14	135.9076	
	Between adjusted means						1	58.0176	58.0176

* Obtained by pooling crude SS and crude CP of both sources and then calculating SS and SCP;
** Calculated as difference between (A + B) line and slopes (pooled) line

$MSS_{E(A)}$ and $MSS_{E(B)}$ are tested by F on $\upsilon = 6, 6$ and $\alpha = 0.05$ (Table value = 4.28); the calculated ratio being 3.886 is suggestive of homogeneity and the validity of H_0. Hence, we can proceed to the next Step.

Note: If > 2 variances have to be tested, Bartlett's test has to be employed (*see* Chapter "**Two-factor analysis of variance**" for details)

Step II: Comparison of slopes of regression lines (H_0: Slopes of the regression lines are same among the different sources)

Comparison of slopes, F = 14.8648 ÷ 5.2521 = 2.830 < 4.75, the table value of $F_{0.05,1,12}$; hence, the slopes are homogenous and lines are parallel again indicating that H_0 is acceptable and we can proceed on to the next Step.

Step III: Comparison of elevations (H_0: Elevations of the regression lines are identical among the different sources)

For comparing elevations, F = 58.0176 ÷ 5.9915 = 9.683 > 4.67, the table value of $F_{0.05,1,13}$; hence, elevations can't be considered homogenous and hence H_0 is rejected.

Therefore, the two regression lines can not be pooled. Had it been possible to pool the lines, the pooled b of 0.8438 will represent the Sources satisfactorily and intercept can be deduced using the "Pooled" values which will be 9.0107.

5.   MULTIPLE COVARIANCE

This is a situation when a particular variable is influenced by > 1 independent variables; for example, weight gain depending on age and initial weight, egg weight depending on age at sexual maturity and egg production, egg shell strength depending on calcium in feed, age of the layer, and temperature, etc.

At the outset, it is easy to note that an animal scientist does control many of the independent variables that are likely to affect the variable in question; for instance, animals of uniform body weight will be allotted at random to treatments; layers of same age (preferably full-sibs) will be studied under the same temperature environment to study effect of calcium, etc. These are generally termed **blocking** or **local control**. Hence, it is not common that a need of multiple covariance analysis does arise. In any case a general scheme will be provided in this publication and for more details, the reader had better refer other publications (for instance Snedecor and Cochran, 1994).

Step I: Let us assume a case of two independent variables, x_1 and x_2. The corrected sums, SSs and SCPs are calculated (for total, treatments and residuals) by usual procedures and tabulated as follows (t = number of treatments; n = number of observations per treatment):

Source	v	Σx_1^2	$\Sigma x_1 x_2$	Σx_2^2	$\Sigma x_1 y$	$\Sigma x_2 y$	Σy^2
Treatments	$t-1$						
Error	$t(n-1)$						
Total	$nt-1$						

Step II: Utilizing the values in the **error line**, partial regression coefficients, b_1 and b_2, with their se, are derived; each of them tested for significance (see Chapter "**Association between variables II**" for details). If both of them are significant, then next step can be taken-up.

Step III: Utilizing (treatment + error) or total values, partial regression coefficients, b_1 and b_2, are recalculated and F test for adjusted means is carried-out as described under **Sections 2.2.4, 3.2** and **3.3**.

Step IV: Adjusted means are calculated on the same lines as under **Sections 2.2.4** and **3.3**. Standard error of difference between any two adjusted means is approximately $\sqrt{\dfrac{MSS_D}{n}}$.

Note: The other aspects like standard errors of partial regression coefficients and error mean square per observation are easier to calculate if matrices are used for deriving multiple regression equation; however, at least the former, can be obtained even when orthogonal polynomials are used for developing multiple regression equation.

19

Analysis of Time Series

As the name goes, **Time series** consists of data collected or referring to a specified time or to a chronological order; for example, month-wise egg production, annual numbers of livestock, prices of commodities at different periods etc. A time series, therefore, relates time (t) with population or temperature or other factors; usually, values of t will be equally spaced *viz.* annual, half-yearly, quarterly, monthly, fortnightly, weekly, hourly, etc. In addition, time series is generally used in Economics to discuss about time-trends. Hence, knowledge on analysis time series has come from economists.

1. COMPONENTS OF TIME SERIES

1.1 Secular Trend (Trend or Long-term Movement)

Trend refers to dynamics over a long period of time (which is ill-defined); for instance, livestock population, egg production, meat production, etc. Since long periods are involved, the fluctuations occurring within each of the periods get cancelled-out and an average tendency is indicated by trend. Trend can assume 0, negative and positive value, depending on the variable in question. The trend need not be linear; it could non-linear (curvilinear) as well.

1.2 Periodic Changes

1.2.1 Seasonal Variation

1.2.1.1 From natural forces
Climate is by far the predominant natural force beyond human control. Variations due to climate, like seasonality in breeding of farm animals like sheep, effect of season on egg production, etc. come under this category.

1.2.1.2 From man-made conventions
This refers to changes in a specific repeatable fashion due to beliefs, habits, customs, etc.; a classical example is egg consumption; which repeatedly slumps during summer months due to wrong belief that eggs are not good during summer.

1.2.2 Cyclic Variation

This category includes variations due to depression, boom, etc. if they occur periodically. Variable falling into this category in animal science is rare.

1.3 Random (Irregular) Movements

These are unexpected or unpredictable changes such as we could see due to natural calamities like cyclone, earthquake, etc.

2. MEASUREMENT OF COMPONENTS OF TIME SERIES

2.1 Secular Trend (Trend or Long-term Movement)

2.1.1 Graphic or Inspection Method

Considering t on x-axis (independent variable), the values of the variable are plotted, a smooth free-hand line/curve is drawn, visually inspected and conclusions are drawn. There is no mathematical measurement involved. This is not commonly used; although, can be very good preliminary method to decide upon further analysis.

2.1.2 Semi-Averages: Trend Line

This method is easy and comparatively more acceptable than graphic method. Let us consider we have n observations of x (independent variable);

1. It is divided into 2 halves; if n is an odd number, $\left(\dfrac{n-1}{2}+1\right)^{\text{th}}$ observation is deleted to get two groups of each with $\frac{1}{2}(n-1)$ observations.
2. Arithmetic mean of both halves is calculated and plotted against $x = \frac{1}{4}(n-1)$ and $\frac{3}{4}(n-1)$, respectively.
3. A line is drawn between the two and extended on either side to touch y-axis and to correspond to nth value. This line is called **trend line** which helps predict intermediate and future values.
4. The actual values are plotted on either sides of the Trend line.
5. If n is an even number, there is no elimination of any observation. Arithmetic average of each half is plotted corresponding to $\frac{1}{2}(n)$ and $\frac{3}{4}(n)$, respectively; which, obviously, will not refer to any of the actual period value in the data.

This method also is not of common application in animal science.

2.1.3 Curve Fitting

The data can be used to fit different types of curves, including linear, multiple regression and non-linear equations. All these aspects are already dealt at length in Chapters 9, 10, 11 and 17. In any case, different types of lines/curves encountered are listed below with remarks for those equations which were not discussed in earlier Chapters:

Line/Curve	Equation	Remarks
Straight line	$y = a + bt$	Changes between successive t's are nearly equal
Second degree polynomial	$y = a + bt + ct^2$	When plotted gives a parabola or a hyperbola
kth degree polynomial	$y = a + b_1 t + b_2 t^2$ $+ \ldots + b_k t^k$	
Exponential curve	$y = ab^t$	Changes between successive t's are by same %; $\log y = \log a + t \log b$
Modified exponential curve	$y = a + bc^t$	Growth curve
2nd degree exponential curve	$y = ab^t c^{t^2}$	$\log y = \log a + t \log b + t^2 \log c$
Gompertz curve	$y = ab^{c^t}$	$\log y = \log a + c^t \log b$; a growth curve
Logistic curve	$y = \dfrac{k}{1 + e^{a+bt}}$	

Note: First three equations can be easily fit by direct method or by use of orthogonal polynomials as described in Chapter "**Association between variables III**"; On logarithmic scale, Exponential curve is similar to a linear equation and 2nd degree Exponential curve to a 2nd degree polynomial; fitting of exponential curve (as an example for calculations on logarithmic scale) and the remaining models are shown in this chapter.

Curve fitting is completely mathematical in nature and hence, is devoid of subjective nature or personal bias. The equations can be used to predict, both within the range as well as beyond the range, depending on variables involved. Rate of change quantized in the process is of high practical utility. However, the method is time-consuming, requires specialized knowledge, the predictions beyond the range of x values used need not be valid every time and it is also not easy to determine the exact equation to be fit for the data.

2.1.3.1 Fitting exponential growth curve

Data on population of population of hens in India (FAO, as quoted by Sreenivasaiah, 2006) is used for fitting an exponential curve.

Year	Time (t)	Hens (m) (y)	Log y	Calculations
1993	1	115	2.0607	$\Sigma t = 66$, $\Sigma \log y = 23.6861$
1994	2	125	2.0969	$\Sigma t^2 = 506$, $\Sigma(\log y)^2 = 51.0404$
1995	3	128	2.1072	$\Sigma t \log y = 144.1115$
1996	4	131	2.1173	$\log y = 2.0445 + 0.0181t$
1997	5	133	2.1239	hence, $y = 110.7899(1.0426)^t$
1998	6	139	2.1430	

(Contd.)

(Contd.)

Year	Time (t)	Hens (m) (y)	Log y	Calculations		
1999	7	146	2.1644	**Predicted values:**		
2000	8	150	2.1761	t	Year	Layers (m)
2001	9	160	2.2041	18	2010	234.757
2002	10	168	2.2253	23	2015	289.206
2003	11	185	2.2672	28	2020	356.284

Note: This equation is the same as compound interest formula; 115.5048 m being the principal (initial population), 4.26% being the rate of interest (growth) and t being the time interval, years; i.e. CI = P{1 + (r ÷ 100)}^{t}; in other words, layer population in India is growing at a rate of 4.26% pa.

2.1.3.2 Fitting a modified exponential curve

For the same data under **Section 2.1.3.1** above, a modified exponential curve can be fit by **method of three selected points** (*see* Appendix 13) as follows:

The three selected points are: t_1 when y_1 was 115 m, t_2 when y_6 was 139 m and t_3 when y_{11} was 185 m. Therefore, t_1, t_2 and t_3 refer to time 1, 6 and 11, respectively; on the same lines, y_1, y_2 and y_3 refer to number of hens at time 1, 6 and 11,

respectively; Then, as per this method, $c = \left[\dfrac{y_3 - y_2}{y_2 - y_1} \right]^{\frac{1}{t_2 - t_1}} = \sqrt[5]{\dfrac{185 - 139}{139 - 115}} = 1.1390;$

$b = \dfrac{(y_2 - y_1)^2}{y_3 - 2y_2 + y_1} \left[\dfrac{y_2 - y_1}{y_3 - y_2} \right]^{\frac{t_1}{t_2 - t_1}} = 22.9874$ and $a = \dfrac{y_1 y_3 - y_2^2}{y_3 - 2y_2 + y_1} = 88.8182$; hence, the

equation is $y_t = 88.8182 + 22.9874(1.1390)^t$. Method of Partial sums (see Appendix 14) can also be used to fit the equation.

Note: The original data can be plotted on a graph paper, a smooth curve drawn manually and any three points, but equidistant, which need not be a part of the actual data can be selected.

2.1.3.3 Fitting of a gompertz curve

A Gomperetz curve is described by $y = ab^{c^t}$ which upon taking logarithms on both sides becomes a modified Exponential curve Log $y = \log a + c^t \log b$; that is $(y = a + bc^t)$ where $y = \log y$, $a = \log a$ and $b = \log b$. For the same data under **Section 2.1.3.1** above, a modified Exponential curve can be fit by **method of Partial sums** (see Appendix 14) as follows: The log y values are already shown in the table above. The data is divided into 3 parts ($n = 3$) viz., $t = 1, 2$ and 3; $t = 4, 5$ and 6; and $t = 7, 8$ and 9. The partial sums (on log scale) are: $S_1 = 6.2648$, $S_2 = 6.3842$ and $S_3 = 6.5446$. Hence, $c = 1.1034$; $b = 0.0326$ ad $a = 1.9724$. That means the equation on logarithmic scale is $y = 1.9724 + 0.0326$ $(1.1034)^t$. On conversion of log units to original scale by taking antilog (in case of a and b) the final equation obtained is: $y = 93.8342(1.0779)^{1.1034^t}$.

2.1.3.4 Fitting a logistic curve

Many methods for fitting a logistic curve are available like three selected points, partial sums, geometric mean (for population values), successive approximation, Yule's and

Hotelling's methods. Of all these, for method of three selected points appears to be very convenient and hence the same is shown below for the data pertaining to egg production of 250 layers. The three selected points are: 2nd, 30th and 58th d after sexual maturity of egg production when the number of eggs produced was 55, 138 and 248, respectively (*see* note under **Section 2.1.3.2**).

Derivation of each of the formulae is given in Appendix 15 for those who are interested to know about them. Only final calculations are shown below (difference between two consecutive points is 28):

$$k = \frac{y_2^2(y_1 + y_3) - 2y_1y_2y_3}{y_2^2 - y_1y_3} = 371.1495; b = \frac{1}{t_2 - t_1}\log_e\left[\frac{(k - y_2)y_1}{(k - y_1)y_2}\right] = -0.0647$$

and $a = \log_e\left(\frac{k - y_1}{y_1}\right) - bt_1 = 1.8782$. Hence, the final equation can be written as

$$y_t = \frac{371.1495}{1 + e^{1.8782 - 0.0647t}}.$$

Note: In this equation, b is always < 0, $k \neq 0$ and $k = y_{max}$

2.1.4 Moving Averages

See **Section 6.1.1** Chapter "**Central tendency**" for a numerical example. Moving averages are mainly used to study trends, particularly of linear nature, and are generally unsuitable for forecasting.

2.1.4.1 Centered moving average

A modification in calculation of moving average is often employed in time series when moving average has to be computed for even number of years; this is referred to as **centered moving average**.

In the above quoted example, price of layer mash from 1975 to 1990 is tabulated along with 3-year and 5-year moving averages. Now, the same data will be utilized to compute 4-year moving average (centered) values:

Year	Price (Rs/Ton) (y)	y + (y+ 4)	(y +1) + (y+5)	4-year moving totals (Not centered)	4-year moving average (Centered)
(1)	(2)	(5)	(6)	(7) = (5)+(6)	(8) = (7) ÷ 8***
1975	1274	5421*	5698**		
1976	1224	5698	6221		
				11119	1389.875
1977	1462	6221	6692		
				11919	1489.875
1978	1461	6692	7204		
				12913	1614.125
1979	1551	7204	7753		
				13896	1737.000

(*Contd.*)

(Contd.)

Year	Price (Rs/Ton) (y)	y + (y+ 4)	(y +1) + (y+5)	4-year moving totals (Not centered)	4-year moving average (Centered)
(1)	(2)	(5)	(6)	(7) = (5)+(6)	(8) = (7) ÷ 8***
1980	1747	7753	8236		
				14957	1869.625
1981	1933	8236	8625		
				15989	1998.625
1982	1973	8625	8931		
				16861	2107.625
1983	2100	8931	9120		
				17556	2194.500
1984	2230	9120	9487		
				18051	2256.375
1985	2322	9487	10111		
				18607	2325.875
1986	2279				
				19598	2449.750
1987	2289				
1988	2597				
1989	2946				

* 1274 + 1224 + 1462 + 1461 = 5421 and ** 1224 + 1462 + 1461 + 1551 = 5698 so on.

*** Divided by 8 because, column (7) is the total of 8 values

2.1.4.2 Weighted moving average

If specific weightages (say $w_1, w_2...w_k$) are available for the moving averages (say m_1,

$m_2....m_k$), respectively, then the weighted moving average is $\dfrac{\sum\limits_{i=1}^{k} w_i m_i}{\sum\limits_{i=1}^{k} w_i}$ which is similar

to the weighted average described in Chapter "**Central tendency**".

2.1.4.3 Spencer's 15 point formula

This procedure requires data of at least 15 years; hence the name. This method incorporates the weights [–3, 3, 4, 3, –3]. The final totals obtained will be divided by 320. Let us consider a hypothetical example:

2.1.4.3.1 Example

The following data refers to prices of broiler mash (Rs/Ton) in India.

Year	Prices	*	*	**	***	****
1	1683					
2	1608					
		7026				
3	1855					
		7352				
4	1880		30918			
		7971				
5	2009		33088			
		8569				
6	2227		35544	177278		
		9196				
7	2453		37854	187871		
		9808				
8	2507		39843	197605	756942	2365.44
		10281				
9	2621		41511	206181	823974	2574.92
		10558				
10	2700		42822	214600	841903	2630.95
		10864				
11	2730		44120	224584	863335	2697.92
		11119				
12	2813		46304	238659	905046	2828.27
		11579				
13	2876		49827	258745	982324	3069.76
		12742				
14	3160		55586	285259		
		14387				
15	3893		62908	316886		
		16878				
16	4458		70634			
		18901				
17	5367		77931			
		20468				
18	5183					
		21684				
19	5460					
20	5674					

Year 1 = 1975 * 4-year moving totals

** 5-year moving totals

*** 5-year moving totals with weights [−3, 3, 4, 3, −3]

**** Total at preceding column ÷ 320

However, Spencer's formula is not commonly used in animal Science. It can have application in studying long-term averages of disease incidence, parasitic infections in a large area.

2.1.5 Progressive Averages

See **Section 6.2** Chapter "**Central tendency**" for a numerical example. Progressive averages, like moving averages, are also mainly used to study trends, particularly of linear nature, and are generally unsuitable for forecasting.

2.2 Seasonal (Periodic) Changes

These are definitely encountered in animal science data; for example, egg prices and demand, occurrence of some of the parasitic and infectious diseases, etc. Hence, it is highly desirable that such variations introduced are eliminated and/or quantized so that actual treatment effects can be studied with more precision. Many methods are available to measure the effect of seasons; salient ones are:

2.2.1 Quantizing Seasonal Effects

2.2.1.1 Average

Much about the averages are already described in Chapter "**Central tendency**". It is easy to calculate weekly, monthly, quarterly, half-yearly or even season-wise averages depending on the type of data collection.

2.2.1.2 Season index

This is the ratio of the average of a particular period (month/quarter/season) to that of the overall average times 100. It is necessary that the number of observations for each of the periods is > 1.

2.2.1.2.1 Example

The following hypothetical data gives month-wise prices of eggs (Rs per 100) over the previous 4 years at Bangalore, Karnataka. Let us develop monthly indices:

Month	Price of eggs (Rs per 100)				Totals	Month average	Month index
	2003	2004	2005	2006			
January	188	195	206	220	809	202.25	116.111
February	189	193	205	210	797	199.25	114.388
March	177	178	200	205	760	190.00	109.078
April	163	170	187	190	710	177.50	101.902
May	115	125	135	140	515	128.75	73.915
June	105	106	110	120	441	110.25	63.294
July	110	115	142	150	517	129.25	74.201
August	140	160	171	180	651	162.75	93.434
September	172	173	200	210	755	188.75	108.360
October	182	184	202	220	788	197.00	113.097

(Contd.)

(Contd.)

Month	Price of eggs (Rs per 100)				Totals	Month average	Month index
	2003	2004	2005	2006			
November	185	192	200	222	799	199.75	114.675
December	190	196	208	225	819	204.75	117.546
			Grand total		8361		1200.001
			Overall average		174.1875		100.000

The month indices are easily understandable; egg prices started declining from March reaching the lowest during June and recovering again by October at Bangalore. The same data can be partitioned into quarters or as per season (depending on the location) and the same calculations can be performed to obtain Quarterly index or Seasonal index, respectively.

2.2.1.2.2 Example

Let us develop indices for periods of 2 months each from the **Example 2.2.1.2.1**:

Year	Period numbers (two months each)						Year total	Year average
	1	2	3	4	5	6		
2003	377	340	220	250	354	375	1916	319.333
2004	388	348	231	275	357	388	1987	331.167
2005	411	387	245	313	402	408	2166	361.000
2006	430	395	260	330	430	447	2292	382.000
Period total	1606	1470	956	1168	1543	1618	8361	348.375
Period average	401.50	367.50	239.00	292.00	385.75	404.50	348.375	
Period index	115.249	105.489	68.604	83.818	110.728	116.111	599.999	

It is apparent that the yearly averages have a linear trend; hence, a linear regression equation is fit (*see* Chapter "**Association between variables I**" for details). The equation is $y = 293.917 + 21.783x$; i.e. per annum there is an increase of Rs 21.78 in the average price of eggs; therefore, for 2 months, the increment will be $(21.78 \div 6)$ = Rs 3.63. By utilizing the linear equation, we can calculate the predicted values, referred to as **trend values**, for each of the years; they are 315.70, 337.48, 359.27 and 381.05, respectively. These values refer to average of the year. Utilizing these trend values, we can calculate the trend values of each of the periods within a year as follows:

The trend values, being average for the year, correspond to a period between periods 3 and 4. It is calculated that per period there is increase of Rs 3.63. That means, the average value between periods 3 and 4 was Rs 315.70 (year 1 or 2003); in half a period, the value would increase (or decrease) by ½ (Rs 3.63) = Rs 1.82. Hence, expected value for period 3 is Rs (315.70 – 1.82) = Rs 313.88 and that of period 4 will be Rs (315.70 + 1.82) = Rs 317.52. From period 3 towards period 1, the price reduces at a rate of Rs 3.63 per period and converse is true for periods 4 towards period 6. Hence, the values for different periods of the year 1 (2003) are 306.62, 310.25, 313.88, 317.52, 321.15 and 324.78, respectively. In the same way, period values of all the years can be calculated which are shown in the table below:

Year	Period numbers (two months each)					
	1	**2**	**3**	**4**	**5**	**6**
2003	306.62	310.25	313.88	317.52	321.15	324.78
2004	328.40	332.03	335.66	339.30	342.93	346.56
2005	350.19	353.82	357.45	361.09	364.72	368.35
2006	371.97	375.60	379.23	382.87	386.50	390.13

Note: The predicted values of periods within a year are not close to the actual values because the trend among periods is not linear but parabolic; the calculations are made to demonstrate the procedure. For period-wise data of each of the years or for the pooled data, parabola can be fit by employing methods explained in Chapter "**Association between variables III**".

2.2.1.3 Ratio to trend method

This is a better method than the Season index method because a suitable curve is fit to the data to obtain a trend line. **Example 2.2.1.2.2** is considered for the purpose. The procedure is as follows:

Step I: Calculation of trend values: Let us develop indices for periods of 2 months each from the **Example 2.2.1.2.2**. As explained under **Section 2.2.1.2.2**, linear regression equation is fit (*see* Chapter "**Association between variables I**" for details) for the Year average values and the equation is utilized to estimate **trend values**.

Step II: Calculation of trend values for periods by employing ratio to trend values: The procedure is same as explained under **Section 2.2.1.2.2**. The equation is $y = 293.917 + 21.783x$; and the trend values are already given above.

Step III: Calculation of trend-eliminated values: Actual values given in Step I will be converted to % of the corresponding values computed in Step II to get the **Trend-eliminated values**; for example, for period 1 of year 1, trend-eliminated value = $(377 \div 306.82) \times 100 = 122.87$ and so on. These are tabulated below along with the adjusted values of Period index:

Year	Period numbers (two months each)					
	1	**2**	**3**	**4**	**5**	**6**
2003	122.87	104.34	66.79	75.09	105.20	110.28
2004	110.19	106.80	70.13	82.60	106.10	114.10
2005	116.72	108.81	68.20	86.28	109.74	110.30
2006	115.18	104.81	68.35	85.94	110.96	114.30
Period total	464.96	424.76	273.47	329.91	432.00	448.98
Period average	116.24	106.19	68.37	82.48	108.00	112.25
Period index (adj)	117.51	107.35	69.12	83.38	109.18	113.47

$k = \{600 \div \Sigma \text{Period averages}\} = 1.0109$; Period index (adj) = Period average $* k$

Note: There are 6 periods and hence, ideally, ΣPeriod averages = 600; hence the correction

2.2.1.4 Ratio to moving average method

2.2.1.4.1 Additive model

Assuming the seasonal effects are additive, we shall now proceed calculating Ratio to Moving Average and Season indices (Adjusted). **Example 2.2.1.2.1** can be considered again for this procedure; only data pertaining to 3 consecutive years will be utilized for demonstration of the method. The principle is to first calculate moving averages to eliminate seasonal trends which are of constant pattern and intensity as well as cyclic variations; this will be followed by calculation of indices.

Step I: Calculation of centered 12 month moving averages and season indices:

Year	Month	Total	12-point moving			Ratio to moving average
			Total	Total*	Average	
(1)	(2)	(3)	(4)	(5)	(6) = (5) ÷ (12)	(7) = {(3) ÷ (6)} × 100
2004	1	195				
	2	193				
	6	178				
	4	170				
	5	125				
	6	106				
			967			
	7	115		1854	154.50	74.43 (−39.50)
			887			
	8	160		1741	145.08	110.28 (14.92)
			854			
	9	173		1703	141.92	121.90 (31.08)
			849			
	10	184		1712	142.67	128.97 (41.33)
			863			
	11	192		1793	149.42	129.49 (42.58)
			930			
	12	196		1950	162.50	120.62 (33.50)
			1020			
2005	1	206		2131	177.58	116.00 (28.42)
			1111			
	2	205		2267	188.92	108.51 (16.08)
			1156			
	3	200		2339	194.92	102.61 (5.08)
			1183			
	4	187		2369	197.42	94.72 (−10.42)
			1186			

(Contd.)

(Contd.)

Year	Month	Total	12-point moving			Ratio to moving average
			Total	Total*	Average	
(1)	(2)	(3)	(4)	(5)	(6) = (5) ÷ (12)	(7) = {(3) ÷ (6)} × 100
	5	135		2315	192.92	69.98 (−57.92)
			1129			
	6	110		2172	181.00	60.77 (−71.00)
			1043			
	7	142		2022	168.50	84.27 (−26.50)
			979			
	8	171		1924	160.33	106.66 (10.67)
			945			
	9	200		1890	157.50	126.98 (42.50)
			945			
	10	202		1905	158.75	127.24 (43.25)
			960			
	11	200		1985	165.42	120.90 (34.58)
			1025			
	12	208		2148	179.00	116.20 (29.00)
			1123			
2006	1	220		2324	193.67	113.60 (26.33)
			1201			
	2	210		2441	203.42	103.23 (6.58)
			1240			
	3	205		2485	207.08	99.00 (−2.08)
			1245			
	4	190		2478	206.50	92.01 (−16.50)
			1233			
	5	140		2406	200.50	69.83 (−60.50)
			1173			
	6	120		2258	188.17	63.77 (−68.17)
			1085			
	7	150				
	8	180				
	9	210				
	10	220				
	11	222				
	12	225				

* Total of two consecutive totals in (4), in an order

Note:

1. Column (7) is the average of two consecutive values, in an order
2. Value in the parentheses indicate {(3) − (6)} designated D_i

Step II: Computation of month indices: From Step I, ratio to moving averages, except the first and the last six, are available which are tabulated as per month and year; it can be noticed that there are at least two values available for each of the months.

Month	2004	2005	2006	Average ratio	Adjusted season index*
1		116.00	113.60	114.80	111.91
2		108.51	103.23	105.87	103.20
3		102.61	99.00	100.81	98.27
4		94.72	92.01	93.37	91.02
5		69.98	69.83	69.91	68.15
6		60.77	63.77	62.27	60.70
7	74.43	84.27		79.35	77.35
8	110.28	106.66		108.47	105.74
9	121.90	126.98		124.44	121.31
10	128.97	127.24		128.11	124.88
11	129.49	120.90		125.20	122.05
12	120.62	116.20		118.41	115.43
				1231.01	1200.01

* Adjusted to total of 1200 by multiplying average ratio with k (0.974809) where k = $\dfrac{1200}{\sum \text{Average ratio}}$ so that each month is equated to 100

Step III: Calculation of **Season Index (Adjusted)**—above Table is self-explanatory. One can't miss the season indices being improved version of the Month indices calculated in **Example 2.2.1.2.1**; however, this procedure is more time-consuming.

2.2.1.4.2 Multiplicative model

Suppose the seasonal trends had multiplicative component, the procedure is modified from **Step I** of the additive model as follows:

Deviation values (D_i) are calculated as {Column (3) – Column (6)} i.e. (Total–Moving Average) which are already available in the table under **Section 2.2.1.3.1 (Step I)**. They are tabulated as per year and month:

Month	2004	2005	2006	Total	Average	Adjusted season index*
1		28.42	26.33	54.75	27.38	25.16
2		16.08	6.58	22.66	11.33	9.11
3		5.08	-2.08	3.00	1.50	-0.72
4		-10.42	-16.50	-26.92	-13.46	-15.68
5		-57.92	-60.50	-118.42	-59.21	-61.43
6		-71.00	-68.17	-139.17	-69.59	-71.81

(Contd.)

(Contd.)

Month	2004	2005	2006	Total	Average	Adjusted season index*
7	−39.50	−26.50		−66.00	−33.00	−35.22
8	14.92	10.67		25.59	12.80	10.58
9	31.08	42.50		73.58	36.79	34.57
10	41.33	43.25		84.58	42.29	40.07
11	42.58	34.58		77.16	38.58	36.36
12	33.50	29.00		62.50	31.25	29.03
					26.66	0.02

* Calculated as (average-k) where k = ΣAverages $\div$ 12 = 2.22 so that ΣAdjusted season indices = 0

It can be appreciated that the results from the multiplicative model is more explicit in the sense that the negative signs directly reveal slump in values (prices in this case) without even a necessity of comparing with other values.

Note: The same procedure is applicable when each year is composed of Quarters or periods of different sizes; but, suitable changes in divisors and expected totals have to be employed.

2.2.1.5 Pearson's link relative (LR) method

Link relative (LR) is the value of one period (Quarter, Season, Two-monthly, etc.) expressed as the % of the preceding period. Let us consider the data from **Example 2.2.1.2.2** converting each value into its average (by halving them because they are the totals of 2 months) to get the following:

Year	1	2	3	4	5	6
2003	188.50	170.00	110.00	125.00	177.00	187.50
2004	194.00	174.00	115.50	137.50	178.50	194.00
2005	205.50	193.50	122.50	156.50	201.00	204.00
2006	215.00	197.50	130.00	165.00	215.00	223.50

Step I: Utilizing these values, LRs are calculated; for example: for period 2 of year 1, LR = (170.00 $\div$ 188.50) $\times$ 100 = 90.19 ...; for period 1 of year 2, LR = (194.00 $\div$ 187.50) $\times$ 100 = 103.47 and so on. It is obvious that there is no LR value for the period located at left-hand top corner of the table. The LRs so calculated are as follows along with subsequent processing:

Year	1	2	3	4	5	6
2003		90.19	64.71	113.64	141.60	105.93
2004	103.47	89.69	66.38	119.05	129.82	108.68
2005	105.93	94.16	63.31	127.76	128.43	101.49
2006	105.39	91.86	65.82	126.92	130.30	103.95
Average	104.93	91.48	65.06	121.84	132.54	106.01
CR	100.00*	91.48	59.52	72.52	96.12	101.90

* 1st CR of 1st Period (assumed); 2nd CR of 1st Period = 106.92; AF = 1.15

Step II: Average of LR is converted to Chain Relative (CR) value by multiplying it with the CR of the preceding period; for the first period, it is taken as 100 and is referred to as **1st CR of 1st period**. CR of the period 2 is (91.48 × 100.00) ÷ 100 = 91.48 itself, CR of period 3 is (91.48 × 65.06) ÷ 100 = 59.52 and so on.

Step III: Calculation of Adjusted CR: When all the periods are over, a **2nd CR of 1st Period** is calculated as (101.90 × 104.93) ÷ 100 = 106.92 which is 6.92 in excess of assumed value of 100 (on which CRs of other periods are calculated). This excess is subtracted equally from all the periods; i.e. 6.92 ÷ 6 = 1.15 is the **Adjustment Factor (AF)** to be subtracted from the CR to get **Adjusted CR**.

2.2.2 Elimination of Seasonal Effects

As discussed already, elimination of seasonal effects greatly helps compare treatments more efficiently. It also helps study cyclic variations in the same data. Elimination of seasonal effects can be done by assuming either additive or multiplicative model.

1. Additive model: Each of the observations, y = Trend effects + Cyclic effects + Season effects + Irregular effects; i.e. $y = T + C + S + I$. Hence, elimination of seasonal effects is simply by subtraction of season effect (season index) from corresponding values.
2. Multiplicative model: $y = TCSI$; therefore, correction is by dividing each value by its corresponding season effect (season index).

2.2.3 Utility of Season Indices

Apart from help elimination of effects for proper comparisons to test other factors, season index is also useful in predicting sales, prices, demand, disease occurrence, etc. depending on the variable in question. Understandably, with the expected values of demand, price and sales, it will be convenient for the manager to plan production and requisite flock schedule, say for instance, in a large poultry concern.

Let us take for example the monthly indices for egg prices calculated under **Section 2.2.1.2.1**. Since season indices are % values, they are converted to season effect by dividing them by 100. Estimated value (price, in this case) is given by the product of season index and season effect (or season index^2 ÷ 100). We shall assume that in January 2007, whole-sale egg prices are Rs 160 per 100; that means, estimated value (111.91 × 1.1191) = Rs 160 or about 125 estimated value equals Rs 160 or each estimated value is Rs 1.28; this factor can be used to multiply the subsequent estimated values to predict price of eggs during the respective seasons.

Month	Season Index	Season effect	Season value	Price Predicted
(1)	(2)	(3) = (2) ÷ 100	(4) = (2) × (3)	(5)
1	111.91	1.1191	125	160*
2	103.20	1.0320	107	137
3	98.27	0.9827	97	124
4	91.02	0.9102	83	106
5	68.15	0.6815	46	59
6	60.70	0.6070	37	47

(Contd.)

(Contd.)

Month	Season Index	Season effect	Price	
			Season value	Predicted
(1)	(2)	(3) = (2) ÷ 100	(4) = (2) × (3)	(5)
7	77.35	0.7735	60	77
8	105.74	1.0574	112	143
9	121.31	1.2131	147	188
10	124.88	1.2488	156	200
11	122.05	1.2205	149	191
12	115.43	1.1543	133	170
Total	1200.01	12.0001		

* Assumed price of 100 eggs during month 1; equated to season value 125 to get Rs 1.28 per season value to multiply rest of the season values to obtain predicted price of 100 eggs.

Prediction of sales can also be done the same way. Conversely, if the total sales or production values are available, the Season value can be used to partition them into different seasonal sales or production.

Note: Ratio to moving average method is the most preferred of all the four methods of measuring seasonal variations (averages, ratio to trend, ratio to moving average and link relative methods).

2.3 Measurement of Cyclic Changes

This category which includes depressions or booms that occur periodically is rare in animal science. Outbreak of avian influenzae for example, was indeed a factor causing "depression"; but, it can't be considered to occur periodically to consider under this category. It can best be grouped in the category of "Irregular Changes". Similarly, a temporary "boom" to poultry production due to "Mad-cow disease" also can not be considered as a regular or periodic effect. Hence, suffice to state that "Harmonic Analysis" is done on data eliminated of trend and seasonal effects to estimate cyclic variations. Readers interested in details are advised to refer to other publications.

2.4 Measurement of Irregular Changes

These include unexpected changes due to Natural calamities such as Earthquake, floods, Tsunami, cyclone, etc. For long-term changes, trend values are calculated between two time–series, usually by Moving Average method for both and the trend values are used (in place of original data) to compute product–moment correlation (*see* Chapter "**Association between variables I**" for details).

For short–term changes, trend values are calculated (by moving average method) for both series and are subtracted from corresponding actual values to get short–time fluctuations isolated. These trend-corrected values are used to compute product–moment correlation.

It is very important to note that it is practically impossible to separate irregular and cyclic changes; therefore, correlation coefficient obtained should be very carefully interpreted, especially if it is significant.

20

Methods of Sampling

The reader is familiar with basic information on Population, Sample, Parameter, Statistic, Estimate, Distribution, Standard error, etc. through the first nine chapters of this publication. Information on sampling theory is available in numerous publications and hence, different methods of sampling and estimation in each of them are outlined in this Chapter. In the discussions that follow, N **represents Population size and** n **sample size**.

1.   METHODS OF SAMPLING

1. **Subjective or judgment sampling:** It is also called **purposive** or **non-probability** or **convenience sampling**; as the name goes, the sample is selected with a specific purpose in view purely on the judgment of the investigator. Obviously, this sample is seldom a representative of the population being violating both Law of Statistical Regularity and Principle of Inertia of Large Numbers. Therefore, on most occasions than not, it will be biased because some of the elements are favored to be in (or out) of the sample. Hence, **this sampling is not recommended for general use** although under extremely exceptional circumstances when the investigator is skilled enough to meticulously plan selection of units, this method can be acceptable; as far as Animal Science field is concerned, we had better avoid this method altogether. Another version of purposive sampling, called **Quota Sampling**, also suffers from the same drawbacks and hence not suitable for experiments in Animal Science.
2. **Probability sampling:** Each unit in the population will have a definite, pre-determined probability of being selected into the sample; variants of this method depend on the probability which could be (a) equal, (b) unequal or (c) proportional to sample size
3. **Mixed sampling:** Selection of units into a sample is partly on the basis of probability and partly on a fixed rule(s) by the investigator. Several variations are possible in this group; hence, the several methods: Simple random, stratified random, systematic, multi-stage sampling, quasi–random, area, simple cluster, multi-stage cluster and quota sampling; of these, the former four methods are employed in Animal Science and therefore, they will be dealt further in the forthcoming sections. It is worth noting that most of the large-scale sampling is by stratified multi-stage random sampling.

2. SIMPLE RANDOM SAMPLING

Each unit has equal chance being included in the sample and hence referred to as **unrestricted** or **simple** random sampling. The unit selected may be replaced to keep the probability of being selected constant at $(1 \div N)$ or not replaced to alter the probabilities every time a sample unit is selected due to reduction in denominator. Many methods of randomization are in vogue; tossing of coin, throwing dice, drawing cards, etc. The best would be allot serial number to each unit, use suitable **random numbers** (2-digit, 3-digit, etc.) and select the unit bearing the number. After the units are selected into the sample, allotment into different treatments can again be by suitable random numbers. With random numbers being available in all scientific calculators, there appears to be no need to opt for an alternative method.

2.1 Estimation

2.1.1 Mean and Variance

They are already provided in Chapters 2 and 3; mean, $\bar{y} = \dfrac{\sum\limits_{i=1}^{n} y_i}{n}$ and variance,

$$s^2 = \frac{\sum\limits_{i=1}^{n} y_i^2 - \dfrac{\left(\sum\limits_{i=1}^{2} y_i\right)^2}{n}}{n-1}$$ where y_i are the individual determinations. Variance of estimated

mean is given by $V(\bar{y}) = s^2\left(\dfrac{1}{n} - \dfrac{1}{N}\right)$; if n is very large, $V(\bar{y}) = \dfrac{s^2}{n}$.

For finite populations, estimate of variance is multiplied by a correction factor $\left(1 - \dfrac{n}{N}\right)$; $\dfrac{n}{N}$ is referred to as **sampling fraction**. Square root of the variance gives se which can be used to set-up confidence intervals for the population mean, μ as $\bar{y} \pm t_{\alpha,(n-1)} se(\bar{y})$.

2.1.2 Sample Size for a Given Precision

Suppose we are interested that the difference between $\bar{y}$ and μ sould not exceed a specific value, say δ at say a significance level α, then, the size of the sample,

$$n = \frac{\left(\dfrac{t_\alpha^2}{\delta^2}\right)\left(\dfrac{s}{\bar{y}}\right)^2}{1 + \dfrac{1}{N}\left(\dfrac{t_\alpha^2}{\delta^2}\right)\left(\dfrac{s}{\bar{y}}\right)^2}$$ where s is the standard deviaton; if N is very large, its reciprocal

will be so low that $\dfrac{1}{N}\left(\dfrac{t_\alpha^2}{\delta^2}\right)\left(\dfrac{s}{\bar{y}}\right)^2 \to 0$; then $n = \left(\dfrac{t_\alpha^2}{\delta^2}\right)\left(\dfrac{s}{\bar{y}}\right)^2$. Now, the obvious question

arises, how to select table value of t because $\upsilon\ (= n-1)$ is required for it. Hence, trial values of n are used and requisite sample size is determined by iteration. Alternatively, t value can be assumed to be 2.0 (value of $t_{0.05,\,60}$); the result will be slight underestimate of n.

2.1.3 Examples

All examples given in all the preceding Chapters, unless otherwise specified, concern Random samples.

2.2 Random Sampling of Attributes

Attributes are the qualitative characteristics; like defective eggs drawn from a consignment, feed bag of improper weight, etc. If P is the Population proportion of the attribute and p is that of a sample, and A out of N in the former and a out of n in the latter do possess the attribute; in other words, P is the ratio of A to N and p of a to n; then, it follows that Q and q are the complementary proportions. Without going to the proof or derivation, the population and sample mean of the attribute is given by $\bar{Y}$ and $\bar{y}$, respectively; population and sample variances by $\dfrac{NPQ}{N-1}$ and $\dfrac{npq}{n-1}$, respectively.

3. STRATIFIED (RANDOM) SAMPLING

It is possible that the population subject for sampling is not homogenous with respect to the variable(s) under investigation. Then, such populations need to be subdivided into more homogenous groups, referred to as **Strata**.

3.1 Allocation of Units

3.1.1 Proportional Allocation

From each of such strata sample(s) is (are) drawn **at random** with proportionate representation from each of the strata. This ensures that, on the whole, each of the units had equal chance to be a part of the sample.

Let us assume that there are k strata of size $N_1, N_2, \dots N_k \dots N_i\ (i = 1, 2, \dots k)$, such

that $\sum\limits_{i=1}^{k} N_i = N$; from each of these strata, a sample of size $n_1, n_2, \dots n_k\ (i = 1, 2, \dots k)$ are

drawn, obviously each of the units can be designated y_{ij}, to mean jth unit in the ith stratum.

As a rule of the thumb, larger the N_i, larger will be the intra-strata variability and

hence, n_i from it should also be larger. As per this procedure, if $\sum\limits_{i=1}^{k} n_i = n$, number of units allocated, $n_i = np_i$ or $\dfrac{n_i}{n} = \dfrac{N_i}{N}$ because p_i is the ratio of N_i to N. This method itself will be optimum if cost of per unit and variance are same in all strata. As the differences between the strata increases, the efficiency of this method of sampling also increases; conversely, Random sampling would be cheaper and easier to undertake if the strata are homogenous.

3.1.2 Neyman's Allocation

While applying the above Rule, cost of collection of data must be borne in mind; if C_T and C_i are the total fixed costs available for estimation of mean with maximum precision and cost per unit in the ith stratum, respectively, and s_i, the standard deviation of the ith stratum, then **Optimum allocation** to obtain maximum precision can be obtained

by $n_i = \left(\dfrac{p_i s_i}{\sqrt{C_i}} \right) \left(\dfrac{C_T}{\sum\limits_{i=1}^{k} p_i s_i \sqrt{C_i}} \right)$; if C_i is same for all strata, then the above formula condenses

as $n_i = n \left(\dfrac{p_i s_i}{\sum\limits_{i=1}^{k} p_i s_i} \right)$ where $n = \sum\limits_{i=1}^{k} n_i$, the total number of units from all strata; this is

popularly known as **Neyman's Allocation**.

3.2 Estimation

3.2.1 Mean and Variance

Mean of the ith stratum is $\bar{Y}_i = \dfrac{\sum\limits_{j=1}^{N_i} y_{ij}}{N_i}$ which is estimated as $\dfrac{\sum\limits_{j=1}^{n_i} y_{ij}}{n_i}$ and that of the entire

population is $\bar{Y} = \dfrac{\sum\limits_{i=1}^{k}\sum\limits_{j=1}^{N_i} y_{ij}}{N} = \dfrac{\sum\limits_{i=1}^{k} N_i \bar{Y}_i}{N} = \sum\limits_{i=1}^{k} p_i \bar{Y}_i$ where p is the ratio of N_i to N. This estimate itself is the unbiased estimate of μ as well.

Variance on the basis of Random Sampling is $V(\bar{y}_{ij}) = \sum\limits_{i=1}^{k} p_i^2 s_i^2 \left(\dfrac{1}{n_i} - \dfrac{1}{N_i} \right)$ which can

be rearranged as $\dfrac{\sum\limits_{i=1}^{k} \dfrac{N_i(N_i - n_i)}{n_i} s_i^2}{N^2}$ where $s_i^2 = \dfrac{\sum\limits_{j=1}^{n_i} y_{ij}^2 - \dfrac{\left(\sum\limits_{j=1}^{n_i} y_{ij} \right)^2}{n_i}}{(n_i - 1)}$ (see Chapter "Dis-

persion" for details of formula of).

3.2.2 Example (Proportional Allocation)

3.2.2.1 Mean Values

Suppose stratified sampling has to be done to select poultry farms from k number of poultry pockets in India each having N_i number of farm units. Therefore, the Population

size is $\sum_{i=1}^{k} N_i = N$. From each of the pockets (stratum), n_i farms will be selected such

that $\sum_{i=1}^{k} n_i = n$. It is reasonable to say that ith pocket contributes $\dfrac{N_i}{N}$ to the population

size; hence, its contribution to a total sample size n should be $n\left(\dfrac{N_i}{N}\right)$ so that it

represents itself in the same proportion among the sample units also. The concept is represented in the following table:

S No. (Stratum)	No of Farms (N_i)	Selected number, $n_i = n\left(\dfrac{N_i}{N}\right)$	Number of layers ('000s) (y_{ij})	$\bar{y}_i = \bar{Y}_i$	$N_i\bar{Y}$	$p_i = \dfrac{N_i}{N}$	$p_i\bar{Y}_i$
1	60	6	2, 3.5, 6.0, 3, 4.5, 5	4.00	240	0.12	0.4800
2	110	11	15, 8, 12, 5, 7, 2.5, 7.5, 9, 12, 20, 16	10.36	1140	0.22	2.2792
3	80	8	12, 5, 7.5, 7.5, 9, 10, 3, 2	7.00	560	0.16	1.1200
4	50	5	5, 3, 8, 2.5, 2.5	4.20	210	0.10	0.4200
5	30	3	8.5, 2.5, 76.00		180	0.06	0.3600
6	170	17	15, 12, 20, 5, 9, 10, 4, 15, 20, 9, 12, 8, 12, 6, 10, 16, 25	12.24	2080	0.34	4.1616
Totals	$N = 500$	$n = 50$	$\sum_{i=1}^{k}\sum_{j=1}^{n_i} y_{ij} = 441$		4410	1.00	8.8208

It can be checked that estimate of mean which obtained as $\sum_{i=1}^{k} p_i\bar{Y}_i$ in the last column

is the same as $\dfrac{1}{N}\sum_{i=1}^{k}\dfrac{N_i}{n_i}\sum_{j=1}^{n_i} y_{ij} = \dfrac{1}{500}\sum_{i=1}^{6} 10 \sum_{j=1}^{n_i} y_{ij} = \dfrac{4410}{500} = 8.82$

3.2.2.2 Variances

Stratum	Number of layers ('000s) (y_{ij})	$\sum_{j=1}^{n_i} y_{ij}$	$\sum_{j=1}^{n_i} y_{ij}^2$	s_i^2	$\dfrac{N_i(N_i - n_i)}{n_i}$	$s_i^2 = \dfrac{N_i(N_i - n_i)}{n_i}$
1	2, 3.5, 6, 3, 4.5, 5	24	106.5	2.10	540	1134.0
2	15, 8, 12, 5, 7, 2.5, 7.5, 9, 12, 20, 16	114	1450.5	26.91	990	26640.9
3	12, 5, 7.5, 7.5, 9, 10, 3, 2	56	475.5	11.93	720	8589.6
4	5, 3, 8, 2.5, 2.5	21	110.5	5.58	450	2511.0
5	8.5, 2.5, 718	127.5	9.75	270	2632.5	
6	15, 12, 20, 5, 9, 10, 4, 15, 20, 9, 12, 8, 12, 6, 10, 16, 25	208	3066.0	32.57	1530	49832.1

$$\sum_{i=1}^{k} \frac{N_i(N_i - n_i)}{n_i} s_i^2 = 91340.1 \text{ and Estimate of variance} = \frac{\sum_{i=1}^{k} \dfrac{N_i(N_i - n_i)}{n_i} s_i^2}{N^2} = 0.365360$$

3.1.3 Example (Neyman's Allocation)
Considering the result from **Example 3.2.2.2**, if cost of allocation of units was not constant; for example, accessibility to farms in different strata costs differently, it can be employed as C_i value (Rs) as shown below:

Stratum	N_i	s_i^2	s_i	p_i	$p_i s_i$	C_i	$\dfrac{p_i s_i}{\div \sqrt{C_i}}$	Allocation (n_i) Proportional	Neyman's	Optimum
1	60	2.10	1.45	0.12	0.1740	7	0.0658	6	2	1
2	110	26.91	5.19	0.22	1.1418	2	0.8074	11	13	12
3	80	11.93	3.45	0.16	0.5520	4	0.2760	8	7	4
4	50	5.58	2.36	0.10	0.2360	4	0.1180	5	3	2
5	30	9.75	3.12	0.06	0.1872	6	0.0764	3	2	1
6	170	32.57	5.71	0.34	1.9414	1	1.9414	17	23	30
Totals	500			1.00	4.2324		3.2850	50	50	50

The estimates of variance for each of the allocation methods are as follows:

Stratum	N_i	s_i^2	s_i	Allocation (n_i)			$\dfrac{N_i(N_i-n_i)}{n_i}$		
				Prop	Neyman's	Opt	Prop*	Neyman's**	Opt
1	60	2.10	1.45	6	2	1	540	1740.00	3540.00
2	110	26.91	5.19	11	13	12	990	820.77	898.33
3	80	11.93	3.45	8	7	4	720	834.29	1520.00
4	50	5.58	2.36	5	3	2	450	783.33	1200.00
5	30	9.75	3.12	3	2	1	270	420.00	870.00
6	170	32.57	5.71	17	23	30	1530	1086.52	793.33
Totals	500			50	50	50			
$\displaystyle\sum_{i=1}^{k}\dfrac{N_i(N_i-n_i)}{n_i}s_i^2$ ***							91340.10	79547.94	90758.92
Estimate of variance $=\dfrac{\displaystyle\sum_{i=1}^{k}\dfrac{N_i(N_i-n_i)}{n_i}s_i^2}{N^2}$							0.3654	0.3182	0.3630
Efficiency: Base: Arbitrary allocation@							100.00	114.83	100.66

@ Same as proportional allocation in this example; but it could be different as well

* Variance can also be calculated as $\dfrac{1}{N^2}\left(\dfrac{N}{n}-1\right)\displaystyle\sum_{i=1}^{k}N_i s_i^2$

** Variance can also be calculated as $\dfrac{1}{N^2}\left[\dfrac{\left(\displaystyle\sum_{i=1}^{k}N_i s_i\right)^2}{n}-\displaystyle\sum_{i=1}^{k}N_i s_i^2\right]$

*** General formula for calculation of variance suitable for all types of allocation.

Calculation of unit cost of sample:

Stratum	C_i	Allocation (n_i)		
		Proportional	Neyman's	Optimum
1	7	6	2	1
2	2	11	13	12
3	4	8	7	4
4	4	5	3	2
5	6	3	2	1
6	1	17	23	30
Total cost, $\displaystyle\sum_{i=1}^{k}C_i n_i$		151	115	91

It is clear from the above that although Neyman's allocation was most efficient as far as reducing the variance is concerned, the optimum allocation was the most economical. It is up to the investigator to choose between 15% increase in efficiency and 16% reduction in costs.

4. SYSTEMATIC SAMPLING

This method of sampling is employed when the units in the population occur in an order over space and time; for instance, daily milk yield, egg production, etc. Let us assume that daily egg production of a hen over 280 d (N) is available. It can be seen as data comprising of 40 (n) weeks (k) or $N = nk$. In simple terms, each of the possible k systematic samples has n units. Therefore, the sampling method is simply to select an initial unit of i at random from the first k units and then choosing every kth unit.

Note: If $N \neq nk$, sample size will differ by 1.

4.1 Estimation

4.1.1 Mean and Variance

Sample mean itself the estimate of μ (Population) and estimate of σ^2 (Population) can be calculated only when number of samples is > 1. If ≥ 2 samples (say m) are available,

estimate of μ is given by the mean of means i.e. Estimate of $\mu = \dfrac{\sum\limits_{i=1}^{m} \bar{y}_i}{m}$ and estimate of

σ^2 by $\dfrac{\sum\limits_{i=1}^{m} \bar{y}_i^2 - \dfrac{(\hat{\mu})^2}{m}}{m(m-1)}$ where $\hat{\mu}$ is the estimate of μ.

Even when $m = 1$, estimation of variance is possible by use of auxiliary variables (*see* Chapter "**Analysis of Covariance**") through (1) ratio method and (2) regression method.

Let us assume that we have the data of export of eggs from a sample of n poultry pockets (let us designate the values, as usual, as y_i's). With this data, we can estimate Population mean, m, simply as the sample mean. But, it is possible get an estimate of population variance, s^2, only if we have data from at least one more sample. This might be expensive and often cumbersome to obtain. Hence, we can introduce another source of information on the same variable; say a private survey of a larger scale by a TV broadcasting channel; the latter can be used as auxiliary variable (let us designate the values as x_i's). Now we have a pair of observation on each of the sample unit (x_i and y_i). Now, the data can be used to estimate s^2 which is demonstrated with a numerical example:

4.1.1.1 Ratio method

This method is ideal if x_i and y_i are linearly related with $a = 0$ (line passing through origin) and y_i is proportional to x_i.

4.1.1.1.1 Example

Poultry pocket	Sample data (y_i)	Private data (x_i)	Ratio, $r_i = (y_i \div x_i)$	Rx_i
1	10	95	0.105	0.680
2	3	60	0.050	0.204
3	8	90	0.089	0.544
4	25	625	0.040	1.700
5	6	70	0.086	0.408
6	14	170	0.082	0.952
7	12	150	0.080	0.816
8	6	75	0.080	0.408
9	18	165	0.109	1.224
Totals	102	1500	0.721	6.936
Crude sum of squares	1534	500500	0.061847	7.093216
Crude sum of cross products	$\sum_{i=1}^{m} x_i y_i = 25495$			

Let us assume that only 8% of the poultry farms were actually involved in this study (i.e. 9 poultry pockets formed 8% of the population or population size, $N = 112$ poultry pockets and total export of 22500 m; the latter representing Population total of x; designated X; therefore, $\mu_x = 200.89$); R, the ratio of y to x is estimated as the ratio of the sum of the former to that of the latter; i.e. $R = \sum_{i=1}^{m} y_i \div \sum_{i=1}^{m} x_i = 0.068$. Assuming that the same ratio exists in the population, estimate of population $\sum_{i=1}^{m} y_i$, designated $Y = RX = 1530$ and that of $\mu_y = Y \div N = 13.66$.

Variance of the Y can be obtained as $\dfrac{N(N-n)}{n(n-1)} \sum_{i=1}^{m} (y_i - Rx_i)^2 = \dfrac{N(N-n)}{n(n-1)}$

$\left[\sum_{i=1}^{m} y_i^2 - 2R \sum_{i=1}^{m} x_i y_i + R^2 \sum_{i=1}^{m} x_i^2 \right]$. This works out to be 51237.7849 and se $\left(\sum_{i=1}^{m} y_i \right) = 226.3576$.

Est (σ^2) or variance of μ_y = Variance of the $Y \div N^2 = 4.0846$ and σ or se of $\mu_y = 2.0211$.

Note: However, some bias is definitely involved in this method; it is desirable that the ratio of bias to se of (estimated mean or total or the ratio) does not exceed 10% of the se of the mean of x. In the

present example, the bias can be estimated as $\dfrac{1}{\bar{x}} \dfrac{\sqrt{\sum_{i=1}^{m} x_i^2 - \dfrac{\left(\sum_{i=1}^{m} x_i \right)^2}{m}}}{\sqrt{m(m-1)}} = 0.3539$ which is > 0.10; hence,

bias is not negligible. Assuming that the bias is negligible, let us find out the efficiency of the ratio estimator. Variance of Y through sample values $= \dfrac{N(N-n)}{n(n-1)}\left[\sum\limits_{i=1}^{m} y_i^2 - \dfrac{\left(\sum\limits_{i=1}^{m} y_i\right)^2}{m}\right] = 60564.00$; when

compared to the same estimate calculated by use of R, gives the efficiency of ratio method over product moment correlation between x_i and y_i as $(60564.0000 \div 51237.7849) \times 100 = 118.20\%$.

4.1.1.2 Regression method

This method is preferred when, although the association between x_i and y_i is linear but $a \neq 0$ (line does not pass through origin). The linear regression line represents $\mu_y = \bar{y} + b(\mu_x - \bar{x})$. As described in Chapter "**Association between variables I**", $b = (SCP_{xy} \div SS_x)$; from **Example 4.1.1.1.1**, $\bar{x} = 166.67$, $SS_X = 250500$, $SS_Y = 378$, $SCP_{XY} = 8495$; $\bar{y} = 11.33$, $\mu_x = 200.89$ and $N = 112$; thus, $b = (8495 \div 250500) = 0.0339$.

Substituting the above values in the linear equation we get, Estimate of $\mu_y = 12.49$ and that of $Y = N \times \mu_y = 1398.89$ (say 1399). Now, with usual meanings for the notations as in Chapter "**Association between variables I**", the estimate of variance

$$(\mu_y) = \left(\dfrac{1}{n-2}\right)\left[SS_Y - \dfrac{(SCP_{XY})^2}{SS_X}\right]\left[\dfrac{1}{n} + \dfrac{(\bar{x}-\mu_x)^2}{SS_X}\right] = 1.4873 \text{ and se } (\mu_y) = 1.2195.$$ Estimate

of variance $(Y) =$ variance $(\mu_y) \times N^2 = 18656.5182$; when compared to the same estimate through sample values, efficiency of the regression method is $(60564.0000 \div 18656.5182) \times 100 = 324.62\%$.

5.   MULTISTAGE SAMPLING

As the name indicates, in this method many stages (usually 2 in case of Animal Science) are involved before a final sample is drawn. For instance, if we want to study egg production of WL; there are many farms, small, medium, and big farm where information has to be collected. So, it is convenient to select large groups as a sample in I Stage (**Primary Sample Units – psu**); from this sample of large groups another sub-sample is drawn which actually forms the sample for study (**Secondary Sample Units, ssu**). This sampling may not be as efficient as Simple Random or Stratified or Systematic sampling; but is definitely convenient and economical. In fact, if all psu are used to draw ssu, it is same as Stratified Sampling. Conversely, if all psu form sample units, it is **Cluster Sampling** which is dealt in the next section.

Let us assume the following: Population size: N, of which n are psu $(i = 1, 2, \dots n)$ each having M_i sampling units of which m_i are selected (all selections in both stages being without replacement) and y_{ij} is the value of jth ssu under ith psu. Obviously, $y_i.$ is the total of ith psu and $y..$ is the total of all psu, Let Y be the Population total (of all N values of Y_{ij}'s) and μ_y, the population mean.

5.1   Estimation

Without indulging in proofs and/or derivations, the following formulae can be used for estimating mean and variance:

5.1.1 Mean

$$\bar{y}_i = \frac{\sum_{j=1}^{m_i} y_{ij}}{m_i} \quad \text{is an unbiased estimate of} \quad \frac{\sum_{j=1}^{M_i} Y_{ij}}{M_i} = \bar{Y}_i; \quad \text{similarly,} \quad \bar{y}. = \frac{N}{M_0}\left(\frac{\sum_{i=i}^{n} M_i \bar{y}_i}{n}\right)$$

$$= \frac{\sum_{i=i}^{n} M_i \bar{y}_i}{n\bar{M}} \quad \text{is an unbiased estimate of } \mu_y; \text{ where } \bar{M} \text{ is the average size of psu determined}$$

as $\dfrac{\sum_{i=i}^{n} M_i}{N}$ or by $\dfrac{M_0}{N}$ when only one psu is used; where M_0 is the total number of units in the psu

5.1.2 Variance

$$\text{Variance of estimate of } \mu_y = \left(\frac{1}{n} - \frac{1}{N}\right)s_{psu}^2 + \frac{\sum_{i=1}^{n}(M_i)^2\left(\frac{1}{m_i} - \frac{1}{M_i}\right)s_{ssu}^2}{nN(\bar{M})^2}, \quad \text{where}$$

$$s_{psu}^2 = \frac{1}{(\bar{M}^2)(n-1)}\left[\sum_{i=1}^{n} M_i^2(\bar{y})^2 - \frac{\left(\sum_{i=1}^{n} M_i \bar{y}\right)^2}{n}\right] \quad \text{and} \quad s_{ssu}^2 = \frac{1}{m_i - 1}\left[\sum_{j=1}^{m_i} y_{ij}^2 - \frac{\left(\sum_{j=1}^{m_i} y_{ij}\right)^2}{m_i}\right].$$

5.1.3 Example

Let us take an example of sampling to estimate number of birds grown at backyard in a State. Let us now consider that 8 Districts (N) form the psu of which 5 Taluks (n) are selected as ssu. From each of these different number of backyard units (M_i) are selected and number of birds (y_{ij}) in the selected backyard units are tabulated below (Total backyard units in the taluk is assumed to be 640 (M_0)):

M_i	y_{ij}	m_i	$\sum_{j=1}^{m_i} y_{ij}$	$\sum_{j=1}^{m_i} y_{ij}^2$	$\bar{y}_i$	$M_i\bar{y}_i$	s_{ssu}^2	$M_i^2\left(\frac{1}{m_i} - \frac{1}{M_i}\right)s_{ssu}^2$
46	20, 8, 16, 30, 12, 5, 10, 8, 12, 15	10	136	2322	13.60	625.6	52.49	8692.34
125	30, 18, 14, 20, 12, 8, 16, 12, 10, 18, 20, 25	12	203	3877	16.92	2115.0	40.27	47401.15
30	6, 8, 10, 8, 16, 12, 6, 10	8	76	800	9.50	285.0	11.14	919.05

(Contd.)

(Contd.)

M_i	y_{ij}	m_i	$\sum_{j=1}^{m_i} y_{ij}$	$\sum_{j=1}^{m_i} y_{ij}^2$	$\bar{y}_i$	$M_i \bar{y}_i$	s_{ssu}^2	$M_i^2\left(\dfrac{1}{m_i}-\dfrac{1}{M_i}\right)s_{ssu}^2$
78	20, 15, 12, 20, 18, 12, 18, 20, 15, 20	10	170	2986	17.00	1326.0	10.67	5659.37
95	20, 16, 20, 14, 18, 25, 30, 26, 12, 20	10	201	4321	20.10	1909.5	31.21	25202.08
374	Totals	50	786	14306		6261.1		87873.99

In this example, $\bar{M} = \dfrac{M_0}{N} = 80$, $\sum_{i=1}^{n} M_i^2 \bar{y}_i^2 = \sum_{i=1}^{n}\left(M_i \bar{y}_i\right)^2 = 10350291.61$; Estimate of μ_y

$= \{6261.1 \div (5 \times 80)\} = 15.65$ (say, 16 birds per backyard unit).

$s_{psu}^2 = \dfrac{1}{6400 \times 4}\left[10350291.61 - \dfrac{(6261.1)^2}{5}\right] = 98.0475$; therefore, estimate of variance of

$\mu_y = \left(\dfrac{1}{5} - \dfrac{1}{8}\right) \times 98.0475 = \dfrac{87873.99}{5 \times 8 \times 80^2} = 7.6968$ and se of $\mu_y = 2.7743$

Note: The Average number of birds on backyard for the entire District ($\bar{y}_D$) can also be estimated; if T_k is the number of Taluks in ith District and $\bar{y}_k$ is the average number of birds for the 4th Taluk, then

$$\bar{y}_D = \dfrac{\sum_{k=1}^{T_k} T_k \bar{y}_k}{\sum_{k=1}^{T_k} T_k} \quad \text{and its variance can be estimated by } V(\bar{y}_D) = \dfrac{\sum_{k=1}^{T_k} T_k^2 V(\bar{y}_k)}{\left(\sum_{k=1}^{T_k} T_k\right)^2}$$

6. CLUSTER SAMPLING

The population (N) is divided into several **clusters** (M) each containing M_i sampling units ($i = 1, 2, \ldots n$) depending on the variable under investigation. Of these clusters, m clusters are selected and from each of the clusters, a simple random sample of n_i experimental units into b blocks is drawn. The individuals selected into these blocks form the experimental units. y_{ij} is the jth observation ($j = 1, 2, \ldots n_i$) of the ith cluster.

Hence, it can be seen that $N = \sum_{i=1}^{n} M_i$. When both M and M_i are not known (which is generally the case), an unbiased estimate of population total can be obtained by $\dfrac{N}{n_i} y_i$.

and estimate of its variance by $\dfrac{N(N - n_i)}{N(n_i - 1)}\left[y_{..}^2 - \dfrac{(y_{..})^2}{n_i}\right]$.

It is easy to note that the population estimates depend only on one cluster and hence, it depends entirely on its homogeneity (heterogeneity); therefore, if differences are high between clusters and/or n_i is large, the estimates suffer severe fall in precision. Therefore, if this sampling is employed, we had better have more number of clusters having a smaller and consistent n_i; further, it is advisable to have n_i among clusters to be approximately same.

7. SAMPLING *VS* COST OF EXPERIMENTATION

This is only an extension of **Section 4.2.3** in Chapter "**One-factor analysis of variance**" involving an RBD with b blocks and t treatments with n observations per cell; since details are already available ANOVA table and further description are given with usual notations:

Source	υ	SS	MSS	EMS
Blocks	$(b-1)$	SS_B	MSS_B	
Treatments	$(t-1)$	SS_T	MSS_T	$\sigma^2 + n\sigma_{BT}^2 + nb\sigma_T^2$
BT Interaction	$(b-1)(t-1)$	SS_{BT}	MSS_{BT}	$\sigma^2 + n\sigma_{BT}^2$
Error	$bt(n-1)$	SS_E	MSS_E	σ^2

It is generally expected that $MSS_{BT} > MSS_T$; hence, the latter (referred to as **experimental error**) is used for testing treatment effects. Variance of treatment mean,

$\sigma_T^2 = \dfrac{\sigma_{BT}^2}{b} + \dfrac{\sigma^2}{nb}$. If p psu and s ssu are drawn from a large population (multi-stage

sampling process), C_B is the cost of experimentation per animal and C_A is the additional cost per observation (animal), the total cost, $CT = C_A p + C_B ps = C_T$. For a given C_T, the

variance is minimum of $s = \dfrac{\sigma^2}{\sigma_{BT}^2}\sqrt{\dfrac{C_A}{C_B}}$ and $p = \dfrac{C_T}{C_A + C_B s}$.

If, $C_A = 0$, $ps = \dfrac{C_T}{C_B} = $ Constant, designated w, then σ_T^2 can be minimized by increasing

p by making $s = 1$ and $p = n$.

In simple terms, **it is wise to take fewer observations per animal** than reducing number of experimental units and making many determinations on each of them unless sampling variation is very high (usually associated with a negative intra-class correlation) or cost per animal is high. A similar conclusion was drawn in **Section 4.2.3** in Chapter "**One-factor analysis of variance**" as well.

21

Statistics in Specific Veterinary Fields

It is generally accepted that the statistical methodology does not change among various scientific fields; Veterinary and Animal Science is no exception to that. All the concepts and procedures described in the Chapters preceding this one are relevant to all fields of Veterinary and Animal Science; only to be carefully chosen depending on the nature of the data proposed to be collected and/or processed.

Notwithstanding the above fact, it is equally important to note that certain procedures and models are, at least, more frequently employed in certain fields; for instance hierarchical design in Animal Breeding, Process control in Animal Nutrition, etc. Therefore, only such topics are taken-up in this chapter so that it will facilitate the reader to effectively locate the desired statistical procedure(s).

1. ANIMAL GENETICS AND BREEDING

The genes in the same locus of homologous chromatids and having only two alternative expressions are referred to as alleles and hence the alleles represent the variants of the gene. When two members of the given pair of alleles are alike, then the individual is said to be homozygote, otherwise heterozygote, with respect to that allele.

However, many and possibly, all genes, can change in different ways giving rise to several alternative states or variants of the gene; these genes are referred to as multiple alleles. Considering 'n' number of alleles at a locus, number of possible genotypes is $\frac{n(n+1)}{2}$ and proportion of individuals belonging to each of the genotypes is referred to as "genotypic frequency" whereas proportion of each allele out of all the genes at that locus gives the "gene frequency".

1.1 Qualitative Genetics

1.1.1 Mendel's Laws and Application of Probability Theory

1.1.1.1 Mendel's I law (or gametic purity or law of segregation)

This states that the characteristics of individual are determined by pairs of genes; but the gametes contain only one gene from each pair. The following Tables demonstrate the use of laws of probability in calculating gene and genotypic frequencies:

1.1.1.1.1 Example

Trait: Shank feathering, Fs Nature: Autosomal, dominant to clean shanks, fs
Case: Both parents being heterozygous

	Male		Female	
Parent's genotype	Fs fs		Fs fs	
Gametes produced	Fs	fs	Fs	fs
Probability of gametes	½	½	½	½
Genotype of offsprings	Fs Fs		Fs fs	fs fs

Therefore, $P(FsFs) = P(Fs)m \times P(Fs)f = ½ \times ½ = ¼$ *,
$P(fsfs) = P(fs)m \times P(fs)f = ½ \times ½ = ¼$ * and
$P(Fsfs) = P(Fs)m \times P(fs)f + P(fs)m \times P(Fs)f = ¼ + ¼ = ½$ ** or
$1 - P(homozygotes) = 1 - ½ = ½$.

	Fs Fs	Fs fs	fs fs
Genotype of the offsprings	Fs Fs	Fs fs	fs fs
Genotypic probability of offsprings	¼	½	¼
Phenotypic probability of offsprings	¾	¼	
Genotypic ratio		1 : 2 : 1	
Phenotypic (Monohybrid) ratio		3 : 1	

* Since the events are independent, multiplicative rule of probability applied
** Both multiplicative and addition rules of probability applicable
Source: Sreenivasaiah, 2006

1.1.1.1.2 Example

Trait: Shank feathering, Fs Nature: Autosomal, dominant to clean shanks, fs
One of the parents being heterozygous, the other homozygote recessive

	Male		Female	
Parent's genotype	Fs fs		fs fs	
Gametes produced	Fs	fs	Fs	fs
Probability of gametes	½	½	0	1
Genotype of offsprings	Fs fs		fs fs	

Therefore, $P(FsFs) = P(Fs)m \times P(Fs)f = ½ \times 0 = 0$ *,
$P(fsfs) = P(fs)m \times P(fs)f = ½ \times 1 = ½$ * and
$P(Fsfs) = P(Fs)m \times P(fs)f + P(fs)m \times P(Fs)f = ½ + 0 = ½$ ** or
$1 - P(homozygotes) = 1 - ½ = ½$.

	FsFs	Fsfs	fsfs
Genotype of the offsprings	FsFs	Fsfs	fsfs
Genotypic probability of offsprings	0	½	½
Phenotypic probability of offsprings	0	1	1
Genotypic ratio		1 : 1	
Phenotypic ratio		1 : 1	

* Since the events are independent, multiplicative rule of probability applied
** Both multiplicative and addition rules of probability applicable
Source: Sreenivasaiah, 2006

1.1.1.2 Mendel's II law (law of independent assortment)

This states that characters are inherited independently of one another. In other words, during the formation of gametes, the members of the individual allelic pairs segregated independently of each other. Following this, one pair of alternative characters is inherited quite independently of each other and probability of the composite genotype when more than one locus is considered is equal to the product of probabilities of its constituents. If an individual is heterozygous to both the loci and hence can produce 4 different types of gametes, it is called a dihybrid genotype.

1.1.1.2.1 Example

Law of independent assortment - Classical

Loci : A and B Nature (both loci): Autosomal, dominant

	Male		Female	
Parent's genotype	Aa	Bb	Aa	Bb
Gametes produced				
'A' locus	A	a	A	a
Probability	½	½	½	½
'B' locus	B	b	B	b
Probability	½	½	½	½
Gametic assortment (as per I Law)				
'A' locus				
AA		½ × ½ = ¼		
Aa		½ × ½ + ½ × ½ = ½		
aa		½ × ½ = ¼		
'B' locus				
BB		½ × ½ = ¼		
Bb		½ × ½ + ½ × ½ = ½		
bb		½ × ½ = ¼		

Therefore, by the multiplicative rule of probability, the genotypic frequency of AABB. AABb, AAbb, AaBB, AaBb, Aabb, aaBB, aaBb and aabb will be 1/16, 2/16, 1/16, 2/16, 4/16, 2/16, 1/16, 2/16 and 1/16

Therefore, $P(A–) = P(AA) + P(Aa) = ¾$, $P(aa) = ¼$ and

$P(B–) = P(BB) + P(Bb) = ¾$, $P(bb) = ¼$

Since the gametes assort independently, by applying multiplicative rule of probability, the following phenotypic frequencies are obtained:

Phenotypic class	Probability
A–B–	9/16
A–bb	3/16
aaB–	3/16
aabb	1/16
Genotypic ratio	1 : 2 : 1 : 2 : 4 : 2 : 1 : 2 : 1
Phenotypic (Dihybrid) ratio	9 : 3 : 3 : 1

Source: Sreenivasaiah, 2006

1.1.1.2.2 *Example*

Law of independent assortment-deviation

Traits: Naked neck (N) and White skin (W) Nature: Autosomal, dominant to neck feathering (n) and yellow skin (w), respectively

	Male		**Female**	
Parent's genotype	Nn Ww		Nn ww	
Gametes produced				
'N' locus	N	n	N	n
Probability	½	½	½	½
'W' locus	W	w	W	w
Probability	½	½	0	1
Gametic assortment (as per I Law)				
'N' locus				
NN	$\frac{1}{2} \times \frac{1}{2} = \frac{1}{4}$			
Nn	$\frac{1}{2} \times \frac{1}{2} + \frac{1}{2} \times \frac{1}{2} = \frac{1}{2}$			
nn	$\frac{1}{2} \times \frac{1}{2} = \frac{1}{4}$			
'W' locus				
WW	$\frac{1}{2} \times 0 = 0$			
Ww	$\frac{1}{2} \times 1 + \frac{1}{2} \times 0 = \frac{1}{2}$			
ww	$\frac{1}{2} \times 1 = \frac{1}{2}$			

Therefore, P(N-) = P(NN) + P(Nn) = ¾ and P(W-) = P(WW) + P(Ww) = ½

Since the gametes assort independently, by applying multiplicative rule of probability, the following phenotypic frequencies are obtained:

Phenotypes	Genotypes	Probability
Naked neck, white skin	N–W–	P(N–) × P(W–) = 3/8 or 6/16
Naked neck, yellow skin	N–ww	P(N–) × P(ww) = 3/8 or 6/16
Normal neck, white skin	nnW–	P(nn) × P(W–) = 1/8 or 2/16
Normal neck, yellow skin	nnww	P(nn) × P(ww) = 1/8 or 2/16
Phenotypic ratio		6 : 6 : 2 : 2

Source: Sreenivasaiah, 2006

1.1.1.3 Epistasis

The concept shown above can be extended to many loci and also for calculating frequencies with epistatic effects.

1.1.1.3.1 Example

Epistasis–Inhibitory gene

Nature: Autosomal, epistatic, I locus: 'II' completely and 'Ii' incompletely masking the expression C locus for color 'C–'

	Male		Female	
Parent's genotype	Ii Cc		Ii Cc	
Gametes produced				
'I' locus	I	i	I	i
Probability	½	½	½	½
'C' locus	C	c	C	c
Probability	½	½	½	½
Gametic assortment (as per I Law)				
'I' locus				
II	½ × ½ = ¼			
Ii	½ × ½ + ½ × ½ = ½			
ii	½ × ½ = ¼			
'C' locus				
CC	½ × ½ = ¼			
Cc	½ × ½ + ½ × ½ = ½			
cc	½ × ½ = ¼			

Therefore, P(C–) = P(CC) + P(Cc) = ¾, P(cc) = ¼ and P(– –) = 1

Since the gametes assort independently, by applying multiplicative rule of probability, the following phenotypic frequencies are obtained:

Phenotypes	Genotypes	Probability
White birds	II– –, – –cc	P(II) X P(– –) + P(– –) X P(cc) – P(IIcc)* = 7/16
Speckled birds	IiC–	P(Ii) X P(C–) = 3/8 or 6/16
Colored birds	iiC–	P(ii) X P(C–) = 3/16
		*Already accounted for under P(II– –)
Phenotypic ratio		7 : 6 : 3

Source: Sreenivasaiah, 2006

1.1.1.3.2 Types of epistasis

Phenotypic ratios are altered when there is epistasis depending on type of association between the two loci. There are several types of epistasis and not all are recorded in animals. Details can be obtained from Sreenivasaiah (2006).

1.1.2 χ^2 Test for Goodness of Fit and Mono- and di-hybrid Ratios

As per Mendel's laws outlined above, when the sample size is large, classical mono-hybrid and dihybrid ratios are expected. This can be checked by χ^2 test. Details of various tests *viz.*, Z, t, F, χ^2 and others are given in Chapter "**Tests of hypotheses**".

1.1.2.1 Example: Monohybrid ratio (phenotypic frequencies)

Shank feathered flock of breeding chicken produced 810 progenies with feathered shanks and 190 with clean shanks; designated O_i, the observed frequencies. We have to check H_0: The number of feathered- and clean-shanked progenies is in the ratio of 3:1 (monohybrid ratio; *see* **Example 1.1.1.1.1**).

Obviously, the expected frequency (E_i) for feathered shanks is 750 and clean shanks

is 250; χ^2 on $(\upsilon = 1) = \sum_{i=1}^{2} \frac{(O_i - E_i)^2}{E_i} = [(810 - 750)^2 \div 750] + [(190 - 250)^2 \div 250] = 19.2$

which is > 3.841, the table value of $\chi^2_{0.05,\ 1}$; hence, H_0 can be rejected. Further, the observed frequencies show more dominant phenotypes indicating that some of the parents were actually homozygous for the dominant allele upsetting the monohybrid ratio.

1.1.2.2 Example: Monohybrid ratio (genotypic frequencies)

This test is simply the extension of the test for phenotypic frequencies shown above; instead of 2 phenotypic classes, there will be 3 genotypic classes with expected

frequencies in the ratio of 1:2:1; hence, χ^2 on $(\upsilon = 2) = \sum_{i=1}^{3} \frac{(O_i - E_i)^2}{E_i}$.

Assuming that in **Example 1.1.1.2.1** out of 810 feathered-shank birds 275 were homozygous and the rest were heterozygous, χ^2 on $(\upsilon = 2)$ will be $[(275 - 250)^2 \div 250]$ + $[(535 - 500)^2 \div 500] + [(190 - 250)^2 \div 250] = 19.35$ which is > 5.99, the table value of $\chi^2_{0.05,\ 2}$ (Appendix 4); hence, H_0 is liable to be rejected (H_0: Genotypic frequency of FsFs, Fsfs and fsfs birds among the progenies is in the ratio of 1:2:1)

1.1.2.3 Example: Dihybrid ratio (phenotypic frequencies)

A breeding flock of shank-feathered white-skinned birds produced the following types of progenies; the expected frequencies based on the classical dihybrid ratio of 9:3:3:1 (*see* **Example1.1.2.1**) are given in parentheses:
H_0: The observed frequencies are in the ratio of 9:3:3:1

Skin color ↓	Shank feathering		Totals
	Present	Absent	
White	1750 (1800)	700 (600)	2450 (2400)
Yellow	660 (600)	90 (200)	750 (800)
Totals	2410 (2400)	790 (800)	3200 (N)

Value in the parentheses indicates expected frequencies

χ^2 (after Yates correction for continuity) = 83.922 which is > 3.841, the table value of $\chi^2_{0.05,1}$ (Appendix 4); hence, H_0 can be rejected.

Note:

1. χ^2 can also be calculated as $\chi^2 = \dfrac{3200 \times \left[|1750 \times 90 - 700 \times 660| - \dfrac{3200}{2}\right]^2}{(2410 \times 790 \times 2450 \times 750)} = 83.922$.

2. The marginal totals can be separately tested for a monohybrid ratio of 3:1 as shown under **Example 1.1.2.1**; in this case, $\chi^2_{skin\ color} = 4.167$ and $\chi^2_{shank\ feathering} = 0.167$; Table value of χ^2 on $\upsilon = 1$ is 3.841 (Appendix 4) and hence, skin color locus appears to be deviating from Classical monohybrid ratio.

1.1.2.4 Dihybrid ratio (genotypic frequencies)

This is similar to monohybrid ratio (genotypic frequencies) as shown in **Example 1.1.2.2** but, by replacing the genotypic ratio to be tested with the observed frequency for each of the genotypic class; however, υ for locating the table value of χ^2 will be (number of genotypic classes-1).

1.1.2.5. Frequency of alleles

Let a characteristic be controlled by a pair of alleles, designated 'A' and 'a' whose expected ratio is m_1 and m_2, respectively (frequencies of f_1 and f_2, respectively). Let us also assume that the observed frequency of the two alleles is a_1 and a_2, respectively. Therefore, the observed probability, $P_o = a_1 \div (a_1 + a_2)$; similarly, expected probability, $P_e = m_1 \div (m_1 + m_2)$. The difference between the observed and the expected probability can be tested (under H_0: $P_o = P_e$) either by $Z = \dfrac{P_o - P_e}{\sqrt{\dfrac{P_o P_e}{N}}}$ or, if a_1 has to be tested directly

with f_1, by $Z = \dfrac{a_1 - f_1}{\sqrt{NP_eQ_e}}$ where $Q_e = (1 - P_e)$. Alternatively, with $N = (f_1 + f_2)$, χ^2 test with

Yates' correction for continuity can be calculated as $\chi^2 = \dfrac{\left[|a_1 m_2 - a_2 m_1| - \dfrac{m_1 + m_2}{2}\right]^2}{m_1 m_2 N}$ on

$\upsilon = 1$.

1.1.2.5.1 Example

Let us test an observed frequency of 156 and 44 for a_1 and a_2, respectively, is in the ratio of 3:1 or not. H_0: observed frequencies are in the ratio of 3:1.

$$\chi^2 = \dfrac{\left[|156 \times 1 - 44 \times 3| - \dfrac{3+1}{2}\right]^2}{3 \times 1 \times 200} = 0.807 \text{ which is } < 3.841, \text{ the table value of } \chi^2_{0.05,1}$$

(Appendix 4) hence, H_0 may be accepted.

Note: Expected frequency (150 and 50, respectively) can be used in place of expected ratio;

$$\chi^2 = \dfrac{\left[|156 \times 50 - 44 \times 150| - \dfrac{150 + 50}{2}\right]^2}{150 \times 50 \times 200} = 0.807$$

1.1.2.6 Heterogeneity among sets of data

In extension of testing frequencies in one sample against expected frequencies, we can also test whether many samples or may be families or over many trials (experiments) follow the expected frequencies or not pertaining to a particular trait.

1.1.2.6.1 Example: Monohybrid ratio (phenotypic)

Let us consider an example of alleles for shank-feathering considered under **Example 1.1.1.1.1** above with expected frequency of 3:1 (mono-hybrid ratio). The following were the results obtained from 10 families for the trait in question; we are required to test the following H_0's:

1. Each of the families is producing progenies at an expected ratio of 3:1
2. All the families belong to the same population (homogeneity)

Hence, for each family χ^2 is calculated as described under **Example 1.1.2.1** above, on $\upsilon = 1$ and added over all the families to get total of χ^2 values on $\upsilon = $ number of families; the latter is designated χ^2_{Total}; both can be tested with a level of significance α. An overall χ^2 considering values pooled over all the families is also calculated and tested on $\upsilon = 1$ and tested with a level of significance α; this is designated χ^2_{Pooled}.

Then, $\chi^2_{Heterogeneity} = (\chi^2_{Total} Pooled - \chi^2_{Pooled})$ on $\upsilon = $ (No of families $- 1$) and α level of significance.

A numerical example (hypothetical) below gives all details of computations:

Family		Frenquencies		n	υ	χ^{2} *	χ^2_{Table} $\alpha = 0.05$
		Feathered shanks	Clean shanks				
1	Observed	40	18	58	1	1.126	3.841
	Expected	43.5	14.5				
2	Observed	26	10	36	1	0.148	3.841
	Expected	27	9				
3	Observed	17	15	32	1	8.167**	3.841
	Expected	24	8				
4	Observed	22	8	30	1	0.022	3.841
	Expected	22.5	7.5				
5	Observed	30	14	44	1	0.916	3.841
	Expected	33	11				
				χ^2_{Total}	5	10.379	11.070
Total	Observed	135	65	200			
	Expected	150	50	χ^2_{Pooled}	1	6.000	3.841
		$\chi^2_{Heterogeneity} = (\chi^2_{Total} - \chi^2_{Pooled})$			4	4.379	9.488

* Calculated without correction for continuity (*see* Chapter **"Tests of hypotheses"**)

** Value > Table value; hence, H_0 (1) in this case may not be accepted

The following conclusions are possible from the above data:

1. Each of the families appears to be producing progenies at a ratio of 3:1 (excepting No 3) – based on individual χ^2 value.

2. All the families put together also appear to be producing progenies at a ratio of 3:1 – based on χ^2_{Pooled} and χ^2_{Total}.
3. All the families appear to be homogenous with respect to this trait-based on $\chi^2_{Heterogeneity}$.

1.1.2.6.2 Example: Backcross data

From the following backcross data, let us calculate heterogeneity χ^2 assuming that both P:p and Q:q loci are expected to be 1:1:

H_0's: Each of the families is producing progenies at an expected ratio of 1:1:1:1 and All the families belong to the same population (homogeneity)

Family		PQ	Pq	pQ	pq	n	υ	χ^2 *	χ^2_{Table} $\alpha = 0.05$
1	Observed	36	20	22	34	112	3	7.143	7.815
	Expected	28	28	28	28				
2	Observed	43	31	27	39	140	3	4.571	7.815
	Expected	35	35	35	35				
3	Observed	22	30	28	20	100	3	2.720	7.815
	Expected	25	25	25	25				
4	Observed	52	42	36	50	180	3	3.644	7.815
	Expected	45	45	45	45				
5	Observed	41	54	58	47	200	3	3.400	7.815
	Expected	50	50	50	50				
					χ^2_{Total}		15	21.748	24.996
Totals	Observed	194	177	171	190	732			
	Expected	183	183	183	183	χ^2_{Pooled}	3	1.913	7.815
		$\chi^2_{Heterogeneity} = (\chi^2_{Total} - \chi^2_{Pooled})$					12	19.835	21.026

* Calculated without correction for continuity (*see* Chapter **"Tests of hypotheses"**)

The following conclusions are possible from the above data:
1. Each of the families appears to be producing progenies at a ratio of 3:1 – based on individual χ^2 value.
2. All the families put together also appear to be producing progenies at a ratio of 1:1:1:1—based on χ^2_{Pooled}.
3. The families appear to be homogenous with respect to this trait-based on $\chi^2_{Heterogeneity}$.

Note: The concept can be extended to dihyrid ratio as well as genotypic frequencies in both mono- and di-hybrid ratios and others where many samples or may be families or over many trials (experiments) are involved.

1.1.3 χ^2 Test for Linkage

Certain genes tend to segregate together and it is referred to as "Linkage" which affects the expected frequency by altering the observed frequency in favor of some and against some of the phenotypes/genotypes.

1.1.3.1 Detection of linkage

Considering two loci 'A' and 'B' with alleles 'A' and 'a' in the ratio of r_1:1 and 'B' and 'b' in the ratio of r_2:1, the expected and observed frequencies are tabulated below:

	Combination				Totals
	AB	**Ab**	**aB**	**ab**	
Ratio	$r_1 r_2$	r_1	r_2	1	
Expected ratio	9	3	3	1	16
Expected frequency (E_i)	$9n \div 16$	$3n \div 16$	$3n \div 16$	$n \div 16$	n
Observed frequency (O_i)	a_1	a_2	a_3	a_4	n

χ^2 on $\upsilon = 3$ is calculated by $\chi^2 = \sum \dfrac{O_i^2}{E_i} - N$ by utilizing observed and expected

frequencies and tested at a set α; if calculated χ^2 is > tabulated value, there is a likelihood of linkage which has to be explored further by calculating χ^2_{Aa}, χ^2_{Bb} and χ^2_{AB}, the latter tests linkage, if any; the method is given below:

	A	**a**	**Totals**	**Ratio**
B	a_1	a_3	R_1	r_2
b	a_2	a_4	R_2	1
Totals	C_1	C_2	N	
Ratio	r_1	1		

Assuming $r_1 = r_2$, we calculate $\chi^2_{Aa} = \dfrac{(C_1 - r_1 C_2)^2}{r_1 N} = \dfrac{(C_1 - rC_2)^2}{rN}$; similarly,

$\chi^2_{Bb} = \dfrac{(R_1 - r_2 R_2)^2}{r_2 N} = \dfrac{(R_1 - rR_2)^2}{rN}$; both on $\upsilon = 1$; in terms of a's, they

are $\chi^2_{Aa} = \dfrac{\left[a_1 + a_2 - r(a_3 + a_4)\right]^2}{rN}$ and $\chi^2_{Bb} = \dfrac{\left[a_1 + a_3 - r(a_2 + a_4)\right]^2}{rN}$. Further, $\chi^2_{Linkage}$,

$\chi^2_L = \dfrac{\left[a_1 + r^2 a_4 - r(a_2 + a_3)\right]^2}{r^2 N}$. The use of these formulae are shown below with an

assumption that $r_1 = r_2 = 3$ or the expected phenotypic ratio is 9:3:3:1.

Note: If, $r_1 \neq r_2$, suitable changes can be easily made in the above formulae.

1.1.3.2 Example

Let us consider an example of two loci, 'A' and 'B' producing the following phenotypic frequencies against an expected ratio of frequencies 9:3:3:1:

H_0's: The observed frequencies are as per the expected ratio of 9:3:3:1; all the families belong to the same population (homogeneity) and there is no linkage between the loci.

			Phenotypic class		
Neck (A locus)	Naked	Naked	Feathered	Feathered	Totals
Skin (B locus)	White	Yellow	White	Yellow	
Observed	770 (a_1)	230 (a_2)	240 (a_3)	60 (a_4)	1300 (n)
Expected	731.25	243.75	243.75	81.25	1300

$\chi^2 = 8.444$ which is $> \chi^2_{0.05, 3} = 7.815$; hence H_0 (that the observed frequencies are as per expected ratio of 9:3:3:1) may be rejected. Now segregation of 'A' and 'a' (A locus) as well as 'B' and 'b' (B locus) can be tested as follows: $\chi^2_{Aa} = \dfrac{\left[(a_1 + a_2) - 3(a_3 + a_4)\right]^2}{3n}$

and $\chi^2_{Bb} = \dfrac{\left[(a_1 + a_3) - 3(a_2 + a_4)\right]^2}{3n}$ on $\upsilon = 1$; in this example, the values of χ^2_{Aa} and χ^2_{Bb} are 2.564 and 5.026, respectively; of these, χ^2_{Bb} is $>$ table value of χ^2 on $\upsilon = 1$ (3.841) (Appendix 4); hence, there is an indication of linkage in locus 'B' which can be calculated

as $\chi^2_L = \dfrac{\left[a_1 - 3a_2 - 3a_3 + 9a_4\right]^2}{9n} = 0.854$ which is < 3.841, table value of χ^2 on $\upsilon = 1$. Since χ^2_{Bb} is $>$ table value, it is reasonable to conclude that locus B is not segregating in the ratio of 3:1. Further, since χ^2_L is $<$ table value, there is no evidence of linkage.

Note: $\chi^2_L = \chi^2_{Total} - (\chi^2_{Aa} + \chi^2_{Bb}) = 8.444 - (2.564 + 5.026) = 0.854$

1.1.3.3 Example

The above concept can be extended on many samples/families/experiments and the same is shown in an example below:

H_0's: Each of the families is producing progenies at an expected ratio of 9:3:3:1; all the families belong to the same population (homogeneity) and there is no linkage between the loci.

			Phenotypic class		Totals
Neck (A locus)	Naked	Naked	Feathered	Feathered	
Skin (B locus)	White	Yellow	White	Yellow	
Family 1	47 (a_1)	8 (a_2)	11 (a_3)	9 (a_4)	75 (n)
Family 2	75 (a_1)	14 (a_2)	14 (a_3)	11 (a_4)	114 (n)
Family 3	65 (a_1)	13 (a_2)	12 (a_3)	11 (a_4)	101 (n)
Totals	187	35	37	31	290

As described under 1.1.3.2, χ^2 values calculated are tabulated below:

	χ^2_{Aa}	χ^2_{Bb}	χ^2_L *
υ	1	1	1
Family 1	0.111	0.218	7.468
Family 2	0.573	0.573	7.895

(Contd.)

(Contd.)

υ	χ^2_{Aa} 1	χ^2_{Bb} 1	χ^2_L * 1
Family 3	0.267	0.083	8.714
χ^2_{Total} on $\upsilon = 3$	0.951	0.874	24.077
χ^2_{Pooled} on $\upsilon = 1$	0.372	0.777	23.946
$\chi^2_{Heterogeneity}$ on $\upsilon = 2$	0.579	0.097	0.131

$$* \chi^2_L = \chi^2_{Total} - (\chi^2_{Aa} + \chi^2_{Bb})$$

In case of each family as well as pooled and total values of χ^2_L were greater than the respective table value at $\alpha = 0.05$; further, $\chi^2_{Heterogeneity}$ was < table value; hence, it is suggestive of the following:

1. All families have come from the same population
2. All families exhibit linkage between A and B loci and therefore,
3. It is likely that the linkage is a population phenomenon

1.1.4 G Test (Log Likelihood Ratio) vs χ^2 Test

Log likelihood ratio is $\sum O_i In\left(\dfrac{O_i}{E_i}\right) = \sum O_i In(O_i) - \sum O_i In(E_i)$; twice this quantity is referred to as **G**, which is distributed similar to χ^2; by converting to $\log_{10}$, we get $G = 4.6052\left[\sum O_i \log(O_i) - \sum O_i \log(E_i)\right]$ which can serve as a test for goodness of fit.

Considering **Example 1.1.3.2** above, G = 9.3542 which is > 7.815, the table value of $\chi^2_{0.05,3}$; hence, H_0 is liable to be rejected.;

1.2 Quantitative Genetics

1.2.1 Calculation of Gene and Genotypic Frequencies (One Locus, Two Alleles)

Total individuals in the population: 5000; Trait: Autosomal, Frizzled plumage (F) incompletely dominant to normal plumage (f); Number of individuals under each genotype:

Calculation of gene and genotypic frequencies
Population considered: Homozygous frizzle (FF): 3042; Heterozygous weakly frizzle (Ff): 1716 and Normal (ff) : 242; Total: 5000

Genotypic frequencies	Gene frequencies
FF = 3042/5000 = 0.6084 = 0.78^2	Total number of genes in the population
Ff = 1716/5000 = 0.3432 = $2 \times 0.78 \times 0.22$	= 5000 × 2 = 10000
ff = 242/5000 = 0.0484 = 0.22^2	Total number of 'F' genes
Total 1.0000	= 3042 × 2 + 1716 = 7800

(Contd.)

(Contd.)

Genotypic frequencies	Gene frequencies
It can be observed that genotypic frequencies can be calculated by knowing the gene frequencies and *vice versa*. For instance, with two alleles at a locus with gene frequencies p (for dominant gene) and q (for recessive gene), the genotypic frequencies are p^2 for homozygous dominant, 2pq for heterozygotes and q^2 for the recessive homozygotes; in other words, the genotypic frequencies are represented by the binominal expansion of $(p+q)^2$	Total number of 'f' genes = 242 x 2 + 1716 = 2200 Frequency of 'F' gene = 7800/10000 = 0.78 (p) = $\sqrt{0.6084}$ Frequency of 'f' gene = 2200/10000 = 0.22 (q) Total = (0.78 + 0.22) = (p + q) = 1.00 p = $\sqrt{(\text{frequency of 'FF' genotype})}$ = $\sqrt{0.6084}$ = 0.78 q = $\sqrt{(\text{frequency of 'ff' genotype})}$ = $\sqrt{0.0484}$ = 0.22

1.2.2 Hardy-Weinberg Equilibrium

In a random mating idealized population, in the absence of mutation, migration and selection, the gene and genotypic frequencies remain unaltered; this all important observation is named after the scientists who first discovered it.

Calculation of gene and genotypic frequencies I generation

Gene and genotypic frequencies

Base population	Reproduced population
Gene frequencies p = 0.78 q = 0.22 Hence, genotypic frequencies are: Homozygous dominant = p^2 = $(0.78)^2$ = 0.6084 or 60.84% of individuals, Heterozygotes = 2pq = 0.3432 or 34.32% of individuals and Homozygous recessive = q^2 = 0.0484 or 4.84% of individuals; Total of all genotypic frequencies = 0.6084+ 0.3432+ 0.0484 = 1.0000.	Gene frequencies: Since p + q = 1, $(p + q)^2 = p^2 + 2pq + q^2 = 1$; $p = (p^2 + \frac{1}{2} \text{ of } 2pq) \div (p^2 + 2pq + q^2)$. Since the denominator is $(p + q)^2 = 1^2$ Frequency of p = $p^2 + pq$ = 0.6084 + ½(0.3432) = 0.78; on the same lines, Frequency of q = $(q^2 + \frac{1}{2} \text{ of } 2pq) \div (p^2 + 2pq + q^2)$ = $q^2 + pq$ = 0.0484 + (0.3432/2) = 0.22

Source: Sreenivasaiah, 2006

Assuming that the population with a genotypic frequency of 0.6084, 0.3432 and 0.0484 with respect to FF, Ff and ff; and gene frequency of 0.78 and 0.22 with respect to F and f underwent a random mating, allowing all matings, the resultant gene and genotypic frequencies are tabulated below.

Calculation of gene and genotypic frequencies II generation				
Type of mating	Frequency of mating	Frequency of offsprings		
Male Female		FF	Ff	ff
FF FF	$p^2 \times p^2 = p^4 = (0.78)^4$	0.3702	–	–
Ff FF FF Ff	$2(p^2 \times 2pq) = 4\,p^3q$ $= 4\,(0.78)^3(0.22)$	0.2088	0.2088	–
FF ff ff FF	$2(p^2q^2) = 2p^2q^2$ $= 2\,(0.78)^2(0.22)^2$	–	0.0589	–
Ff Ff	$2pq \times 2pq = 4\,p^2q^2$ $= 4\,(0.78)^2(0.22)^2$	0.0294	0.0589	0.0294
Ff ff ff Ff	$2(pq \times q^2) = 4\,pq^3$ $= 4\,(0.78)\,(0.22)^3$	–	0.0166	0.0166
ff ff	$q^2 \times q^2 = q^4 = (0.22)^4$	–	–	0.0024
Total	$p^4 + 4p^3q + 6p^2q^2 + 4pq^3 + q^4$ $= (p^2 + 2pq + q^2)^2 = (p + q)^4 = 1$	0.6084	0.3432	0.0484

Source: Sreenivasaiah, 2006

Again, it can be seen that in an idealized population, gene and genotypic frequencies follow Hardy-Weinberg equilibrium. Conversely, if a random mating population continues to produce same gene and genotypic frequencies, then the population is said to be in Hardy-Weinberg equilibrium and it remains so, only as long as the Idealized conditions are met.

1.2.2.1 Sex-linked genes

In case of sex-linked genes, equilibrium is not achieved in one random mating but at each generation, difference in the gene frequency between the sexes is halved. In other words, if an allele is more frequent in female at the beginning, in the subsequent generation, it will be more abundant in males. That means, if base generation $(p_f - p_m)$ = x, then, Generation I $(p_f - p_m) = (-)\,\tfrac{1}{2}$ x, Generation II $(p_f - p_m) = \tfrac{1}{4}$ x and Generation III $(p_f - p_m) = (-)\,1/8$ x and so on. Therefore, after about seven generations, $(p_f - p_m)$ will be approximately zero indicating the reaching of equilibrium frequency.

Another important difference in case of sex-linked genes is that the genotypic frequencies p^2, $2pq$ and q^2 applied only to the homogametic sex (female in all animals and male, in case of poultry) whereas, for heterogametic (hemizygous) sex (male in all animals and female, in case of poultry), genotypic frequency is the same as equilibrium frequency of each allele.

1.2.3 *Gene and Genotypic Frequencies of Quantitative Traits*

Assuming a locus A, with alleles 'A' and 'a' with complete dominance, whose frequencies are p and q, respectively, in an idealized large population, genotypic frequencies are:

$(pA + qa)^2 = p^2 AA + 2pq\ Aa + q^2\ aa$; and the phenotypic are

Dominant allele, $A = p^2 + 2pq$ and recessive allele, $a = q^2$.

In case of quantitative traits, the alleles will have equal effects and assuming p = q = ½ and that gene action is additive with the addition of 'A' gene to the phenotype causing one unit increase in phenotype whereas that of 'a' gene causing no change in the phenotypic value, the phenotypic values will be : AA = 2, Aa = 1 and aa = 0 whose frequencies in an idealized population will be p^2 = ¼ , $2pq$ = ½ and q^2 = ¼, respectively.

Extending the same to two unlinked, non-interacting loci (A and B) with equal gene frequencies (pA = qA = pB = qB = ½) and equal additive effects (a = b = 0 and A = B = 1), the phenotypic values will be 4, 3, 2, 1 and 0 with phenotypic frequency of 0.0625, 0.2500, 0.3750, 0.2500 and 0.0625, respectively (see table below).

From the results obtained for two loci, it can be noticed that with 'n' number of unlinked, non-interacting loci, with equal allelic frequency and equal additive effects at each locus, 3^n distinct genotypes and $(2n + 1)$ distinct phenotypes are possible. Further, the phenotypic array can be found by expanding the trinomial $(\frac{1}{4} + \frac{1}{2} + \frac{1}{4})^n$ and the frequency of individuals whose phenotype will be exactly 'k' units, f(k), will be given by

$$f(k) = \frac{(2n)!}{k!(2n-k)!}\left(\frac{1}{2}\right)^{2n} \text{ or } {}^{2n}C_k\left(\frac{1}{2}\right)^{2n}.$$

Gene and genotypic frequencies–quantitative trait				
Genotype	Phenotypic value	Frequency	Phenotypic Class	Freq
AABB	4	$p^2A.p^2B = (\frac{1}{2})^4 = 0.0625$	4	0.0625
AABb	3	$p^2A.2pBqB = (\frac{1}{2})^2.(\frac{1}{2}) = 0.1250$	3	0.2500
AaBB	3	$2pAqA.p^2B = (\frac{1}{2}).(\frac{1}{2})^2 = 0.1250$		
AAbb	2	$p^2A.q^2B = (\frac{1}{2})^2.(\frac{1}{2})^2 = 0.0625$		
AaBb	2	$2pA.qA.2pBqB = (\frac{1}{2}).(\frac{1}{2}) = 0.2500$	2	0.3750
aaBB	2	$q^2A.p^2B = (\frac{1}{2})^2.(\frac{1}{2})^2 = 0.0625$		
Aabb	1	$2pAqA.q^2B = (\frac{1}{2}).(\frac{1}{2})^2 = 0.1250$	1	0.2500
aaBb	1	$q^2A.2pBqB = (\frac{1}{2})^2.(\frac{1}{2}) = 0.1250$		
aabb	0	$q^2A.q^2B = (\frac{1}{2})^4 = 0.0625$	0	0.0625

Source: Sreenivasaiah, 2006

A close perusal of frequencies of different phenotypic classes indicates that:
1. As 'n' increases, number of distinct phenotypes increases arithmetically whereas that the genotypes increases geometrically.
2. At intermediate gene frequencies (p = q = ½), the frequency of extreme phenotypes are relatively rare.
3. Individuals can differ genotypically but still they can have the same phenotypes which, in fact, is unique to quantitative traits.

In case of complete dominance in all the 'n' loci, 3^n distinct genotypes and $(n + 1)$ distinct phenotypes are possible. Assuming that phenotypic value of aa = bb = cc = dd = ... nn = 0 and that of AA = Aa = BB = Bb = ... NN = Nn = 2, the phenotypic array can be obtained by expanding the bi-nominal $(\frac{3}{4} + \frac{1}{4})^n$. Further, frequency of individuals whose phenotype will be exactly '2k' units with k lying between 0 and n can be obtained by

$$f(2k) = \frac{n!}{(n-k)!}\left(\frac{3}{4}\right)^k\left(\frac{1}{4}\right)^{n-k} \text{ or } {}^nP_k\left(\frac{3}{4}\right)^k\left(\frac{1}{4}\right)^{n-k}$$

Even with dominance, as 'n' increases, the number of phenotypic classes increases arithmetically whereas, frequency of one extreme class is high whereas that of the other is low.

In any case, it is noticeable that as 'n' increases, the phenotypic expression shows a continuous distribution. Since dominance is a rare phenomenon in polygenes, the frequency of the extreme classes will be low and that of the intermediate phenotypes will be high. Thus, when plotted on a graph, the frequencies follow, on most occasions, a symmetrical or Normal distribution.

Under realistic situations, most of the quantitative traits are controlled by more than two pairs of alleles but exact number cannot be known. Neither equal allelic frequency at each locus need be always true nor their effects equal and additive. In addition, when 'n' is large, linkage cannot be ruled out and environmental effects, more often than not, cannot be disregarded.

However, generalizations drawn on idealized populations are the best available as far as quantitative traits are concerned. Therefore, it is generally assumed and/or agreed that quantitative traits are continuously (Normally) distributed with intermediate phenotypes being most common and extreme phenotypes least common.

1.2.4 Average Effect of Gene (a)

Considering recessive dwarf gene (dw) in a population with the frequency of the dominant allele (DW) which does not depress body weight, p, as 0.7 and that of dw gene, q, as 0.3; and the day-old body weight of normal (DWDW and DWdw) as 40 g and that of dwarf chicks (dwdw) as 28 g, it is understandable that the day-old body weight is dependent on number of DW genes.

Therefore, a regression equation can be fit (*see* Chapter "**Association between variables I**") with day-old weight as the dependent variable (y) on number of DW genes (x). As per the Hardy–Weinberg law, frequency of homozygous dominants, heterozygotes and homozygous recessives will be 0.49 (i.e. 0.7^2), 0.42 (i.e. $2 \times 0.7 \times 0.3$) and 0.09 (i.e. 0.3^2), respectively. Keeping these in view, a linear regression equation is fit (Fig. 21.1).

Population mean of DW genes = 1.40 and population mean of body weight = 38.92 g. The y values can be considered to be the phenotypic averages from large populations which nullify the net environmental effect so that the values measured represent those without error and thus reflect the genotypic values directly.

No. of DW genes (x_i)	Chick weight (g) (y_i)	f_i	$f_i x_i$	$f_i y_i$	$f_i x_i^2$	$f_i y_i^2$	$f_i x_i y_i$
0	28	0.09	0.00	2.52	0.00	70.56	0.00
1	40	0.42	0.42	16.80	0.42	672.00	16.80
2	40	0.49	0.98	19.60	1.96	784.00	39.20
Σ 3	108	1.00	1.40	38.92	2.38	1526.56	56.00

Corrected sum of cross products = $56 - \{(1.40 \times 38.92) \div 1.00\} = 1.512$

Corrected sum of squares of x = $2.38 - (1.40^2 \div 1.00) = 0.42$

Regression coefficient, $b_{yx} = 1.512 \div 0.42 = 3.60$ g/DW gene

Intercept of the line = $\{38.02 - (3.60 \times 1.40)\} \div 1.00 = 33.88$ g

Regression equation is y = 33.88 + 3.60 x; predicted values of x when y assumes a value of 0, 1 and 2 are 33.88, 37.48 and 41.08 g, respectively as against corresponding actual values of 28, 40 and 40 g.

Corrected sum of squares of y = $1526.56 - (38.92^2 \div 1.00) = 11.7936$

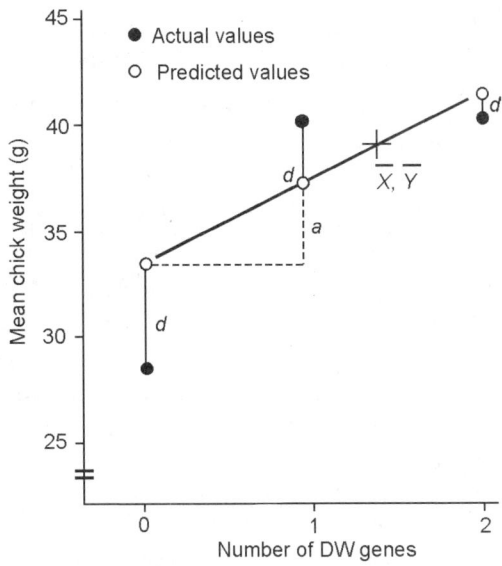

Fig. 21.1: Average effect of gene and breeding value

The population mean body weight (38.92 g) obtained is closer to normal birth weight (38 g). This is because the normal chicks represent $p^2 + 2pq = 0.91$ i.e., 91% of the population. The actual mean chick weight was 38.96 g which was 0.04 g more than the calculated mean weight which may be due to errors in the determination of the chick weight itself.

Regression coefficient, b_{yx}, indicates changing mean value of y per unit change in x; that is, change in the mean chick weight per single substitution of dw gene with DW gene; this is referred to as **Average effect of gene substitution**, designated a, which, in this example, is 3.60 g. The average of the gene or gene substitution is defined as deviation of the phenotypic mean of the progeny from that of population mean, where the progeny obtained one gene from its parents and the other is coming at random from the population.

1.2.5 *Breeding Value*

BV of an individual is the value of the individual judged by the mean value of its progeny. An individual contributes 50% of genes to its progenies produced over several mating and if each gene has an average effect of a, the total effect contributed is Σa. However, as only half the genes of its progeny is contributed by the individual, the BV = $2\Sigma a$. The points on the regression line (Fig. 21.1) represent the BV of individuals with 0, 1 and 2 DW genes.

1.2.5.1 Calculation of breeding value

Calculation of BV for each of the parents with 0, 1 and 2 DW genes is shown below. It is conspicuous that the BV of the parents in actual values is nothing but the points of the regression line. Therefore, there is a difference between the actual mean value (genotypic value) and the BV (the corresponding points on the regression line) which is designated d in Fig.21.1. The deviation between genotypic value and BV is referred to as **dominance deviation** for the respective genotype.

		Parents	
	dwdw	**DWdw**	**DWDW**
Alleles transmitted	All dw	Half each DW and dw	All DW
Frequency of alleles from parents	DW = 0 dw = 1	DW = ½ dw = ½	DW = 1 dw = 0
Frequency of alleles from population	DW = 0.7 dw = 0.3	DW = 0.7* dw = 0.3	DW = 0.7 dw = 0.3
Type of progeny	DWdw dwdw	DWDW DWdw dwdw	DWDW DWdw
Frequency	0.70 0.30	0.35 0.50 0.15	0.70 0.30
Chick weight (g)	40 28	40 40 28	40 40
Mean chick weight of progeny (g)	0.7 × 40 + 0.3 × 28 = 36.4	0.35 × 40 + 0.5 × 40 + 0.15 × 28 = 38.2	0.7 × 40 + 0.3 × 40 = 40.0
Mean chick weight as a deviation from population mean (g); i.e. 'a'	36.4 – 38.92 = (–) 2.52	38.2 – 38.92 = (–) 0.72	40.0- 38.92 =1.08
Breeding value (2Σa), g	(–) 5.04	(–) 1.44	2.16
Breeding value in actual units (Population mean +2Σa), g	38.92 – 5.04 = 32.88	38.92 – 1.44 = 37.48	38.92 + 2.16 = 41.08
Breeding value predicted from regression line, g	33.88	37.48	41.08

* Half the frequency of the gametes combines with DW and the other half with dw

Sreenivasaiah, 2006

1.2.5.2 Calculation of additive, genotypic and phenotypic variances

Population mean, P* = 38.92 g	Genotypes of individuals		
	dwdw	**DWdw**	**DWDW**
Frequency (f)	0.09	0.42	0.49
Genotypic value (G), g	28.00	40.00	40.00
Breeding value (A), g	33.88	37.48	41.08
(A – P*), g	(–) 5.04	(–) 1.44	2.16
$f(A - P^*)^2$	2.286144	0.870912	2.286144
$\Sigma f(A - P^*)^2 = V(A)$		5.4432**	
(G – A)	(–) 5.88	2.52	(–) 1.08
$f(G - A)^2$	3.111696	2.667168	0.571536
$\Sigma f(G - A)^2 = V(D)$		6.3509	
(G – P*) i.e. row 4 + row 6	(–) 10.92	1.08	1.08
$f(G - P^*)^2$	10.732176	0.489888	0.571536
$\Sigma f(G - P^*)^2 = V(G)$ which is same as Corrected $\Sigma f_i y_i^2$ from Table under 1.2.4 above		11.7936	

** Can also be calculated as variance of breeding values i.e.

$V(A): [\Sigma f_i A_i^2 - (\Sigma f_i y_i)^2] \div \Sigma f_i = [1520.2096 - (38.92)^2] \div 1.00 = 5.4432$

Sreenivasaiah, 2006

It has been shown above that BV refers to transmitting ability of an individual and hence refers to additive genetic variance. If A, G and P* refer to BV, genotypic value and Population mean, the calculation of V(G), V(A) and V(P) are shown below with an assumption that variance due to environment (V(E)) is zero and hence, V(P) = V(G).

It can be seen from that V(G) = V(A) + V(D). If there is no dominance, that means V(D) = 0, then it is easy to conclude that magnitude of V(A) is dependent on deviation of BV of each genotype from Population average and the frequency of each of the genotypes in the population. Similarly, V(D) is dependent on deviation of genotypic value from BV and genotypic frequency. Hence, changes in genotypic frequency can alter both V(A) and V(D), and in turn V(G). When many loci are involved, variance due to epistasis (V(EP)) is also a possibility. Statistically, it is possible to estimate V(A) and the deviation V(P) – V(A); the latter accounting for the sum of V(D), V(EP) and V(E).

In the above example, with V(E) = 0, **Heritability**, h^2 = V(A) ÷ {V(A) + V(D)} or V(A) ÷ V(G) = 5.443 ÷11.7936 = 0.4615

1.2.6 *Heritability*

Considering a trait X with the mean value of X* and variance V(X), the V(X) refers to the observed variance or phenotypic variance, V(P). But, as discussed earlier P = G + E and hence, it is essential to know what proportion of V(P) or V(X) is due to genetic effects or genotypic variance, V(G). It is equally important to know the proportion of differences between two individuals that can be transmitted to the next generation. In other words, if an individual with a phenotypic superiority of 'a' units is selected, what proportion of this superiority is expectable in its offsprings? In still simpler terms, how reliable is the phenotype of the individual in predicting its genetic worth?

Heritability narrow sense, designated h^2, is one of the most useful estimates for animal breeders. In other words, h^2 indicates the proportion of V(P) attributable to V(A) or is the proportion of differences among individuals expected, on average of the population, to be transmitted to their progeny. It follows therefore that h^2 is the proportion of superiority of the selected parents that is expected to be realized in their progeny. Estimation of h^2 is also possible as the regression of BV on phenotypic value, V(P); the coefficient of determination (R^2) is the proportion of variability in BV that is attributable to its linear association with V(P); in other words, $R^2_{AP} = h^2$. If h^2 is large, it indicates that an animal which is above average phenotypically is likely to be correspondingly superior genetically and *vice versa*. That means, high h^2 suggests that phenotype is a reliable indicator of genotype and *vice versa* (details can be obtained from Sreenivasaiah, 2006).

1.2.6.1 Estimation of heritability

1.2.6.1.1 *Heritability in broad sense*

Although, this estimate has little practical utility, its estimation necessitates a genetically uniform Population in which V(G) is likely to be zero so that V(P) of such population estimates V(E). However, in livestock, severe loss in fitness traits at high inbreeding coefficient precludes this method of estimation. But, monozygotic twins as may be available in case of cattle, sheep, etc. (not in poultry) can be considered genetically uniform.

Variance calculated from a normal genetically variable population estimates V(P). Then, by definition, heritability in broad sense is the ratio of V(G) to V(P); the numerator can be estimated as V(P) – V(E). Therefore, heritability in broad sense =1 – V(E) ÷V(P); in other words, it is equal to 1 –, the ratio of V(P) in genetically uniform population to that in genetically variable population.

1.2.6.1.2 Heritability in narrow sense

1.2.6.1.2.1 Response to selection

By definition, h^2 is the superiority of selected parents transmitted to the next generation. If mean of the selected individuals was 'S' units superior to that of the base population from which they are selected (selection differential), and the mean of the reproduced population was 'R' units superior to that of the base population (response), then h^2 = R ÷ S. In livestock population, including poultry, as the males form a smaller proportion, S is calculated separately for males and females, and averaged. h^2 calculated by this method is referred to as **realized h^2**. If S and R over several generations are known, h^2 can be estimated as regression of R on S.

Calculation of realized h^2 (mean body weight, kg)		
Population	Males	Females
Base population	1.80	1.50
Selected population	2.20	1.70
Selection differential	0.40	0.20
Mean selection differential	0.30	
Reproduced population	1.90	1.60
Response	0.10	0.10
Mean response	0.10	
Realized h^2	0.10 ÷ 0.30 = 0.33	

Sreenivasaiah, 2006

1.2.6.1.2.2 Resemblance among relatives

Any relationship can be used provided it is amenable to the following steps:
1. Quantification by correlation (r) or regression (b) coefficient
2. Explanation as to how much a relationship can cause more resemblance than those chosen strictly at random and
3. Equating the observed resemblance to theoretical causes so that h^2 can be estimated with minimum bias

1.2.6.1.2.2.1 Direct relationship

1.2.6.1.2.2.1.1 Offspring with one of the parents

The same trait is estimated at the same stage of life-cycle in both offspring and parent. Normally, offspring (O) – dam (D) relationship is commonly used because number of sires used in livestock breeding is low. If V(P) among dam and offsprings are homogeneous, either r_{OD} or b_{OD} can be calculated. But, as dams are subjected to selection, V(P) reduces among them. Therefore, if the relationship is linear, b_{OD} is a better statistic. If sire is known, numerator and denominator for calculation of b_{OD} can be obtained under each sire and then pooled to get intra-sire b_{OD}. On the same lines, if the data is stratified as per treatments or locations, etc., "intra-class r_{OD} or b_{OD} can be computed (*see* Chapter "**Association between variables I**").

Sire and dam contribute 50% of genes to their offspring; in other words, covariance of offspring with any of the parent estimates $\frac{1}{2}V(A)$ + other Genetic effects like variance due to interaction, maternal influence (parent is dam), etc. Since b_{OD} is the ratio of covariance$_{OD}$ to variance among the dams, it estimates only $\frac{1}{2}h^2$; in other words, $h^2 = 2b_{OD}$

If x_i and y_i are the values of a trait recorded on ith dam and offspring, respectively, the following are calculated: $\sum_{i=1}^{n} x_i$, $\sum_{i=1}^{n} x_i^2$, $\sum_{i=1}^{n} y_i$ and $\sum_{i=1}^{n} x_i y_i$. They are designated, A, B, C and D, respectively. Then, $b_{OD} = \dfrac{D - (A)(C)/n}{B - A^2/n}$ and $h^2 = 2b_{OD}$ and variance (h^2)

$$2\left(\sqrt{\dfrac{\dfrac{SS_Y}{SS_X} - b_{yx}^2}{(n-2)}} \right)$$ (van Vleck, 1979).

Note: r_{xy} can also be used to estimate h^2 analogous to b_{xy}; but it is not a common practice.

1.2.6.1.2.2.1.2 Example

From **Example 3.2.2.1** Chapter "**Association between variables I**", we have the following values: $n = 12$, A = 74.9, B = 499.03, C = 76.8, D = 510.03 and b_{yx} or $b_{OD} = 0.9759$; therefore, h^2 exceeds the theoretical limit of + 1 in this case primarily because of small sample size. When values of many samples are pooled, such discrepancies do not arise. Method for pooling of b_{yx} values is given in Chapter "**Association between variables I**". In this example, SS_Y and SS_X were 30.9200 and 31.5292, respectively;

hence, Variance of $h^2 = 0.106$ and variance of $h^2 = 2*se(b_{yx}) = 2\left(\sqrt{\dfrac{SS_Y - b(SCP_{XY})}{SS_X(n-2)}} \right) = 0.112$

(van Vleck, 1979).

1.2.6.1.2.2.1.3 Offspring with mid-parent

Mid-parent values are not always practicable because of less number of sires in animal breeding. If mid-parent values are used, pooled mean (P) = $\frac{1}{2}$ of mean of dams (D) + $\frac{1}{2}$ of mean of sires (S); since each of them contribute $\frac{1}{2}$ of genes (V(P)) to the next generation and they are unrelated, V(P) = $\frac{1}{4}$ V(D) + $\frac{1}{4}$ V(S). Further, assuming variances are homogeneous, V(D) = V(S) = V(P), it is clear that V(P) = $\frac{1}{2}$ V(D) or $\frac{1}{2}$ V(S) or $\frac{1}{2}$ V(P) itself. Since it is known that covariance estimates $\frac{1}{2}$ V(A), the regression coefficient b_{OD} = covariance ÷ variance = $\frac{1}{2}$ V(A) ÷ $\frac{1}{2}$ V(P) which is nothing but V(A) ÷ V(P) = h^2. Therefore, regression coefficient calculated by using mid-parent values is itself the value of h^2; use of mid-parent values is preferred because it is less influenced by maternal effects although interaction effects cannot be ruled out.

Note: No numerical example given since it is same as regression between offspring with one of the parents.

1.2.6.1.2.2.2 Collateral relationship

In the forthcoming sections on estimation of h^2 and correlations, notations already introduced in Chapters "**One-factor analysis of variance**", "**Two-factor analysis of variance**", "**Analysis of more than two factors**" and "**Analysis of covariance**" will be used.

1.2.6.1.2.2.2.1 Paternal half-sibs

Resemblance of half-sibs to that among individuals related by an average amount for the population is the criterion. This is estimated by analysis of variance (ANOVA) method. Data in the form of maternal half-sibs is available at least in poultry. The following calculations have to be made:

If X_{ij}'s are the observations on the jth half-sib ($j = 1, 2, 3, 4, \ldots n$) under ith sire ($i = 1, 2, 3, 4, \ldots s$), n_i is the number of observations under ith sire, $X_{i.}$ is the total of ith sire, n. is the total number of observations and X.. is the grand total, by using standard statistical procedures (*see* Chapter "**One-factor analysis of variance**"), the following are obtained:

$$\text{Total crude SS, TSS} = \sum_i^s \sum_j^{n_i} x_{ij}^2, \text{ Total SS} = \sum_i^s \sum_j^{n_i} x_{ij}^2 - \frac{(x_{..})^2}{n_.}, \text{ SS due to Sires, } SS_S =$$

$$\sum \frac{(x_{i.})^2}{n_i} - \frac{(x_{..})^2}{n_.}, \text{ within sires SS, } SS_W = TSS - SS_S; \text{ and number of half-sib families, } k =$$

$$\frac{1}{s-1}\left(n_. - \frac{\sum_i^s n_i^2}{n_.} \right)$$

V(S) can be calculated as $(MS_S - MS_w) \div k$, and V(P) = V(S) + V(E) and intra-class correlation, $r_I = V(S) \div V(P)$.

Probability that to half-sibs inherit copy of the particular gene from their sire is ½ and therefore, the Probability that both of them will inherit the same gene is ½ x ½ = ¼ because the events are independent. It follows therefore that V(S) = ¼ V(A) or V(A) = 4 V(S); hence, $h^2 = 4$ V(S) ÷ V(P) or $h^2 = 4$ r_I.

ANOVA of half-sib relationship

Source	v^*	Sum of squares (SS)	Mean sum of squares (MSS)**	Expected mean sum of squares (EMS)
Between sires	S – 1	SS_S	MS_S	V(E) + kV(S)
Within sires	n. – S	SS_W	MS_W	V(E)

* v indicates degrees of freedom
** Calculated as (SS ÷ v)

1.2.6.1.2.2.2.2 Example

The data pertains to weight gain up to 6 weeks of age (x_{ij}, kg) by broilers (Progenies, p; $k = 1, 2, \ldots p$) as stratified by sire ($i = 1, 2, s$).

	Sire 1			Sire 2			Sire 3	
1.90	1.90	2.03	2.05	2.00	1.98	2.00	1.45	1.93	1.73
1.43	2.00	1.91	2.10	2.11	1.66	1.79	1.68	1.49	1.44
1.62	1.74	1.68	1.79	1.76	1.73	2.12	1.79	1.66	1.59

(Contd.)

(Contd.)

Sire 1			Sire 2			Sire 3			
1.99	1.64	1.88	1.68	1.83	1.57	1.56	1.94	1.72	1.63
1.51	1.59	1.54	2.06	1.67	1.79	1.70	1.53	1.44	1.38
1.29	2.00	1.76	1.66	1.80	2.00	1.63	1.42	1.33	1.77
		1.89	2.03	1.97	1.53	1.33	1.33	1.47	1.84
								1.64	1.67

Totals $n_i = 19$, $x_{i.} = 33.30$ $n_i = 21$, $x_{i.} = 38.77$ $n_i = 30$, $x_{i.} = 49.00$

$n. = 70$, $x.. = 121.07$, $x^2.. $ (or $\displaystyle\sum_{i=1}^{s}\sum_{j=1}^{p} x_{ij}^2) = 212.7343$; $\displaystyle\sum_{i=1}^{s} n_i^2 = 1702$; $k = 22.84$; Total SS = 3.3351, SS due to sires, $SS_S = 0.5736$, SS within sires, $SS_W = 2.7615$

Source	υ	SS	MSS
Sires	2	0.5736	0.2868
Within sires	67	2.7615	0.0412
Total	69	3.3351	

Therefore, $V(S) = 0.0108$, $V(W) = 0.0412$, $V(P) = 0.0520$, $r_1 = 0.2077$ and $h^2 = 0.8308$.

Estimate of variance of $h^2 = \dfrac{1}{4}\left(\dfrac{2(n.-1)(1-r_1)^2 \{1+(k-1)r_1\}^2}{k^2(n.-S)(S-1)} \right)$ which works – out to be 0.0095 in this example.

1.2.6.1.2.2.2.3 Full-sibs

Litter-mates, progeny from repeat-mates or single-sire pedigree mating (which is very popular in poultry) can yield data of full-sibs. Full-sibs get 50% of genes each from sire and dam and hence their resemblance estimates 50% of V(A) of which 25% is from sire and the other 25% is from dam component. In other words, V(S) and variance (dams), V(D) account for ¼ V(A) each. They can be estimated by ANOVA (see Chapter "**Analysis of variance for more than two factors**").

The preliminary calculations for obtaining ANOVA table are as follows:

Assuming that several sires (i = 1, 2, 3, … s) where each mated to several dams (j = 1, 2, 3, … d) and each dam produced several progenies (k = 1, 2, 3, … p). The value of each progeny for the trait in question represented by X_{ijk} is tabulated as per sire and dam.

Let $x_{ij.}$ be the total of the jth dam under ith sire (designated A), $x_{i..}$ be the total of ith sire (designated B), $x_{...}$ the grand total (designated C), n_{ij} the number of observations under jth dam under ith sire, $n_{i.}$ be the number of observations under ith sire and $n_{..}$ be the total number of observations. The following re calculated from the data:

Total crude SS $= \displaystyle\sum_{i}^{s}\sum_{j}^{d}\sum_{k}^{p} x_{ijk}^2$ designated T; SS due to sires, $SS_S = \displaystyle\sum_{i}^{s} \dfrac{B^2}{n_{i.}} - \dfrac{C^2}{n_{..}}$, SS

due to dams within sires, $SS_{D/S} = \displaystyle\sum_{i}^{s}\sum_{j}^{d} \dfrac{A^2}{n_{ij}} - \sum_{i}^{s} \dfrac{B^2}{n_{i.}}$, SS between progeny within dam within sire, $SS_{P/D/S} = T - (SS_S + SS_{D/S}) = T - \sum_i^s \sum A^2 \over n_{ij}$, $E = \sum_i^s {\sum_j^d n_{ij}^2 \over n_{i\cdot}}$, $F = \sum_i^s \sum_j^d n_{ij}^2$,

$G = \sum_i^s n_{i\cdot}^2$, $k_1 = {(n_{\cdot\cdot} - E) \over (D - S)}$, $k_2 = {\left(E - {F \over n_{\cdot\cdot}}\right) \over (S - 1)}$ and $k_3 = {\left(n_{\cdot\cdot} - {G \over n_{\cdot\cdot}}\right) \over (S - 1)}$

ANOVA of full-sib relationship

Source	v*	SS	MSS**	EMS
Sires	S-1	SS_S	MS_S	$V(E) + K_2 V(Dam) + K_3 V(S)$
Dams within sires	S(D-1)	$SS_{D/S}$	$MS_{D/S}$	$V(E) + K_1 V(Dam)$
Progenies within dams within sires	SD(P-1)	$SS_{P/D/S}$	$MD_{P/D/S}$	$V(E)$

* v indicates degrees of freedom
** Calculated as (SS ÷ v)

From EMS, $V(E) = MS_{P/D/S}$, $V(Dam) = (MS_{D/S} - MS_{P/D/S}) \div k_1$
$V(S) = \{MS_S - MS_{P/D/S} - (k_2 \div k_1)(MS_{D/S} - MS_{P/D/S})\} \div k_3$
If $k_1 = k_2$, $V(S) = (MS_S - MS_{D/S}) \div k_3$

Note: k_1, k_2 and k_3 represent number of progenies per dam, per dam within sire and per sire, respectively.

After obtaining the variance components, $V(P) = V(S) + V(Dam) + V(E)$; since $V(S)$ and $V(Dam)$ each estimates ¼ $V(A)$,

4 $V(S) = V(A)$ and 4 $V(Dam) = V(A)$; hence

h^2(sire component), $h^2_S = 4 \times \{V(S) \div V(P)\}$,

h^2(dam component), $h^2_D = 4 \times \{V(Dam) \div V(P)\}$ and

h^2(sire + dam components), $h^2_{S+D} = \{2 \times (V(S) + V(Dam)) \div V(P)\}$

Errors in the computing correlation of relationship are estimated by multiplying the calculated correlation with the reciprocal of the theoretical genetic relationship among the individuals considered. Value of reciprocal increases as the denominator reduces and therefore, as theoretical genetic relationship among the relatives considered reduces, error in estimation is magnified. Half-and full-sibs are, by far, the most popularly used relationships for estimating h^2.

1.2.6.1.2.2.2.4 Example

Let us assume that in the **Example 1.2.6.1.2.2.2.2** above, data on dams are also available as follows: then, each of the observation now pertains to weight gain up to 6 weeks of age (x_{ijk}, kg) by broilers (Progenies, p; $k = 1, 2, \ldots p$) as stratified by sire ($i = 1, 2, s$) and dam ($j = 1, 2, \ldots d$):

Dams	Sire 1			Sire 2			Sire 3			
	1	2	3	4	5	6	7	8	9	10
	1.90	1.90	2.03	2.05	2.00	1.98	2.00	1.45	1.93	1.73
	1.43	2.00	1.91	2.10	2.11	1.66	1.79	1.68	1.49	1.44
	1.62	1.74	1.68	1.79	1.76	1.73	2.12	1.79	1.66	1.59
	1.99	1.64	1.88	1.68	1.83	1.57	1.56	1.94	1.72	1.63
	1.51		1.54	2.06	1.67	1.79	1.70	1.53	1.44	1.38
	1.29		1.76		1.80	2.00	1.63	1.42	1.33	1.77
			1.89		1.97	1.53		1.33		1.84
			1.59			1.66		1.64		1.67
			2.00			2.03				1.47
										1.33
n_{ij}	6	4	9	5	7	9	6	8	6	10
$x_{ij.}$	9.74	7.28	16.28	9.68	13.14	15.95	10.80	12.78	9.57	15.85
Totals	$n_{i.} = 19, x_{i..} = 33.30$			$n_{i.} = 21, x_{i..} = 38.77$			$n_{i.} = 30, x_{i..} = 49.00$			

$$S = 3, D = 10, P = 70; n.. = 70, x... = 121.07, x^2... \ (or \ \sum_{i=1}^{s}\sum_{j=1}^{d}\sum_{k=1}^{p} x_{ijk}^2 \ ) = 212.7343; \sum_{i=1}^{s}\sum_{j=1}^{d} n_{ij}^2$$

$= 524, \sum_{i=1}^{s} n_{i.}^2 = 1702$; Total SS = 3.3351; SS due to sires, $SS_S = 209.9728 - 209.3992 =$ 0.5736; SS due to dams within sires, $SS_{D/S} = 210.4251 - 209.9728 = 0.4523$; SS due to progenies within dams within sires, $SS_{P/D/S} = 212.7343 - 210.4251 = 2.3092$; E = 22.2476, F = 524, G = 1072; $k_1 = 6.82$, $k_2 = 7.38$ and $k_3 = 27.34$. Now, variance components can be obtained:

Source	υ	SS	MSS
Sires	2	0.5736	0.2868
Dams/sires	7	0.4523	0.0646
Progenies/dams/sires	60	2.3092	0.0385
Total	69	3.3351	

$V(E) = MS_{P/D/S} = 0.0385$, $V(Dam) = (MS_{D/S} - MS_{P/D/S}) \div k_1 = 0.0038$, $V(S) = \{MS_S - MS_{P/D/S} - (k_2 \div k_1)(MS_{D/S} - MS_{P/D/S})\} \div k_3 = 0.0071$; $V(P) = 0.0494$, $h^2_S = 4 \times \{V(S) \div V(P)\} = 0.5749$, $h^2_D = 4 \times \{V(Dam) \div V(P)\} = 0.3077$ and $h^2_{S+D} = \{2 \times (V(S) + V(Dam)) \div V(P)\} = 0.4413$

1.2.6.1.3 h^2 of threshold characters

Phenotypic expression of threshold characters is discrete; for instance, hatchability which can be recorded as discrete values only whereas the underlying distribution can be conveniently assumed to be normal. Therefore, h^2 can be estimated by assuming different numerical values to the alternate expression and carrying out ANOVA with data on full- and half-sibs. Alternatively, realized h^2 can be calculated with some modifications based on the assumption that the underlying distribution is a Standard Normal Deviate with mean = 0 and SD = 1.

1.2.6.1.3.1 An example

Incidence of disease in the affected population (population mean = 0 and SD = 1) was 7%; this corresponds to 1.48 s units (Appendix 1). The mean incidence was 3.5% corresponding to 1.92 s units. In a related population the corresponding values were 12% (1.18 s units) and 6% (1.67 s units). Keeping these in view,

S = (Mean of the affected population—Mean of the base population)

= 1.92 – 0.00 = 1.92 s units.

R = (Mean of the related population—Mean of the base population); since both are 0,

R = (Incidence in base population—Incidence in related population)

= 1.48 – 1.18 = 0.30 s units.

R/S = 0.156. The genetic relationship between parent and offspring is one half and therefore $h^2 = 2(R/S) = 0.312$

Another method has also been suggested. If P_i values are the survival of paternal half-sib families, and P* is the average survival, it is easy to visualize that, if the trait is not heritable, each of the P_i's will be the same as P* and if it is heritable, families differ from P*. The difference can be tested by χ^2. Subsequently, if S is the number of paternal half-sib families each having k (effective number) of individuals, h^2 is calculated as:

$$h^2 = \frac{1}{\text{Genetic relationship}}\left(\chi^2 - \frac{(S-1)}{k(S-1)}\right).$$

1.2.7 Repeatability

Certain traits are expressed more than once in a lifetime; for example, egg weight. For such traits, V(E) has two components namely permanent and temporary sources of environmental variation designated $V(E)_{PMT}$ and $V(E)_{TMP}$, respectively. That means, $V(E) = V(E)_{PMT} + V(E)_{TMP}$. Those environmental causes that affect the trait every time the trait is expressed constitute $V(E)_{PMT}$; for instance, a permanent damage in yolk formation results in a permanent reduction in egg weight. On the other hand, factors that do not affect the trait every time form $V(E)_{TMP}$; for instance, effect of high temperature during a particular phase of egg production. Therefore, for repeatable traits, $V(P) = V(G) + V(E)_{PMT} + V(E)_{PMT} = V(A) + V(D) + V(EP) + V(E)_{PMT} + V(E)_{TMP}$.

Repeatability, designated R, is defined as a proportion of V(P) for a trait attributable to permanent differences among individuals. Since V(G) and $V(E)_{PMT}$ constitute permanent differences, R is the ratio of {V(G) + $V(E)_{PMT}$} to V(P). Traits which are repeated may be influenced by the same genes each time they are expressed and so-called permanent environmental influence. $V(E)_{PMT}$ may not be always permanent; in spite of these, R is a useful tool to the animal breeders.

1.2.7.1 Estimation of repeatability

1.2.7.1.1 Product-moment correlation coefficient

If only two records per individual are available, repeatability is simply the product-moment correlation between the two records (*see* Chapter "**Association between** variables I"). In other words, repeatability is the ratio of covariance between the two records to the geometric mean of the variances of the two records. If x_{i1} and x_{i2} refer to two records of ith individual among 'n' individuals, then

$$R = \cfrac{\displaystyle\sum_{i=1}^{n} x_{i1} x_{i2} - \cfrac{\left(\displaystyle\sum_{i=1}^{n} x_{i1}\right)\left(\displaystyle\sum_{i=1}^{n} x_{i2}\right)}{n}}{\left[\sqrt{\displaystyle\sum_{i=1}^{n} x_{i1}^2 - \cfrac{\left(\displaystyle\sum_{i=1}^{n} x_{i1}\right)^2}{n}}\,\sqrt{\displaystyle\sum_{i=1}^{n} x_{i2}^2 - \cfrac{\left(\displaystyle\sum_{i=1}^{n} x_{i2}\right)^2}{n}}\right]}$$

1.2.7.1.2 With > 2 records per individual

1. Sum of squares and cross products are calculated for all possible combinations within a sub-class (i.e. individual) and pooled to finally obtain repeatability value by the formula given above.
2. With many records per animal, repeatability can be calculated by the method of half-sib analysis with only changes in terminologies; V(S) is termed variance between sub-class or individuals (V(B)) and V(E) is referred to as variance within subclass or individuals (V(W)), The intra-class correlation (r_I) gives the estimate of repeatability directly; $r_I = R = V(B) \div (V(B) + V(W))$.

1.2.7.2 Examples

1.2.7.2.1 Product-moment correlation coefficient

Let us take-up **Example 5.5.1.1** Chapter "**Association between variables I**" concerning lactation yield of twins.

Twin No.	1	2	3	4	5	6	7	8	9	10	Sum	Crude SS
Yields (kg)	12.5	8.5	13.0	8.0	9.5	10.8	16.4	13.0	9.0	10.6	111.3	1299.71
	13.5	8.0	11.5	8.3	9.4	11.2	15.7	12.9	8.8	10.0	109.3	1251.53

Total crude SCP = 1165.29 and $r_{xy} = 0.647$ and $b_{yx} = 0.986$; hence, R = 0.647. Note that b_{yx} is not accurate in estimating R; however, if many sample values are pooled, the pooled b_{yx} will be a reliable estimate. Similarly, r_{xy} can also be pooled over several samples (see Chapter "**Association between variables I**" for details).

1.2.7.2.2 Variance component analysis

From **Section 4.2** Chapter "**One-factor analysis of variance**", the following ANOVA table is reproduced:

Source	υ	SS	MSS	EMS
Total	29	1.2917		
Hens	4	1.2333	0.3083	$\sigma^2 + k\sigma_A^2$
Error	25	0.0584	0.0023	σ^2

The data were on cholesterol content in 6 eggs each (k) from 5 hens (B) making totally 30 observations ($n.$); $\sigma_A^2 = 0.051$; hence, $R = \dfrac{0.051}{(0.051 + 0.0023)} = 0.957$; method of calculating weighted number of observations per animal is also given in the Chapter referred to above.

$$\text{Variance of R} \approx \frac{2(n. - 1)(1 - R)^2 \left[1 + (k - 1)R\right]^2}{k^2 (n. - B)(B - 1)} = 0.0010 \text{ and se} = 0.032$$

Note: For pooling of R from many samples, sample-wise values of σ^2 and σ_A^2 can be tabulated along with respective variance. Average of σ^2, σ_A^2 and variance calculated; the average values of σ^2 and σ_A^2 are used to compute pooled R and its variance.

1.2.8 Correlations

In practical situations, many quantitative traits are associated with each other. For example, body weight with egg weight, age at sexual maturity with egg production, etc. These associations can be due to genetic and/or environmental causes.

1.2.8.1 Types of correlations

1.2.8.1.1 Phenotypic correlation (r_p)

This measures linear association between two traits. In other words, it predicts deviation from population mean in one trait of an individual as a function of its deviation from the population mean of the other when both the measured in terms of their standard deviation units. As in the case of V(P), r_p also can be partitioned into genetic and environmental components.

1.2.8.1.2 Genetic correlation (r_g)

This measures the extent to which the same genes, are grossly linked genes, cause simultaneous variation in two different traits or the extent to which individuals genetically above average in one trait are genetically above, equal or below average for a second trait. Analogous to h^2, r_g can be of two types:

1.2.8.1.2.1 Genotypic correlation

Similar to h^2 (broad sense)—theoretically, it is the correlation that would exist if environmental conditions affecting the two traits are exactly the same ever since the conception till the two traits are measured; but it is unrealistic to accept that environment can cause no variation in either of the traits. Hence, this is of less practical value and also requires specialized populations for computation.

1.2.8.1.2.2 Additive genetic correlation

This is analogous to h^2 (narrow sense) and is very useful to estimate genetic merit of individuals and predict correlated response to selection. This is designated by r_g and it refers to correlation between individuals for the two traits considered.

1.2.8.1.3 Environment correlation (r_e)

If the same environmental effect causes simultaneous variation in both traits, a correlation results; which is referred to as r_e. For example, increased light during growing period causes early sexual maturity, increased egg production and reduced egg weight. In real sense, r_e is not purely environmental but also includes dominance and epistatic effects because it is calculated as a deviation from r_g (which takes into account additive effects and a small portion of epistatic effects). Therefore, r_e is the net effect of environmental and non-additive genetic factors causing the two traits to vary simultaneously in either positive or negative direction.

1.2.8.2 Estimation of correlations

1.2.8.2.1 Phenotypic correlation

Phenotypic correlation, r_p, Can be calculated as a simple product-moment correlation (*see* Chapter "**Association between variables I**"). However, sums of cross products and sums of squares can be calculated within various groups and later on, pooled to get a more reliable estimate of r_p.

1.2.8.2.2 Environmental correlation

By using the formula $r_p = r_g h_x h_y + r_e e_x e_y$, r_e can be estimated. e_x and e_y can be estimated by using the formula $h^2_X + e^2_X = 1$ and $h^2_Y + e^2_Y = 1$.

1.2.8.2.3 Genetic correlation

1.2.8.2.3.1 Through correlated response to selection

It has been shown that $R = h^2 S$ and it is more relevant to convert in terms of the corresponding s to obtain "standardized selection differential" or "intensity of selection" designated 'i'. Hence, $i = S \div s$ or $S = i*s$. Keeping this in view, r_g can be calculated from correlated response (CR) to selection. Let h be $\sqrt{h^2}$. Considering a trait X, $R_X = h^2_X S_X = h^2_X i_X SD(P_X)$; considering trait Y, $R_Y = h^2_Y S_Y = h^2_Y i_Y SD(P_Y)$

If the traits are genetically correlated, selection in trait X should bring a change in V(A) component of trait Y. Therefore, CR_Y = Regression of additive genetic component of trait on the phenotype of trait X times S_X. In other words, $CR_Y = b_{AyPx} S_X$; Further, b_{AyPx} is the product of change in A_X per unit change in P_X and change in A_Y per unit change in A_X. That means, $b_{AyPx} = b_{AxPx} \cdot b_{AyAx}$. Therefore, $CR_Y = b_{AxPx} \cdot b_{AyAx} S_X$ and

$$r_g = \frac{CR_Y}{h_X h_Y SD(P_Y) i_X} \cdot$$

Alternatively, if CR_Y and CR_X due to direct selection in trait X and trait Y, respectively are estimated simultaneously in different selection lines from the same base population,

and substituting suitably for CR's and R's, we get $r_g = \sqrt{\left(\frac{CR_X}{R_X}\right)\left(\frac{CR_Y}{R_Y}\right)}$.

If CR_X and R_X, and CR_Y and R_Y differ in sign, the negative square root and if they have positive signs, positive square root gives r_g. However, in practice, CR of only one trait is commonly available; in such cases $r_g = \left(\frac{CR_Y h_Y}{R_Y h_X}\right)$ (details of derivations can be obtained from Chapman, 1985, Sreenivasaiah, 2006)

1.2.8.2.3.2 *From covariance among relatives*

1.2.8.2.3.2.1 *Parent-offspring relationship*

Usually dam-offspring data are used because of limited number of sires. Relationship between dam and daughter is ½ i.e. $CoV(A_X A_Y) = ½$. With traits X and Y between dams (P) and daughter (O), the possible covariances are $CoV(P_X O_X)$, $CoV(A_X A_Y)$, $CoV(P_Y O_X)$ and $CoV(P_Y O_Y)$. Ignoring dominance, epistasis and maternal influence, and assuming $CoV(P_X O_Y) = CoV(P_Y O_X) = CoV(A_X A_Y) \div 2$ and $CoV(P_X O_Y) = V(A_X) \div 2$ and $CoV(P_Y O_Y) = V(A_Y) \div 2$. After rearrangement of terms (Chapman, 1985, Sreenivasaiah, 2006) we get $r_g = \dfrac{CoV(A_X A_Y)}{\sqrt{(SD(A_X))(SD(A_Y))}}$; further, b_{yx} can also be employed by suitable substitutions in the above formula.

1.2.8.2.3.2.2 *Paternal half-sibs*

Data on two traits X and Y are utilized to perform analysis of covariance analogous to ANOVA for such data while calculating r_I and h^2. Since half-sibs share ¼ of common additive genes, intra-class correlation obtained by covariance components $(r_{I(XY)})$ is multiplied by 4 to estimate r_g i.e. $r_g = 4\ r_{I(XY)}$.

Let x_{ij} and y_{ij} represent jth value under ith sire (total sires = s) in respect of traits X and Y, respectively with number of half-sibs per sire being n_i and total number of parental half-sibs being n.; $x..$ and $y..$ be the grand totals. Let $A = \sum\limits_{i}^{s} \sum\limits_{j}^{n_i} x_{ij} y_{ij}$ and $B =$

$\sum\limits_{i}^{s} \dfrac{(x_{i.})(y_{i.})}{n_i}$, then SCP due to sires, $SCP_S = B - \dfrac{(x..)(y..)}{n.}$, SCP within sires, $SCP_W = A -$

B and number of half–sib progenies per sire $= k = \dfrac{1}{s-1}\left(n. - \sum\limits_{i}^{s} \dfrac{n_i^2}{n.}\right)$

Analysis of covariance (ANACOVA) for half-sib relationship				
Source	$v*$	Sum of cross products	Mean sum of cross products**	Estimated mean sum of cross products (EMCP)
Between sires	$S - 1$	SCP_S	MCP_S	$CoV_W + kCoV_S$
Within sires	$n. - S$	SCP_W	MCP_W	CoV_W

* v indicates degrees of freedom
** Calculated as $(SCP \div v)$

$CoV_S = (MCP_S - MCP_W) \div k$, $r_{IXY} = CoV_S \div (CoV_S + CoV_W)$ and finally $r_g = 4\ r_{IXY}$.

1.2.8.2.3.2.2.1 *Example*

Let us consider the same **Example 1.2.6.1.2.2.2** above for Trait X and consider corresponding feed intake as Trait Y. Since variance components of Trait X are already available, calculations of variance components for Trait Y and covariance components will be shown below:

ANOVA for Trait X: Refer **Example 1.2.6.1.2.2.2**

Sire 1

Trait	X	Y	X	Y	X	Y
	1.90	4.6	1.90	4.6	2.03	4.9
	1.43	3.4	2.00	4.8	1.91	4.6
	1.62	3.9	1.74	4.2	1.68	4.0
	1.99	4.8	1.64	3.9	1.88	4.5
	1.51	3.6	1.59	3.8	1.54	3.7
	1.29	3.1	2.00	3.9	1.76	4.2
					1.89	4.5
Totals	$n_i. = 19$, $x_i.. = 33.30$, $y_i.. = 79.0$; $y^2_{ijk} = 333.24$; $x_{ijk}y_{ijk} = 140.301$					

Sire 2

Trait	X	Y	X	Y	X	Y
	2.05	4.3	2.00	4.2	1.98	4.2
	2.10	4.4	2.11	4.4	1.66	3.5
	1.79	3.8	1.76	3.7	1.73	3.6
	1.68	3.5	1.83	3.8	1.57	3.3
	2.06	4.3	1.67	3.5	1.79	3.8
	1.66	3.5	1.80	3.8	2.00	4.2
	2.03	4.3	1.97	4.1	1.53	3.2
Totals	$n_i. = 21$, $x_i.. = 38.77$, $y_i.. = 80.4$; $y^2_{ijk} = 311.26$; $x_{ijk}y_{ijk} = 149.709$					

Sire 3

Trait	X	Y	X	Y	X	Y	X	Y
	2.00	4.5	1.45	3.3	1.93	4.3	1.73	3.9
	1.79	4.0	1.68	3.8	1.49	3.4	1.44	3.2
	2.12	4.8	1.79	4.0	1.66	3.7	1.59	3.6
	1.56	3.5	1.94	4.4	1.72	3.9	1.63	3.7
	1.70	3.8	1.53	3.4	1.44	3.2	1.38	3.1
	1.63	3.7	1.42	3.2	1.33	3.0	1.77	4.0
	1.64	3.7	1.33	3.0	1.47	3.3	1.84	4.1
					1.33	3.0	1.67	3.8
Totals	$n_i. = 30$, $x_i.. = 49.00$, $y_i.. = 110.3$; $y^2_{ijk} = 411.89$; $x_{ijk}y_{ijk} = 182.968$							

ANOVA for Trait Y:

$n. = 70$, $y.. = 269.7$, $y^2.. $ (or $\sum_{i=1}^{s}\sum_{j=1}^{p} y_{ij}^2$) $= 1056.39$; $\sum_{i=1}^{s} n_i^2 = 1702$; $k = 22.84$; Total SS $=$ 17.2744, SS due to sires, $SS_S = 2.7116$, SS within sires, $SS_W = 14.5628$

Therefore, V(S) = 0.0498, V(W) = 0.2173, V(P) = 0.2671, $r_I = 0.1864$ and $h^2 = 0.7456$.

Source	v	SS	MSS
Sires	2	2.7116	1.3558
Within sires	67	14.5628	0.2173
Total	69	17.2744	

Estimate of variance of $h^2 = \dfrac{1}{4}\left(\dfrac{2(n_.-1)(1-r_1)^2\{1+(k-1)r_1\}^2}{k^2(n_.-S)(S-1)}\right)$ which works – out to be

0.0084 in this example.

ANACOV for traits X and Y:

$n_. = 70$, $x_{..} = 121.07$, $y_{..} = 269.7$, $x_{ij}y_{ij} = 472.978$; $= 1702$; $k = 22.84$; Total SCP = 6.5126, SS due to sires, $SS_S = 0.5829$, SS within sires, $SS_W = 5.9297$. The ANACOV table will be:

Source	v	SCP	MSCP
Sires	2	0.5829	0.2915
Within sires	67	5.9297	0.0885
Total	69	6.5126	

$CoV_S = 0.0089$, $CoV_W = 0.0885$; $CoV_P = 0.0974$; $r_{IXY} = 0.0914$ and finally $r_g = 0.3656$.

1.2.8.2.3.2.3 Full-sibs

Data on full-sibs are frequently available from poultry breeding experiments. In such cases, ANOVA is performed separately for traits X and Y as described under estimation of h^2 by utilizing relationship between full-sibs and variance components $V(S)_X$, $V(Dam)_X$, $V(E)_X$ and $V(S)_Y$, $V(Dam)_Y$, $V(E)_Y$ as well as k_1, k_2 and k_3 values are obtained.

Covariance components are calculated (ANACOV) analogous to variance component analysis performed by calculating h^2 by utilizing relationship between full-sibs. Finally, rg is computed as the ratio of covariance to geometric mean of SD of traits X and Y. The following are assumed:

1. x_{ijk} and y_{ijk} are the kth observation under jth dam under ith sire (P progenies per dam within sire)
2. $x_{ij.}$ and $y_{ij.}$ are the dam totals (D dams per sire)
3. $x_{i..}$ and $y_{i..}$ are the sire totals (total sires S)
4. $x_{...}$ and $y_{...}$ are the grand totals
5. n_{ij} is the number of observations under jth dam under ith sire
6. $n_{i.}$ is the number of observations under ith sire and
7. $n_{..}$ is the total number of observations

The following are calculated:

$A = \sum\limits_i^s \dfrac{(x_{i..})(y_{i..})}{n_{i.}}$, $B = \sum\limits_i^s \sum\limits_j^d \dfrac{(x_{ij.})(y_{ij.})}{n_{ij}}$, Crude SCP, $C = \sum\limits_i^s \sum\limits_j^d \sum\limits_k^p x_{ijk}y_{ijk}$, SCP between sires, $SCP_S = A - \dfrac{(x_{...})(y_{...})}{n_{..}}$, SCP between dams within sires, $SCP_{D/S} = B - A$ and SCP

between progenies within dam within sire, $SCP_{P/D/S} = C - B$.

Further, $E = \displaystyle\sum_i^s \dfrac{\displaystyle\sum_j^d n_{ij}^2}{n_{i.}}$, $F = \displaystyle\sum_i^s \displaystyle\sum_j^d n_{ij}^2$, $G = G = \displaystyle\sum_i^s n_{i.}^2$, $k_1 = \dfrac{(n_{..} - E)}{(D - S)}$, $k_2 = \dfrac{\left(E - \dfrac{F}{n_{..}}\right)}{(S - 1)}$ and

$k_3 = \dfrac{\left(n_{..} - \dfrac{G}{n_{..}}\right)}{(S - 1)}$.

From EMCPs, $CoV(E) = MCP_{P/D/S}$, $CoV\,(Dam) = (MCP_{D/S} - MCP_{P/D/S}) \div k_1$
$CoV\,(S) = \{MCP_S - MCP_{P/D/S} - (k_2 \div k_1)(MCP_{D/S} - MCP_{P/D/S})\} \div k_3$
If $k_1 = k_2$, $V(S) = (MCP_S - MCP_{D/S}) \div k_3$

Note: k_1, k_2 and k_3 represent number of progenies per dam, per dam within sire and per sire, respectively.

ANACOVA for full-sib relationship

Source	υ*	Sum of cross products	Mean sum of cross products**	Estimated mean sum of cross products***
Between sires	S-1	SCP_S	MCP_S	$CoV_E + k_2 CoV_D + k_3 CoV_S$
Between dams within sire	S(D-1)	$SCP_{D/S}$	$MCP_{D/S}$	$CoV_E + k_1 CoV_D$
Between progenies within dam within sire	SD(P-1)	$SCP_{P/D/S}$	$MCP_{P/D/S}$	CoV_E

* υ indicates degrees of freedom
** Calculated as (SCP ÷ υ)
*** Designated EMCP

Utilizing the variance components of traits X and Y and covariance components between them, various correlation coefficients are calculated as follows:

Covariance	Components		Correlation coefficients
	Variance		
	Trait X	Trait Y	
CoV_S	$V(S)_X$	$V(S)_Y$	$r_{g(s)} = CoV_S / \sqrt{(V(S)_X)(V(S)_Y)}$
CoV_D	$V(D)_X$	$V(D)_Y$	$r_{g(d)} = CoV_D / \sqrt{(V(D)_X)(V(D)_Y)}$
CoV_E	$V(E)_X$	$V(E)_Y$	$r_{g(e)} = CoV_E / \sqrt{(V(E)_X)(V(E)_Y)}$
CoV_P	$V(P)_X$	$V(P)_Y$	$r_{g(p)} = CoV_P / \sqrt{(V(P)_X)(V(P)_Y)}$

1.2.8.2.3.2.3.1 *Example*

Let us consider the same **Example 1.2.6.1.2.2.4** above for Trait X and consider corresponding feed intake as Trait Y. Since variance components of Trait X are already available, calculations of variance components for Trait Y and covariance components will be shown below:

ANOVA for Trait X: Refer **Example 1.2.6.1.2.2.4**

Sire 1

Dams	1		2		3	
Trait	X	Y	X	Y	X	Y
	1.90	4.6	1.90	4.6	2.03	4.9
	1.43	3.4	2.00	4.8	1.91	4.6
	1.62	3.9	1.74	4.2	1.68	4.0
	1.99	4.8	1.64	3.9	1.88	4.5
	1.51	3.6			1.54	3.7
	1.29	3.1			1.76	4.2
					1.89	4.5
					1.59	3.8
					2.00	3.9
n_{ij}	6		4		9	
$x_{ij\cdot}/y_{ij\cdot}$	9.74	23.4	7.28	17.5	16.28	38.1
$y^2_{ijk}/x_{ijk}y_{ijk}$	93.54/38.907		77.05/32.044		162.65/69.350	
Totals	$n_{i\cdot} = 19$, $x_{i\cdot\cdot} = 33.30$, $y_{i\cdot\cdot} = 79.0$					

Sire 2

Dams	4		5		6	
Trait	X	Y	X	Y	X	Y
	2.05	4.3	2.00	4.2	1.98	4.2
	2.10	4.4	2.11	4.4	1.66	3.5
	1.79	3.8	1.76	3.7	1.73	3.6
	1.68	3.5	1.83	3.8	1.57	3.3
	2.06	4.3	1.67	3.5	1.79	3.8
			1.80	3.8	2.00	4.2
			1.97	4.1	1.53	3.2
					1.66	3.5
					2.03	4.3
n_{ij}	5		7		9	
$x_{ij\cdot}/y_{ij\cdot}$	9.68	20.3	13.14	26.5	15.95	33.6
$y^2_{ijk}/x_{ijk}y_{ijk}$	83.03/39.595		101.43/49.942		126.80/60.172	
Totals	$n_{i\cdot} = 21$, $x_{i\cdot\cdot} = 38.77$, $y_{i\cdot\cdot} = 80.4$					

(Contd.)

(Contd.)

Sire 3

Dams	7		8		9		10	
Trait	X	Y	X	Y	X	Y	X	Y
	2.00	4.5	1.45	3.3	1.93	4.3	1.73	3.9
	1.79	4.0	1.68	3.8	1.49	3.4	1.44	3.2
	2.12	4.8	1.79	4.0	1.66	3.7	1.59	3.6
	1.56	3.5	1.94	4.4	1.72	3.9	1.63	3.7
	1.70	3.8	1.53	3.4	1.44	3.2	1.38	3.1
	1.63	3.7	1.42	3.2	1.33	3.0	1.77	4.0
			1.33	3.0			1.84	4.1
			1.64	3.7			1.67	3.8
							1.47	3.3
							1.33	3.0
n_{ij}	6		8		6		10	
$x_{ij.}/y_{ij.}$	10.80	24.3	12.78	28.8	9.57	21.5	15.85	35.7
$y^2_{ijk}/x_{ijk}y_{ijk}$	99.67/44.287		105.18/46.669		78.19/34.813		128.85/57.199	
Totals			$n_i = 30,\ x_{i..} = 49.00,\ y_{i..} = 110.3$					

ANOVA for Trait Y:

$$S = 3, D = 10, P = 70; n.. = 70, y... = 269.7, y^2... \text{ (or } \sum_{i=1}^{s}\sum_{j=1}^{d}\sum_{k=1}^{p} y^2_{ijk}) = 1056.39; \sum_{i=1}^{s}\sum_{j=1}^{d} n^2_{ij} =$$

$524, \sum_{i=1}^{s} n^2_{i.} = 1702$; Total SS = 17.2744; SS due to sires, $SS_S = 1041.8272 - 1039.1156 =$

2.7116; SS due to dams within sires, $SS_{D/S} = 1043.8776 - 1041.8272 = 2.0504$; SS due to progenies within dams within sires, $SS_{P/D/S} = 1056.3900 - 1043.8776 = 2.4231$; E = 22.2476, F = 524, G = 1072; $k_1 = 6.82$, $k_2 = 7.38$ and $k_3 = 27.34$. Now, variance components can be obtained:

Source	v	SS	MSS
Sires	2	2.7116	1.3558
Dams/sires	7	2.0504	0.2929
Progenies/dams/sires	60	12.5124	0.2085
Total	69	3.9520	

$V(E) = MS_{P/D/S} = 0.2085$, $V(Dam) = (MS_{D/S} - MS_{P/D/S}) \div k_1 = 0.0124$, $V(S) = \{MS_S - MS_{P/D/S} - (k_2 \div k_1)(MS_{D/S} - MS_{P/D/S})\} \div k_3 = 0.0355$; $V(P) = 0.2564$, $h^2_S = 4 \times \{V(S) \div V(P)\} = 0.5538$, $h^2_D = 4 \times \{V(Dam) \div V(P)\} = 0.1934$ and $h^2_{S+D} = \{2 \times (V(S)+V(Dam)) \div V(P)\} = 0.3736$.

ANACOV for Traits X and Y:

$S = 3$, $D = 10$, $P = 70$; $n.. = 70$, $x... = 121.07$, $\dot{y}... = 269.7$; $k_1 = 6.82$, $k_2 = 7.38$ and $k_3 =$

27.34. Crude SCP, $C = \sum_i^s \sum_j^d \sum_k^p x_{ijk} y_{ijk} = 472.978$, Total SCP $= 6.5126$, $A = \sum_i^s \dfrac{(x_{i..})(y_{i..})}{n_{i.}}$

$= 467.0483$, $B = \sum_i^s \sum_j^d \dfrac{(x_{ij.})(y_{ij.})}{n_{ij}} = 467.9714$, SCP between sires, $SCP_S = A - \dfrac{(x_{...})(y_{...})}{n_{..}} =$

0.5829, SCP between dams within sires, $SCP_{D/S} = 467.9714 - 467.0483 = 0.9231$ and SCP between progenies within dam within sire, $SCP_{P/D/S} = 472.9780 - 467.9714 = 5.0066$.
Now, ANACOV can be laid as follows:

Source	v	SCP	MSCP
Sires	2	0.5829	0.2915
Dams/sires	7	0.9231	0.1319
Progenies/dams/sires	60	5.0066	0.0834
Total	69	6.5126	

From EMCPs, $CoV(E) = MCP_{P/D/S} = 0.0834$, $CoV(Dam) = (MCP_{D/S} - MCP_{P/D/S}) \div k_1$
$= 0.0071$, $CoV(S) = \{MCP_S - MCP_{P/D/S} - (k_2 \div k_1)(MCP_{D/S} - MCP_{P/D/S})\} \div k_3 = 0.0057$,
$CoV(P) = 0.0962$

Utilizing the variance components of traits X and Y and covariance components between them, various correlation coefficients are calculated as follows:

Components			Correlation coefficients
Covariance	Variance		
	Trait X	Trait Y	
0.0057	0.0071	0.0355	$r_{g(s)} = 0.3590$
0.0071	0.0038	0.0124	$r_{g(d)} = 1.0343$
0.0834	0.0385	0.2085	$r_{g(e)} = 0.9309$
0.0962	0.0494	0.2564	$r_{g(p)} = 0.8548$

Note:
1. Genetic correlation coefficient, r_g, also lies within -1 to $+1$; however, values > 1 in the above table is primarily due to small number of sires and dams considered in the example.
2. On the same lines described above, h^2 and r_g can be computed utilizing any relationship provided the genetic relationship can be mathematically explained and quantized.

1.2.9 Inbreeding Coefficient (F_x)

Inbreeding coefficient of an individual X (F_x) is the probability of an individual being an identical homozygote; in other words, F of an individual is the probability that a pair of alleles carried by the gametes (that combined to produce the individual) were identical by descent. It can also be viewed as the relationship between the parents that produced it; i.e. the **Co-ancestry (f)** which is defined as the probability that the two gametes taken one each from each of the parents contain alleles that are identical by descent; also referred to as **coefficient of parentage**. Hence, for calculation of F, its pedigree tree has to be available indicating relationships that are likely to contribute common alleles.

1.2.9.1 Estimation of F_x

1.2.9.1.1 Number of generations to each of the common ancestor

In this method, number of generations (separate paths) that have elapsed between the common ancestor and each of the parents of the individual in question is found and designated n (number of generations from the common ancestor to each of the parents should be separately counted; i.e. if n_1 and n_2 are the number of generations from common ancestor to each of the parents of the individual X, then $n = (n_1 + n_2)$. Since each of the generations is an independent event, multiplication rule of probability is applicable.

Another factor has to be considered; the parent(s) itself (themselves) may be inbred. Therefore, if F_{com} is the inbreeding coefficient of the common parent A, then,

$$F_X = \frac{1}{2}\sum\left[\left(\frac{1}{2}\right)^n (1+F_{com})\right]; \text{ if } F_{com} = 0, \ F_X = \frac{1}{2}\sum\left(\frac{1}{2}\right)^n. \text{ The summation applies over all}$$

the common ancestors. This method is called the Wright's method (after Wright, 1921).

Alternatively, $\sum\left(\frac{1}{2}\right)^{n_1+n_2+1}(1+F_{com})$ can also be employed to get the same value of F_X.

1.2.9.1.2 By coefficient of parentage (R_{XY})

The following rules are followed in calculation of R_{XY} assuming that individual X is born to Y and Z:

1. Parent with offspring: ½(parent with itself + between parents)
2. Individual (X) with itself: ½ × (1 + F_X)
3. Individual (X) with another individual (T) other than its parents: is ¼ of the coefficients among the 4 possible parents: if A and B are the parents of T, $R_{XT} = ¼ \times (R_{YA} + R_{YB} + R_{ZA} + R_{ZB})$ and finally
4. $F_X = R_{YZ}$; i.e. inbreeding coefficient of an individual is the coefficient of parentage between its parents.

This method is called the Male'cot's method (after Male'cot, 1948).

Note: Derivation of the above formulae is available in many Publications on population Genetics.

1.2.9.1.3 Example

Let us consider the following pedigree (arrow) chart for calculation by both the above methods:

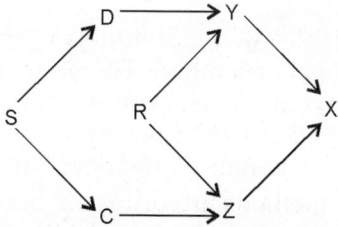

Fig. 21.2: Pedigree (arrow) chart

It is very clear that individual X has two common ancestors in R and S; the latter likely to pass on common alleles through C and D. The calculation of F_X is as follows under the assumption that $F_R = 0.5$ and $F_S = 0.25$:

Wright's method common ancestor	n_1	n_2	n	F_{com}	$\left(\dfrac{1}{2}\right)^n (1 + F_{com})$	$\sum \left(\dfrac{1}{2}\right)^{n_1 + n_2 + 1} (1 + F_{com})$
R	1	1	2	0.25	0.31250	0.156250
S	2	2	4	0.50	0.09375	0.046875
Total	3	3	6		0.40625*	0.203125

$$* F_X \text{ is } \frac{1}{2}\sum\left(\frac{1}{2}\right)^n (1 + F_{com}) = 0.203125$$

In case of Malecot's method, a table to calculate all possible R_{XY} is prepared (according to hierarchy; starting from the oldest to the youngest in the pedigree) and calculations are made as per the rules given above till coefficient of parentage between the parents of the individual is reached:

x 64	S	D	C	R	Y	Z
S	48	24	24	0	12	12
D		32	12	0	16	6
C			32	0	6	16
R				40	20	20
Y					32	13

Note: All values are multiplied by 64 to get integers

$R_{SS} = \frac{1}{2}(1 + F_S) = 0.75$; R_{SD} and R_{SC} are the parent offspring relationships $= \frac{1}{2}(1 + R_{SS}) = 0.375$; R_{SR} is the relationship between unrelated individuals and hence, is 0; $R_{SY} = \frac{1}{2}(R_{SD} + R_{SR}) = 0.1875$ and $R_{SZ} = \frac{1}{2}(R_{SR} + R_{SC}) = 0.1875$; R_{DD} is relationship of individual with itself $= \frac{1}{2} \times (1 + F) = 0.5$; R_{DC} is the relationship between an individual with another which is not its parent/offspring $= \frac{1}{4}(4$ relations between the parents; of these, on R_{SS} is 0.75; others are 0) $= 0.1875$; and so on. Finally $F_X = R_{YZ} = 0.203125$.

1.2.9.2 Detrimental effects of inbreeding

Many books on Population genetics give details of detrimental effects of inbreeding. However, special reference regarding conservation of wild animals *vis-à-vis* inbreeding is made in **Section 6.1** of this Chapter.

1.2.10 Index Selection

Selection is a process in which certain individuals in the population are referred to others for the production of next generation. Therefore, new gene(s) is(are) not introduced in the selection process, but frequency of the more desirable genes is increased. Selection can be effected among individuals within a population (intra—population selection) or individuals from different populations (inter-population selection).

Inter-population selection methods are primarily based on h^2 value of the trait in question (Individual, Sire–family, Dam–family selection) and in case of Osborne index, deviations of the individual, sire and dam family means from the overall mean is weighted with economic values.

In selection methods where more than one trait is selected, multivariate analytical methods are useful (*see* **Chapter "Multivariate analysis"** for details). Multivariate technique is particularly employed in construction of selection index which is outlined below:

If b_j and d_j are the weightage and phenotypic value of trait j (j = 1, 2, ... k) as a deviation from overall mean (i.e. $d_i = X_i - \mu$), where μ is the population (overall) mean,

then selection index, $I = \sum_{j=1}^{k} b_j d_j$ and in terms of vectors of weighatges (b) and d,

$I = b^T d$.

Obviously, the index I is the predictor of the True value (T) of the individual and hence, it should have the following properties:

1. $E(I - T)^2$ i.e. expected or average squared difference, is minimal.
2. The probability of selecting one of the largest sample values of T is maximal by selecting the largest value of the index criteria; in other words, r_{TI} is high and very close to unity.
3. The property of selecting the higher merit of any two individuals is maximal.
4. Genetic progress in any round of selection is maximal

For instance, considering two traits X_1 and X_2, the factors involved in selection index (I) are shown in a path diagram below. k_i's are partial regression coefficients of T (not

I) on $X_i\left(b_i = \dfrac{\sigma_{X_i}}{\sigma_T}\right)$; G_i's are measures of genetic source of variation in X_i's; E_i's, G_i's and

X_i's are used to represent deviation from their respective means; e_i's and g_i's are standardized influence/path coefficients/standard partial regression coefficients; $r_{e_1 e_2}$ is the environmental and $r_{g_1 g_2}$, the genetic correlation. d_i's are standardized partial regression coefficients and are usually function of relative economic values (V_i's) so

that $d_i = \dfrac{V_i \sigma_{g_i}}{\sigma_T} = \dfrac{V_i g_i \sigma_{X_i}}{\sigma_T}$.

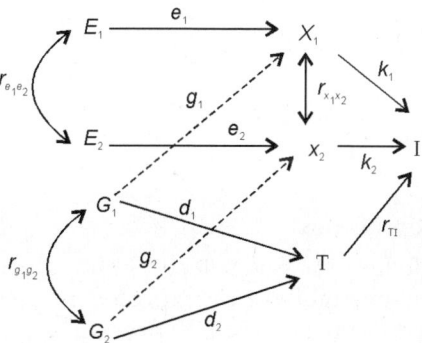

V_i's are weighting factors for G_i's to establish the theoretical aggregate genetic value (T); that is T = $V_1 G_1 + V_2 G_2$..

b_i's can be obtained by solving the following simultaneous equations:

$k_1 + k_2 r_{X_1 X_2} = r_{X_1 T}$ (Equation 1) and $k_1 r_{X_1 X_2} + k_2 = r_{X_2 T}$ (Equation 2) and in terms of path

coefficients, $r_{X_1 T} = g_1 \left(d_1 + r_{g_1 g_2} d_2 \right) = \dfrac{g_1 \left(V_1 g_1 \sigma_{X_1} + V_2 g_2 \sigma_{X_2} \right)}{\sigma_T}$.

By substituting $k_i = \dfrac{b_i \sigma_{X_i}}{\sigma_T}$ and multiplying both sides by σ_{X_1} and σ_T in Eqn. 1 and σ_{X_2}

and σ_T in Eqn. 2, the equations 1 and 2 can be written as $b_1 \sigma_{X_1}^2 + b_2 \sigma_{X_1 X_2} = \sigma_{X_1 T}$

and $b_1 \sigma_{X_1 X_2} + b_2 \sigma_{X_2}^2 = \sigma_{X_2 T}$. By solving the above simultaneous equations, b_i's for the index I are obtained.

Further, if P and A denote phenotypic and additive genotypic covariance matrices, then $\sigma_I^2 = \sigma \left(b^T X, b^T X \right) = b^T P b$. On the same lines, $\sigma_A^2 = \sigma_A \left(b^T X, b^T X \right) = b^T G b$. This

follows that heritability, $h_I^2 = \dfrac{b^T G b}{b^T P b}$ and if i is the intensity of selection, $R_I = i h_I^2 \sigma_I$

$= i \left(\dfrac{b^T G b}{\sqrt{b^T P b}} \right)$. Realized h^2 can be calculated as regression of R_I on cumulative selection differential.

The simultaneous equations can also be extended to any number of variables as follows:

$b_1 \sigma_{X_1}^2 + b_2 \sigma_{X_1 X_2} + b_3 \sigma_{X_1 X_3} + b_4 \sigma_{X_1 X_4} \ldots\ldots + b_n \sigma_{X_1 X_n} = C \sigma_{X_1 T}$

$b_1 \sigma_{X_2 X_1} + b_2 \sigma_{X_1}^2 + b_3 \sigma_{X_2 X_3} + b_4 \sigma_{X_2 X_4} \ldots\ldots + b_n \sigma_{X_2 X_n} = C \sigma_{X_2 T}$

$\ldots\ldots\ldots\ldots\ldots\ldots\ldots\ldots\ldots\ldots\ldots\ldots\ldots\ldots\ldots\ldots\ldots\ldots\ldots\ldots$

$\ldots\ldots\ldots\ldots\ldots\ldots\ldots\ldots\ldots\ldots\ldots\ldots\ldots\ldots\ldots\ldots\ldots\ldots\ldots\ldots$

$b_n \sigma_{X_n X_1} + b_2 \sigma_{X_n X_n} + b_3 \sigma_{X_n X_3} + b_4 \sigma_{X_n X_4} \ldots\ldots + b_n \sigma_{X_n}^2 = C \sigma_{X_n T}$

where $C = \sigma_I^2 / \sigma_{TI}$ and $\sigma_{X_i X_j}$ are covariances between X_i and X_j. The above equations are solved by matrix inversion.

The r_{TI} can also be calculated as $r_{TI} = \sqrt{\dfrac{\sigma_{TI}^2}{\sigma_T^2 \sigma_I^2}}$; since $\sigma_I^2 = \sigma_{TI}$

$r_{TI} = \sqrt{\dfrac{\sigma_{TI}}{\sigma_T^2}} = \sqrt{\dfrac{\sum_i b_i \sigma_{X_i T}}{\sigma_T^2}}$

1.2.10.1 Restricted selection index

Restrictions can be included optimizing selection for a given genotype, subject to the conditions that no genetic change will be expected to occur in one or more of the traits. Best Linear Unbiased Prediction (BLUP) procedure is normally used (*see* Section 1.2.10.2 below).

An exhaustive description of selection methods is beyond the scope of this book. However, the details can be obtained from several publications exclusively on selection methods, in general, and selection index, in particular. Selection index has become a very popular method especially for improving characters known for low heritability.

1.2.10.2 Best linear unbiased predictor (BLUP)

BLUP is generally employed in animal breeding to predict breeding value accurately by taking into account all the information from the pedigree and also the environmental deviation due to fixed effects (mixed model).

In mixed models, this can be represented as $y = M\beta + N\alpha + e$ where y is the phenotypic value whose expectation is given by $M\beta$, M and N are the incidence matrices, α and β are the random and fixed effects; the former assumed to be distributed Normally with mean 0 and variance σ_a^2, and e, the error or residuals assumed to be distributed Normally with mean 0 and variance σ_e^2. Hence, variance covariance of y is given by: $V = NAN'\sigma_a^2 + I\sigma_e^2$ where A and I are the numerator relationship and identity matrices, respectively. Then BLUP $(\alpha) = \hat{\alpha} = AN'\sigma_a^2 V^{-1}\left(y - M\hat{\beta}\right)$ where $\hat{\beta}$ is the BLUP (β) given by $\left(M'V^{-1}M\right)^{-1} M'V^{-1}y$.

Through a Mixed Model Equation (MME), solutions for BLUP can be obtained without V^{-1} as follows: $\begin{bmatrix} \hat{\beta} \\ \hat{\alpha} \end{bmatrix} = \begin{bmatrix} M'M & M'N \\ N'M & N'NA^{-1}\alpha \end{bmatrix}^{-1} \begin{bmatrix} N'y \\ M'y \end{bmatrix}$ where $\alpha = \dfrac{\sigma_e^2}{\sigma_a^2} = \dfrac{1-h^2}{h^2}$.

BLUP accuracy

If $C = \begin{bmatrix} M'M & M'N \\ N'M & N'NA^{-1}\alpha \end{bmatrix}^{-1}$, and diagonal for animal$_i$ is C^{ii}, then, accuracy of estimated breeding value (EBV) $= \sqrt{1 - C^{ii}\alpha}$ and selection response, $R = i\sigma_{EBV}$.

1.3 Modern Genetics

1.3.1 Linkage Analysis

1.3.1.1 Recombination fraction (θ)

Recombination fraction, θ is the P(the two genes were on the same haploids before meiosis but are found on different haploids after meiosis). Hence, θ is directly proportional to the distance between the two genes. In general, therefore, closer the loci, lesser the value of θ. When two genes are on different chromosomes or distance between them on the same chromosome is large, then $\theta = \frac{1}{2}$ (i.e. $\theta \leq 0.5$). Hence, if location of one gene is known, the location of the other is a function of θ between them.

Unit of distance between genes is **Morgan**, designated **M**; that means, two genes are said to be θM apart (cM = centi – Morgans). If x is the distance between two genes and θ, their cross – over probability, both measured in M, **Haldane Map Function**, $\theta(x) = \dfrac{1}{2}\left(1 - e^{-2|x|}\right)$. If $x = 0.5$M (or 50 cM), then $\theta = 0.316$ (or 31.6%) and $x \to 0$, $\theta \to x$.

Note: The following can be deduced from the above discussion:

1. cM is also defined as 1% chance that a marker at the genetic locus on a chromosome will be separated from a marker at the second locus due to crossing over in a single generation; it is also referred to as **map unit (mu)**, the measure of distance between two linked genes corresponding to a recombinant frequency of 1%.

2. 50 cM distance means that the genes will re-assort when an odd number of crossing–over happen; it happens 31.6% of times.

1.3.1.1.1 Example

Let us consider two loci A and B and identify recombinants (R) and non–recombinants (NR) over two generations:

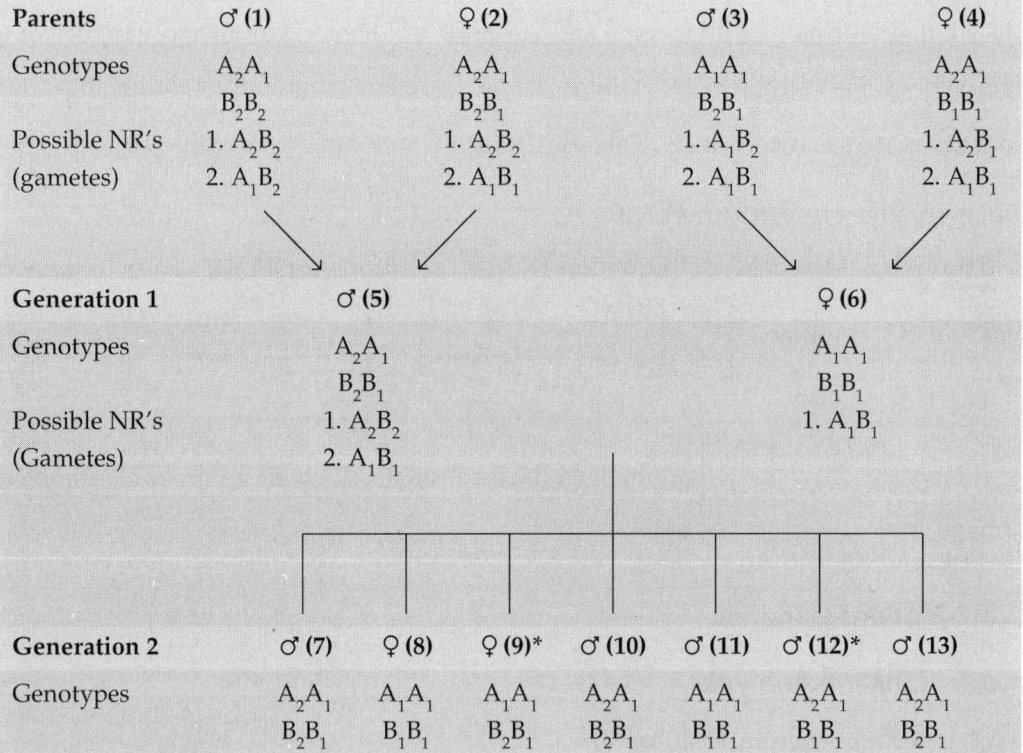

(*Adapted from:* Strachan and Read, 2004)

In case of ♀ (6), it is obvious that it is not possible to identify the source of A_1 for sure and hence it can't be classified as either R or NR. Therefore, Generation I does not provide complete information and hence, Generation II is considered wherein out of 7 progenies, Two are recombinant (individuals 9 and 12) giving a recombination frequency is (2 ÷ 7).

Note: Recombinant frequency is not synonymous to θ because it refers only to the ratio of R to (NR + R) in a sample/population; hence, if the data on entire population is available, it may be numerically equivalent to θ

Theoretically, considering the individual ♂ (5), probability of a sperm receiving A_1 receives B_1 = probability of a sperm receiving A_1 receives B_2; in other words P(NR) =

$P(R) = \frac{1}{2}$ when one pair of loci is considered. When many loci are involved, double or multiple cross-over can not be ruled-out. In any case, $P(R)$ reduces because the loci are independent and the probability follows multiplicative rule. Obviously, recombinant fraction will always be ≤ 0.5.

1.3.1.1.2 Marker

Any mendelian character which is polymorphic so that a randomly selected individual has a high probability of being heterozygous and that can be scored (counted) easily and economically by using readily available material (such as blood cells, serum etc) can be referred to as a **Marker**.

It follows that heterozygosity of a marker can used as a measure of informativeness; if $A_1, A_2, A_3, \ldots A_n$ marker alleles with gene frequency of $p_1, p_2, p_3, \ldots p_n$, the proportion of individuals who will be heterozygous will be $1 - \sum_{i=1}^{n} p_i^2$ because, frequency of homozygotes to each of the markers will be $p_1^2, p_2^2, p_3^2, \ldots p_n^2$, respectively or $\sum_{i=1}^{n} p_i^2$

When a gamete can be identified whether it is recombinant or not, such meiosis is considered **informative meiosis**. Meiosis will not be informative when (a) Parent is homozygous for the markers and (b) 50% cases when both parents have the same heterozygous genotype.

Polymorphism information content (PIC) gives weightage when both parents are heterozygous thereby producing progenies half of which are heterozygous; making the mating uninformative. PIC can be calculated as $1 - \sum_{i=1}^{n} p_i^2 - \sum_{i=1}^{n} \sum_{j=i+1}^{n} 2p_i p_j$. For X –

linked markers, PIC = heterozygosity and for autosomal markers with equal allelic frequency, heterozygosity = ½ and PIC = 0.375

1.3.1.2 LOD score

LOD score (also referred to as Z) is the logarithm of odds ratio of linkage. In other words, ratio of likelihood that the loci are linked (with a recombination fraction θ) to that of likelihood that they are not linked ($\theta = 0.5$). LOD score is calculated over a range of θ values; in a set of families, since the families are independent, P(linkage) follows multiplicative rule of probability. Further, LOD being logarithm, it becomes additive.

Note:
1. If LOD is positive, it indicates presence of linkage and *vice versa*.
2. Most likely θ is the one at which LOD is maximum
3. If there is no R, LOD will be maximum at $\theta = 0$
4. If LOD < –2.0 linkage can be rejected
5. LOD values between –2.0 and 3.0, indicates evidence of linkage as inconclusive
6. Threshold for accepting linkage with 5% chance of error is LOD = 3.0 which corresponds to 1000 : 1 odds ($\theta = 0.05$ statistically).
7. It is generally accepted that the confidence interval is the θ at which LOD score will be 1 unit below the peak LOD value.

1.3.1.2.1 Example: Dominant gene for disease

1.3.1.2.1.1 Case I

Disease gene (dominant) is nearer to A_1; hence, genotype $(A_1\text{—})$ will be diseased (progeny 1, 3 and 4 below); but it was found that individual (6) also was diseased; hence, 1 to 5 are NR and 6 is R.

$$A_2A_5\,(\sigma)\times A_1A_6\,(\female)$$
$$\downarrow$$

$A_1A_2\,(\female)$	(σ)	$(\female)$	(σ)	(σ)	$(\female)$	$(\female)$
$\times\quad\rightarrow$	A_1A_3	A_2A_3	A_1A_4	A_1A_4	A_2A_4	A_2A_3
$A_3A_4\,(\sigma)$	(1)	(2)	(3)	(4)	(5)	(6)*

(*Adapted from:* Strachan and Read, 2004)

1.3.1.2.1.1.1 Calculation of LOD

R=1, NR = 5; Overall likelihood = $(1-\theta)^5\,\theta$; likelihood of no linkage = $(½)^6$. Therefore,

$LOD(Z) = \log\left(\dfrac{(1-\theta)^5\,\theta}{(0.5)^6}\right)$; Z value can be calculated for different values of θ:

θ	0	0.1	0.2	0.3	0.4	0.5
Z	$-\infty$	0.577	0.623	0.509	0.299	0

1.3.1.2.1.2 Case–II

A_1A_2 $(\female)$ was found diseased but since the genotype of the parents is unknown, there is equal probability of obtaining A_1 or A_2 gene with disease. Obviously, either 1 to 5 are NR and 6 is R or *vice versa*.

$$????\,(\sigma)\times????\,(\female)$$
$$\downarrow$$

$A_1A_2\,(\female)$	(σ)	$(\female)$	(σ)	(σ)	$(\female)$	$(\female)$
$\times\quad\rightarrow$	A_1A_3	A_2A_3	A_1A_4	A_1A_4	A_2A_4	A_2A_3
$A_3A_4\,(\sigma)$	(1)	(2)	(3)	(4)	(5)	(6)

(*Adapted from:* Strachan and Read, 2004)

1.3.1.2.1.2.1 Calculation of LOD

If A_1 is marker for disease, NR = 5 and R = 1, $L(\theta) = \dfrac{(1-\theta)^5\,\theta}{(0.5)^6}$; conversely, if A_2 is the

marker for the disease, NR = 1 and R = 5, $L(\theta) = \dfrac{(1-\theta)\theta^5}{(0.5)^6}$. Therefore, overall likelihood

follows additive rule of probability being mutually exclusive events. Consequent on this, overall likelihood $= \dfrac{1}{2}\left[\dfrac{(1-\theta)^5\theta}{(0.5)^6} + \dfrac{(1-\theta)\theta^5}{(0.5)^6}\right]$ and the LOD for different values of θ will be:

θ	0	0.1	0.2	0.3	0.4	0.5
Z	$-\infty$	0.276	0.323	0.222	0.076	0

Note: To test whether a marker (say M_1) is associated with the disease or not when the parents (heterozygous to the marker) can either be diseased or healthy but produce [3] 1 diseased offspring and to find the number of parents who transmit the marker to their affected offspring: if a is the number of times a heterozygous parent transmits the marker to affected offspring and b is the number of times it transmits the other allele, then **transmission disequilibrium test (TDT)** $= \dfrac{(a-b)^2}{(a+b)}$ which is distributed as χ^2 on $\upsilon = 1$.

1.3.1.2.2 Example: Recessive gene for a disease

A marker with 4 alleles (1 to 4) close to the D locus with D being dominant, d recessive and dd expressing disease is considered.

$D_1d_4\,(\male)$

$\quad$ X $\qquad \rightarrow \quad D_1D_1$ or D_1d_1 or $d_1D_1\,(\male)$, disease–free

$D_1d_4\,(\female)$ $\qquad d_4d_4\,(\female)$ diseased; $d_4d_4\,(\male)$ diseased

$\qquad\qquad\qquad D_1d_4$ or D_1D_4 or D_4D_1 or D_4d_1 or d_4D_1 (all $\female$s) disease–free

(*Adapted from*: Yang, 2002)

Since both $\male$ and $\female$ offsprings are affected with parents being disease free, the parents must be heterozygous (D_1d_4). Consequent on this, gametes D_1 and d_4 from either parents are NR and D_4 and d_1 are R.

If θ is the recombinant fraction, $P(d_1) = P(D_4) = \theta/2$ and $P(D_1) = P(d_4) = (1-\theta)/2$. Assuming that both parents are D_1d_4, probability of all possible genotypes in the offsprings can be calculated as follows:

$\female\,(D_1d_4)$				$\male\,(D_1d_4)$			
		Gametes		D_1	d_4	D_4	d_1
		Probability		$(1-\theta)/2$	$(1-\theta)/2$	$\theta/2$	$\theta/2$
Gametes	Probability	Notation		f_1	f_2	f_3	f_4
D_1	$(1-\theta)/2$	m_1		$(1-\theta)^2/4$	$(1-\theta)^2/4$	$\theta(1-\theta)/4$	$\theta(1-\theta)/4$
d_4	$(1-\theta)/2$	m_2		$(1-\theta)^2/4$	$(1-\theta)^2/4$	0	0
D_4	$\theta/2$	m_3		$\theta(1-\theta)/4$	0	0	$\theta^2/4$
d_1	$\theta/2$	m_4		$\theta(1-\theta)/4$	0	$\theta^2/4$	0

Hence, in the above example, likelihood that a male offspring is not diseased $=$

$$P(D_1D_1 + D_1d_1 + d_1D_1) = \frac{(1-\theta)^2}{4} + \frac{\theta(1-\theta)}{2}; \text{similarly, likelihood that a female offspring}$$

is not diseased $= P(D_1d_4 + D_1D_4 + d_4D_1 + D_4D_1 + D_4d_1 + d_1D_1) = \frac{(1-\theta)^2}{2} + \frac{\theta(1-\theta)}{2} + \frac{\theta^2}{2}$

and likelihood of a female or male offspring being diseased $= \dfrac{(1-\theta)^2}{4}$.

Total P (all the three categories) = product of individual probabilities; i.e.,

$$\left[\frac{(1-\theta)^2}{4} + \frac{\theta(1-\theta)}{2}\right]\left[\frac{(1-\theta)^2}{2} + \frac{\theta(1-\theta)}{2} + \frac{\theta^2}{2}\right]\left[\frac{(1-\theta)^2}{4}\right].$$

Using the notations indicated in the above table, $L(f,m) = (m_2 f_2)^2 \left[f_1 m_1 + f_1 m_4 + f_4 m_1\right]$ $\left[f_1(m_2 + m_3) + f_2 m_1 + f_3(m_1 + m_4)\right]$

Note: Similar calculations are possible with the assumption that (a) parents are both d_4D_1 (b) $\male D_1d_4 \female$ D_4d_1 (c) $\male D_4d_1 \female D_1d_4$.

1.3.1.2.3 Sex-linked recessive disease gene

It is well known that genetic information of the heterogametic sex does not apply to the heterogametic offspring. Let us consider d as recessive disease gene against D dominant allele for healthy status in the following pedigree information:

1.3.1.2.3.1 Example

? Heterogametic sex (D_1) Offsprings

       X $\rightarrow$ Homogametic, disease free $(D_1d_2$ or $D_1D_1)$

?? Homogametic sex   Heterogametic, disease free (D_1)

     $(D_1d_2$ or $d_1D_2)$ Heterogametic, disease free (D_1)

                                   Heterogametic, diseased (d_2)

                                   Heterogametic, diseased (d_2)

The pedigree clearly indicates that a) the homogametic offspring can't provide any information and b) homogametic parent is either D_1d_2 or d_1D_2 (P = ½ for both); in case of the former, all heterogametic offsprings are NR and in case of the latter, all heterogametic offsprings are R. Consequent on this, $L(\theta) = \dfrac{\theta^4 + (1-\theta)^4}{2}$

Note: Linkage analysis of large pedigrees is more complex and often requires computer programs. Further details can be obtained from books dedicated to such topics.

1.3.1.2.4 Affected sib-pairs to locate a gene

In case of unaffected sib-pairs, genotype with regard to the trait can't be predicted for certain and hence, it does not serve the purpose of estimating θ. Therefore, if R_p is the disease risk in the Population, R_o is risk in the offspring, R_s is risk in the sibling and R_m

is risk in the monozygotic twin given that one of them is affected, then $R_m = 4R_s - 2R_o - R_p$ and P(Both sibs are affected) $= R_s \times R_p$ (proofs of these equations are beyond the scope of this publication). Let G_t be the genotype of two sibs, I_t be the **Identical by descent (IBD)** at the trait locus and I_m be IBD at marker locus. The following table gives $P(I_t = j \mid I_m = i)$ where i = 2, 1 and 0 where $\Psi = \theta^2 + (1 - \theta)^2$:

I_m		I_t		
		$j = 2$	$j = 1$	$j = 0$
	i = 2	Ψ^2	$2\Psi(1 - \Psi)$	$(1 - \Psi)^2$
	i = 1	$\Psi(1 - \Psi)$	$\Psi^2 + (1 - \Psi)^2$	$\Psi(1 - \Psi)$
	i = 0	$(1 - \Psi)^2$	$2\Psi(1 - \Psi)$	Ψ^2

1.3.2 Quantitative Trait Locus (QTL)

1.3.2.1 Sib-pair study

Considering 2 alleles of a single gene at locus 'B', a as the additive effect, d as the dominance when effects are non-additive, genotypes, their frequency and phenotypic value are tabulated below:

Genotype	BB	Bb	bb
Frequency	p^2	$2pq$	q^2
Phenotypic value	$\mu_{BB} + \varepsilon_{BB}$	$\mu_{Bb} + \varepsilon_{Bb}$	$\mu_{bb} + \varepsilon_{bb}$
Genotypic effect	a	d	$-a$

Note:

1. If d = 0, the alleles are additive; if d > 0, 'B' is dominant; if d < 0, 'b' is dominant; if d = a or d = −a, it is total dominance.

2. If μ is the overall mean, $E(X) = p^2(\mu + a) + 2pq(\mu + d) + q^2(\mu - a)$ which can be simplified as $E(X) = \mu + ap^2 + 2pqd - aq^2$

If a marker is linked to the gene which has to be located, it is expected that sibs sharing the same marker will have the same phenotypic value. Let us consider a pair of sibs whose phenotypic values are X and Y for a trait with S_m number of common alleles (0, 1 and 2 in this case because of single gene being involved). Obviously, if the marker is linked to the gene in question, the phenotypic difference between the sibs ($|X - Y|$) must be maximum when $S_m = 0$ and *vice versa*. In other words, S_m and $|X - Y|$ are negatively correlated. This follows that a negative correlation coefficient (*r*) is suggestive of existence of linkage for n number of sib-pairs.

To convert $|X - Y|$ to positive values, let $\Delta_j^2 = |X_j - Y_j|^2$; further, with only S_m being observable, as per Bayes' Theorem (*see* **Chapter "Probability"**), $E(\Delta^2 \mid S_m) =$

$$\sum_{G_t} \sum_{I_t} \sum_{I_m} E(\Delta^2 \mid G_t) P(G_t \mid I_t) P(I_t \mid I_m) P(I_m \mid S_m) \text{; and assuming that the markers are highly}$$

polymorphic [i.e., $I_m = S_m$, $P(I_m \mid S_m) = 1$ and $P(I_t \mid I_m)P(I_m \mid S_m)$ vanish]. Hence, $E(\Delta^2 \mid S_m) =$

$$\sum_{G_t} \sum_{I_t} \sum_{I_m} E(\Delta^2 \mid G_t) P(G_t \mid I_t).$$

1.3.2.1.1 Calculation of $P(G_t|I_t)$

	Terms involved	$P(G_t|I_t)$
$P(Bb,BB|I_t = 1)$	P(IBD on father's side and non–IBD from mother's side) * P(IBD is B) * P (non-IBD's are B and b) + symmetric term for the mother's side	$\frac{1}{2}*p*2pq + \frac{1}{2}*p*2pq = 2p^2q$
$P(Bb,Bb|I_t = 1)$	P(IBD on father's side and non–IBD from mother's side) * P(IBD is B) * P (non-IBD's are b and b) + P(IBD on father's side and non–IBD from mother's side) * P(IBD is b) * P(non-IBD's are B and B) + symmetric term for the mother's side	$\frac{1}{2}(p*q^2 + q*p^2) + \frac{1}{2}(p*q^2 + q*p^2) = pq$

Note: On the same lines other $P(G_t|I_t)$ can be derived

1.3.2.1.2 Calculation of $E(\Delta^2|I_t)$

$E(\Delta^2 | I_t = 2, 1$ and $0)$ can be calculated by the formula $\sum_{G_t} E(\Delta^2|G_t) * P(G_t|I_t = 2,1,0)$ for each I_t separately.

G_t	$E(\Delta^2|G_t)$	$P(G_t|I_t = 0)$	$P(G_t|I_t = 1)$	$P(G_t|I_t = 2)$
BB, BB	σ^2	$(p^2)^2 = p^4$	p^3	p^2
bb, bb	σ^2	$(q^2)^2 = q^4$	q^3	q^2
Bb, Bb	σ^2	$(2pq)^2 = 4p^2q^2$	pq	$2pq$
Bb, BB	$(a-d)^2 + \sigma^2$	$4p^3q$	$2p^2q$	0
Bb, bb	$(a+d)^2 + \sigma^2$	$4pq^3$	$2pq^2$	0
bb, Bb	$4a^2 + \sigma^2$	$2p^2q^2$	0	0
Total		1	1	1
$E(\Delta^2|I_t)$		$\sigma^2 + 2\sigma^2_a + 2\sigma^2_d$	$\sigma^2 + \sigma^2_a + 2\sigma^2_d$	σ^2

1.3.2.1.3 Calculation of $E(\Delta^2|S_m)$ or $E(\Delta^2|I_m)$

$E(\Delta^2|Sm) = $; the values of $P(I_t | I_m)$ are available in table under **Section 1.3.1.2.4** above. Similarly, $E(\Delta^2| I_t)$ are available in table under **Section 1.3.2.1.2** above. Accordingly, calculation of $E(\Delta^2 | S_m)$ is shown below (assuming that the marker is highly polymorphic, I_m and S_m are used synonymously):

Ψ^2	$2\Psi(1-\Psi)$	$(1-\Psi)^2$
$\Psi(1-\Psi)$	$\Psi^2 + (1-\Psi)^2$	$\Psi(1-\Psi)$
$(1-\Psi)^2$	$2\Psi(1-\Psi)$	Ψ^2

is considered as a 3×3 matrix of $P(I_t | I_m)$ elements with columns corresponding to I_m = 0, 1 and 2, respectively. It is multiplied to a (3×1) column vector of $E(\Delta^2| I_t)$ elements with rows corresponding to $I_t = 0$, 1 and 2, respectively; i.e.,

$$\sigma^2 + 2\sigma^2_a + 2\sigma^2_d$$
$$\sigma^2 + \sigma^2_a + 2\sigma^2_d$$
$$\sigma^2$$

to get another column (3 × 1) vector whose elements will be $E(\Delta^2 | S_m)$:

$$\sigma^2 + 2\Psi\sigma^2_a + 2\Psi(2 - \Psi)\sigma^2_d$$
$$\sigma^2 + \sigma^2_a + 2(\Psi^2 - \Psi + 1)\sigma^2_d$$
$$\sigma^2 + 2(1 - \Psi)\sigma^2_a + 2(1 - \Psi^2)\sigma^2_d$$

The rows of the above column vector are designated m_i (i = 0, 1 and 2, respectively) and assuming that $d = 0$, calculation of m_i or $E(\Delta^2 | S_m)$ can be made by $m_i = \sigma^2 + 2\psi\sigma^2_a +$ $(1 - 2\psi)\sigma^2_a * i$. To test H_0: $\theta = \frac{1}{2}$, in terms of θ, $m_i = 2[1 - 2\theta(1 - \theta)]\sigma^2_a + \sigma^2 - (1 - 2\theta)^2 \sigma^2_a * i$.

Under the assumption that $d = 0$ (additive effects), it is possible explore the relationship between Δ^2 and $E(\Delta^2 | S_m)$ through a linear regression equation: $\Delta^2 = \alpha +$ $\beta I_m + \varepsilon$ and obtain $\beta = (1 - 2\Psi)\sigma^2_a$. To test H_0: $\beta = 0$ (equivalent of $\theta = \frac{1}{2}$) against H_1: $\beta < 0$ it is important to note that Δ^2 is not normally distributed; t – test with $\alpha = 0.001$ is considered to be roughly equivalent to LOD score of 3.0 is therefore considered satisfactory to accept existence of linkage.

1.3.2.1.4 Example

Family	Parental mating type	Sib 1		Sib 2		S_m	I_m	$\Delta^2 = \|x - y\|^2$
		Markers	x*	Markers	y*			
1	12 × 13	12	55	12	58	2	2.0	9
2	11 × 34	13	54	14	64	1	0.5	100
3	12 × 34	13	65	14	60	1	1.0	25
4	11 × 12	12	57	12	51	2	1.5	36
5	12 × 23	12	58	23	50	1	0	64

* Value of the quantitative trait   *Adapted from*: Yang, 2002

The values in the table above are used to obtain a linear regression equation (see **Chapter "Association between variables I"** for details): $\Delta^2 = 81.6 - 34.8I_m + \varepsilon$ with a standard error of β of 16.809 to yield $t = (-) 2.07$ which is not significant at $\alpha = 0.001$ (table value of $t_{0.001, 3} = 10.214$, *see* **Appendix 3**) indicating that H_0 is liable to be accepted.

Note: If markers are less polymorphic and F_m is the full marker information of the sibs,

$\hat{I}_m = E(I_m | F_m) = 2P(I_m = 2 | F_m) + P(I_m = 1 | F_m)$. In animal breeding, large number of offsprings from the same parents under the same environment is common facilitating selection of parents and control of environment.

1.3.2.2 Interval mapping

Assuming that the trait is affected by one gene in two pure-breeds with similar markers (M_1 and M_2) at known locations, θ_1 and θ_2 as recombination frequency, $\theta_1 + \theta_2 - 2\theta_1\theta_2$ $= \theta_{12} \equiv r$ (if r is small, $r \approx \theta_1 + \theta_2$), the distance between M_1 and M_2, interval mapping of QTL is outlined below:

1.3.2.2.1 Additive model

Let 'G' is the genotype and 'y_G' is the phenotypic value which are normally distributed with mean μ_G, variance σ^2.

1.3.2.2.1.1 Example

Parents:	θ_1		θ_2		θ_1		θ_2		F_1		θ_1		θ_2
	M_1	G	M_2	X	M_1	G	M_2	$\rightarrow$	M_1		G		M_2
	11	BB	11		22	bb	22		12		Bb		12

Backcross:	F_1 X Parent (BB)	$\rightarrow$	M_1		G	M_2
		Case 1)	11		Bg_2	11
		Case 2)	12		Bg_2	12
		Case 3)	11		Bg_2	12
		Case 4)	12		Bg_2	12

(*Adapted from*: Yang, 2002)

Obviously, g_2 can be either 'B' or 'b' and it determines the phenotypic value; if $y_i = \mu + a\xi_i + \varepsilon_i$, $\xi_i = 1$ if $g_2 = 'B'$ and $\xi_i = 0$ if $g_2 = 'b'$. It is clear from the condition of markers that in Case–1, $P(g_2 = 'B') = 1$ (no recombination indicated by markers), in Case–2, $P(g_2 = 'B') = 0$ (recombination indicated by markers) and in Cases 3 and 4, it is intermediate. The probabilities of $g_2 = 'B'$ with given marker conditions in terms of θ_1 and θ_2 is tabulated below:

Marker			$P_m \equiv P(g_2 = 'B' \mid m_i)$	
M_1	M_2	(m_i)	Actual	When θ_1 and θ_2 are small
11	11	(11/11)	$(1 - \theta_1)(1 - \theta_2)/[(1 - \theta_1)(1 - \theta_2) + \theta_1\theta_2]$	1
12	12	(12/12)	$\theta_1\theta_2/[(1 - \theta_1)(1 - \theta_2) + \theta_1\theta_2]$	0
11	12	(11/12)	$(1 - \theta_1)\theta_2/ [(1 - \theta_1) \theta_2 + (1 - \theta_2)\theta_1]$	$\theta_2/(\theta_1 + \theta_2)$
12	11	(12/11)	$(1 - \theta_2)\theta_1/[(1 - \theta_1) \theta_2 + (1 - \theta_2)\theta_1]$	$\theta_1/ (\theta_1 + \theta_2)$

Source: Yang, 2002

Density function of y_i, $f(y_i \mid m_i) = p_{m_i}^* \phi(\mu + a, \sigma^2) + (1 - p_{m_i})\phi(\mu - a, \sigma^2)$ and likelihood

function will be $L[\mu, a, \sigma^2 \mid (y_i, m_i)] = \prod_{i=1}^{n} f(y_i \mid m_i)$. Further, LOD score with a given θ_1

for H_0: $\beta \neq 0$ will be $\log_{10} L(\bar{\mu}^*, \bar{a}^*, \hat{\sigma}^2) - \log_{10} L(\bar{\mu}, \bar{\sigma}^2)$ where the first part of the equation contains maximum likelihood estimates (mle) based on model $y_i = \mu + a\xi_i + \varepsilon_i$ and the second part are the mle of $y_i = \mu + a\xi_i + \varepsilon_i$ under H_0: a = 0.

LOD scores are calculated along the length of the chromosome and highest LOD indicates the location of QTL.

If the x_i's indicate location of markers M_i, location of the gene is at x, $\theta_1 \approx x - x_2$, $\theta_2 \approx x_3 - x$ and if θ_1 known, the distances can be converted into recombination fractions by employing Haldane's transformation thus:

$$\theta_1 = \frac{1}{2}\left(1 - e^{-2|x - x_2|}\right) \text{ and } \theta_2 = \frac{1}{2}\left(1 - e^{-2|x - x_3|}\right).$$

1.3.2.3 Non-additive model

Let all the genotypes BB, Bb and bb designated G = 1, 2 and 3 considered in F_2, then

$f(y_i \mid m_i) = \sum_{G=1}^{3} \phi(\gamma_G, \sigma^2) * P(G_i \mid m_i)$. Gametic frequency for the parents in F_1 (**Example**

1.3.2.2.1.1) and $P(G_1 \mid m_i)$ will be as follows:

Haploid		Diploid (m_i = 11/11)	
$M_iG_iM_i$	$P(G_i \mid m_i)$	G_i	$P(G_i \mid m_i)^*$
1B1 or 2b2	$(1 - \theta_1)(1 - \theta_2)/2$	BB	$[(1 - \theta_1)(1 - \theta_2)/2]^2$
1B2 or 2b1	$(1 - \theta_1)\theta_2/2$	Bb	$[2\theta_1\theta_2(1 - \theta_1)(1 - \theta_2)]$
2B1 or 1b2	$\theta_1(1 - \theta_2)/2$		
1b1 or 2b2	$(\theta_1\theta_2)/2$	bb	$[(\theta_1\theta_2)/2]^2$
Total, $\sum_{i=1}^{3} P[G_i \mid (11/11)]$		$[1 - (\theta_1 + \theta_2 - 2\theta_1\theta_2)]^2/4 = (1 - r)^2/4$	

* Conditional probability, $P(G_i \mid m_i) = P(G_i \mid m_i)/ \sum_{i=1}^{3} P[G_i \mid (11/11)]$

On the same lines as in case of additive model, Density function of

$$y_i, \ f(y_i \mid m_i) = \sum_{i=1}^{3} \phi(\gamma_g, \sigma^2) * P(G_i \mid m_i)$$

and likelihood function will be

$$L[\mu, a, d, \sigma^2 \mid (y_i, m_i)] = \prod_{i=1}^{n} f(y_i \mid m_i).$$

Further, LOD score with a given θ_1 for H_0: $\beta \neq 0$ will be

$$\log_{10} L(\bar{\mu}^*, \bar{a}^*, \bar{d}^*, \hat{\sigma}^2) - \log_{10} L(\bar{\mu}, \bar{\sigma}^2)$$

where the first part of the equation contains maximum likelihood estimates (mle) based on model $y_i = \mu + a\beta_i + \varepsilon_i$ and the second part are the mle of $y_i = \mu + a\xi_i + \varepsilon_i$ under H_0: a = d = 0.

Consequent on the above, $E(y_i \mid m_i)$ can be calculated as $\mu + f(y_i \mid m_i)$:

G_i	γ_g	Conditional $P[G_i \mid (11/11)]$
BB	a	$(1 - \theta_1)^2(1 - \theta_2)^2/(1 - r)^2$
bb	−a	$(\theta_1\theta_2)^2/(1 - r)^2$
Bb	d	$[2\theta_1\theta_2(1 - \theta_1)(1 - \theta_2)]/(1 - r)^2$

Note:

1. Sum of the product of γ_g and conditional $P[G_i \mid (11/11)]$ over all the G_i's gives $f(y_i \mid m_i)$ and $E(y_i \mid m_i) = \hat{i} + f(y_i \mid m_i)$.

2. On the same lines $E(y_i \mid m_i)$ for other types of marker combinations viz., (11/12), (11/22), and (12/12) can be calculated; those of (22/22), (22/12), 922/11), (12/11) and (12/22) can be obtained by symmetry.

Adapted from: Yang, 2002

1.3.2.4 Others

Estimation of breeding value, Marker Assisted Selection (MAS), Simulation study and others require use of matrix algebra and computers; hence are not included in this publication. Similarly, other applications of Modern Genetics like development of Phylogenetic tree, Forensic evidence, etc., are not in the scope of this publication.

2. ANIMAL NUTRITION

2.1 Statistical Process Control (SPC)

SPC is applicable at several stages of process of feed manufacturing; *viz.* receiving, grinding, batching, conditioning, pelleting and composition of final product. For this purpose, several tools are available; most popular being Frequency Histogram, Control Charts, Pareto Chart and Cause and Effect diagram.

2.1.1 Frequency Histogram

All Animal Science workers will be definitely familiar with development of a frequency histogram; further, almost all books on Statistics will give the details; hence, it is not detailed here. In any case, if there is doubt in fixing the number of classes (k), it can be obtained as $1 + 3.322 \log N$ where N is the total number of frequencies (observations).

2.1.1.1. Example

A feed manufacturer obtained 50 loads of GNC (guaranteed to contain 40% CP) and the protein content of each of the loads (lots) was 40.50 40.25 41.30 40.90 41.52 42.30 40.56 40.98 41.73 42.09 40.99 41.25 40.88 41.57 42.65 41.56 42.03 40.78 40.38 41.00 40.20 40.40 43.00 43.00 42.10 42.95 41.06 41.35 41.95 41.78 41.56 41.21 40.63 40.26 40.78 41.23 41.48 41.07 41.13 40.82 41.06 40.21 40.22 40.43 40.23 40.78 41.21 40.62 40.22 40.50

The values ranged from 40.20 to 43.00%. The number of classes in this case is $1 + 3.322 \times \log 50 \approx 7$. Hence, the range of 2.8% is divided into 7 classes of 0.4% each. The frequency distribution of the above data will be: ·

Class interval	Class value (x_i)	Frequency (f_i)
40.20 – 40.59	40.40	14
40.60 – 40.99	40.80	9
41.00 – 41.39	41.20	11
41.40 – 41.79	41.60	7
41.80 – 42.19	42.00	3
42.20 – 42.59	42.40	2
42.60 – 43.00	42.80	4

Mean protein content calculated (*see* Chapter "**Central tendency**") is $\dfrac{\sum\limits_{i=1}^{k} f_i x_i}{\sum\limits_{i=1}^{k} f_i}$ =

$(2059.20 \div 50) = 41.184\%$ and s calculated (*see* Chapter "**Dispersion**")

$$\text{is } \sqrt{\dfrac{\displaystyle\sum_{i=1}^{k} f_i x_i^2 - \dfrac{\left(\displaystyle\sum_{i=1}^{k} f_i x_i\right)^2}{\displaystyle\sum_{i=1}^{k} f_i}}{\displaystyle\sum_{i=1}^{k} f_i - 1}} = 0.736\% \text{ which appears to be within reasonable limits because}$$

CV is only 1.79%. But, what is conspicuous is: about 54% of samples had a protein content > 41% (after giving leverage of 1% above the guaranteed value). Therefore, if rations are formulated using the guaranteed value of 40%, the compounded feed will have excess protein proportionate to the level of GNC in the formula. To put in other terms, the ration formula can be modified to **reduce** GNC levels and save on cost of GNC. Hence, the frequency distribution is helping economic analysis, in Statistical terms **process control**, of feed manufacture.

Note: The above frequency table can be drawn into a histogram

2.1.1.2 Economic analysis

If x is the % composition of CP in GNC, and y is the rate (Rs per quintal) of GNC, value of 1% protein through GNC is Rs (y ÷ x).

Note: If GNC has x% protein, to increase protein content of the ration by 1%, (100 ÷ x) kg (per quintal) or (1000 ÷ x) kg per ton of GNC has to be added. Assuming that GNC costs Rs y per ton or Rs (y ÷ 1000) per kg, cost involved to increase 1% protein in the ration is {(1000 ÷ x) × (y ÷ 1000)} = Rs (y ÷ x) per ton.

Let us now find out the economic analysis of the above aspect considering that the label protein content was 23.0, the feed mill had 24.0 percent protein target (to ensure 23% at consumers' level) and about 1000 tons of this feed was manufactured per month:

Following are the protein content in 40 lots of compounded Broiler Starter feed: 24.32 23.90 25.00 24.68 23.97 24.78 24.32 25.12 24.76 24.66 25.88 24.89 24.47 25.09 25.76 24.32 24.63 23.20 25.75 25.12 25.90 25.25 24.20 23.75 26.00 23.23 23.53 23.46 24.39 24.59 24.30 25.20 25.72 24.22 24.18 24.20 23.20 25.10 25.79 24.33. The data is converted into a frequency distribution table with $k = 7$ and class width of 0.4.

Boundaries	Class value	Frequency (f_i)	Probability	Extra CP%**	Cost of protein (Rs per % per Ton)	Total cost (Rs)***
23.20 – 23.59	23.40	5	0.125	–	–	–
23.60 – 23.99	23.80	3	0.075	–	–	–
24.00 – 24.39	24.20	10	0.250	0.2		12500
24.40 – 24.79	24.60	7	0.175	0.6		26250
24.80 – 25.19	25.00	6	0.150	1.0	Rs 250	37500
25.20 – 25.59	25.40	2	0.050	1.4		17500
25.60 – 26.00	25.80	7	0.175	1.8		78750
Totals		40	1.000			172500

* $\dfrac{f_i}{\displaystyle\sum_{i=1}^{k} f_i}$; ** Difference between class value and target CP; y = Rs 10000 and x = 40%;

*** Product of probability, extra CP%, cost per % per ton and total production

In simple terms, cost of over-fortifying (extra protein) calculated for each class (bar of the histogram) above the target protein level of 24% by:

(% frequency÷100) × (% protein over – target) × (protein cost) × (tons/month). For

example; for class value of 25%, cost of over–fortifying is $\dfrac{\left(\dfrac{6}{40}\times100\right)}{100} \times 1.00 \times 250 \times$

Rs 1000 = Rs 37500 as shown in the table by utilizing probabilities.

It is easy to see in practical terms: The table clearly indicates that out each ton of feed manufactured, 0.25 ton had 0.2% extra CP, 0.175 Ton had 0.6% extra CP ..... 0.175 ton had 1.8% extra CP; over and above the targeted value which itself was 1% above the label value. Therefore, that much of cost on protein is a loss to the Manufacturer. It is working out to be a substantial amount of Rs 1,72,500 per 1000 tons or Rs 172.50 per ton. That means, there is scope for changing the ration formula depending on the protein content of GNC and make considerable improvements in profit.

Note: No deduction was taken for feed falling below the targeted 24% since the label protein content was 23%.

2.1.2 Control Chart

Another control point in SPC is bagging process of the compounded feed; which is generally a Machine–operation. Let us consider that in each lot of compounded feed, 5 bags at random are weighed (Expected weight 50 kg).

2.1.2.1 Example (bag weight, kg):

Lot No	Bag 1	Bag 2	Bag 3	Bag 4	Bag 5	Mean	Range
1	50.03	50.13	50.50	50.01	50.00	50.13	0.50
2	50.02	50.17	50.25	50.13	50.01	50.12	0.24
3	50.00	49.98	50.00	50.01	48.56	49.71	1.45
4	50.02	50.15	50.23	50.17	49.95	50.10	0.28
5	48.98	46.53	49.76	49.88	50.00	49.03	3.47
6	52.16	51.87	51.00	50.64	50.09	51.15	2.07
7	50.00	50.13	50.64	50.72	50.24	50.35	0.72
8	52.13	51.68	50.07	50.12	50.33	50.87	2.06
9	50.13	49.95	49.86	51.00	50.22	50.23	1.14
10	50.17	50.11	50.07	50.03	50.00	50.08	0.17
11	50.26	50.00	50.18	50.42	49.75	50.12	0.67
12	50.13	49.74	49.12	48.95	48.64	49.32	0.30
13	50.00	50.12	50.11	50.06	50.17	50.09	0.17
14	50.08	50.12	50.21	50.16	50.13	50.14	0.15
15	50.02	50.11	50.06	50.14	50.12	50.09	0.12
16	50.06	50.02	50.10	50.11	50.07	50.07	0.09
17	50.10	50.11	50.03	50.02	50.05	50.06	0.09

(Contd.)

(Contd.)

Lot No	Bag 1	Bag 2	Bag 3	Bag 4	Bag 5	Mean	Range
18	50.03	50.04	50.07	50.12	50.08	50.07	0.09
19	50.10	50.00	50.00	50.10	50.06	50.05	0.10
20	50.02	50.07	50.08	50.04	50.00	50.04	0.08
					Total	1001.82	13.96
					Average	50.091	0.698

Note: When there are no sub-samples (Ex: Protein content in every batch of feed), moving range is used in place of Range (*see* Chapter "**Central tendency**"). As in the case of **Example 3.1.1** above, if mean and s are calculated, they will be within reasonable limits; 50.091 ± 0.441 kg (CV = 0.88%). But upon developing Control Charts for Mean and Range, we can appreciate the actual consequences.

With the above data, we can calculate the Upper and Lower Control Limits for the mean (designated UCL_M and LCL_M) and the Upper Control Limit for the range, designated UCL_R.

A simplified method for calculating control limits involves the use of factors for calculating control limits. The complete table is published by the American Society for Quality Control (Part is provided in Appendix 12); The A_2 column provides a list of factors used to calculate the UCL_M and LCL_M for data sets with sub-samples. The D_4 column is used to calculate the UCL_R. The d_2 column is used to calculate the UCL_M and LCL_M for data sets that contain only one measurement per sampling.

In the current example, factor from Appendix 12 under the column titled D_4 for n = 5 is 2.114. Designating average of means (50.091 kg) as M and average of ranges (0.698 kg) as R, the upper control limit of Range $(UCL_R) = D_4{}^*R$. Hence, $UCL_R = 2.114 \times 0.698 = 1.476$; $UCL_M = M + A_2 \times R$; $LCL_M = M - A_2 \times R$. $A_2 \times R = 0.577 \times 0.698 = 0.403$ and hence, $UCL_M = 50.091 + 0.403 = 50.494$ and $LCL_M = 50.091 - 0.403 = 49.688$

2.1.2.2 Interpretation of control chart

The control limits are set at three standard deviations (since, under Normal distribution, $\mu \pm \sigma = 68.26\%$, $\mu \pm 2\sigma = 95.46\%$, $\mu \pm 3\sigma = 99.73\%$ observations; *see* Chapter "**Continuous probability distributions**"). In other words, the probability of weights beyond control limits (either sides) is 0.27 out of 100 or about 3 out of 1000 which is very low ($p = 0.003$); hence, even if the Control Chart shows any point away from UCLM and LCLM, it suggests that the process is **out of Control** for having such a rare event occurring in the manufacturing process which can not be accepted to be due to any assignable cause. Similarly, even if seven consecutive values fall above or below the "Mean" line but within UCLM and LCLM, respectively, the process is considered **out of control**. The logic is very simple; it is well known that the probability of obtaining male or female chick from a fertile egg is ½; but, the probability of getting 7 chicks belonging to the same sex consecutively when 7 eggs hatch is $(½)^7 = 0.007813$ (about 8 out of 1000).

In the current example, the following conclusions are possible:

1. The upper and lower control limits on either side of mean is only about 0.4 kg suggesting over–filling is within a reasonable limit
2. At the same time, the customers may complain of under-filling because, the lower control limit is 0.312 kg less than the expected weight and at least 3 out of 20 bags are definitely below 50 kg

3. Bag weight measurement is not uniform as indicated by the chart
4. The process is out of control since the chart has crossed the UCLM and LCLM twice. It may be due to incorrect calibration of the bagging machinery or an error by the personnel in the process.

Note: Control chart only gives when the event occurred but not its cause.

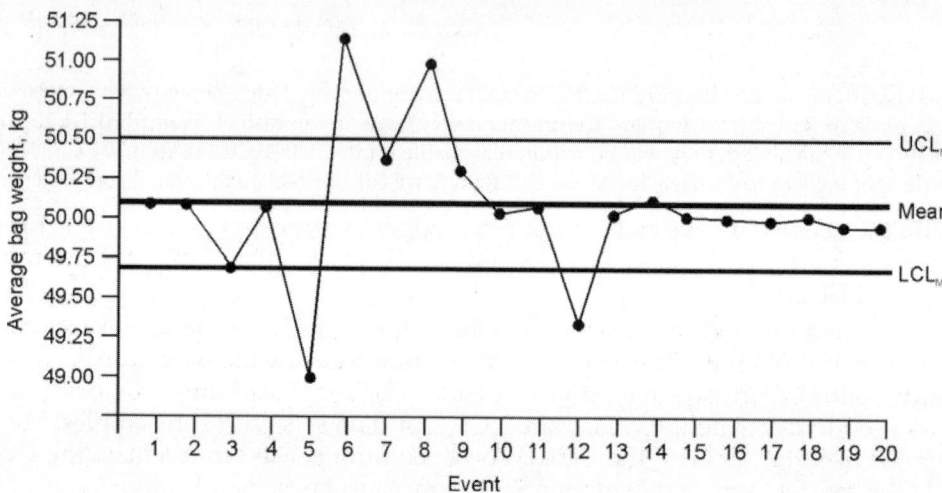

Fig. 21.3: Control chart for bag weight

2.1.3 Range Chart

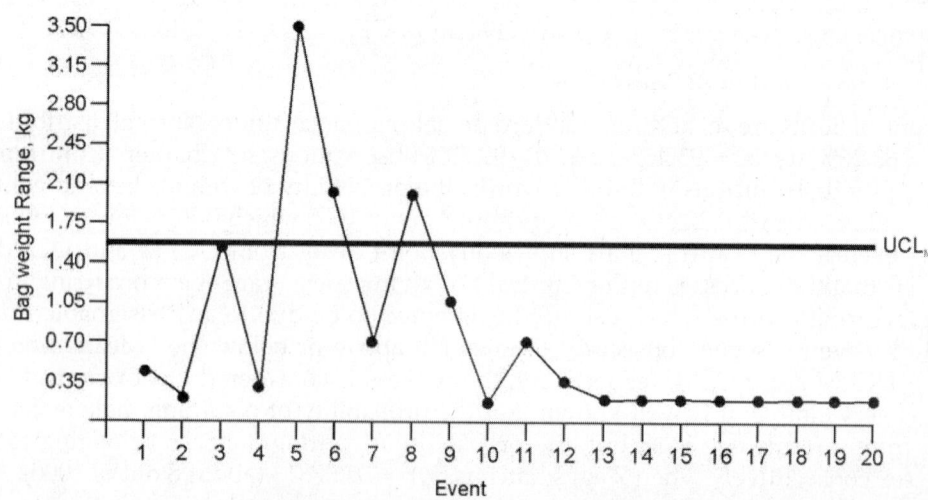

Fig. 21.4: Range control chart for bag weights

2.1.3.1 Interpretation of range control chart

In the range control chart also, three values were above the upper control limit, again, indicating the process was out of control.

2.1.4   Pareto Chart

A Pareto chart is a special type of frequency histogram that records the most frequent problem as the first bar, the next most frequent problem as the next bar, and so on. This procedure helps prioritize problem solving activities.

2.1.4.1 Example

The following is the data from a Feed Manufacturing Company based on the feed–back from their customers regarding Broiler feeds (Starter and Finisher; pellets) over one–year period arranged in the descending order of frequency:

Defect		Cumulative	
Description	Number	Number	Percentage
Clumps of molasses	29	29	38.67
Pellets not of uniform size	17	46	61.33
Too much powder	12	58	77.33
Bad odor	11	69	92.00
Moldy	6	75	100.00

The above data (last column) plotted as a histogram is called pareto chart.

2.1.5   Cause and Effect Diagram

The cause and effect diagram is a picture or graph showing relationship(s) between various problem(s) and possible cause(s) thereon; it is also referred to as a **Fishbone Diagram**. The main causes (bones) in a feed mixing unit usually concern with 1. Material 2. Machine 3. Environment 4. Method and 5. Operator.

2.1.5.1 Example

Let us consider **Example 3.1.1.2** again. It can be seen that the range in protein value was from 23.20 to 26.00% (2.80%); that means there is a probability, no matter how small or big, that excess protein is given away. Considering that the protein cost worked out was Rs 250 per % per ton, the manufacturer is continuously giving away money.

To solve this problem, representatives from all stages of feed manufacture (say feed–mill supervisor, lab analyst, ration formulation expert, veterinarian, etc.) meet and use the cause and effect diagram as a guide to locate the source and solution to the problem. Obviously, a wide range in GNC protein content between lots will be discovered rations will be based on 1 percent GNC protein increments. Further, the protein content of different lots of GNC in the receiving point will be evaluated and communicated at once to the ration formulating unit to make suitable corrections to save upon GNC cost. It is expected that variation in finished product protein content ceases and the company can make additional profit due to proper identification and rectification of the problem.

2.2   Switch (Cross)-over and Switch-back Experiment

Discussion on these designs used frequently in large animal feeding trials is given in **Section 3** Chapter **"Three-factor analysis of variance"**.

3. POULTRY SCIENCE

Statistical methods in the field of Poultry Science mostly involve continuous variables which can be subjected to analyses described in relevant chapters. However, mathematical models for egg production curve need a special mention. Several models have been and are being proposed to fit an equation to egg production curve. These changes in models have arisen primarily due to changes in egg production pattern of hens subjected to breeding for improved production. Wood's (Wood, 1967), McMillan's (McMillan *et al.*, 1970), McNally's (McNally, 1971) and Yang (1989) models are popularly fit in addition to Exponential, Modified Exponential, Growth curves, etc.; procedure for fitting latter three equations is given in Chapter "**Analysis of time series**".

3.1 McMillan's Model

The algebraic equation is $Y(T) = A\left[1 - e^{-B(T-C)}\right]e^{-DT}$ where $Y(T)$ is the egg production at time T; the partial regression coefficients A, B, C and D have special significance in this model; *viz.*, A is the potential maximum egg production, B is the rate of increase in egg production, C is the initial period of laying (T_0), D is the rate of decrease in egg production and e the base of Natural logarithm. Let T_{max} be the period when the egg production curve attained maximum value; then, constants A and D are computed for the period $T \geq T_{max}$ by logarithmic transformation of $Y(T) = Ae^{-DT}$ as $\log_e Y(T) = \log_e A - DT$ which is simply a linear equation (*see* Chapter "**Association between variables I**"). The constants B and C are then calculated by utilizing values corresponding to $1 \leq T < T_{max}$ by (Natural) logarithmic transformation of $Y(T) = A\left[1 - \beta e^{-BT}\right]$ to get $\log_e\left[\dfrac{A - F}{A}\right] = \log_e \beta - BT$ where $F = Y(T)e^{DT}$ and $\beta = e^{BC}$ which is once again a simple linear regression equation (*see* Chapter "**Association between variables I**").

Note: $e^{-B(T-C)} = e^{-BT} \times e^{BC}$ and $\beta = e^{BC}$ is assumed for calculations.

After the constants are calculated, the following can be estimated:

1. $T_{max} = C + \dfrac{1}{B}In\left(\dfrac{B+D}{D}\right)$;

2. $Y(T)_{max} = \dfrac{ABD^{\frac{D}{B}}}{e^{CD}(B+D)^{\left(1+\frac{D}{B}\right)}}$;

3. $Y(T)_{0-\infty} = \dfrac{Ae^{-CD}}{D\left(1+\dfrac{D}{B}\right)}$ or $Y(T)_{0-\infty} = \dfrac{1}{D}\left(1+\dfrac{B}{D}\right)^{\frac{D}{B}}Y(T)_{max}$

4. k, Egg development rate (instantaneous) = B + D and

5. Egg production between any two periods, T_1 and T_2 (T_2 can be the last period

studied) is $Y(T)_{T_1,T_2} = Y(T)_{0-\infty} \left[\left\{ 1 + \dfrac{D}{B} \left(1 - e^{-B(T_1-C)} \right) \right\} \right] - e^{-D(T_2-T_1)} \left\{ 1 + \dfrac{D}{B} \left(1 - e^{-B(T_2-C)} \right) \right\}$

where $Y(T)_{0-\infty} = \dfrac{Ae^{-CD}}{D\left(1+\dfrac{D}{B}\right)}$

3.2   McNally' Model

This model is described by $Y(T) = At^B e^{-CT + D\sqrt{T}}$. On (Natural) logarithmic transformation to $\log_e Y(T) = \log_e A + B\log_e T - CT + D\sqrt{T}$ which can be easily solved as a multiple regression equation (*see* Chapter "**Association between variables II**"). Matrix method can be employed because a 3×3 can be easily inversed on a scientific calculator itself.

3.3   Wood's Model

This model is described by $Y(T) = AT^B e^{-CT}$. On (Natural) logarithmic transformation to $\log_e Y(T) = \log_e A + B\log_e T - CT$ which can be easily solved as a multiple regression equation (*see* Chapter "**Association between variables II**"). This model was actually proposed for describing the lactation curve. After obtaining the equation, the following can also be calculated: 1. $T_{max} = \dfrac{B}{C}$, 2. $Y(T)_{max} = A\left(\dfrac{B}{C}\right)^B e^{-B}$ and 3. $Y(T)_{0-\infty} = \dfrac{A(B+1)}{C^{B+1}}$

which are period of maximum production, maximum production and total production, respectively. Matrix method can be employed because a 2×2 can be easily inversed on a scientific calculator itself.

3.4   Yang's Model

This model as proposed by Yang *et al.*, 1989 is described by $Y(T) = \dfrac{Ae^{-BT}}{1+e^{-C(T-D)}}$ where B is the rate of decrease in egg production, $\dfrac{1}{C}$ is the variation in sexual maturity, D is the mean number of weeks in test till sexual maturity (or age at sexual maturity) and A is the scale parameter. This model can not be converted into a linear form by any transformation. Therefore, assistance by computer is required to obtain the constants.

3.5   Example

Weekly Hen-day egg production (%, HDEP) data of a large flock of White Leghorns is utilized to fit Wood's, McMillan's, McNally's and Yang's models as described above. The data along with predicted values from each of the models is given below:

McMillan's model: $Y(T) = 120.3692 \left[1 - e^{-0.5234(T - 19.6459)} \right] e^{-0.0103T}$

Ageweeks	Hen-day egg production,%				
		Predicted			
	Actual	McMillan's	McNally's	Wood's	Yang's
19	5	*	27.8	28.0	6.9
20	18	16.6	31.4	31.7	16.1
21	34	49.2	35.1	35.6	32.9
22	54	68.0	38.9	39.4	55.1
23	71	78.6	42.7	43.3	74.1
24	89	84.4	46.4	47.2	85.0
25	92	87.4	50.2	51.0	89.6
26	91	88.8	53.9	54.7	91.0
27	90	89.2	57.5	58.3	90.9
28	89	89.1	60.9	61.8	90.3
29	88	88.6	64.2	65.1	89.5
30	88	88.0	67.4	68.2	88.6
31	87	87.2	70.3	71.1	87.7
32	86	86.4	73.0	73.8	86.8
33	85	85.6	75.6	76.3	85.9
34	85	84.8	77.8	78.5	85.0
35	84	83.9	79.9	80.5	84.1
36	83	83.1	81.7	82.2	83.2
37	82	82.2	83.2	83.7	82.4
38	82	81.4	84.5	84.9	81.5
39	81	80.6	85.5	85.9	80.7
40	80	79.7	86.3	86.6	79.8
41	79	78.9	86.9	87.1	79.0
42	78	78.1	87.2	87.4	78.2
43	78	77.3	87.2	87.4	77.4
44	77	76.5	87.1	87.3	76.6
45	76	75.7	86.7	86.9	75.8
46	75	75.0	86.2	86.4	75.0
47	75	74.2	85.4	85.6	74.2
48	74	73.4	84.5	84.7	73.4
49	73	72.7	83.4	83.7	72.6
50	72	71.9	82.2	82.5	71.9
51	72	71.1	80.8	81.2	71.1
52	71	70.5	79.3	79.7	70.4
53	70	69.7	77.7	78.2	69.7
54	69	69.0	76.0	76.6	68.9
55	69	68.3	74.2	74.9	68.2

(Contd.)

(Contd.)

Ageweeks	Hen-day egg production,%				
		Predicted			
	Actual	McMillan's	McNally's	Wood's	Yang's
56	68	67.6	72.4	73.1	67.5
57	67	66.9	70.4	71.2	66.8
58	66	66.2	68.4	69.3	66.1
59	66	65.6	66.4	67.4	65.4
60	65	64.5	64.3	65.5	64.7
61	64	64.2	62.3	63.5	64.1
62	63	63.6	60.2	61.5	63.4
63	63	62.9	58.1	59.5	62.7
64	62	62.2	56.0	57.5	62.1
65	61	61.6	53.9	55.5	61.4
66	60	61.0	51.8	53.5	60.8
67	60	60.4	49.8	51.5	60.2
68	59	59.9	47.7	49.6	59.5
69	58	59.1	45.7	47.7	58.9
70	57	58.5	43.8	45.8	58.3

McNally's model: $Y(T) = 0.0008T^{2.9665} e^{-0.1491T + 1.0451\sqrt{T}}$

Wood's model: $Y(T) = 0.0004T^{4.4636} e^{-0.1045T}$

Yang's model: $Y(T) = \dfrac{121.373e^{-0.01T}}{1 + e^{-0.959(T-21.7)}}$

Visual inspection of the results clearly indicates that McMillan's and Yang's models were most suitable followed by McNally's and Wood's models. This can also be verified by the predictions yielded by each of the above models which are summarized below:

Parameter	Actual	Prediction models			
		McMillan's	McNally's	Wood's	Yang's
T_{max}, Weeks	25	23.6	42**	42.7	26**
$Y(T)_{max}$, %	92	89.2	87.2**	87.5	91**
Y(T) up to 70 weeks, %	72.3	73.5	67.1*	67.9*	71.0*
Y(T) up to 70 weeks, Number	263.2*	259.3*	244.2*	247.1*	258.4*

* Calculated by utilizing relevant values

** By inspection of predicted values

However, the suitability of each of the above models for describing the egg production can be determined based on Coefficient of determination (R^2) (*see* Chapter

"**Association between variables I**" Section 3.2.2.1.1.2 for details), Mean absolute error (MAE), Mean square error (MSE) and Akaike Information Criterion (AIC) which can be calculated as follows:

$$R^2 = 1 - \frac{(\text{Residual Sum of Squares})^2}{(\text{Corrected Sum of Squares})^2} = 1 - \frac{\sum\left(Y(T) - Y(\hat{T})\right)^2}{\sum\left(Y(T) - \overline{Y(T)}\right)^2},$$

$$\text{MAE} = \frac{\sum\left|Y(T) - Y(\hat{T})\right|}{n}, \text{MSE} = \frac{\sum\left(Y(T) - Y(\hat{T})\right)^2}{n - p}.$$

and $\text{AIC} = n\log_e(\text{MSE}) + 2p$ where $Y(T)$ is the actual, $Y(\hat{T})$ the predicted and $\overline{Y(T)}$ the mean egg production value, n the number of observations and p the number of parameters.

Goodness of fit is indicated by higher R^2 and lower MAE, MSE and AIC values. The above models yielded the following Goodness of fit values:

Goodness of fit criterion	Prediction models			
(HDEP, weekly data)	McMillan's	McNally's	Wood's	Yang's
R^2, %	94.93	36.84	37.12	99.60
Mean absolute error, MAE	1.41	11.52	11.20	0.70
Mean square error, MSE	11.91	255.16	237.62	1.19
Akaike Information Criterion, AIC	136.82	296.18	290.48	16.88

Recently, Ganesan *et al* (2010), utilizing daily egg production data of 481 White Leghorns (WL) from 19th to 70th week of age, fit the above four non-linear models separately for daily, weekly, fortnightly and monthly HDEP values. The suitability of each of the above models for describing the egg production was determined based on R^2, MAE, MSE and AIC. It was found that the modified compartmental model by Yang *et al.*, (1989) was the best to predict the daily, weekly and monthly HDEP of WL with R^2 values of 92.2%, 95.3% and 98.5%, respectively and McMillan's model was found to be the best to predict the fortnightly HDEP of WL with R^2 values of 97.4%. The fitted models were validated using the egg production data of another 460 white leghorns and similar findings were observed.

Goodness of fit criterion	Prediction models			
(HDEP, weekly data)	McMillan's*	McNally's	Wood's	Yang's
R^2, %	97.40	86.10	63.10	95.30
Mean absolute error, MAE	1.96	4.04	6.45	2.50
Mean square error, MSE	7.03	36.65	95.07	12.41
Akaike Information Criterion, AIC	60.70	202.50	251.9	144.00

* Fortnightly data Ganesan *et al.*, 2010

3.6 Akaike Information Criterion (AIC)

AIC is a measure of the goodness of fit of an estimated statistical model as a relative measure of the information lost when a given model is used to describe the actual dependant variable. In other words it estimates difference between bias and variance. The complement of information lost, the information gain was described by Kullback and Leibler (1951) and hence known as the Kullback–Leibler divergence (also information divergence, information gain, relative entropy, or KLIC). Considering two probability distributions P (actual) and Q (theoretical, model), KLIC measures the expected number of additional information required to represent samples from P based on Q. In other words amount of information the model (or Q) does not describe or the amount of information lost due to the prediction model. Obviously, amount of information lost from Q to estimate P need not be the same from P to estimate Q. Further, lower the amount of information lost, better is the model.

In view of the above, the AIC = 2k − 2 ln(L) where k is the number of parameters in the statistical model, and L is the maximized value of the likelihood function for the estimated model, Residual Sum of Squares, $RSS = \sum_{i=1}^{n} \hat{\varepsilon}_i^2$. Assuming that errors in each of the models under test are a) unknown but equal and b) Normally and independently distributed, $AIC = 2k + n\left[\ln\left(\dfrac{2\pi RSS}{n}\right) + 1\right]$ where n is the number of observations.

The term is constant and hence does not influence the ranking of the models. Therefore, ignoring the term, $AIC = 2k + n\left[\ln\left(\dfrac{RSS}{n}\right)\right]$ Further, the term $\left(\dfrac{RSS}{n}\right)$ is given by MSE and hence, $AIC = n\left[\ln(MSE)\right] + 2k$.

If k is increased, the model becomes more complicated; but increases the goodness of fit. Therefore, AIC discourages inordinate increase in k by the term $2p$. This follows that a model which can yield lowest AIC with least k will be the best model.

It is also important to note that the absolute value of AIC has no meaning by itself but ranks the models depending on relative loss of information while describing the original probability distribution. In other words, AIC indicates as to how close the estimated values by the given model to the original ones.

3.6.1 Fitting Mathematical Models–Outline of Procedure

3.6.1.1 McMillan's model

First constants A and D are computed for the period $T \geq T_{max}$ (25 weeks) by logarithmic transformation of $Y(T) = Ae^{-DT}$ as $\log_e Y(T) = \log_e A - DT$; $\Sigma \log_e Y(T) = 197.7713$, $\Sigma \log_e Y(T)^2 = 851.1636$, $\Sigma T = 2185$, $\Sigma T^2 = 111895$, $\Sigma T \log_e Y(T) = 9310.2989$, therefore, $\log_e Y(T) = \log_e 4.7906 - 0.0103T$ or A = 120.3692.

In the next stage, 6 records pertaining to $T < T_{max}$ are utilized. For these records, F is calculated as $Y(T)e^{DT} = Y(T)e^{0.0103T}$:

$T < T_{max}$	Y(T)	$F = Y(T)e^{0.0103T}$	$\log_e\left(\dfrac{A-F}{A}\right)$
19	5	6.0808	−0.0518
20	18	22.1176	−0.2030
21	34	42.2101	−0.4318
22	54	67.7337	−0.8272
23	71	89.9793	−1.3765
24	89	113.8587	−2.9326

Values in last column designated "K"

Now, utilizing K values, a log–linear regression equation $K = \log_e \beta - BT$ where $\beta = e^{BC}$ is fit: $\Sigma T = 129$, $\Sigma T^2 = 2791$, $\Sigma K = -5.8229$, $\Sigma K^2 = 11.4095$, $\Sigma TK = -134.3523$, therefore, or $BC = 10.2832$. Since $B = 0.5234$, $C = 19.6459$. In other words, the egg production, theoretically, began at 19.6 weeks of age.

With the above, all the constants of the model are obtained: $A = 120.3692$, the potential maximum egg production, $B = 0.5234$, the rate of increase in egg production, $C = 19.6459$, the initial period of laying (T_0) and $D = 0.0103$, the rate of decrease in egg production

Note: The constants, especially of this model are of biological significance and can be used in selection of breeding birds and to compare treatments; as for instance, effect of cage *vs* deep–litter systems of rearing (Sreenivasaiah *et al.*, 1985) and seasons of hatching (Sreenivasaiah and Krishnamurthy, 1986) on egg production of Japanese quails.

3.6.1.2 McNally's model

Considering all the 72 records (N), the following are calculated: (a) $\Sigma\log_e Y(T)$, (b) $\Sigma\log_e T$,

(c) ΣT, (d) $\sum \sqrt{T}$, (e) $\sum \log_e Y(T)\log_e T - \dfrac{\left(\sum \log_e Y(T)\right)\left(\sum \log_e T\right)}{N}$,

(f) $\sum T\log_e Y(T) - \dfrac{\left(\sum T\right)\left(\sum \log_e Y(T)\right)}{N}$, (g) $\sum \sqrt{T}\log_e Y(T) - \dfrac{\left(\sum \sqrt{T}\right)\left(\sum \log_e Y(T)\right)}{N}$,

(h) $\sum \left(\log_e T\right)^2 - \dfrac{\left(\sum \log_e T\right)^2}{N}$, (i) $\sum T\log_e T - \dfrac{\left(\sum T\right)\left(\sum \log_e T\right)}{N}$,

(j) $\sum \sqrt{T}\log_e T - \dfrac{\left(\sum \sqrt{T}\right)\left(\sum \log_e T\right)}{N}$, (k) $\sum T^2 - \dfrac{\left(\sum T\right)^2}{N}$,

(l) $\sum T\sqrt{T} - \dfrac{\left(\sum T\right)\left(\sum \sqrt{T}\right)}{N}$ and (m) $\sum T - \dfrac{\left(\sum \sqrt{T}\right)^2}{N}$.

The values in the present example are a = 218.54, b = 194.04, c = 2314, d = 341.59, e = 1.9642, f = 41.2400, g = 4.5631, h = 7.1308, i = 284.59, j = 22.2496, k = 11712, l = 903.0950 and m = 70.0822. After deriving the Normal equations (see Chapter "**Association between variables II**" for details), LHS and RHS of the matrix will be:

$$\begin{bmatrix} h & i & j \\ i & k & l \\ j & l & m \end{bmatrix} \text{ and } \begin{bmatrix} e \\ f \\ g \end{bmatrix}, \text{ respectively. Inverse of LHS matrix obtained was:}$$

$$\begin{bmatrix} 136.5673873 & 3.84006122 & -92.84111839 \\ 3.84006122 & 0.121218994 & -2.781193415 \\ -92.84111839 & -2.781193415 & 65.32841049 \end{bmatrix} \text{ and RHS was } \begin{bmatrix} 1.9642 \\ 41.2400 \\ 4.5631 \end{bmatrix}. \text{ On multi-}$$

plication of inverse matrix with RHS, $\begin{bmatrix} 2.9665 \\ -0.1491 \\ 1.0451 \end{bmatrix}$ indicating the constants B, C and D of

the model were obtained. Finally, constant A is obtained by substituting values of B, C and D with average values of a, b and c (calculated above) in $\log_e Y(T) = \log_e A + B$

$\log_e T - CT + D\sqrt{T}$. In this example, $\log_e A = -7.1002$ and hence, $A = 0.0008$.

3.6.1.3 Wood's model
Similar to McNally's model, the following are calculated considering all the 72 records:

(a) $\Sigma\log_e Y(T)$, (b) $\Sigma\log_e T$, (c) ΣT, (d) $\sum\log_e Y(T)\log_e T - \dfrac{\left(\sum\log_e Y(T)\right)\left(\sum\log_e T\right)}{N}$,

(e) $\sum T\log_e Y(T) - \dfrac{\left(\sum T\right)\left(\sum\log_e Y(T)\right)}{N}$, (f) $\sum\left(\log_e T\right)^2 - \dfrac{\left(\sum\log_e T\right)^2}{N}$,

(g) $\sum T\log_e T - \dfrac{\left(\sum T\right)\left(\sum\log_e T\right)}{N}$ and (h) $\sum T^2 - \dfrac{\left(\sum T\right)^2}{N}$.

The values in the present example are a = 218.54, b = 194.04, c = 2314, d = 1.9642, e = 41.2400, f = 7.1308, g = 284.59 and h = 11712. After deriving the Normal equations (*see* Chapter "**Association between variables II**" for details), LHS and RHS of the matrix will be:

$$\begin{bmatrix} f & g \\ g & h \end{bmatrix} \text{ and } \begin{bmatrix} d \\ e \end{bmatrix}, \text{ respectively. Inverse of LHS matrix obtained was:}$$

$$\begin{bmatrix} 4.639405275 & -0.112732953 \\ -0.112732953 & 0.002824682 \end{bmatrix} \text{ and RHS was } \begin{bmatrix} 1.9642 \\ 41.2400 \end{bmatrix}. \text{ On multiplication of inverse}$$

matrix with RHS, $\begin{bmatrix} 4.4636 \\ -0.1045 \end{bmatrix}$ indicating the constants B and C of the model were

obtained. Finally, constant A is obtained by substituting values of B and C with average values of a, b, c and d (calculated above) in $\log_e Y(T) = \log_e A + B\log_e T - CT$. In this example, $\log_e A = -7.8035$ and hence, $A = 0.0004$.

3.6.1.4. Yang's model

As indicated earlier, Yang's model was fit using computer facility.

3.7 Other Models

Several models have been and are being proposed for predicting egg production. Many of these require Computers for calculations; for instance, Grossman and Koops, 2001

proposed a model as $Y(T) = mk_1 \left[\dfrac{1-e^{-T}}{1+e^{-T}} \right] - m(k_1 - k_2) \left[\dfrac{1-e^{-T}}{1+e^{-(T-C_2)}} \right]$ where m is the

maximum egg production, k_1 and k_2 are rate of increase and decrease in egg production, respectively, and c_2 is the point of inflection between increasing and decreasing rates.

4. VETERINARY EPIDEMIOLOGY

4.1 Sample Size Determination

Calculation of sample size required for various tests is provided in the relevant Chapters. However, in Epidemiology, the sample size is determined by factors such as sensitivity, specificity, type of sampling, etc. (which are not factors for general tests of hypotheses). Hence, they are summarized below:

4.1.1 For Disease Detection

Sample size required for various tests of hypotheses has already been provided in Chapter "**Tests of hypotheses**". However, sample size, n, recommended for detecting

a disease in a population is $\left[1 - (1-p)^{\frac{1}{n}} \right] \left(N - \dfrac{d-1}{2} \right)$ where p is the probability of finding

at least one case at a set α (generally 0.05, occasionally 0.01), d the number of detectable cases in the population of size N and sensitivity of the test is 100%. If sensitivity is < 100%, $d = (d*\text{Sensitivity}) \div 100$. It is also assumed that the test does not give false positive results.

4.1.1.1 Example

If one is interested to detect TB in a large herd of cattle ($N = 5000$) where the disease is expected in 4% of cattle ($d = 200$) by tuberculin test whose sensitivity is 40% at $\alpha = 0.05$ (or $p = 0.95$), sample size required is 72.86 or 73 animals.

4.1.1.2 Maximum number of positive cases

If all the n animals tested clean (negative) for a screening test, then maximum number of positives (d) can be estimated by (replacing n in place of d in the above formula):

$$\left[1 - (1-p)^{\frac{1}{n}} \right] \left(N - \dfrac{n-1}{2} \right).$$

4.1.1.2.1 Example

In a large abattoir, 500,000 broilers were slaughtered and all the 10% of the chicken screened (sensitivity 90%) for *Campylobacter* were found negative. Now, we can set α

at 0.05 ($p = 0.95$) and estimate the maximum number of positives by the above formula as 297.99 (i.e. 298); since the sensitivity is only 90%, the maximum number of positives increases to $(298 \times 100) \div 90 = 331.11$ or 331 birds or a prevalence of $(331 \div 500000) \times 100 = 0.066\%$.

4.1.2 To Estimate Association between Exposure and Disease

If p_n is the relative frequency of exposure among non-diseased animals, R is the minimal magnitude of risk measure, r is the ratio between non-diseased animals to diseased animals (number of controls), Z_α and $Z_{(1-\beta)}$ table values of Z with usual meanings, then sample size, n, required to assess risk is

$$n = \frac{1}{(p_e - p_n)} \left[Z_\alpha \left(\sqrt{\left(1 + \frac{1}{r}\right) p_e' q_e'} \right) + Z_{1-\beta} \left(\sqrt{\left(p_e q_e + \frac{p_n q_n}{r}\right)} \right) \right]^2 \quad \text{where } p_e' = \frac{(p_e + r p_n)}{(1+r)}$$

and $q_e' = 1 - p_e'$; p_e is the relative frequency of exposure calculated as $\frac{p_n R}{1 + p_n (R-1)}$.

4.1.2.1 Example

Suppose we want to know the association between litter condition and coccidiosis in broilers with estimated p_n of 20% (0.20; $q_n = 0.80$) and R is at least 5. If r is 0.1, Z_α and $Z_{(1-\beta)}$ are 1.96 and 0.75, respectively, then $p_e = 0.56$, $q_e = 0.44$, $p'_e = 0.26$ and $q'_e = 0.74$. By substituting these, sample size required to estimate association between litter condition and coccidiosis in broilers as 10.21 or 10. Hence, 10 cases and $10 \times R = 50$ controls have to be included for investigation.

4.1.3 To Estimate Disease Prevalence

4.1.3.1 Simple random, systematic and stratified sampling

If P_{exp} = expected prevalence and α = precision required (usually 0.05), then

$$n = \frac{1.96^2 P_{exp}(1 - P_{exp})}{\alpha^2}.$$

4.1.3.2 Cluster sampling

If MSS_C is the mean sum of squares between clusters, $n.$ is the total number of animals sampled over c samples or clusters (each containing n animals), p' is the estimate of overall prevalence from the sample, m is the number of diseased animals in each cluster, N is the Population size, C is the number of clusters in population, c is the number of

clusters in the sample, $K_1 = \frac{C-c}{C}$, $K_1 = \frac{N-n.}{N}$ and $V = P'^2 \left(\sum_{i=1}^{c} n_i^2 \right) - 2P' \left(\sum_{i=1}^{c} n_i m_i \right) + \sum_{i=1}^{c} m_i^2$

then, $MSS_C = c \left[\frac{K_1 c V}{n_.^2 (c-1)} - \frac{K_2 P'(1-P')}{n_.} \right].$

4.1.3.2.1 One-stage cluster sampling

With the notations as above, $c = \dfrac{1.96^2 \left\{ nMSS_C + P_{exp}\left(1 - P_{exp}\right) \right\}}{n\alpha^2}$ and if C is not very large,

$$c_{adj} = \frac{Cc}{(C+c)}.$$

4.1.3.2.2 Two-stage cluster sampling

If $n'.$ is the total number of animals to be sampled, $c = \dfrac{1.96^2 n'_. MSS_C}{n'_. \alpha^2 - 1.96^2 P_{exp}\left(1 - P_{exp}\right)}$

and if C is not very large, $c_{adj} = \dfrac{Cc}{(C+c)}$; if N is not very large, c =

$\dfrac{1.96^2 Nn'_. MSS_C}{Nn'_. \alpha^2 - 1.96^2 \left(N - n'_.\right)P_{exp}\left(1 - P_{exp}\right)}$. When c is fixed, $n'_. = \dfrac{1.96^2 cP_{exp}\left(1 - P_{exp}\right)}{c\alpha^2 - 1.96^2 MSS_C}$ and if c is

not very large $n'_. = \dfrac{1.96^2 CcP_{exp}\left(1 - P_{exp}\right)}{Cc\alpha^2 - 1.96^2 MSS_C \left(C - c\right)}$ and if N is not very large, adjusted $n'_. =$

$\dfrac{Nn'_.}{\left(N + n'_.\right)}$

4.1.4 Confidence Intervals

4.1.4.1 Random, systematic and stratified sampling

For any of the estimates, S_n, S_p, etc. (unless otherwise specified) se

is $\sqrt{\dfrac{\text{Estimate}\left(1 - \text{estimate}\right)}{n}}$ and confidence intervals as Estimate $\pm$ se*Z where Z is the

table value of Standard Normal Deviate (at set α and $\upsilon = n - 1$ where n is the sample size). *See* Chapters "**Tests of hypotheses**" and "**Methods of sampling**".

4.1.4.2 Cluster sampling

For cluster sampling, 5% confidence intervals are given by $P' \pm 1.96\left(\dfrac{c}{n_.}\sqrt{\dfrac{V}{c(c-1)}}\right)$

where $V = P'^2 \left(\displaystyle\sum_{i=1}^{c} n_i^2\right) - 2P'\left(\displaystyle\sum_{i=1}^{c} n_i m_i\right) + \displaystyle\sum_{i=1}^{c} m_i^2$.

4.2 Measurement of Disease Frequency

Definitions of **Prevalence** and **Incidence** are given in Chapter "**Probability**", To recapitulate, prevalence is the ratio of number of diseased animals at the given moment to the total animals at risk at the same moment; incidence is the number of new cases recorded during a specified period. **Cumulative Incidence (CI)** is the ratio of total animals that actually were diseased to that of all animals at risk (including the affected ones) during the given period; the ratio of new cases of disease per unit time is referred to as **Incidence Rate (IR,** or simply *r***)** or **Force of morbidity** or **Velocity of occurrence of new cases per unit time**. The units can be animal-year or animal-week, etc.

4.2.1 Example

In the following example, number of new cases of coccidiosis in a broiler farm of 1000 birds is given:

Weeks	New cases	CI	Animal–weeks (diseased)*
1	0	0	0
2	0	0	0
3	0	0	0
4	10	0.01	35
5	50	0.06	225
6	90	0.15	495
7	40	0.19	260
8	10	0.20	75
Total	200	0.20**	1090

* Calculated assuming that the disease was contracted, on average, by mid-week; therefore, animal weeks (diseased) for 4th week = 10*3.5 = 35.

** Probability that a broiler, at random, can contact coccidiosis during 8-week period

Obviously, 800 animals were disease-free and hence, contributed $800 \times 8 = 6400$ animal weeks (healthy). Therefore, $r = 1090 \div 6400 = 0.1703$ animals per animal-week.

Note: Only animal-weeks contributed by healthy birds is taken in the denominator because only they are at risk of disease (coccidiosis in this example). Animal-week value can be converted to animal-year value by multiplying with 52.

CI and *r* are related by the exponential decay formula $CI = 1 - e^{-rt}$ where *t* is the time unit; if expected CI < 0.10, then $CI \approx rt$. For instance, if we say that **incidence density** (the number of events per unit animal-year, *r*) of rabies in dogs is 2 per 1000 per annum, it means out of 1000 dogs completing one animal-year each, 2 had rabies ($r = 0.002$); this can be used to calculate **cumulative incidence (CI)** say for the next 10 years ($t = 10$) by the above formula $CI = 1 - e^{-(0.002*10)}$ which works out to be 19.80 (say 20) per 1000. Since CI < 0.02, $CI \approx r * t = 0.02$ or 20 per thousand.

If prevalence is designated, P, it is related to *r* by $\dfrac{P}{(1-P)} = rD$ where D is the duration of the disease. The denominator (1 – P) represents proportion of population that is healthy and hence is liable to contact the disease. If P < 0.05, $P \approx r*D$.

Note: P, CI and *r* of the entire population carry a prefix "Crude" while those of specific subgroup (such as class, sex etc.) will carry a prefix "Specific".

4.2.2 Ratios/Rates in Epidemiology

Ratio/Rate	Numerator	Denominator
Risk Ratios/Rates		
True rate, TR	Number acquiring the risk	ANR*ITC
Risk rate, RR	Number acquiring the risk	Initial ANR – ½ of withdrawals
Morbidity		
Morbidity rate	Number diseased	Number in Population at risk
Crude true prevalence	Number developing disease during the period	ANR*ITC
Real prevalence	Apparent prevalence + Specificity – 100	Sensitivity + Specificity – 100
Prevalence immune	Number immune	Number in Population
Attack rate, AR	Number of animals developing diseases following exposure	Total number exposed
Secondary Attack rate (SAR)	Total number exposed to first case (proband) that develop disease within the incubation period	Total number exposed to the proband
Mortality		
Crude mortality (True) rate	Total deaths in the duration considered	ANR*ITC
Cause–specific mortality (True) rate	Number of deaths due to a specific disease under study	ANR*ITC
Risk of death due to specific disease	Total deaths due to the disease during the period after diagnosis	Total animals acquiring the disease
Case-fatality rate (CFR)	Number of deaths due to a cause	Total number affected by that cause
Survival rate	Newly diagnosed cases– Number of deaths during the study period	Newly diagnosed cases during the study period
Age/Breed/Sex/Cause–specific death rates	Number of deaths due to the specific category	ANR
Neonatal mortality rate (in domestic mammals, NMR)	Deaths within 4 weeks of birth	Total number of live births
Calf mortality rate (CFR) in cattle	Number of calves dying up to weaning	Total number of calves born
Fetal death rate, FDR	Total fetal deaths	Total live births
Maternal mortality rate (domestic mammals)	Number of dams dying due to puerperal causes	Number of live births

(Contd.)

(Contd.)

Ratio/Rate	Numerator	Denominator
Proportional mortality rate, PMR	Deaths due to specific cause	Total deaths from all causes
Perinatal mortality rate	Number of deaths within few days around birth	Total born into the population
Population studies		
Prevalence ratio, PR	Diseased among exposed	Diseased among unexposed
Cumulative incidence, CI	Total animals that actually were diseased	All animals, including the affected, at risk
Incidence rate, IR	Number of new cases of a disease	ITC
Area incidence ratio	Number of new cases of a disease	Unit geographical area in which study is made*ITC
Vaccine efficacy, VE	$(AR_{Unvaccinated} - AR_{vaccinated})$	$AR_{vaccinated}$
Zoonosis incidence ratio, ZIR	New cases of zoonosis in animal species at the time	Average human population
Replacement rate	Number introduced	Average herd inventory
Removal rate	Number sold/culled/dead	Average herd inventory
Culling rate	Number culled	Average number in the herd
Vital statistics		
Crude live birth rate	Number of live births	Average Population
General fertility rate	Number of live births	Average number of females of reproductive age
Crude death rate	Number of deaths	Average Population
Pregnancy rate	Number pregnant	Number of females bred

* All the rates can be multiplied by 10^x where x can take values between 2 to 6 to interpret as per 100 to per million accordingly. Otherwise, they are simply ratios or rates. For VE, $x = 2$; Death rate is the sum of mortality due to all diseases during the study period.

4.2.2.1 Example

For instance, in a large dairy farm with 500 cows, 10 cows developed chronic mastitis (CM) and had a lifetime loss of ½ of the milk yield, 300 cows calved of which 8 were culled due to mastitis; In addition, 16 more were culled due to other reasons and were replaced by 30 new purchases. In the farm 6 animals died of which 4 had Downer's syndrome (DS). Totally 20 cows had Downer's of which 4 had mastitis. In addition to these, 75 other cows had ≥ 1 other disease(s). Assuming that Downer's is a short – duration ailment only among cows soon after calving whereas mastitis lifetime affliction let us calculate various morbidity and mortality rates (ITC = 1):

Let us tabulate the above information:

Herd size at the beginning		Events during the period of one year				6 Died	Other diseases
	CM	300 Calved					
500	10	256 Normal	8 CM	16 Misc	20 DS		
							75
			24 Culled	4 CM	12 recovered	4 died	2 Misc
30 Purchased		Herd size at the end of one year 500					

CM Chronic mastitis; DS Downer's syndrome

1. Morbidity (DS) RR = 20 ÷ {(300 + 30) – ½ × 4 died} = 0.0610 pa
2. Mortality (DS) RR = 4 ÷ {(300 + 30) – ½ × (4 died + 8 culled)} = 0.0123 pa
3. Case fatality rate (DS) = 4 ÷ 20 = 0.25 pa
4. Proportional mortality rate (DS) = 20 ÷ (75 others + 10 CM + 20 DS) = 0.1904 pa
5. Morbidity (CM) RR = 14 ÷ [ITC × {(500 – 10) + (490 – 6 deaths – 18 culls – 14 cases + 30 additions)} ÷ 2] = 0.0285 pa
6. Crude mortality rate, True rate: The farm started with 500 animals and after ITC of 1 year had 500 – 24 culls – 6 deaths + 30 new additions = 500 animals. Hence, average number of animals = 500. Therefore, Crude mortality rate, True rate = 6 ÷ (500 × 1) = 0.0120 pa
7. Proportional mortality rate (CM) = (10 + 4) ÷ (500 – 20) = 0.0292 pa
8. Culling rate (in continuation of (6) above) = 24 ÷ (500 × 1) = 0.0480 pa

If ITC was x and we need to calculate RR for an ITC of y, assuming a constant RR,

$$RR = 1 - \left(1 - RR_x\right)^{y/x}$$

4.2.2.2 Example

Ten animals were observed for a specific disease for one year (ITC); 4 showed disease during 1st 3 months (0.25 year) and 2 more in the next 3 months (0.5 year). That means, 4 animals were disease – free throughout; 3 for 0.25 year and 2 for 0.50 year. Hence, ANR = 4 × 1 + 4 × 0.25 + 2 × 0.5 = 6.0; ITC = 1 and 6 animals acquired the disease; therefore, TR = 6 ÷ 6 = 1 animal pa. Since there were no withdrawals, RR = 6 ÷ 10 = 0.6; assuming RR as constant, RR after 5 years will be = 0.9961 or 99.61%.

Note: When RR < 0.15, (TR – RR) can be ignored and in a dynamic Population, RR is the ratio of number of animals acquiring the disease to ANR.

	Vaccinated	Not vaccinated	Not known	Totals
Disease +	8 (a)	412 (b)	80 (c)	500 (a + b + c)
Disease –	492 (d)	88 (e)	170 (f)	750 (d + e + f)
Totals	500 (a + d)	500 (b + e)	250 (c + f)	1250 (n)

4.2.2.3 Vaccine efficacy, VE

$$VE(\%) = \frac{\frac{b}{b+d} - \frac{a}{a+c}}{\frac{b}{b+d}} \times 100 = \left(1 - \frac{AR_{Vaccinated}}{AR_{Unvaccinated}}\right) \times 100 = (1 - RR) \times 100 = 80.05 \text{ in}$$

the above example. Proportion of cases in vaccinated individuals (PCV) is given

by $\frac{P_{Vac} - (P_{Vac} \times VE)}{1 - (P_{Vac} \times VE)}$ where P_{Vac} is the proportion of Population vaccinated. In the above

example, $P_{Vac} = 0.40$, VE = 0.80 and hence, PCV = 0.1176 or 11.76%.

4.3 Disease Detection

None of the tests available for disease diagnosis is perfect or 100% fool-proof or **Valid** in statistical terms. The validity of a test is measured in terms of **Sensitivity (S_n)** and **Specificity (S_p)**. These are already defined in terms of probability in the Chapter "Probability"; however, in Animal Scientists' point of view, Sensitivity, S_n, is the ratio of number of diseased animals detected by the test to that of total number of animals actually diseased and Specificity, S_p, on the other hand, is the complement of S_n being the ratio of number of healthy animals detected as healthy by the test to that of total number of healthy animals.

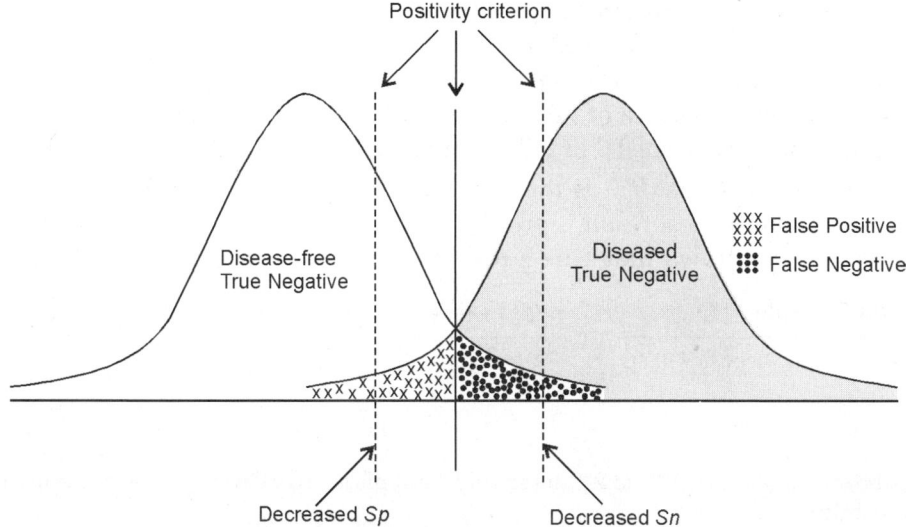

Fig 21.5: Disease detection by predictive value method (**Source:** Knapp and Miller, 1992)

4.3.1 Example

Let us revisit the **Example 4.1.2.1** in Chapter "**Probability**": Tuberculin test used to diagnose TB in animals; it was assumed that the test identifies 60% of diseased and 35% of normal animals as positive. Say 200 animals (100 each of diseased and healthy category) were tested by this method; the following will be the numbers:

Tuberculin skin-test		Actual		
		Diseased, D+	Healthy, D–	Total
Test result	Diseased, +	60 (a)	35 (b)	95 (R_1)
	Healthy, –	40 (c)	65 (d)	105 (R_2)
	Total	100 (C_1)	100 (C_2)	200 (n)

Then $S_n = a \div C_1 = 0.60$ or 60% and $S_p = d \div C_2 = 0.65$

4.3.2 Predictive Value (PV)

Positive predictive value, designated PV^+ is the proportion of animals tested positive when they were actually diseased; $\dfrac{a}{R_1}$ which, in terms of P, S_n and S_p will be

$\dfrac{PS_n}{PS_n + (1-P)(1-S_p)}$. Its complement, the proportion of animals tested negative when

they were actually healthy is referred to as PV^-; $\dfrac{d}{R_2}$ which, in terms of P, S_n and S_p will

be $\dfrac{(1-P)S_p}{P(1-S_n) + (1-P)S_p}$

Given: Sensitivity = 0.60, Specificity = 0.65, P = 0.08; therefore, $PV^+ = (0.60 \times 0.08) \div$ [(0.60 × 0.08) + (0.35 × 0.92)] = 0.1297 and $PV^- = (0.65 \times 0.92) \div$ [(0.65 × 0.92) + (0.40 × 0.08)] = 0.9492 which indicates that the Tuberculin test is more efficient to predict absence rather than presence of TB in milch animals. In other words, it is not reliable for diagnosis of presence of TB in milch animals.

It is easy to notice that PV^+ is the conditional probability that the animal has the disease given that the test result is positive, i.e. $p(D+ \mid T+)$ and on the same lines $PV^- = p(D^- \mid T^-)$. It follows that **true prevalence** is $p(D+)$ which can be calculated

as $\dfrac{p(T^+) - p(T^+ \mid D^-)}{1 - \{p(T^+ \mid D^-) + p(T^- \mid D^+)\}}$ or $\dfrac{p(T^+) + S_p - 1}{S_n + S_p - 1}$

Note:
1. The above formulae for PV^+ and PV^- are simply the application of Bayes' rule as shown in Chapter "**Probability**".
2. Apparent prevalence, $P_a = R_1 \div n$ and True prevalence, $P = C_1 \div n$; they are 0.475 and 0.500, respectively in the above example.
3. S_p can be calculated indirectly as $1 - \{$(Number of false positives) $\div (n - $number of actually diseased among test positives)$\}$ i.e. $1 - \{b \div (n - a)\}$; in the above example, it works out to be 0.75.
4. PV is directly proportional to probability of presence of the disease.
5. Generally, prevalence will be < 0.20

4.3.3 Receiver-Operator Characteristic (ROC) Curve

ROC curve is a parabola with S_n as a function of $(1 - S_p)$ as shown below.

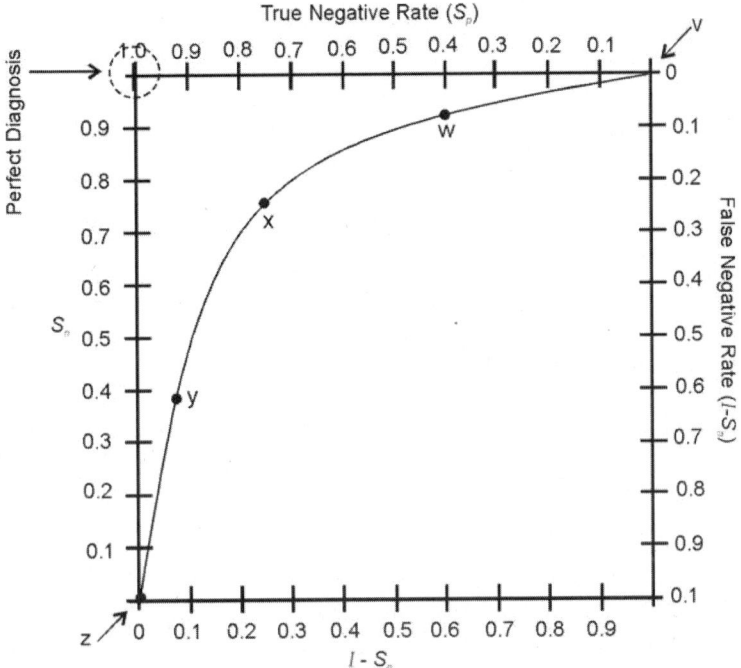

Fig. 21.6: Receiver-operator characteristic (ROC) curve (**Source:** Knapp and Miller, 1992)

4.3.3.1 Interpretation and uses of ROC curve

The left-hand top corner is the ideal (perfect) requirement for a diagnostic test because at that point a) all diseased and disease-free are correctly detected b) none of the disease-free is labeled diseased and *vice versa*. ROC curve can be used as follows:

1. When cost of false positive and false negative test is same, test criterion can be chosen closest to the left-hand top corner, i.e. *x*.
2. When false negative is not desired test criterion is set at *z*
3. When false positive is not desired, test criterion is set at *w* or *v*
4. For comparing two screening tests, the area under the curve is the criterion; larger the accurate. If the curve is a straight line making 45° at the origin, it gives no information; more it curves towards the left-hand top corner, more area it covers under it and more accurate it becomes.

4.3.4 Improving PV

Improvement of PV of a test can be achieved by (a) screening only high–risk population which obviously is expected to increase the conditional probability $p(T+ \mid D+)$ and/or (b) employing > 1 screening tests for the same disease simultaneously which not only increase the conditional probability $p(T+ \mid D+)$ but also reduce the conditional probability $p(T- \mid D+)$.

4.3.4.1. Example

Let us consider that two screening tests were used to diagnose a disease in sheep population and the following were the combination of results obtained:

Screening test result		Disease status	
I	II	+	−
+	−	50	120
−	+	130	150
+	+	680	50
−	−	140	9680
		1000	10000

Let us rearrange the above data into 2 × 2 contingency tables as per tests conducted independently, both together (parallel) and test 2 after test 1 (series) so that the changes in S_n and S_p can be easily appreciated:

	Test 1		Test 2		Test 1 and 2 (Parallel)		Test 1 and 2 (Series)	
Disease status	+	−	+	−	+	−	+	−
Test +	730	170	810	200	860	320	680	50
Test −	270	9830	190	9800	140	9680	320	9950
Totals	1000	10000	1000	10000	1000	10000	1000	10000
S_n $(a \div C_1)$	0.730		0.810		0.860		0.680	
S_p $(d \div C_2)$		0.983		0.980		0.968		0.995

If increasing predictive value (sensitivity) is the criterion, both the tests had better be run simultaneously (parallel) and positive result in any or both the tests counted for presence of disease. It can be noticed in the above example that sensitivity increased to 86% from 73 and 81% when the tests were conducted parallel. There was, however, a slight reduction in specificity.

On the other hand, if the tests are conducted separately over a period of time, it becomes necessary that only those which are positive in both the tests can be considered diseased. Therefore, sensitivity reduces. But, if specificity of the test is the criterion, as negative result in any one of the tests is considered absence of disease, using tests in series is preferable. However, on most practical situations, sensitivity becomes more important and hence, to increase PV it is better to rum both the tests simultaneously.

4.3.5 Herd-Level Diagnosis

Extending the rules of probability, it can be stated that an animal from a disease-free herd has a probability of $(1 - S_p)$ of being declared positive, popularly referred to as **False-positive**. Therefore, if S_p is < 1, there is definitely a possibility, high or low, that an animal is declared positive even though it is not actually so; at once even one animal is found positive, the herd is declared positive. It follows that, if n animals are sampled from a negative herd and tested by a test of S_p < 1, S_p of the test, as far as herd is concerned, reduces further as $(S_p)^n$. Considering the tuberculin test from the **Example 2.2.1** above, and n as low as 10, its S_p reduces to $0.65^{10} = 0.01$ indicating a very poor herd specificity of Tuberculin test.

On the same lines, S_n of a test at herd level is dependent on apparent prevalence, designated P_a by the formula $1 - (1 - P_a)^n$ where $P_a = $; $(1 - P_a)$ is the probability of testing one animal as negative, therefore, $(1 - P_a)^n$ is the probability of n animals tested as negative and $1 - (1 - P_a)^n$ is the probability of testing at least one animal as positive which is the sufficient condition to declare the herd as positive. Assuming $P = 0.08$, $P_a = 0.37$ and for $n = 10$, herd sensitivity = 0.99 indicating that this test has a tendency of declaring 99 out of 100 herds positive for TB! This must be considered with caution because, for the same conditions, herd specificity is only 0.01.

4.3.6 *Comparison of Agreement between Tests*

A new test developed can be tested against the test(s) already in use by application of Kappa statistic (*see* **Section 3.4.2** Chapter **"Tests of Hypotheses"**).

4.3.6.1 Example

		Test 1		
		Disease +	Disease –	
Test 2	Disease +	60 (*a*)	35 (*b*)	95 (R_1)
	Disease –	40 (*c*)	65 (*d*)	105 (R_2)
		100 (C_1)	100 (C_2)	200 (*n*)

It can be noticed that *a* and *d* are concordant and *b* and *c* are discordant pairs. Hence, Observed proportion of agreement $(O_A) = (a + d) \div n = 0.625$. Expected proportion of

agreement $(E_A) = \left(\dfrac{R_1}{n} \times \dfrac{C_1}{n}\right) + \left(\dfrac{R_2}{n} \times \dfrac{C_2}{n}\right) = \dfrac{R_1 C_1 + R_2 C_2}{n^2} = 0.5$; $(O_A - E_A) = 0.125$.

Maximum possible agreement beyond chance $= 1 - E_A = 0.5$. Now, the Kappa statistic,

$\kappa = \dfrac{O_A - E_A}{1 - E_A} = 0.25$. Complete agreement is indicated if $\kappa = 1$ and *vice versa*. No stan-

dards are available for interpretation for intermediate values of κ between 0 and 1; however, the following are generally accepted for epidemiological results:

Range of κ values	Intensity of agreement
> 0.81	Almost perfect
0.61 – 0.80	Substantial
0.41 – 0.60	Moderate
0.21 – 0.40	Fair
≤ 0.20	Poor

Source: Thrusfield, 1995

Note: The κ statistic can be applied for comparing the agreement between a new test *Vs* standard test or two clinicians diagnosing reasons for a particular ailment among the same cases etc.

4.3.7 *Repeatability of a Test*

A diagnostic test can be evaluated by checking how far the results are repeatable, and hence, reliable by conducting the test more than once followed by comparison of the results.

4.3.7.1 Test conducted twice (McNemar's change test)

This is a modified χ^2 test on $\upsilon = 1$ using discordant observations applicable when total number of discordant observations is > 10; otherwise, Fisher's exact test is resorted to (*see* Chapter **"Tests of hypotheses"**).

4.3.7.1.1 *Example*

Number of individuals under different combination of test result which was conducted twice is given below to assess its reliability:

H_0: There is no difference in 1st and 2nd time test results

$$\chi^2 = \frac{(|b-c|-1)^2}{b+c} = 0.213$$ which is < 3.841, the table value of $\chi^2_{0.05,\ 1}$; hence, H_0 is acceptable and the test has a high reliability.

		1st time		
		+	−	
2nd time	+	60 (*a*)	35 (*b*)	95 (R_1)
	−	40 (*c*)	65 (*d*)	105 (R_2)
		100 (C_1)	100 (C_2)	200 (*n*)

4.3.7.2 Test conducted ≥ 3 times (Cochran's Q test)

H_0: There is no difference in the test result over different test runs

$$\text{Cochran's } Q = \frac{(k-1)\left\{k\sum G_i^2 - \left(\sum G_i\right)^2\right\}}{k\sum L_i - \sum L_i^2} = 0.33$$ which is distributed as χ^2 on $\upsilon = (k-1)$

Animal	Test run (k = 5)					Total (+), Li
	1	2	3	4	5	
1	+	−	+	+	−	3
2	+	+	+	+	+	5
3	−	+	+	−	+	3
4	+	+	−	−	+	3
5	−	−	−	+	+	2
6	+	+	+	+	−	4
7	−	+	−	−	−	1
8	+	+	+	−	−	3
9	+	+	−	+	+	4
10	−	−	+	+	+	3
Total (+), $\sum G_i$	6	7	6	6	6	$\sum L_i$ or $\sum G_i = 31$
Sum of squares (+)						107, $\sum L_i^2$
$\sum G_i^2 = 193$						

i.e. 4. The calculated value is < table value 9.49 and hence the H_0 is acceptable and test is a reliable one. *See* **Section 7** Chapter "**Two-factor analysis of variance**" also.

4.3.8   *Sero-diagnosis*

Diagnosis of a disease by using serum samples to detect disease specific antibodies has been in vogue for many decades now. Serum will be diluted on a geometric series

$(x_i$'s$)$ *viz.* 2, 4, 8, 16, 32 ... so that $\log_2 (x_i)$'s will be 1, 2, 3, 4, 5 ... ($i = 1, 2, 3 ... n$) with a

mean on $\log_2$ scale as $\dfrac{\displaystyle\sum_{i=1}^{n} \log_2 x_i}{n}$ which can be transformed to the original scale by

taking antilog on a suitable base; 2 in this case. If the initial dilution is 1:10 followed by dilution on $\log_2$ scale, we get dilutions 1/10, 1/20, 1/40, ... which on converting to $\log_{10}$, will become values with a difference of $\log_{10}3$ (or 0.3020) between any two consecutive dilutions (d). Therefore, to calculate mean, the sum is first divided by 10 and then antilog is taken on $\log_2$ scale.

Criterion for diagnosis is the highest dilution that gives a test reaction (positive). While referring to the dilution, usually the numerator is ignored and only the denominator is mentioned referring as **titer**. Concentration of antibodies is directly proportional to the titer. Since the dilutions are in an order, the data is Ordinal (*see* Chapter "**Introduction**"). If each dilution is tested once, it is referred to as single serial dilution assay; otherwise, multiple serial dilution assay. In the latter, usually each dilution is tested at least 5 times; in other words, 5 animals or test material for each dilution so that dilution to get at least 50% of the end-point (test result) can be calculated (*see* **Section 4: Veterinary pharmacology and toxicology** wherein 10 animals are used for each of the dosages to estimate LD_{50}).

Note: Since logarithm of zero is indeterminable, sero-negatives are excluded

4.3.8.1 Example

Let us assume that sero-prevalence of a particular disease was studied and number of serum samples testing positive for a test (out of $n = 5$) are tabulated below. It is required to estimate the titer at which 50% of animals are likely to give a positive test.

ΣP, the sum of proportions from highest dilution showing negative result = 1.0 + $0.8 \times 2 + 0.6 + 0.4 + 0.2 = 3.8$. Now, $\log_{10} ED_{50} = L - d\left(\sum P - 0.5\right) = -0.438 = 1/2.742$.

Titer*	Log$_{10}$(titer)	Positives	Negatives	Proportion negative (P)**	1 − P
1	0.0	0	5	1.0	0.0
2	−0.3	0	5***	1.0	0.0
4	−0.6	1	4	0.8	0.2
8	−0.9	1	4	0.8	0.2
1	−1.2	2	3	0.6	0.4
32	−1.5	3	2	0.4	0.6
64	−1.8	4	1	0.2	0.8
128	−2.1	5	0	0.0	1.0
256	−2.4	5	0	0.0	1.0
512	−2.7	5	0	0.0	1.0

* All are reciprocals; numerator ignored;

** Number of negatives $\div n$;

*** Log of highest dilution wherein none is positive (L); $d = 0.3$, the log–dilution factor; $\Sigma P(1 - P) = 0.96$

That means, 0.1 ml has 2.742 ED_{50}'s and hence, 1 ml has 27.42 ED_{50}'s. Estimate of standard error can be obtained by $se\left(\log_{10} ED_{50}\right) = \dfrac{d\sqrt{n-1}}{\sqrt{\sum P(1-P)}} = 0.625$. This method is popularly known as **Spearman–Karber titration**.

4.3.9 Sero-conversion in Populations

If p is the probability of getting infected in one year and P_y is the proportion of population that is infected by the age of y years, then $P_y = 1 - (1-p)^y$; taking logarithms on both sides and rearranging the terms, we get $p = 1 - Antilog\left[\dfrac{\log(1-P_y)}{y}\right]$ which is referred to as **sero-conversion rate**.

4.3.9.1 Example

Let us consider the following data on sero-prevalence of a certain disease in cattle and estimate the sero-conversion to assess the proportion of animals of different ages getting exposed to/affected by the disease: (assumed that large number of animals of each age is screened to assess sero-prevalence)

Age (years, y)	1	2	3	4	5	6
P_y	0.20	0.28	0.31	0.40	0.47	0.55
p^*	0.200	0.151	0.116	0.120	0.119	0.125

* Calculated by the formula $p = 1 - Antilog\left[\dfrac{\log(1-P_y)}{y}\right]$

Note: If several samples are tested, they can be compared by t–test or other appropriate tests described in earlier chapters after suitable transformation of data.

4.4 Population Studies

For the discussion below, 2×2 contingency table with the same notations indicated above are assumed.

4.4.1 Prevalence Ratio (PR)

This is the ratio of diseased among exposed to diseased among unexposed. If (R_1) individuals are exposed of which a are diseased and (R_2) individuals are unexposed of which c are diseased, then $PR = \dfrac{a/R_1}{c/R_2}$ or $\dfrac{aR_2}{cR_1}$. It is very clear by the formula that if PR = 1, there is equal chance that both exposed and unexposed animals can contract disease, if PR > 1, exposure increases risk of disease and conversely, if PR < 1, exposure could reduce disease risk. PR is calculated in cross-sectional studies undertaken at a particular moment.

4.4.1.1 Example

Suppose in a cross-sectional study involving 500 poultry units (250 in endemic and 250 in disease-free areas) were investigated to study the occurrence of a disease ad the following results are obtained:

	Disease occurrence		
	Yes	No	Total
Endemic	210 (a)	40 (b)	250 (R_1)
Disease-free	25 (c)	225 (d)	250 (R_2)
Total	235 (C_1)	265 (C_2)	500 (n)

PR = 8.4 indicating that endemic areas are potential areas of disease occurrence.

4.4.2 Odds Ratio (OR)

From **Section 1.4.1**, (C_1) are diseased and (C_2) are disease-free. If these two groups are considered as sampling units (as in case-control studies), OR of exposure,

$$OR_{exp} = \frac{a/c}{b/d} = \frac{ad}{bc}.$$ Similarly, in cohort studies (involving group of individuals that either do or do not possess a factor that influences the occurrence of disease) OR of

disease, $OR_{dis} = \frac{a/b}{c/d} = \frac{ad}{bc}$ which is same as OR_{exp}.

Note: OR_{exp} or OR_{dis} is designated OR.

4.4.2.1 Example

From the **Example 1.4.1.1** above, OR = 47.25 which indicates that probability of an unit in an endemic area getting infected is about 47 times that in a disease–free area.

4.4.3 Cumulative Incidence Ratio (CIR) and Disease Odds Ratio

PR and OR from a cohort study are the CIR and OR_{dis}, respectively.

4.4.3.1 Incidence rate ratio (IRR)

This is a synonym of rate ratio (RtR), incidence density ratio (IDR) and relative risk (RR). If t_1 and t_0 are the total time at risk in exposed and unexposed groups, respectively,

$$IRR = \frac{a/t_1}{c/t_0} = \frac{at_0}{ct_1}.$$ This is employed in dynamic populations wherein there is conti-

nuous entry and exit of animals from the groups.

4.4.3.1.1 *Example*

From the **Example 1.4.1.1** above, if we assume time units as shown below, IRR calculated is 6.72:

	Endemic area	Disease-free area	Total
Diseased	210 (a)	25 (c)	235
Time at risk, week-units	260 (t_1)	208 (t_0)	468 (n)

4.5   Data Analysis (Crude)

Mainly involves construction of confidence limits (intervals); First order Taylor's series (asymptotic method) is generally used to construct confidence intervals for OR. As in case of 2 × 2 contingency table χ^2 test, minimum cell frequency is 5. Violation of this rule compels use of exact methods. OR ranges from > 0 to ∞, but most times, the value hovers around 1.0. Hence, OR is highly skewed to the right (*see* Chapter "**Dispersion**") and does not follow normal distribution; therefore, it is transformed to natural logarithmic scale (*In* i.e. $\log_e$). Then confidence intervals are constructed analogous to any other statistic as: $\log_e OR \pm Z\sqrt{Var(\log_e OR)}$. The values on Natural logarithms can be retransformed by raising lower and upper-limit values to the base e separately. As indicated in Chapter "**Tests of Hypotheses**", value of Z is 1.96 and 2.58 for α of 0.05 and 0.01, respectively.

$$\text{Variance} (\log_e OR) = \frac{1}{a} + \frac{1}{b} + \frac{1}{c} + \frac{1}{d}; \text{Variance} (\log_e CIR) = \frac{b}{aR_1} + \frac{d}{cR_2}; \text{Variance} (\log_e IRR)$$

$$= \frac{1}{a} + \frac{1}{b}.$$ These can be employed to estimate confidence intervals.

4.5.1   Example

We shall consider **Example 1.4.1.1** above for calculation of 95% confidence intervals of OR: Z = 1.96

	Disease occurrence		
	Yes	No	Total
Endemic	210 (a)	40 (b)	250 (R_1)
Disease-free	25 (c)	225 (d)	250 (R_2)
Total	235 (C_1)	265 (C_2)	500 (n)

OR = 47.25; $\log_e OR = 3.8555$; Variance $(\log_e OR) = \frac{1}{210} + \frac{1}{40} + \frac{1}{25} + \frac{1}{225} = 0.0742$ and se($\log_e OR$) = 0.2724; confidence intervals = 3.8555 ± 1.96 × 0.2724; the 95% Confidence limits are 3.5831 and 4.1279 which upon retransformation ($e^{3.5831}$ and $e^{4.1279}$) will be 35.9849 and 62.0475, respectively.

Note:

1. Confidence interval doesn't include OR value of 1.0 even though it is mathematically included; obviously because, OR value of 1.0 indicates there is no difference between endemic and disease – free areas as far as disease occurrence is concerned.

2. Since (Natural) logarithmic transformation is involved, confidence intervals will not be symmetrical about the OR on original scale.

3. By appropriate modifications, $\log_{10}$ can be used in place of ln i.e. $\log_e$

4. Association between the attributes can be tested by χ^2 test as described in Chapter "**Tests of hypotheses**".

4.5.2 Mantel-Haenszel OR (OR_{MH})

In biological experiments, confounding is not uncommon because several factors operate on a variable at a time and it is, on most occasions, not possible to control and/or consider all factors. For instance, occurrence of a disease in endemic areas in chicks with high or low maternal antibodies (Ab); milk fever *vs* condition of the animal (fat/normal) over parity. Clearly, maternal antibodies and disease occurrence, body condition and parity are confounded.

4.5.2.1 Example

	Disease occurrence, low maternal Ab			Disease occurrence, high maternal Ab		
	Yes	No	Total	Yes	No	Total
Endemic	210 (a_1)	40 (b_1)	250	10 (a_2)	240 (b_2)	250
Disease-free	25 (c_1)	225 (d_1)	250	5 (c_2)	245 (d_2)	250
Total	235	265	500 (n_1)	15	485	500 (n_2)

OR values: Low maternal Ab: 47.25 (35.9849 to 62.0475); High maternal Ab: 2.042 (1.5004 to 2.7790) which indicates that even with high maternal Ab, chicks in endemic areas have double the risk of disease occurrence than those in disease-free areas.

Let us combine the data as follows:

	Disease occurrence (Pooled)		
	Yes	No	Total
Low maternal Ab	235 (a)	265 (b)	500 (R_1)
High maternal Ab	15 (c)	485 (d)	500 (R_2)
Total	250 (C_1)	750 (C_2)	1000 (n)

OR = 28.673 (26.555 to 30.963); similarly, keeping row titles as above, if the data of only endemic area were to be analyzed OR = 126.000 (110.208 to 144.060) or the data of only disease-free area were to be analyzed OR = 5.444 (4.248 to 6.983) both indicating high risk involved in endemic areas which is more magnified when maternal Ab levels are low.

Therefore, an unbiased estimate of OR is required giving weightage to maternal Ab levels; this can be obtained by Mantel-Haenszel OR by the formula given in **Section 3.2.4.2.2** Chapter "**Tests of hypotheses**" which is reproduced here:

$$OR_{MH} = \frac{\sum_{i=1}^{k}(a_i d_i \div n_i)}{\sum_{i=1}^{k}(b_i c_i \div n_i)} = \frac{210\times225/500 + 10\times245/500}{40\times25/500 + 250\times245/500} = 47.29 \text{ confirming that chicks in}$$

endemic areas are highly susceptible for the disease. If the data are tabulated with maternal Ab levels as rows, we get:

$OR_{MH} = 131.444$ indicating the importance of maternal antibodies in control of disease occurrence.

Disease occurrence	Endemic			Disease-free		
	Yes	No	Total	Yes	No	Total
Low maternal Ab	210 (a_1)	40 (b_1)	250	25 (a_2)	225 (b_2)	250
High maternal Ab	10 (c_1)	240 (d_1)	250	5 (c_2)	245 (d_2)	250
Total	220	280	500 (n_1)	30	470	500 (n_2)

4.5.2.2 Adjusting OR for confounding (mantel extension test)

See **Section 3.2.4.4.3** Chapter "Tests of hypotheses" for details.

4.5.3 OR with Independent Variable in > 2 Categories

Hitherto the discussion was on both dependant and independent variables being Binomial/binary. But, if we consider different classes of independent variable with a binary data of disease occurrence for each, then OR is calculated keeping one of them as reference.

4.5.3.1 Example

The data below pertains to number sick piglets at different ages:

Utilizing the independent variable values (age in this example) as x_i's and $\log_e OR$ as y_i's, suitable regression equation (linear, quadratic, cubic, etc.) can be fit. In this

	Age (months)					
	1	2	3	4	5	6
Diseased	30	45	48	36	15	2
Healthy	70	55	52	64	85	98
Total	100	100	100	100	100	100
OR	1.00*	1.91	2.15	1.31	0.41	0.05
$\log_e OR$**	0	0.65	0.77	0.27	−0.89	−3.00
se(OR)	0.10	0.09	0.09	0.09	0.13	0.56

* Calculated with itself as reference

** Regression coefficient (b) in logistic equation because $OR = e^b$

example, $\log_e OR$ values apparently show a parabolic trend and hence, a quadratic equation is fit which is: $y = -1.508 + 1.7901x - 0.3379x^2$; attaining a theoretical maximum $\log_e OR$ of 0.8628 (OR = 2.37) at 2.65 weeks of age; that means, at around 19th day of age they are most susceptible to disease.

4.5.4 Other OR

Odds that an exposed to risk factor (E+) will have the disease (D+) i.e. OR(D+ | E+) = $(a \div b)$; this is useful in Cohort/Experimental studies. Similarly, odds that a non-exposed will have disease, OR(D+ | E−) = $(c \div d)$ and OR for matched pair samples (case-control studies) is given by $(b \div c)$. In case-control studies, exposure OR among cases is $(a \div c)$ and among controls is $(b \div d)$. In all studies, OR of disease/prevalence is $(ad \div bc)$.

4.5.5 Standardization of Rates

When rates are evaluated at various strata, standardization is required against population rates.

4.5.5.1 Direct standardization

Let us assume that occurrence of avian influenza (AI) is studied in birds eared in confinement and free-range and the following are recorded:

	AI occurrence		Total	Incidence
	Yes	No		
Free-range	235 (a)	265 (b)	500 (R_1)	0.47
Confinement	15 (c)	485 (d)	500 (R_2)	0.03
Total	250 (C_1)	750 (C_2)	1000 (n)	

Further, the data was stratified into broilers and layers under each row classification as follows:

	Total	Observed rate	AI +	Incidence	Standardized rate
Free-range					
Broilers	250	0.3	85	0.34	½(0.3 + 0.06) = 0.18
Layers	250	0.7	150	0.60	½(0.7 + 0.08) = 0.39
Confinement					
Broilers	250	0.06	5	0.02	½(0.3 + 0.06) = 0.18
Layers	250	0.08	10	0.04	½(0.7 + 0.08) = 0.39

Adjusted rates = Σ[Observed incidence × Standardized rate]

Free-range	0.34 × 0.18 + 0.60 × 0.39 = 0.2952 or 29.52%
Confinement	0.02 × 0.18 + 0.04 × 0.39 = 0.0192 or 1.92%

4.5.5.2 Indirect standardization

Indirect standardization becomes essential especially when each of the strata is further subdivided into categories based on age, sex, etc.

4.5.5.2.1 Example

Antibody levels for a certain disease in cattle as per age groups were evaluated (over many samples for each age group) in two areas and the results are as follows:

Age, years	Observed proportions, P_i		Population rates, R_i
	Area 1, P_1	Area 2, P_2	
2.0–3.9	0.20	0.30	0.15
4.0–5.9	0.25	0.45	0.22
6.0–7.9	0.40	0.15	0.40
8.0–9.9	0.10	0.08	0.15
≥ 10.0	0.05	0.02	0.04
Total cases studied	5000	6000	
Reactors	1250	1500	
Crude rate	0.25	0.25	
$\sum P_i R_i$	0.2620	0.2168	
Standardized reactor rate*	0.9542	1.1531	
Adjusted rate**	0.1718	0.2076	

Average reactor rate for population is 0.18; * Crude rate $\div \sum P_i R_i$; ** Standardized rate × Average reactor rate for population

Note: As per the adjusted rates, antibody levels were higher in area 2 than in area 1 although crude rates were identical.

4.5.6 Dose-Disease Relationship: Logistic Curve

Fitting a logistic curve is already discussed under **Section 2.1.3.4** Chapter "**Analysis of time series**". In epidemiological studies, the dependent variable (y; usually row titles) is usually binary (yes/no, present/absent, etc. given values 1 and 0, respectively) and the independent variable continuous.

4.5.6.1 Example: categorized binary variable

Suppose occurrence of coccidiosis in broilers at 10 doses of oocysts is experimentally studied and the following result was obtained:

Dose	1x	2x	3x	4x	5x	6x	7x	8x	9x	10x
Diseased	0	3	6	8	10	62	70	86	95	98
No disease	100	97	94	92	90	38	30	14	5	2
Total	100	100	100	100	100	100	100	100	100	100
Probability	0	0.03	0.06	0.08	0.10	0.62	0.70	0.86	0.95	0.98
Predicted*	0.01	0.02	0.06	0.16	0.36	0.62	0.82	0.91	0.95	0.96

* from the logistic equation calculated below; $R^2 = 90.71\%$, $r = 0.95$

Now, the binary values are **categorized** and hence become continuous. With this, logistic curve can be fit with dose 1, 2..10 (x_i) predicting probability of disease occurrence (y_i): Considering 3rd, 6th and 9th set of values as three equidistant

$$\text{points}, k = \frac{y_2^2 (y_1 + y_3) - 2y_1 y_2 y_3}{y_2^2 - y_1 y_3} = 0.9700; b = \frac{1}{t_2 - t_1} \log_e \left[\frac{(k - y_2) y_1}{(k - y_1) y_2} \right] = -1.0970$$

and $a = \log_e\left(\dfrac{k - y_1}{y_1}\right) - bt_1 = 6.0101$. Hence, the final equation can be written as:

$$y_t = \frac{0.9700}{1 + e^{6.0101 - 1.0970t}}.$$

Note: In this equation, b is always < 0, $k \# 0$ and $k = y_{max}$; since y_i's are probabilities, $k \le 1$. Without going into mathematical details, OR $= e^b = e^{1.0970} = 2.9952$.

4.5.6.2 Example: 2 × 2 Table

Logistic regression equation can also be fit on data from a 2 × 2 table. Let us take **Example 1.4.1.1** discussed above for this purpose with binary values indicated):

(y_i)	Disease occurrence (x_i)		Total
	Yes (1)	No (0)	
Endemic (1)	210 (a)	40 (b)	250 (R_1)
Disease-free (0)	25 (c)	225 (d)	250 (R_2)
Total	235 (C_1)	265 (C_2)	500 (n)

Probability of occurrence of disease given that the area is endemic, $y(1) = 210 \div 235 = 0.8936$; Probability of not occurrence of disease given that the area is endemic, $y(0) = 40 \div 265 = 0.1509$. logit of $y(1) = In\left(\dfrac{y(1)}{1 - y(1)}\right) = 2.1281$; similarly, logit of $y(0)$

$$= In\left(\frac{y(0)}{1 - y(0)}\right) = -1.7276.$$

Since logit $y(x) = a + bx$; $y(1) = a + b*1 = 2.1281$ or $b = 2.1281 - a$; further, $y(0) = a + b*0 = a = -1.7276$; and $b = 2.1281 + 1.7276 = 3.8557$. Value of b can be used to calculate OR as $e^b = 47.26$ which is same as calculated earlier. By utilizing the logistic equation fit, probabilities and values predicted for the same data is given below to verify the accuracy:

(y_i)	Disease occurrence (x_i)	
	Yes (1)	No (0)
Endemic (1)	$y(1) = \dfrac{e^{a+b}}{1 + e^{a+b}} = 0.8936$ (210)	$y(0) = \dfrac{e^a}{1 + e^a} = 0.1510$ (40)
Disease-free (0)	$1 - y(1) = \dfrac{1}{1 + e^{a+b}} = 0.1064$ (25)	$1 - y(0) = \dfrac{1}{1 + e^a} = 0.8491$ (225)

Value in the parentheses indicates total predicted frequencies

4.5.7 Measures of Association

Statistical associations can be tested by χ^2 or McNemar's test or t-test or, when the data is quantitative (continuous), product-moment correlation itself. For instance, if paired t-test comparing milk yields of normal and FMD-affected dams is significant in favor of normal dams, it is also suggestive that FMD decreases milk yield because of association between the two traits.

Further, in a 2 × 2 contingency table, correlation coefficient, r, can be estimated by $r = \dfrac{ad - bc}{\sqrt{R_1 R_2 C_1 C_2}}$ which is also same as $\left(\chi^2 \div \sqrt{n}\right)$ on $\upsilon = 1$.

In a 2 × 2 contingency table, several probabilities can be calculated regarding causation of disease:

Exposure to etiology	Disease occurrence D+	D–	Total
Exposed (E+)	210 (a)	40 (b)	250 (R$_1$)
Not exposed (E–)	25 (c)	225 (d)	250 (R$_2$)
Total	235 (C$_1$)	265 (C$_2$)	500 (n)

$p(E+) = R_1 \div n = 0.5$; $p(D+) = C_1 \div n = 0.47$; $p(\text{disease and exposed}) = a \div n = 0.42$; $p(\text{disease among exposed}) = a \div R_1 = 0.84$; $p(\text{disease among not exposed}) = c \div R_2 = 0.10$; $p(\text{exposed among diseased}) = a \div C_1 = 0.89$; $p(\text{exposed among not diseased}) = b \div C_2 = 0.15$

Epidemiological measures of association for independent proportions in 2 × 2 tables with notations as indicated above are:

Measure	Formula	Suitability of measure Case-control studies	Cross-sectional studies	Cohort/ Experimental studies
Strength				
Relative risk, RR	$aR_2 \div cR_1$	No	Yes	Yes
Population RR, RR$_{Pop}$	$C_1 R_2 \div cn$	No	Yes	No
Odds ratio, OR	$ad \div bc$	Yes	Yes	Yes
OR$_{Pop}$	$dC_1 \div cC_2$	Yes*	Yes*	No
Effect				
Attributable rate, AR	$(a \div R_1) - (c \div R_2)$	No	Yes	Yes
Attributable fraction, AF	$AR \div (a \div R_1)$ or $(RR - 1) \div RR$	No	Yes	Yes
Estimated AF	$(OR - 1) \div OR$	Yes	No	No
Total effect (importance)				
Population AR, PAR	$(C_1 \div n) - (c \div R_2)$ or $(R_1 \div n)*AR$	No	Yes**	No
Population AF, PAF	$PAR \div (C_1 \div n)$ or $(RR_{Pop} - 1) \div RR_{Pop}$	No	Yes	No
Estimated PAF	$1 - (cR_2 \div dC_1)$ or $(OR_{Pop} - 1) \div OR_{Pop}$	Yes*	No	No

* When controls represent non–diseased population;
** When disease frequency is available

Note: AR is also referred to as risk difference or excess risk or rate difference; AF is also referred to as simple etiological fraction and PAF as total etiological fraction *adapted from Martin et al., 1993*

4.5.7.1. Example

Let us calculate various measures of association from the following data on occurrence of ascites in dogs on only vegetarian diet:

H_0: There is no association between diet and ascites

	Ascites+	Ascites–	Total	Ascites rate
Vegetarian diet	210 (a)	40 (b)	250 (R_1)	0.84
Normal diet	25 (c)	225 (d)	250 (R_2)	0.10
Total	235 (C_1)	265 (C_2)	500 (n)	0.47
p(Ascites among Vegetarian dogs) = 0.8936				

$$\chi^2 = \frac{n\left[|ad-bc|-\dfrac{n}{2}\right]^2}{R_1 R_2 C_1 C_2} = 271.827$$ which is > 3.841, table value of $\chi^2_{0.05,1}$ indicating that

the diet and ascites are related (H_0 rejected). Other epidemiological measures of association and their interpretation are:

Measure	Value	Interpretation
RR	8.40	Risk of ascites is 8 times higher in vegetarian dogs
OR	47.25	Risk of ascites is 47 times higher in vegetarian dogs
RR_{Pop}	4.70	Risk of ascites increases with vegetarian diets
OR_{Pop}	7.98	Same as above
AR	0.74	Ascites in vegetarian dogs is 74 per 100
AF	0.88	88% of ascites in dogs is due to vegetarian diet
PAR	0.37	37% of ascites is because of diet
PAF	0.88	88% of ascites in population is due to vegetarian diet

4.5.8 Measuring Interaction

Although additive and non-additive models are possible, the former is most commonly employed. Considering two factors x and y, if I_{00}, I_{01}, I_{10} and I_{11} are the rates of incidence when both factors were absent, only x was present, only y was present and when both factors were present, respectively, then risk attributable to $x = I_{10} - I_{00}$, and to $y = I_{01} - I_{00}$. If $(I_{11} - I_{00})$ is equal to sum of the risks attributable to x and y, then there is no interaction; i.e. $(I_{11} - I_{00}) = (I_{10} - I_{00}) + (I_{01} - I_{00})$. By dividing both sides by I_{00} and rearranging terms $RR_{xy} = (RR_x - 1) + (RR_y - 1) = 1 + \Sigma(RR_i - 1)$; by extending to j factors, we get $RR_{xy} = 1 + \sum_{i=1}^{j}(RR_i - 1)$.

4.6 Survival Analysis

4.6.1 Definitions

4.6.1.1. Survivor function, S(t)

S(t) is the probability that an animal will not show the event before time t; $S(t) = P(T > t)$. It is logical to say that survivor function can't increase but, generally decreases gradually.

4.6.1.2 Hazard function, h(t)

This is near complement of S(t); it gives the probability per unit time that the event occurs in the next period of time given the animal doesn't have the event already.

Hence, h(t) is a rate function $= \lim\limits_{\Delta t \to 0} \dfrac{P(t \leq T < t + \Delta t \mid T \geq t)}{\Delta t}$. When h(t) is plotted against

t, different types of curves result: Exponential, increasing or decreasing Weibull, Lognormal, etc. It is also obvious that being a probability per unit time, $0 \leq h(t) \leq \infty$ but never negative. Weibull's decreasing function (survival function) is $S(t) = e^{-(at)^p}$ and

Weibull's increasing function (hazard function) is $h(t) = ap(at)^{p-1}$ where a and p are scale and shape parameters, respectively. When $p = 1$, Weibull's function becomes the Exponential function

Note: $h(t) = \dfrac{1}{S(t)} \left[\dfrac{\partial}{\partial t} S(t) \right]$.

4.6.1.2.1 Example

To test the efficacy of a coccidiostat in preventing deaths due to coccidiosis, 250 broilers each were put on the treated and untreated groups for 6 weeks. Number of birds surviving at the end of the week (actually the number of birds died is given which indicates that they survived till that time; the rest continued to survive which will be automatically accounted for at the last period) is given below:

Weeks	Treated No	Treated Time at risk, weeks	Untreated No	Untreated Time at risk, weeks
1	0	0	0	0
2	0	0	0	0
3	0	0	0	0
4	1	4	25	100
5	5	25	60	300
6	3	18	48	288
7	3	21	27	189
8	238	1904	90	720
Total	250	1972 weeks	250	1597 weeks
Mean		7.89 weeks		6.69 weeks
Failures	12		160	
h_i		$12 \div 1972 = 0.006$		$160 \div 1597 = 0.100$
			Hazard Ratio, HR $= 0.006 \div 0.100 = 0.060$	

The values of failures, survivors and total can be formed into a 2 × 2 contingency table and tested for significance by χ^2 or by log-rank or Wilcoxon test (*see* Chapter "**Tests of hypotheses**" for details). The calculated χ^2 on $\upsilon = 1$ is 83.841 which is > 3.841 the table value of $\chi^2_{1, 0.05}$; hence, H_0: Survival functions do not differ is rejected and concluded that the survival functions differ significantly.

4.6.1.3 Average hazard rate

This is defined as the number of failures per unit time at risk; $h_i = \dfrac{\sum\limits_{i=1}^{k} \text{failures}_i}{\sum\limits_{i=1}^{k} t_i}$ where

k represents number of periods ($i = 1, 2 \dots K$) in hours, days, weeks, etc. In the example, it is weeks and $k = 6$.

4.6.1.4 Hazard ratio (HR)

HR is the ratio of average hazard rates in question; if HR = 1, the treatment has no effect, if it is > 1, the treatment corresponding to the numerator has a significant promoting effect on the disease occurrence and *vice versa*. In the present example, the HR was < 1 and hence, coccidiostat has helped reduce occurrence of coccidiosis.

4.6.2 Estimation of HR

4.6.2.1 Cox exponential hazard model

This is a simple Exponential equation $y = e^{bx}$; hence $\log_e y = bx$. This is the reason that, for validity of this model, hazards in both the groups must be proportional in time.

4.6.2.2 Weibull regression

Procedure for fitting this equation is beyond the scope of this publication and one had better use the computer software for this purpose.

4.7 Clinical Trials

4.7.1 Vaccinal Efficacy

4.7.1.1 Example

The following are the results of application of a new vaccine against FMD in cattle:

	Disease present	Disease absent	Total
Not vaccinated	146 (*a*)	78 (*b*)	224 (R$_1$)
Vaccinated	23 (*c*)	253 (*d*)	276 (R$_2$)
Total	169 (C$_1$)	331 (C$_2$)	500 (*n*)

$$\text{Proportion of cattle exposed, } p_{\text{exp}} = \frac{\dfrac{a}{R_1} - \dfrac{c}{R_2}}{\dfrac{a}{R_1}} = \frac{\text{Prevalence among exposed} - \text{Prevalence among unexposed}}{\text{Prevalence among exposed}} = $$

0.8721; that means 87.21% of FMD in those cattle which are not vaccinated is attributable to the fact that they are not vaccinated; in simple terms, the new FMD vaccine can prevent 87.21% of disease in cattle; hence referred to as **vaccinal efficacy**.

The above data can also be tested by χ^2 on υ 1 by methods already given in Chapter "**Tests of hypotheses**" under H$_0$: There is no difference between vaccinated and not vaccinated groups as far as FMD disease presence is concerned; the calculated value of $\chi^2 = 178.567$ which is > 3.981, the table value at $\alpha = 0.05$. Hence, H_0 is rejected.

4.7.2 Efficacy of an Ectoparasiticide

Percent efficacy is 100 times the ratio of reduction in mean number of ectoparasites per animal due to treatment to that of number of ectoparasites per animal in the control group (C); if T is the number of ectoparasites per animal in the treated group, % efficacy

$$= \frac{C - T}{C} \times 100.$$

4.8 Epidemic Curve

Number of infected animals as a function of time gives the epidemic curve. The nature of curve depends on number of animals a) infected b) susceptible and c) immune. However, it is also required that the period of infection is short, incubation period is constant and all the infected develop the disease and become infectious for the next stage and become immune in the meantime so that mathematical predictions are possible. Under these conditions and assumptions, the occurrence of disease becomes a binomial event or a chain of binomial events; thus the model is referred to as **Chain–Binomial model** which is described by $C_{t+1} = S_t\left(1 - q^{C_t}\right)$ where t is usually the incubation period, C_{t+1} is the number of infectious cases in time $(t + 1)$, S_t is the number of susceptible animals in time t and q is the probability of an animal **not** making contact with the infectious agent (p being its complement). This model is popularly known as **Reed-Frost model.**

4.8.1 Example

Let us assume that there is only one bird infected of *Avian influenzae* among 1000 birds, none exposed earlier and hence not immune. If $p = 0.02$ ($q = 0.98$), it means $C_t = 1$ and 20 out of 1000 susceptible will come in contact with the infection; therefore, at time $t + 1$, $C_{t+1} = 1000 \times (1 - 0.98^1) = 20$ infectious cases; obviously for the next period only $(1000 - 20)$ susceptible are left and $C_{t+2} = 980 \times (1 - 0.98^{0.20}) \approx 326$. In the next period 654 susceptible are left and $C_{t+3} = 654 \times (1 - 0.98^{0.326}) \approx 653$ (only one bird left susceptible). That means, the disease spreads so rapidly to involve all susceptible by the third period itself. It should be noted that number of immune animals is the cumulative total of infected animals till the period in question. In the above example, the number of birds immune (I_t) by time t, $t + 1$ and $t + 2$ will be 20, 346 and 999, respectively. If mortality and/or culling is involved this formula needs modification. The above results can be tabulated as follows:

Time, t	C_t	S_t	I_t	Totals	p	pS_t
0	1	1000	0	1001	0.02	20.00
1	20	980	1	1001	0.02	19.60
2	326	654	21	1001	0.02	13.08

Note: Epidemic can occur if $pS_t > 1$ and declines if $pS_t < 1$

4.8.2 Density *vs* Disease Occurrence

The occurrence of a disease, especially infectious one, is likely to be higher if more number of susceptible is available; in other words when animal density is higher. This can be tested by χ^2 test for trend (*see* **Sections 3.2.4.4.2** and **3.2.4.4.3,** Chapter **"Tests of hypotheses"** also).

4.8.2.1 Example

The following data refers to occurrence of IBD in poultry farms as per number of birds (all values in '000):

H_0: Number of birds affected and density of birds are not associated

Number of birds per farm	Mid-value, x_i	Number affected Observed (a_{i1})	Number affected Expected $(E_i) =$ $(R_i C_1' \div N)$	Total number at risk (R_i)	% affected $= 100^*(a_{i1} \div R_i)$
≤ 1	0.5	1.0	0.096	10	1.0
1–5	3.0	2.5	0.483	50	5.0
5–10	7.5	8.0	9.668	1000	0.8
10–50	30.0	4.0	4.834	500	0.8
≥ 50	75.0	2.0	2.417	250	0.8
$j = 5$		17.5×10^3 (C_1)	17.498×10^3	1810×10^3 (N)	

$$C_2 = N - C_1 = 1792.5 \times 10^3; \quad \sum_{i=1}^{j} x_i^2 R_i = 1912952.5 \times 10^9; \quad \sum_{i=1}^{j} x_i R_i = 41405 \times 10^6;$$

$$\sum_{i=1}^{j} x_i (a_{i1} - E_i) = -62.302 \times 10^6. \text{ Now, } \chi^2 = \frac{N^2 (N-1) \left[\sum_{i=1}^{j} x_i (a_{i1} - E_i) \right]^2}{C_1 C_2 \left[N \sum_{i=1}^{j} x_i^2 R_i - \left(\sum_{i=1}^{j} x_i R_i \right)^2 \right]} = 419.74 \text{ is}$$

> 3.481, the table value of $\chi^2_{0.05,1}$; hence, the H_0 is liable to be rejected and hence, density of birds does influence occurrence of disease.

4.9 Summary of Statistical Methods in Epidemiology

Many other statistical applications described in other preceding Chapters are possible on epidemiological data; for instance, correlation and regression analysis, analysis by time series (cyclical/seasonal/secular trends) etc. In addition, modeling (beyond the scope of this publication) based on differential calculus, stochastic (probability) and simulation models can also be employed. Different non-parametric tests applicable and specific tests of associations in different epidemiological studies are separately tabulated below as a ready reference:

Nature of data	Test (s)
	Single sample
Nominal	Binomial test, χ^2 goodness of fit
Ordinal	Komolgov-Smirnov test, Run test, Change point test*
Interval/Ratio	Test for distributional symmetry
	Two samples—matched/related
Nominal	McNemar's change test
Ordinal	Sign test, Wilcoxon signed rank test
Interval/Ratio	Permutation test*
	Two samples—independent
Nominal	Fisher's exact test, χ^2 tests
Ordinal	Median test, Wilcoxon-Mann Whitney test, Robust rank-order test(U)*, Komolgov-Smirnov test, Siegel-Tukey test
Interval/Ratio	Permutation test*, Moses rank-like test*
	Multiple samples—related
Nominal	Cochran's Q test
Ordinal	Friedman's ANOVA by ranks, Page test*
	Multiple samples—independent
Nominal	χ^2 test
Ordinal	Median test, Kruskal-Wallis ANOVA, Jonckheere test(J)*
	Non-parametric tests
Nominal	Cramer's coefficient*, Φ coefficient, κ coefficient, λ test*
Ordinal	Spearman's rank correlation coefficient, Kendall's rank-order correlation coefficient, Kendall's partial rank-order correlation coefficient*, Kendall's coefficient of concordance, Kendall's coefficient of agreement, Correlation between k judges*
Interval/Ratio	γ statistic, G, Somer's index of asymmetric association*

* Not included and/or beyond the scope of this publication
Adapted from: Thrusfied, 1995

The table below summarizes tests for analyzing associations and differences in data obtained from different types of epidemiological studies:

| Type of study | Matched data | | Independent data | |
	Counts	Interval/Ratio	Counts	Interval/Ratio
	Measuring strength of association			
Cross-sectional	Not applicable			OR, RR_t
Case-control	OR	r_{xy} / b	OR, RR_t	r_{xy} / b
Cohort/Experimental	OR	r_{xy} / b	OR, RR	

(Contd.)

(Contd.)

Type of study	Matched data		Independent data	
	Counts	Interval/Ratio	Counts	Interval/Ratio
		Testing significance		
Cross-sectional	Not applicable			
Case-control	McNemar's	r_{xy}/b	χ^2	r_{xy}/b
Cohort/Experimental	McNemar's	r_{xy}/b		
		Analyzing differences—Proportions		
Cross-sectional	Not applicable			
Case-control	McNemar's	Not applicable	χ^2	Not applicable
Cohort/Experimental	McNemar's	Not applicable		
		Analyzing differences—Interval/Ratio		
Two treatments	Paired t test		Pooled t test	
Multiple treatments	ANOVA, RBD		ANOVA, CRD	

Adapted from: Knapp and Miller, 1992

5. VETERINARY PHARMACOLOGY AND TOXICOLOGY

5.1 Drug Elimination

Drug elimination from the body follows either a linear fashion (0 – Order) or exponential fashion (I – Order). Obviously, for 0 – order elimination, linear regression equation, of plasma concentration (y_i) against time (t_i) can explain the kinetics. For I – Order elimination, y_i's are converted to logarithmic scale to make the association linear and linear equation is fit (*see* Chapter "**Association between variables I**" for details). It is very clear that b_{yx} will be negative and indicates the quantum of drug (actual or log units) eliminated per unit time (usually hours).

5.1.1 Half-Life (t½)

Half-life is the time required to reduce the plasma concentration of a drug to ½ in its **original scale** (because, ½ log $y \neq$ ½ y). Half-life can be calculated for both drug distribution as well as its elimination; the former preceding the latter event for all drugs. Time taken for a two-fold decrease has been shown to be mathematically proportional to $\log_e 2$ (or *In* 2 or 0.693147); hence, t½ is the ratio of $\log_e 2$ and k; where k is the elimination/distribution rate constant, as the case may be. Considering drug elimination, if V is the volume of distribution and Cl, the clearance, $k = (V \div Cl)$ and

therefore, t½ $= \log_e(2)\dfrac{V}{Cl}$.

Note: At every t½, 50% of the drug left is cleared.

5.1.2 Drug Given Repeatedly

It is well known that a drug is generally repeated over time to maintain a steady plasma concentration by countering its elimination. Hence, steady-state plasma concentration is the ratio of dose rate to clearance rate which follows that dose rate is the product of target plasma steady concentration (C_{st}) and clearance rate. The following two considerations are important in dose determinations:

1. Does all the drug administered reach plasma?; for instance, with oral administration, it is not. Therefore, if only F (bioavailability) fraction of the drug administered reaches plasma, dose rate must be increased by replacing Cl with $(Cl \div F)$. To sum-up: Dose rate $= \dfrac{C_{st}Cl}{F}$. This is simply a linear relationship between dose and C_{st} which is generally true for drugs following I – Order kinetics.

2. In case of drugs following I – Order kinetics in the beginning and then changing over to 0 – Order kinetics, Dose – Rate $= \dfrac{V_{max}C}{k_m + C}$ where V_{max} is maximum rate of drug elimination, C, the plasma concentration and k_m, the plasma concentration when elimination rate is half maximal or half of maximum value.

5.2 Dose *vs* Response

In highly generalized terms, dose-response relationship is hyperbolic; if E is the observed effect at a concentration of C and EC_{max} and EC_{50} are the concentrations producing maximum and 50% of maximum effects, then, $E = \dfrac{E_{max}C}{C + EC_{50}}$.

5.2.1 Median Effective/Lethal Dose

Estimation of LD_{50} or Median Lethal or Semi-lethal dose is an important aspect in pharmacodynamics. A drug under test for toxicity, is administered to a group of experimental (lab) animals. The dosage is given in such a way that each dosage is a product of a constant (**dose factor**) and the preceding dose so that on the logarithmic scale, the difference between any two consecutive doses becomes same in an experiment.

5.2.1.1 Example

A particular drug was under trial for toxicity and the following dosages (l = 5) were employed on 10 lab animals (n) each. The mortality was recorded as % of the total animals employed for the particular dosage. We now need to calculate the dose that can cause 50% mortality among lab animals.

Note: Dose factor (d) is 3 in this case and therefore, on logarithmic transformation, the difference between two consecutive dosages is log 3 = 0.4771.

Dosage level (l)	Dose, ppm	Log dose, (x_i)	Number of deaths (a)	% Dead, (y_i)	Number survived	$a*l$
1	333.3	2.5229	0	0	10	0
2	1000	3.0000	3	30	7	6
3	3000	3.4771	5	50	5	15
4	9000	3.9542	7	70	3	28
5	27000(H)	4.4313	10	100	0	50
Totals		17.3855	25 (A)	250	25 (C)	99 (B)

$$\sum_{i=1}^{l} x_i^2 = 62.7274; \ \sum_{i=1}^{l} y_i^2 = 18300; \ \sum_{i=1}^{l} x_i y_i = 983.7790; \ \bar{x} = 3.4771 \ (3000 \ \text{ppm}); \ \bar{y} = $$

50%; $SS_X = 2.2763$; $SS_Y = 5800$; $SCP_{XY} = 114.5040$; $a = -124.9118$; $b_{yx} = 50.3039$; $MSS_e = (SS_Y - b_{yx} \times SCP_{XY}) \div (k-2) = 13.3341$; table value of $t_{3,0.05} = 3.182$, $\mathrm{Var}(b_{yx}) = MSS_e \div SS_X = 5.8578$

Transformation of dose on to logarithmic scale results in linear association between log dose (x_i) and % Death (y_i). Therefore, a linear equation is fit for the above data (see Chapter "**Association between variables I**" for details): $y_i = -124.9118 + 50.3039 x_i$. But, what is needed is dose at which there will be 50% deaths; in other words, we have to predict the value of independent variable (inverse prediction). Hence, by rearranging

terms in the linear equation, $x_i = \dfrac{(y_i - a)}{b_{yx}}$. Now, by putting $y_i = 50$ (for LD_{50} or median

lethal or semi-lethal dose) we get $x_i = 3.4771$ on log units which on retransformation to original scale gives the median lethal dose as 2999.85 or 3000 ppm.

This is a rare case where independent variable is predicted for a known value of dependent variable (Inverse prediction). If $k = b_{yx}^2 - t_{\alpha,(n-2)}^2 \mathrm{var}(b_{yx}) = 2471.1714$, confidence limits can be obtained by solving

$$\bar{x} + \frac{b_{yx}(y_i - \bar{y})}{k} \pm \frac{t}{k} \sqrt{MSS_e \left[\frac{(y_i - \bar{y})^2}{SS_x} + k\left(1 + \frac{1}{l}\right) \right]}$$

at set α (*see* **Section 3.2.2.2** Chapter "**Association between variables I**"). Since $y_i = \bar{y}$

in the present case, 95% confidence limits will be $\bar{x} \pm \dfrac{t}{k} \sqrt{MSS_e \left[k\left(1 + \dfrac{1}{l}\right) \right]} = 3.4771 \pm$

0.2560 log units. In original scale, the values will be 3000 ± 1747.5 ppm

$(se = \dfrac{1}{k} \sqrt{MSS_e \left[k\left(1 + \dfrac{1}{l}\right) \right]} = 0.0805$ or 559.2 ppm$)$. In original scale, $s = se^2$ and therefore,

on log scale $s = 2*se = 0.161$; in original scale $s = 1137.7$ ppm (*see* Chapter "**Transformations**" for procedure of retransformation of se/s values on log scale to original scale).

Note: Same procedure can be adapted to estimate effective concentration (EC_{50}) or median effective dose (ED_{50}) is calculated with % effectively treated on the y-axis; the ratio of LD_{50} to ED_{50} is called the **Therapeutic Index (TI)**. Similarly, tissue-culture infection dosage ($TCID_{50}$), egg infection dosage (EID_{50}), egg lethal dose (ELD_{50}) and plaque forming units (pfu) are also estimated.

5.2.2 Arithmetic Method

The result in **Example 1.2.1.1** can be solved by an arithmetic method given by Cornfield and Mantel (1950):

$$\log LD_{50} = \log H - \log d \left(\frac{A}{n} - 0.5 \right) = \log(27000) - \log(3)* \{(25 \div 10) - 0.5\} = 3.4771 \ \text{or}$$

3000 ppm. $\log se = \dfrac{\log d}{n} \sqrt{\dfrac{C}{n-1}} = 0.0795$ or 552.2 ppm and 95% confidence intervals are given by log $LD_{50} \pm 2*(\log se)$ or 3.4771 ± 0.159 on log scale; on re-transformation, the 95% confidence limits are 3000 ± 1122.9 ppm. Further,

$$\log s = \frac{\log d}{n^2}\sqrt{n(2B-A)-A^2-\frac{n^2}{12}} = 0.158;$$ on retransformation, the s is 1115.6 ppm

Note:

1. SD is generally se^2; therefore, on log scale it will be $2*\log se$ as in the present example.

2. The difference in 95% confidence limits between regression method and arithmetic method is due to the coefficient of se employed; in the former method, table value of t at $\alpha = 0.05$ and $\upsilon = (l-2)$ i.e. 3.182 is employed whereas, in the latter the table value is assumed as 2. It is interesting that the se value by both methods is similar (0.0805 Vs 0.0795).

5.2.3 Logistic Equation

The values of dosage vs lethality (%) can be directly used to fit a logistic equation and inverse prediction made to calculate the value of dosage when lethality is 50%. If the dosages are equally spaced, method of three points can be used to fit the equation manually (*see* Chapter "**Analysis of time series**" for details); else, computer aid may be required.

6. WILDLIFE MANAGEMENT

6.1 Population Dynamics

Change in size of Population of wild animals has been found to follow an exponential trend; where N_t is the size at time t, N_{t+1} is the expected size after a lapse of a unit of time, and r, the rate of change (can be positive or negative). Usually, base of Natural logarithm is used in such equations because it has been found that most processes in nature change in proportion to $\log_e 2$ ($= 0.693147$).

By rearrangement of terms, $r = \log_e\left(\dfrac{N_{t+1}}{N_t}\right)$; for instance, let us assume that

population of a certain wild species doubled in a year; therefore, $\left(\dfrac{N_{t+1}}{N_t}\right) = 2$ or $r = $

$\log_e 2 = 0.693$ per annum; conversely, if the population had halved a year, $r = \log_e \frac{1}{2} = -0.693$ per annum.

By extending the above concept, if N_0 is the population at the beginning and N_t

after the lapse of time t, and $r = t\log_e\left(\dfrac{N_t}{N_0}\right)$. Further, if intermediate values, say

monthly data in a year or yearly data over many years is available, a simple linear equation can be fit to $N_t = N_0 e^{rt}$ by taking $\log_e$ on both sides to obtain an equation analogous to $y = a + bx$; i.e. $\log_e N_t = \log_e N_0 + rt$. Obviously, the regression coefficient is the rate of growth, r; the maximum rate of growth of a species is popularly referred to as **intrinsic rate of growth** designated r_m.

Note: It is generally agreed that r of vertebrates fluctuates around a mean value of zero.

For any species, r_m varies with body size as per $1.5W^{-0.36}$ where, W is the mean adult weight (kg).

6.1.1 Fecundity Rate (m$_x$)

In wild animals, fecundity is measured as number of females born per annum as per classes (say age groups) and designated m_x.

Age, years (x$_i$)	Sample size (f$_i$)	Pregnant/Lactating (B$_i$)	Fecundity ($m_x = B_i \div 2f_i$)*
x_1	f_1	B_1	m_{x1}
x_2	f_2	B_2	m_{x2}
x_3	f_3	B_3	m_{x3}
.	.	.	.
.	.	.	.
.	.	.	.
x_k	f_k	B_k	m_{xk}

*$2f_i$ in the denominator to indicate that same number of males in the population.

6.1.2 Mortality Rate (q$_x$) and Life Table

This is the complement of fecundity rate which measures number of animals that die during a year; this also is given as per classes (age groups).

Age, years (x$_i$)	Survivors		Mortality	
	Number (f$_i$)	Proportion ($p_i = f_i \div f_1$)	Proportion ($d_i = p_i - p_{i+1}$)	Rate $q_x =$ ($p_i - p_{i+1}$) or $d_i \div p_i$
x_1	5000(f_1)	1.00(p_1)	0.60(d_1)	0.60
x_2	2000(f_2)	0.40(p_2)	0.15(d_2)	0.375
x_3	1250(f_3)	0.25(p_3)	0.15(d_3)	0.60
x_4	500(f_4)	0.10(p_4)	.	.
.	.	.	.	.
.	.	.	.	.
x_k	f_k	p_k	d_k	q_k

Note: p_i values represent survival up to the age x_i

The above table is also referred to as **life table**. However, in the above case each animal has to be identified by banding, marking, etc. which is practically difficult. An indirect way is possible by assessing age of a living population which is as follows:

Approximately at about middle of the season of births, if age of an unbiased sample of a population of the species in question is taken, it is reasonable to assume that the sample does reflect the population parameters adequately. The same procedure to calculate the mortality as shown above can be used. On the same lines, unbiased sample of deaths (collection of skulls or other remains) can be used for indirect estimation of mortality rate.

6.1.3 Equation of Population Dynamics

The above parameters can be combined to develop the equation of population

dynamics: $\sum_{i=1}^{k} p_i m_{x_i} e^{-rx} = 1$. If p_i and m_{xi} remain constant, then frequencies in different age groups in the Population can be described by: $S_x = p_x e^{-rx}$ also called Stable Age Distribution. When $r = 0$, Stable Age Distribution is known as Stationary Age Distribution.

6.2 Herbivores

Herbivores primarily depend on plants for food; the latter depends on land and rainfall. A multiple regression equation (*see* Chapter "**Association between variables II**" for details) can be fit for growth of plant biomass (y) as a function of land (x as well as x^2) and rainfall (R). To set the minimum levels for the biomass to grow, y can be set to zero and R calculated (isocline of zero growth).

6.2.1 Functional Response

This describes consumption by animals depending on the availability of resource. If I is the intake per d, I_{max} is the maximum (satiating) intake per d, V is the volume (level) of resource, then the intake follows an exponential decay form $I = I_{max}\left(1 - e^{-bV}\right)$; the regression coefficient (b) indicates the reduction in V per d or **grazing efficiency**; the reciprocal of b is the value of V at which 63% $(1 - e^{-1})$ of satiating intake is consumed. Let us consider this equation for two species as reported by Short (1987):

Species	Weight	I_{max}	b	$I_{max}/W^{0.75}$
Kangaroo	35 kg	892 g/d	−0.012	62.0 g/d
Rabbit	2 kg	102 g/d	−0.007	60.6 g/d

Note: When I_{max} was considered on absolute weights, the species appeared to differ considerably; but when considered on **metabolic body size ($W^{0.75}$)**, both species are simply comparable as far as satiating intake is concerned!

6.2.2 Numerical Response

This studies the effect of resource on animal numbers. Generally, like functional response, numerical response also is an asymptote (reaching a plateau and remaining so in spite of extra resource available) and is describes by an exponential equation $r = -a + c\left(1 - e^{-dV}\right)$ where r is the rate of growth, a is the maximum rate of decrease which is countered by c; therefore $(c - a) = r_m$, the maximum rate of increase; d is the **Demographic efficiency**, the ability of the population to withstand shortage of resources and grow. If $r_m = x$, **Intrinsic rate of increase** is e^x and on % basis it will be $(e^x - 1) \times 100$. For example, if $r_m = 0.25$ for a species, $e^x = 1.284$ or 28.4% increase per annum.

6.3 Competition within and between Species

Most of these follow exponential form and such equations can be fit by procedure shown in Chapter "**Analysis of time series**".

6.4 Predators

6.4.1 Functional Response

This refers to response of predators as a function of density of prey.

6.4.1.1 Type I

Number of prey caught increases directly with prey density (linear association). In other words, % prey eaten remains almost constant regardless of prey density.

6.4.1.2 Type II

Number of prey caught increases to an asymptote with prey density; or, % prey population consumed reduces as prey density increases.

6.4.1.3 Type III

When number of prey caught is plotted against prey density, a sigmoid curve is obtained; that means, at low prey density, the increments in number of prey caught are slower which increase at intermediate prey densities and again plateau at higher prey densities. If % prey eaten is plotted against prey density, it increases rapidly till intermediate prey density and falls rapidly thereafter.

6.4.2 Numerical Response

Predator population changes its reproduction and migration (immigration and emigration) patterns depending on the prey density which is referred to as numerical response. Generally, predator density increases to an asymptote with prey density.

6.4.3 Consumption of Prey

6.4.3.1 Sharing

It is extremely difficult to give a satisfactory mathematical model for the way the killed prey is shared by the predators due mainly to factors such as behavior, numbers involved, hunger, previous meal, prey density, idiosyncrasies and many others which are by themselves beyond total mathematical analysis. In any case, a very simple model assuming only two females in a habitat sharing a kill one after another is given below:

Suppose P = shared kill per unit time, kg/s; W = weight, kg; E = encounter rate/s, it follows that $P = W*E$ kg/s.

Many factors determine each of W and E; for instance, W depends on:

1. Proportion of meat edible, factor C_e; always < 1, generally 0.75 analogous to dressing % in meat animals
2. Amount of meat eaten by the female that has killed the prey, W_f
3. Amount of meat eaten by scavengers before the second arrives, W_{sc}
4. Proportion of meat for each of the females after II joins the I female; factor C_p, assumed to be equal for both and obviously < 1
5. Amount of meat left-over after both predators have eaten, W_s

Let us consider each of the above factors one by one; Out of W kg of kill, C_e*W is available as edible (contents of the gastrointestinal tract for instance is not edible); of this W_f would have been eaten by the first female soon after killing the prey; therefore, $C_e \times W - W_f$ is left of which W_{sc} would have been consumed by scavengers leaving $C_e \times W - W_f - W_{sc}$; of this, both females $C_p \times (C_e \times W - W_f - W_{sc})$; C_p generally considered as 0.50. Finally some portion of the kill is left as unused, designated, W_{left}. Therefore, the total weight of W kg is partitioned as $[C_p(C_eW - W_f - W_{sc}) - W_{left}]$.

Similarly, E depends on:
1. Prey density, N/m^2
2. Capture rate per female, K/s and
3. Searching rate, S/s
4. Time available, T

Therefore, $E = N \times K \times S \times T$ per m^2.

Now, substituting for W and E in the equation $P = W \times E$, we get $P = [C_p(C_eW - W_f - W_{sc}) - W_{left}]NKST$. To compare prey intake by various species, P is divided by adult female body weight (BW, kg) of the predator to get weighted P or $P_w = (P \div BW)$.

6.4.3.1.1 Example

Suppose a lioness hunted a buffalo weighing about 560 kg (W). Of this ¾ (C_e) only is edible (420 kg) and the lioness who hunted the prey ate away 60 kg soon after hunting (W_f) and left. This was followed by a pack of Hyena scavenging 20 kg of the kill to leave 340 kg of the meat. This is followed by another lioness joining the first one and eat, sharing equally ($C_p = ½$), 140 kg each, leave-out 60 kg (W_{left}). Assuming prey density as 0.0005 per m^2 (N), capture rate per female is 0.0006/s (K), searching rate is 0.002/s (S) and time available is 3 hours (10800 s, T), we can estimate shared kill per unit time i.e. P as $[C_p(C_eW - W_f - W_{sc}) - W_{left}]NKST = 0.0007$ kg/s or 61.6 kg/d.

6.4.3.2 Eaten by the predator itself

This is rare in wild animals; but domestic animals like cats do eat their prey without sharing. Again, a mathematical model is difficult; but one on extremely generalized assumptions is given below:

As in case of shared kill, P is a function of W and K or $P = W \times K$; of these, W is a function of 1) proportion of meat edible, factor C_e (because, some portion may decompose and only C_e times the original amount will be edible; $C_e < 1$) and 2) amount of meat eaten by scavengers, W_{sc}

Therefore, $P = (C_e - W_{sc}) \times K$. As in case of shared kill, to compare prey intake by various species, P is divided by adult female body weight (BW, kg) of the predator to get weighted P or $P_w = (P \div BW)$.

It is also adequately recorded that wild animals eat maximum at the first time and subsequently at a much reduced rate; if we assume that two females do meet, considering that E is the encounter rate and S is the searching rate (both independent), the probability that two females meet over time T (s) is $E \times S \times T$. With this, if W_{max} is the maximum weight a female can eat per unit time (kg/s) and W_{min} is the minimum weight a female has to eat for survival (kg/s), the maximum value of W_f can be estimated as follows:

1. When $S \times N < 1$: $W_f = TW_{max} + W_{min}\dfrac{(1-T)}{SN}$

2. When $S \times N > 1$: $W_f = \dfrac{W_{max}}{SN}$

6.4.3.3 Total weight consumed by a predator

We have to consider yet another factor; the predator always will have a variety in its meal. Therefore, assuming that its meal consists of different prey weighing $X_1, X_2 \ldots$

X_i ($i = 1, 2 \ldots k$) kg forming $Y_1, Y_2 \ldots Y_i$ (%) of the meal, then the total weight consumed

by the predator is given by $\dfrac{\sum\limits_{i=1}^{k} X_i Y_i}{\sum\limits_{i=1}^{k} Y_i}$

6.4.3.3.1 Example

Suppose a lion kills a wildebeest weighing 120 kg, a zebra weighing 200 kg, a buffalo weighing 560 kg and a gazelle weighing 10 kg and eats 25, 20, 20 and 30 % of the prey, respectively, the total meat consumed is given by:

$$\frac{\left(120 \times 25 + 200 \times 20 + 560 \times 20 + 10 \times 30\right)}{\left(25 + 20 + 20 + 30\right)} = 194.7 \text{ kg.}$$

The following values are reported for wild animals (Turner and Bateson, 2000): W_{max} = 20% and 8% BW per d for large smaller felids, respectively. W_{min} as % of BW is 3.5 (Lion), 3.8 (Tiger), Jaguar (3.9), Leopard (8.1), Cheetah (7.1) etc. C_e is considered ¾ to obtain edible body weight of the prey (similar to dressing % in meat animals) and C_p as ½ considering both females equal. Value of searching rate, S can be assessed as S_p*R where S_p is the speed the predator can travel (in m/s) and R (in m) is the range which the species can survey for another female from a random point in the habitat. The value of R depends on the type of habitat; but, for smaller species, half of those values for larger species are used.

6.5 Counting Animals

6.5.1 Sampling: Transects vs Quadrats

Transects are imaginary lines oriented at right angles so that rows form transects, running across the grain of the country, up the slope, across a river (than parallel) to cover as much variability as possible but variation between transects is as minimum as possible. Quadrats are also imaginary lines to form 4 units for sampling. Obviously, quadrats are likely to result in higher variability than transects. Sampling in either case is preferred to be strictly random or restricted random sampling to systematic sampling.

The following notations will be used for various estimates:

Y and y for number of animals in a region of size A and a sample, respectively

A and a for area of the region and a sample, respectively

D or d for estimate of density

n for number of sampled units

se(Y), se(D) for standard error of Y and D, respectively

If an area A sq km is divided into n transects each of area a sq km, then sampling intensity = ($na \div A$). If each of the units had y_i animals, the following formulae are used for estimation:

Model	Density
Simple	$$D = \dfrac{\sum\limits_{i=1}^{n} y_i}{\sum\limits_{i=1}^{n} a_i}$$
se, with replacement	$$se(D) = \left(\dfrac{1}{a}\right)\sqrt{\dfrac{\sum\limits_{i=1}^{n} y_i^2 - \dfrac{\left(\sum\limits_{i=1}^{n} y_i\right)^2}{n}}{n(n-1)}}$$
se, without replacement	FPC*se with replacement
Ratio	Same as simple estimate
se, with replacement	$$se(D) = \left(\dfrac{n}{\sum\limits_{i=1}^{n} a_i}\right)\sqrt{\dfrac{\sum\limits_{i=1}^{n} y_i^2 + D^2\sum\limits_{i=1}^{n} a_i^2 - 2D\sum\limits_{i=1}^{n} a_i d_i}{n(n-1)}}$$
se, without replacement	FPC*se with replacement
PPS	$$d = \dfrac{1}{n}\sum\limits_{i=1}^{n} \dfrac{y_i}{a_i}$$
se, with replacement	$$se(d) = \sqrt{\dfrac{\sum\limits_{i=1}^{n}\left(\dfrac{y_i}{a_i}\right)^2 - \dfrac{\left[\sum\limits_{i=1}^{n}\left(\dfrac{y_i}{a_i}\right)\right]^2}{n}}{n(n-1)}}$$

In all cases, actual number estimates can be obtained by $Y = AD$ and $se(Y) = A*se(D)$ using the corresponding A and D values; **finite population correction**, FPC $= \sqrt{1 - \dfrac{\sum\limits_{i=1}^{n} a_i}{A}}$; which, being near unity on most occasions, is ignored.

If observations of animals are made from a distance involving angles and radial distance of the animal from the observer, the latter designated r, suppose k number of animals is sighted and L is the length of line of march, then $D = \dfrac{1}{2L}\sum k\left(\dfrac{1}{r}\right)$. Alternatively, if Δ is the arbitrary distance perpendicular from the line of march, $k1$ and $k2$ are number of animals on either side of the line-transect at distances 0 to Δ and Δ to 2Δ, respectively, then $D = \dfrac{3k_1 - k_2}{4L\Delta}$

6.5.2 *Indirect Methods*

6.5.2.1 Index method

If I_1 and I_2 are the indices of population size before and after C number of animals was removed, Y_1, population size at the time of $I_1 = I_1 \times C \div (I_1 - I_2)$. Proportion of population removed, $p = (I_1 - I_2) \div I_1$, $q = (1 - p)$; hence, $Var(Y) = Y^2 \left(\dfrac{q}{p}\right)^2 \left(\dfrac{1}{I_1} + \dfrac{1}{I_2}\right)$ and $se(Y) = \sqrt{Var(Y)}$.

6.5.2.2 Change of ratio method

Suppose the entire population is divisible into two distinct classes, x and y (on age, sex, etc.) making proportions of p_1 and $(1 - p_1)$, respectively, from which C_x individuals are removed or added from class x causing a change of proportions to p_2 and $(1 - p_2)$, respectively, then the population size before manipulation is give by $\dfrac{C_X - p_2 C}{p_2 - p_1}$ where $C = (C_x + C_y)$.

6.5.2.3 Mark and recapture method

In this method, some animals in a sample are marked and released. After a known time, another sample is taken and the ratio of marked to unmarked animals is taken as the criterion to estimate population size. Several models are available for this method; the Petersen model with Bailey's correction is as follows:

If M animals in a sample were marked and later on, out of n animals captured m were marked, the population size (Y) after Bailey's correction is given by $\dfrac{M(n+1)}{(m+1)}$

with an estimate of se as $\sqrt{\dfrac{M^2(n+1)(n-m)}{(m+1)^2(m+2)}}$. It is well recognized that the distribution of the estimates is highly skewed and hence, se value is not generally used to construct confidence limits; instead, if $a = (m \div n)$, 95% confidence limits of a are $\pm 1.96 \sqrt{\dfrac{a(1-a)}{n}}$

where 1.96 is the value of normal deviate at $á = 0.05$. Since $Y = (M \div a)$, confidence limits of Y can be set-up by dividing M by upper and lower confidence limits of a.

6.5.2.4 Frequency of capture model

In this model capturing is taken-up many times, usually on successive days; number of times the same animal is caught is recorded and a frequency distribution table is made as follows:

Number of times same animal captured (i)	1	2	......	k
Number of animals, (f_i)	f_1	f_2	......	f_k

It is obvious from the above table that $\sum_{i=1}^{k} f_i$ is the number of animals that are caught

at least once. In other words, the population has at least $\sum_{i=1}^{k} f_i$ animals. If f_0 is the

number of animals that are not caught even once, then $Y = f_0 + \sum_{i=1}^{k} f_i$. Many distributions

are employed to estimate f_0; for instance, Poisson, geometric, negative-binomial etc.

6.5.2.5 Method of two-counts

Suppose two independent surveys are conducted, to estimate the number of animals, nests, etc. may be aerial and ground, the following are the possibilities (frequencies):

		II Survey		
		Counted	Missed	Totals
I Survey	Counted	B	S_2	R_1
	Missed	S_1	M	R_2
		C_1	C_2	N

By application of Rules of Probability (*see* Chapter "**Probability**"), probability of counting in the I Survey, $P_1 = (B \div R_1)$; in the II Survey, $P_2 = (B \div C_1)$, $M = S_1 \times S_2 \div B$ and estimate of Population size, $Y = R_1{}^*C_1 \div B$ which after correction for bias will be

$Y = \{(R_1 + 1) \times (C_1 + 1) \div (B + 1)\} - 1$ with a variance estimate of $\dfrac{S_1 S_2 (R_1 + 1)(C_1 + 1)}{(B+1)^2 (B+2)}$.

6.6 Consequences of Inbreeding

Basic concept of inbreeding is outlined in **Section 1.2.9**. Many books on population genetics give details of detrimental effects of inbreeding. One of such effects is reduction in effective Population size (N_e) from N to $\{N \div (1 + F)\}$. In domestic animals which are specifically bred by careful planning, problems of Ne are fewer; however, wild populations follow poisson distribution and hence high variability is expected.

For instance, in a stable population, an average of a male and female will replace each parent; hence, family size, $m = 2$ with variance, $V_m = 2$ because it is a Poisson variate. Obviously, probability of 0,1,2,3,4,5 offsprings (r) are 0.135, 0.271, 0.271, 0.180, 0.090 and 0.036, respectively (*see* **Section 2**, Chapter "**Discrete probabilty distributions**" for details). N_e can be estimated as $\dfrac{4N - 2}{V_m + 2}$; hence, if variance is ≈ 2, $N_e = N$; else, it starts reducing rapidly.

Wild populations vary in size as well; if N is the number of adults in the previous generation, and m is the mean family size (a poisson variate), then $N_e = \dfrac{Nm - 1}{\left(m - 1 + \dfrac{V_m}{m}\right)}$;

it can be noted that if $m = 2$, again $N_e = \dfrac{4N - 2}{V_m + 2}$. Dividing both sides by N we get an idea of N_e as a proportion of original population size.

6.6.1.1 Example

In Asiatic lions, it is reported (Frankham *et al.*, 2002) that $m = 1.65$, $V_m = 32.65$. Hence, by the above equation we can estimate that $(Ne \div N) = 0.081$; that means only about 8% of the adults represent the population or only 8% of the adults contribute to the next generaton. Obviously, this triggers a vicious cycle of inbreeding, loss of hetero-zygosity (genetic diversity), further reduction in N_e. It will not be surprising that the population of Asiatic lions may become extinct if proper conservation strategies are not taken-up.

6.7 Testing of Hypotheses and Analysis of Data

These methods are described in separate chapters of this publication; depending on the nature of data, suitable method can be chosen and applied.

7. GENERAL GUIDELINES FOR CHOOSING ANALYTICAL METHOD

The following table gives a general idea as to which type of data is suitable for different statistical procedures. More importantly, it helps plan the experiment depending on the type (distribution) of data expected so that sample size, type of test(s), level of significance, power (accuracy) of test, etc. can be planned **before** conduct of an experiment. It is in the fitness of things to once again reiterate that **data has to be obtained on a well planned statistical design and one should not attempt fitting a design on the data already collected.**

Distribution	2 samples	> 2 samples	Agreement/ Association
Categorical	χ^2, Z, Fisher's exact test, McNemar's test	χ^2, Cochran's Q test	Kappa statistic
Count/continuous, non–normal	Mann-Whitney test, Wilcoxon rank-sum test, Wilcoxon signed-rank test	Kruskal-Wallis or Friedman's ANOVA by ranks	Spearman's rank correlation coefficient
Continuous, normal	Independent sample or Paired t test	ANOVA with or without repetition values	Pearson's product-moment correlation coefficient

22

Multivariate Analysis

1. INTRODUCTION

At the outset it is necessary to note that multivariate analyses involve matrices of higher order, iterations, inequalities etc. and hence use of computers is mandatory. Several softwares are available with specific package on multivariate analysis. The reader is advised to buy the requisite software which also includes instructions and/or tutorials along with examples. Further, several publications are also available on use of computer–based programs for multivariate analyses. Hence, only concepts involved in multivariate analyses will be highlighted in this chapter.

As the name suggests "Multivariate analysis" deals with analysis of the data involving more than 1 variable which could be either independent or correlated to one another. If the variables are correlated, the statistical treatment becomes more complex depending on number, nature, intensity (ies), and magnitude (s) of such correlation (s). Such associations between variables are given due weightage in the analytical procedures and hence, the variables are considered as random variables for developing the analytical models/techniques.

In most multivariate methods, all the variables involved are assumed to have a joint (combined) probability distribution which, in turn, is assumed to be Normal although it may not be appropriate especially with nominal and/or ordinal data. The reasons why Normal distribution is assumed are essentially the same as in case of univariate analysis (see **Chapter "Continuous probability distributions", Section 1.4**).

Interestingly, most real situations, especially with animal experimentations, involve multiple variables. For instance, let us assume that one has to evaluate a broiler farm. The information on floor space, ventilation, vaccination, feed intake, weight gain, feed efficiency, livability, welfare, microenvironment, etc. are obtained on the farm. It can be noticed that each of the variables listed is random and variables like weight gain and feed efficiency are related as is livability. Similarly, ventilation is related to growth and livability, etc. Not all the variables need be metric; for instance, data on welfare could be ordinal and/or nominal. It is reasonable to consider as many variables as possible to obtain information so as to reduce cost of experimentation as well and also to help more appropriate conclusions.

Further, analyzing only growth data without feed consumption/feed efficiency/livability has a very limited value. In the same way, many other interrelationships are too strong to be analyzed separately. Therefore, multivariate analysis becomes mandatory.

In simple terms, multivariate analysis involves the analysis of combination of random and inter-related variables in a single or multiple relationship(s), as the case may be. To be specific, if the interrelationships are so strong that the variables can not be considered separately, multivariate analysis becomes more appropriate but not by mere number of variables.

It follows that when data on many variables are available, one can think of univariate analysis for each of the variables in question. Such treatment is not only cumbersome but also fails to recognize combined play of all the variables in unison thereby weakening the conclusion (s) drawn. Therefore, it is necessary to recognize a combination of variables that play a major role and consider all of them together including any association (s) *inter se* and draw conclusion (s) under an assumption of multivariate normality.

In most methods, the model is fit and tested utilizing a sample/part data and the same is validated on the main/another set of data.

2. MEANS, VARIANCES AND COVARIANCES

In multivariate distributions, more than 1 (possibly) p correlated random variables $(y_1, y_2 \dots y_p)$ are involved where $E(y_i) = \mu_i$. Obviously more than 1 means $(\mu_1, \mu_2 \dots \mu_p)$ and variances $(\sigma_{11}, \sigma_{22} \dots \sigma_{pp})$ result. The former is usually represented in the form of a column vector y. Since the variables could also be correlated, the variances and covariances (σ_{ij}) are represented in the form of $n \times n$ matrix M with the diagonal elements being variances.

$$y = \begin{bmatrix} y_1 \\ y_2 \\ \cdot \\ \cdot \\ \cdot \\ y_p \end{bmatrix} \text{ and matrix } M = \begin{bmatrix} \sigma_{11} & \sigma_{12} & \cdots & \sigma_{1p} \\ \sigma_{21} & \sigma_{22} & \cdots & \sigma_{2p} \\ \cdot & \cdot & \cdots & \cdot \\ \cdot & \cdot & \cdots & \cdot \\ \sigma_{p1} & \sigma_{p2} & \cdots & \sigma_{pp} \end{bmatrix} \text{ where } = E[(y_i - \mu_i)(y_j - \mu_j)] = E(y_i y_j) - \mu_i \mu_j.$$

Since $i = j$ and $\sigma_{ij} = \sigma_{ji}$, variance-covariance matrix M is square symmetric and assumed to be positive.

Notes: In multivariate analysis, all variables are generally designated y_i's because it is not necessary that one or some of them need be dependent on others.

Variance which is generally designated σ_i^2 is designated σ_{ii} to facilitate understanding while working with matrices.

Total variance is given by $\sum_{i=1}^{p} \sigma_{ii}$ and **generalized variance** = determinant of M or

Det $|M|$; both measuring overall variability in y and with their own limitations.

Pearson's (product–moment) correlation coefficient between the variables's (*see* Chapter "Association between variables I", Section 4" for details) is represented by matrix $R = \begin{bmatrix} \rho_{11} & \rho_{12} & \cdots & \rho_{1p} \\ \rho_{21} & \rho_{22} & \cdots & \rho_{2p} \\ \cdot & \cdot & \cdots & \cdot \\ \cdot & \cdot & \cdots & \cdot \\ \rho_{p1} & \rho_{p2} & \cdots & \rho_{pp} \end{bmatrix}$. Naturally, the diagonal elements will be unity and R

is also square symmetric. Since $\rho_{ij} = \dfrac{\sigma_{ij}}{\sqrt{\sigma_{ii}\sigma_{jj}}}$, matrix R can be represented

as $(M_D)^{-\frac{1}{2}}(M)(M_D)^{-\frac{1}{2}}$ where M_D is the diagonal element of M wherein the diagonal elements are variances, the non-diagonal elements are zero and $M_D = (M_D)^{\frac{1}{2}}(M_D)^{\frac{1}{2}}$.

2.1   Partial Correlation Coefficient

If the (joint) probability distribution (density) function of a vector y (i.e., $y_1, y_1, \ldots y_p$), is denoted by $f(y)$ then marginal distribution y_1 denoted $f(y_1)$is a subvector of y, i.e.,

$\begin{bmatrix} y_1 & \cdots & y_{p_1} \end{bmatrix}$. To obtain $f_1(y_1)$, matrix y has to be subdivided as $y = \begin{bmatrix} y_{1_{p_1}} \\ y_{2_{(p-p_1)}} \end{bmatrix}$ (each

element being a column vector with p_1 and $p - p_1$ elements, respectively) and y_2 has to be integrated out from $f(y)$. Then conditional distribution of y_2 when y_1 has been fixed,

denoted by $f^*(y_2/y_1)$ is given by $\dfrac{f(y)}{f_1(y_1)}$. If is designated y_i (a $p_1 \times 1$ vector) and $y_{2_{(p-p_1)}}$ is

designated y_j [a $(p - p_1) \times 1$ vector], then Pearson's correlation coefficient between them is the partial correlation coefficient between two components of y_1 i.e., y_i and y_j (being conditional on y_j).

Obviously, with partitioning of y as shown above, matrix (M) will be subdivided as

follows: $M = \begin{bmatrix} M_{11} & M_{12} \\ M_{21} & M_{22} \end{bmatrix}$ where M_{11} is a $p_1 \times p_1$, M_{12} is a $p_1 \times p - p_1$, M_{21} is a $p - p_1 \times p$

and M_{22} is a $p - p_1 \times p - p_1$ variance-covariance matrix.

If $M(y_1/y_2)$ is $p_1 \times p_1$ is the variance-covariance matrix y_1 for given y_2, then, population correlation coefficient between y_i and y_j where i and j take the values from $1, 2 \ldots p_1$ is

given by: $\rho_{ij.p_{1+1}, \ldots p} = \dfrac{M_{ij}}{\sqrt{M_{ii}M_{jj}}}$ and matrix of all partial correlation coefficients, P

contains elements $\rho_{ij.p_{1+1}, \ldots p; i,j = 1, 2 \ldots p_1}$. P can be obtained by $M_{Dij}^{-\frac{1}{2}}M_{Dij}M_{Dij}^{-\frac{1}{2}}$ where indicates diagonal elements.

Further, it will be more useful to find strength of correlation between two variables among many variables in consideration after eliminating the effects of other variables. In other words, correlation coefficient between y_i and y_j where i and j take the values from $1, 2 \ldots p$ conditional on all y_k such that $k = 1, 2, \ldots p$ and $k \neq i$ and $k \neq j$. This can be achieved by calculating maximum correlation coefficient between one of the variables (say y_1) with the linear combination of rest of the variables (say y_2, a $p-1 \times 1$

vector) by computing $\dfrac{\left[M_{12}M_{22}^{-1}M_{21}\right]^{1/2}}{M_{11}^{1/2}}$ where $y = \begin{bmatrix} y_{1_{p_1}} \\ y_{2_{(p-p_1)}} \end{bmatrix} = \begin{bmatrix} M_{11} & M_{12} \\ M_{21} & M_{22} \end{bmatrix}$. This correlation coefficient is the multiple correlation coefficient and its square is the population coefficient of determination which indicates the proportion of variance explained by the regression involved (same as R^2 explained in Chapter "Association between variables I, Section 3.2.2.1.1.2")

If the random variable y_1 is replaced by a random vector, the multiple correlation coefficient is referred to as **Canonical correlation coefficient**.

3. MULTIVARIATE NORMALITY

Extending the concept of normal distribution explained in Chapter "**Continuous Probability distributions**", **Section 1**, the density function is defined by

$$f(y) = \dfrac{1}{(2\pi)^{p/2}\,M^{1/2}}e^{-\frac{1}{2}(y-\mu)'M^{-1}(y-\mu)}$$ where μ is the mean and M is the variance-covariance

matrix. This is also generally denoted by $y \sim N_p\,(\mu,\,M)$. Further, it follows that

$$\bar{y} \sim N_P\left(\mu, M/n\right).$$

3.1 Sampling from Multivariate Normal Distribution (MND)

Sample means and variances from a univariate Normal population are distributed as $N \sim (\mu, \sigma^2)$ and χ^2, respectively. Sample means and variance–covariance matrix from a Multivariate Normal population are distributed as $N_P \sim (\mu, M/n)$ and Wishart distribution (after John Wishart, 1928); the latter being a distribution of non-negative, matrix-valued random variables or "Random matrices"; in simple terms distribution of variance-covariance matrices designated as $(n-1)V \sim W_p[(n-1), M]$ meaning $\upsilon = (n-1)$ and expectation $(n-1)M$ where V is an unbiased estimator of M; the

former estimated as $V = \dfrac{1}{(n-1)}\sum_{i=1}^{n}(y_i - \bar{y})(y_i - \bar{y})' = \dfrac{1}{(n-1)}\left[\sum_{i=1}^{n}y_iy_i' - n\bar{y}\bar{y}'\right]$ and it

contains $p(p+1)/2$ number of random variables. Further, sample mean $\bar{y}$ and V are statistically independent.

Note: Superscript " ' " indicates transpose of the matrix involved

Let Y be an $n \times p$ data matrix as follows: $Y = \begin{bmatrix} y_{11} & y_{21} & \cdots & y_{p1} \\ y_{12} & y_{21} & \cdots & y_{p2} \\ \cdot & \cdot & \cdots & \cdot \\ \cdot & \cdot & \cdots & \cdot \\ y_{1n} & y_{2n} & \cdots & y_{pn} \end{bmatrix}$ and column vector

$$U_C = \begin{bmatrix} 1 \\ 1 \\ \cdot \\ \cdot \\ 1 \end{bmatrix}$$ with all elements as unity, then obviously sample means form another column

vector $\overline{Y} = \dfrac{1}{n} Y' C_U$. Replacing for $\overline{Y}$ with this vector in the equation for V, and further

rearrangement of the terms, $V = \dfrac{1}{n-1}\left(Y'Y - n\overline{y}\,\overline{y}' \right)$. Further, that $(n-1)V \sim W_p(n-1, M)$ is true has been established.

Variance-covariance matrix V, also possesses following properties: $(n-1)s_{ii} \div \sigma_{ii} \sim$
$\chi^2(n-1)$ for $i = 1, 2 \dots p$ $V = \begin{bmatrix} V_{11} & V_{12} \\ V_{21} & V_{22} \end{bmatrix}$ and $M = \begin{bmatrix} M_{11} & M_{12} \\ M_{21} & M_{22} \end{bmatrix}$ then $V_{11.2} = V_{11} - V_{12} V_{22}^{-1} V_{21}$,

$M_{11.2} = M_{11} - M_{12} M_{22}^{-1} M_{21}$, $V_{22.1} = V_{22} - V_{21} V_{11}^{-1} V_{12}$ and $M_{22.1} = M_{22} - M_{21} M_{11}^{-1} M_{12}$

$(n-1)V_{11} \sim W_{p1}[(n-1), M_{11}]$

$(n-1)V_{22} \sim W_{p2}[(n-1), M_{22}]$

$(n-1)V_{11.2} \sim W_{p1}[(n-p+p_1-1), M_{11.2}]$

$(n-1)V_{22.1} \sim W_{p2}[(n-p_1-1), M_{22.1}]$

V_{11} and $M_{22.1}$ are independently distributed

V_{22} and $M_{11.2}$ are independently distributed

If s^{ii} and σ^{ii} are the ith diagonal elements of V^{-1} and M^{-1}, respectively, then $(n-1)\sigma^{ii}/s^{ii} \sim \chi^2(n-p)$

If K is an arbitrary but fixed vector such that $K \neq 0, (n-1)\dfrac{K'VK}{K'MK} \sim \chi^2(n-1)$ and

$(n-1)\dfrac{K'M^{-1}K}{K'V^{-1}K} \sim \chi^2(n-p)$

If F is an arbitrary matrix of size $p \times q$ such that $p \leq q$, then $(n-1)FVF' \sim W_z[(n-1), FMF']$; if $p > q$, probability density for the matrix is not obtainable.

On the same lines, if V_1 and V_2 are two independent variance-covariance matrices following Wishart distribution on $\upsilon = (n_1 - 1)$ and $(n_2 - 1)$, respectively and V_i's are unbiased estimators of M; then, $\beta_1 = (V_1 + V_2)^{-\frac{1}{2}} V_1 (V_1 + V_2)^{-\frac{1}{2}}$ and $\beta_2 = V_2^{-\frac{1}{2}} V_1 V_2^{-\frac{1}{2}}$ follow matrix variate β type 1 and β type 2 distribution, respectively designated as $\beta_p\left(\dfrac{n_1-1}{2}, \dfrac{n_2-1}{2}\,\text{Type 1}\right)$ and $\beta_p\left(\dfrac{n_1-1}{2}, \dfrac{n_2-1}{2}\,\text{Type 2}\right)$, respectively.

Note: "$-\frac{1}{2}$" indicates square root of the matrix.

Details of proof for the above are beyond the scope of this publication.

3.2   Assumptions of MND

Of the many assumptions made, the following are most important:

3.2.1   Normality

This essentially refers to the shape and properties of the curve analogous to univariate (Gaussian) Normal distribution which forms the basis for all tests of hypothesis *viz.*, t, F, etc. Interestingly, even if each of the variates confirm to Normal distribution, all the variates together need not be MND; but conversely, if MND is true, each of the variates do follow Normal distribution.

3.2.1.1 Tests of Normality

Testing of Normality is more complicated than for univariate distribution. However, tests based on skewness and kurtosis are easy and quick to perform (*see* Section 3.1 above and Section 3.3.4 for calculation of skewness and kurtosis). $z_{Skewness} = \dfrac{Skewness}{\sqrt{6/n}}$ and $z_{Kurtosis} = \dfrac{Kurtosis}{\sqrt{24/n}}$ can be used usually with a critical value of ± 2.58 (or 1% significance level). Specific tests for testing normality of multivariate distribution are also available; for instance, Shapiro-Wilks test and modified Kolmogorov-Smirnov test.

3.2.2   Homoscedasticity

It is assumed that the variance of dependent variable(s) across the different independent (predictor) variables is (are) uniform. This can be tested either graphically or by statistical tests. The latter for non-metric variables is Levene test and for metric variables, equality of variance-covariance matrix can be tested by Box's M test. Heteroscedasticity, if detected, can be remedied by employing suitable transformations depending on type of relationship involved.

3.2.3   Linearity

In multivariate methods where correlations are involved *viz.*, Multiple/Logistic Regression, Factor Analysis and Structural Equation Modeling, linear relationship is assumed. This can be tested graphically or more appropriately by examining the magnitude of R^2 through regression analysis. Non-linearity can also be remedied by suitable transformation depending on the type of association between the variables.

3.2.4   Prediction Errors are Uncorrelated

In multivariate analytical methods on dependence, errors in assessing dependent variable must be uncorrelated and should have a mean 0. If all the errors are either positive or negative, the accuracy of prediction reduces. This error can result due to the differences in response of groups for the same factor(s) and same group at different times. Careful observation of the data collected can reveal such possibility(ies). Remedy for this kind of error is by including/excluding such causes in the multivariate analysis itself.

3.2.5 Transformations

Description of transformation methods can be obtained in publications on detailed multivariate analysis; however, a general transformation(s) that could be employed is tabulated below (also *see* **Chapter "Transformations"**):

Error	Description		Transformation
Non-normality	Flat distribution		Inverse $(1/y)$
	Positively skewed		Log y, $\sqrt{y}$
Heteroscedasticity	Cone shaped distribution; cone open to	Right	Inverse $(1/y)$
		Left	$\sqrt{y}$
	Frequency counts		$\sqrt{y}$
	Proportions		2 Arcsine $\sqrt{y}$
	Proportional change		Log y
Non-linearity (y = dependent variable, x = independent variable)	Line bulged towards	Right hand top corner	y^2, x^2
		Right hand bottom corner	Log $y, -1/y, \sqrt{y}, x^2$
		Left hand top corner	Log $x, -1/x, \sqrt{x}, y^2$
		Left hand bottom corner	Log $y, -1/y, \sqrt{y}$, Log $x, -1/x, \sqrt{x}$

Adapted from: Hair *et al.*, 2010

3.2.6 Non-Metric Data: Dummy Variables

In multivariate analysis, non-metric data are not uncommon; for instance, sex of the animals, overall acceptance of a product, liking a particular farm enterprise, etc. Each of such variables can be converted to metric scale by introducing a dummy variable. For example, if male and female are coded x_1 and x_2, respectively, x_1 can be assigned a value 1 if it is male and 0 if it is not. Similarly, x_2 can be assigned a value 1 if it is female and 0 if it is not. Likewise, any number of dummy variables can be introduced. Hence, a variable which takes the value 1 or 0 depending on whether it possesses a particular character or not, respectively is called a "Dummy variable". However, there are other alternatives of dummy variables in which they take values (–) 1 and 1 (effects coding) or 1, 0 and 0 (indicator coding), etc. Such changes depend on the number and nature of such non-metric variables. In case of indicator coding a dummy variable may get 0 for all the characters under consideration.

Use of dummy variables is common in multiple regression and discriminant analysis because the constants (coefficients) indicate quantitative (metric) relationship.

3.3 Multivariate Sampling Statistics and their Distributions

It is shown above that $\bar{y} \sim N_P\left(\mu, \frac{M}{n}\right)$ and $(n-1)V \sim W_P(n-1, M)$. Therefore, any linear combination of $\bar{y}$ like $K'\bar{y}$ given that K is non-zero follows a multivariate Normal distribution with mean $K\mu$ and variance $\frac{K'MK}{n}$. In addition, $(n-1)\frac{K'VK}{K'MK} \sim \chi^2(n-1)$ with $\bar{y}$ and V being independently distributed.

3.3.1 t-Test

In view of the above, extending the concept of t-test (*see* Chapter "**Tests of hypothesis**"),

$$t = \frac{K'(\bar{Y} - \mu)}{\sqrt{K'MK/n}} = \frac{\sqrt{n}K'(\bar{Y} - \mu)}{\sqrt{K'MK}} \text{ follows } t\text{-distribution on } \upsilon = (n-1).$$

3.3.2 z-Test

To test the H_0 = Population vector (μ) is equal to given vector (μ'), since

$$\bar{y} \sim N_P\left(\mu, \frac{M}{n}\right), z = \frac{(\bar{y} - \mu)}{\sqrt{M/n}} = \sqrt{n}M^{-1/2}(\bar{y} - \mu) \text{ and } z \sim N_P(0, I) \text{ where } z \text{ is the Standard}$$

Normal Deviate and I is the identity matrix.

Note: Since for each of the variables, z is distributed with mean 0, variance 1, identity matrix is indicated.

3.3.2.1 Case–1: $H_0: \mu = \mu'$ (when M is known)

$$\sum_{i=1}^{p} z_i^2 = z'z = \left[\sqrt{n}M^{-1/2}(\bar{y} - \mu')\right]'\left[\sqrt{n}M^{-1/2}(\bar{y} - \mu')\right] = n(\bar{y} - \mu')' M^{-1}(\bar{y} - \mu') \text{ and } z'z \text{ follows}$$

$\chi^2 \sim$ on $\upsilon = p$.

3.3.2.2 Case–2: $H_0: \mu = \mu'$ (when M is not known): Hotelling's T^2

By replacing M in the equation under Section 3.2.2.1 by V, we get the Statistic

$$T^2 = n(\bar{y} - \mu')' V^{-1}(\bar{y} - \mu'); \text{ however, } n \geq p \text{ to allow inverse of } V.$$

Finally, $\dfrac{n-p}{p(n-1)}T^2$ follows F distribution with $\upsilon_1 = p$ and $\upsilon_2 = n - p$.

3.3.3 Maximum Likelihood Estimates (MLE)

MLE of μ and M is given by $\bar{y}$ and $\dfrac{n-1}{n}V$, respectively (proof for this aspect is beyond the scope of this publication).

3.3.4 *Mardia's Skewness and Kurtosis of Multivariate Distribution*

3.3.4.1 When μ and *M* are known

$$\beta_{1,p} = E\left\{ \left(\overline{y} - \mu' \right)' M^{-1} \left(x - \mu' \right) \right\}^3 \quad \text{where } x \text{ is independent of } y \text{ and}$$

$$\beta_{2,p} = E\left\{ \left(\overline{y} - \mu' \right)' M^{-1} \left(x - \mu' \right) \right\}^2 .$$

Generally, for a multivariate normal distribution, $\beta_{1,p} = 0$ and $\beta_{2,p} = p(p + 2)$.

3.3.4.2 When μ and *M* are not known

From a sample of size n, $\beta_{1,p}$ and $\beta_{2,p}$ can be estimated as

$$\beta_{1,p} = \frac{1}{n^2} \sum_{i=1}^{n} \sum_{j=1}^{n} \left\{ \left(y_i - \overline{y} \right)' V^{-1} \left(y_j - \overline{y} \right) \right\}^3 \quad \text{and} \quad \beta_{2,p} = \frac{1}{n} \sum_{i=1}^{n} \left\{ \left(y_i - \overline{y} \right)' V^{-1} \left(y_i - \overline{y} \right) \right\}^2 .$$

In addition, d_i, is the **Mahalonobis distance** between y_i and $\overline{y}$ estimated by a sample is

given by $d_i = \sqrt{\left(y_i - \overline{y} \right)' V^{-1} \left(y_i - \overline{y} \right)}$, and $\beta_{2,p} = \frac{1}{n} \sum_{i=1}^{n} d_i^4$.

Note: Several Statistical software are available for testing Normality of multivariate data which assess based mainly on Skewness and Kurtosis. Readers interested in such details need to refer books dedicated on these topics.

3.3.5 *Akaike Information Criterion (AIC)*

AIC is a measure of the goodness of fit of an estimated statistical model as a relative measure of the information lost when a given model is used to describe the actual dependant variable. In other words it estimates difference between bias and variance. The complement of information lost, the information gain was described by Kullback and Leibler (1951) and hence known as the Kullback–Leibler divergence (also information divergence, information gain, relative entropy, or KLIC). Considering two probability distributions P (actual) and Q (theoretical, model), KLIC measures the expected number of additional information required to represent samples from P based on Q. In other words amount of information the model (or Q) does not describe or the amount of information lost due to the prediction model. Obviously, amount of information lost from Q to estimate P need not be the same from P to estimate Q. Further, lower the amount of information lost, better is the model.

In view of the above, the AIC = 2k – 2 ln(L) where k is the number of parameters in the statistical model, and L is the maximized value of the likelihood function for the

estimated model, residual sum of squares, $RSS = \sum_{i=1}^{n} \hat{\varepsilon}_i^2$. Assuming that errors in each of the models under test are (a) unknown but equal and (b) normally and independently distributed, $AIC = 2k + n\left[\ln\left(\dfrac{2\pi RSS}{n}\right) + 1\right]$ where n is the number of observations.

The term $n[\ln(2\pi)]$ is constant and hence does not influence the ranking of the models. Therefore, ignoring the term, $AIC = 2k + n\left[\ln\left(\dfrac{RSS}{n}\right)\right]$ Further, the term $\left(\dfrac{RSS}{n}\right)$ is given by MSE and hence, $AIC = n[\ln(MSE)] + 2k$.

If k is increased, the model becomes more complicated; but increases the goodness of fit. Therefore, AIC discourages inordinate increase in k by the term $2p$. This follows that a model which can yield lowest AIC with least k will be the best model.

It is also important to note that the absolute value of AIC has no meaning by itself but ranks the models depending on relative loss of information while describing the original probability distribution. In other words, AIC indicates as to how close the estimated values by the given model to the original ones.

4. CLASSIFICATION OF MULTIVARIATE ANALYTICAL METHODS

Object of study	Type of variables involved		Analytical method
Dependence	Relationship among > 1 dependent and independent variables		Structural equation modeling
	Single relationship among > 1 dependent variables	Independent and dependent variables–metric	Canonical correlation
		Independent variable–non-metric	Multiple analysis of variance
		Dependent variable–non-metric	Canonical correlation with dummy variables*
	1 dependent and > 1 independent variables	Single relationship	Dependent variable–metric	Multiple regression, conjoint analysis
		Dependent variable–non-metric	Multiple discriminant analysis, linear probability models

(Contd.)

(Contd.)

Object of study	Type of variables involved		Analytical method
Interdependence (no variable designated as dependent/ independent)	Relationship among variables		Factor analysis, confirmatory factor analysis**
	Relationship among cases/respondents		Cluster analysis
	Relationship among objects	Measurement metric	multidimensional scaling
		Measurement non-metric	Multidimensional scaling, correspondence analysis

* Non-metric variable(s) is (are) are assigned values 1 or 0 depending on whether it possesses a particular character or not, respectively.

** Principal component and principal factor analysis

Nature of variables involved in multivariate analyses			
Dependent variable	Nature	Nature of independent variables, $x_1, x_2, \ldots x_n$	Analytical method
$y_i = y_1, y_2, \ldots y_n$	Metric/non-metric	Metric/non-metric	Canonical correlation
$y_i = y_1, y_2, \ldots y_n$	Metric	Non-metric	Multiple analysis of variance
y	Non-metric	Metric	Multiple discriminant analysis
y	Metric/non-metric	Metric/non-metric	Multiple regression analysis
y	Metric/non-metric	Non-metric	Conjoint analysis
$y_i, i = 1, 2, \ldots m$	Metric	$x_{ij}, i = 1, 2 \ldots m, j = 1, 2 \ldots n;$ Metric/non-metric	Structural equation modeling

Types of data are outlined in Chapter **"Introduction"**, Section 3

Various publications are available giving exhaustive treatment to each of the above methods and hence, readers are advised to approach such dedicated publications for detailed information. However, only concepts involved in the above multivariate techniques and their suitability to Animal Science data will be outlined in this Chapter.

5. MULTIVARIATE ANALYTICAL METHODS

The most common multivariate analytical methods in vogue are tabulated below:

Multivariate analytical methods to study dependence			
Method	**Main objective**	**Use**	**Example**
Multiple regression analysis (MRA)	Quantitative effect of each of the independent variables on the dependent variable by least square analysis	Determines weightage for each of the independent variables	Construction of selection index for identifying parents for breeding; especially in poultry and cattle breeding
Canonical correlation (CCR)	Extension of MRA involving many independent and dependent variables each of them being either metric or non-metric	Correlations among and between dependent and independent variables	Study of views of a commercial hatchery with regards to selected metric and non-metric variables *vis-à-vis* opinion of several established hatcheries on the same variables
Conjoint Analysis (CJA)	Similar to MRA; independent variables are non-metric	Identification of set of most desired non-metric variables	Evaluation of animal products based on known criteria each at known levels and develop a most suitable product design
Multiple discriminant analysis (MDA)	Similar to MRA but the dependent variable is non-metric and independent variables are (assumed to be) metric	When dependent variable is dichotomous (men/ Women) or multichotomous (income groups, social classes, etc), determines weightage for each of the independent variables	Comparison of two villages/groups in respect of their response towards an existing/new scheme
Logistic regression analysis (LRA) or *logit* analysis	Similar to MRA except that the dependent variable is non-metric but non-metric independent variable(s) can also be employed	Characterization of groups based on selected criterion	Study of successful *vs* unsuccessful poultry/ dairy farmers utilizing the past records of their farming.

(Contd.)

(Contd.)

Multivariate analytical methods to study dependence

Method	Main objective	Use	Example
Multivariate analysis of variance and covariance (MANOVA)	To remove intangible effects of independent variables on dependent variables	Accurate assessment of relationship between dependent variables with independent variables	In promotion of products in market; for instance to compare the effect of two types of advertisement boards to promote an animal product say sausage, cutlets, etc.
Structural equation modeling (SEM) and confirmatory factor analysis (CFA)	Factor analysis of scale items followed by MRA using factor scores	Assessment of simultaneous relationship along with elimination of measurement error	To assess welfare and efficiency of personnel in farming/marketing, etc.

Multivariate analytical methods to study interdependence

Method	Main objective	Use	Example
Factor analysis (FA) and Principal factor analysis (PFA); Principal component analysis (PCA)	Identifying variables that are most important so that other variables can be ignored with little loss of information	Reduces cost of experimentation, time and labor involved; simplifies data collection. A common factor can be formed by combining the selected variables	Survey data on experiences in dairy/poultry farming, implementation of animal husbandry schemes, etc.
Cluster analysis (CSA)	Unlike MDA, classification of a bigger entity into smaller mutually exclusive homogenous groups with respect to interdependent variables	Facilitate MDA which can be performed after cluster formation	Identification of reason(s) why a particular farming is preferred and then discriminate which of the factors was the most important. Identify distinct clusters which are homogenous within themselves
Multidimensional scaling (MDS) or perceptual mapping	Represent independent variables in the form of multidimensional distances with respect to each of the dependent variables	Identify similarities or otherwise among independent variables with respect to dependent variables	Identify why a particular feed/vaccine/product/farming is in most demand and which of them are similar/dissimilar

(Contd.)

(*Contd.*)

Multivariate analytical methods to study interdependence			
Method	Main objective	Use	Example
Correspondence Analysis (CRA)	Similar to MDS on non-metric variables	Quantification of qualitative data and subsequently, factor analysis and MDA can be performed	Similar to MDS on non-metric variables; the data is mainly in the form of contingency table

5.1 Multivariate Methods to Study Dependence

5.1.1 Multiple Regression Analysis (MRA)

The model is described by: $y_i = a + b_1 x_1 + b_2 x_2 + \ldots\ldots + b_n x_n + e_i$ where y is the dependent variable and x_i's are the independent variables, b_i's are the weightages and e_i is the error associated with y_i. If any or many of the variables is (are) non-metric, it (they) will be suitably modified by use of dummy variable(s). This model has already been discussed in Chapter "**Association between variables II**"

It is easy to visualize that employing each of the x_i's, simple linear regression equation can be developed (*see* Chapter "**Association between variables I**" for details) and the square of the correlation coefficient between y and x is the coefficient of determination (R^2) which gives the proportion of variation in y explained by its association with x.

However, when the number of x_i's increase, correlations between x_i's (referred to as multicollinearity) reduces the predictive power of each of the x_i's to the extent of their multicollinearity although, the overall R^2 of the multiple regression equation increases. In simple terms, overall $R^2 \neq$ summation of R^2s of each of the x_i's with y. Sometimes, correlation among two of the x_i's may be so high that one of them can be conveniently deleted from the MRA without affecting the overall R^2. Hence, the researcher must use utmost care in selecting x_i's. Obviously, it is preferable to select x_i's in such a way that correlations among x_i's (multicollinearity) is as low as possible and each of them has an R^2 as high as possible with y.

The multiple regression equation not only predicts the value of independent variable but also estimates the relative importance of each of the x_i's in predicting y. For instance, in a selection index, y can be the phenotypic value of a trait in question, x_i's can be sire family value, dam family value, economic value, etc. and b_i's will be the relative weightages. If many x_i's have high relationship, a derived x_i may replace the related x_i's in order to offset the reduction in R^2 of the MRA.

Analogous to linear regression model, MRA also assumes linearity of association of each of the x_i's with y and x_i's are metric in nature. If there is any deviation in this assumptions, suitable transformations must be employed on the x_i('s) as indicated in Section 3.2.5 above.

Minimum sample size required depends on the trait in question and its variability. However, generally, sample size desirable increases as the number of constants increases and level of significance (α) decreases. At least 5 and preferably 20 to 25 observations per x_i is advisable. If step-wise MRA is planned, 50 observations per x_i are desirable. To ensure satisfactory conclusions, as a general rule, υ for error sum of squares or error degrees of freedom [which is total observations less (the total number of parameters/constants or number of x_i's +1)] should be increased.

5.1.1.1 Non-linear components

In MRA even curvilinear effects can be accommodated (*see* Chapter "**Association between variables III**" for details"); generally, effects up to cubic form (3rd degree polynomial) are considered if change(s) in R^2 brought about by such form(s) is (are) considerable. Initially, only linear components are considered; later on, higher degree polynomials are introduced till no more significant change is achieved. Whether higher degree component(s) has (have) to be considered or not depends mainly on the improvement in R^2 *vis-à-vis* loss of υ and increments in multicollinearity component(s). It is up to the prerogatives of the researcher.

5.1.1.2 Interaction (moderator) effects

When one of the x_i's may change the relationship between another x_i and y, it is referred to as interaction or moderator effect. In a set of variables, there can be more than one moderator effects as well. As in case of non-linear effects, depending on the increase in R^2 due to consideration of interaction effect(s) at the cost of υ (one per interaction effect) and increments in multicollinearity component(s), interaction between two x_i's can also be considered. If such effects(s) are added to the MRA, the model will have additional independent variable, x_{ij} where $i \neq j$ and $i, j = 1, 2 \dots n$.

5.1.1.3 Assumptions for MRA

Understandably, the first assumption is the linearity of relationship between y and x_i's and the second being the error terms have a constant variance (homoscedasticity) and are distributed Normally and independently. These are applicable to individual relationship of y with each of the x_i's and also the whole relationship.

The graphical representation of the data helps diagnose any violation(s) from the assumptions; if any deviations are detected, suitable modification(s) in the x_i('s) is (are) mandatory.

5.1.1.4 Estimation of the model

The estimation of the multiple regression equation can be either by addition or deletion of one x_i at a time and assessing the change in R^2. Alternatively, modern computers allow all possible x_i's (including interactions and non-linear components, if any) to be considered at a time followed by elimination of one x_i at a time; all in quick time. After studying the R^2 values, final equation is determined. The general procedure is as per that outlined in Chapter "**Association between variables II**".

5.1.1.5 Testing of the model

Testing of the model is by ANOVA and F ratio as described in Chapter "**Association between variables II**", Section 1.1.2.1.

It is expected that additional x_i always increases R^2 regardless whether that x_i is really a predictor variable or not. This is particularly true when n is less and is close to the number of x_i. As n increases, such effects minimize; hence, minimum number of observations is suggested as given under Section 5.1.1 above. In any case, adjusted R^2 values are given by the computer based on n as against number of x_i's (in other words by giving weightage to υ of error mean square) which can be used to compare regression equations with different n and/or x_i.

Standard error of each of the partial regression coefficients as well as that of multiple regression equation is given by the computer. Depending on the level of significance (α) set by the researcher (which is generally 0.05 and sometimes 0.01), confidence intervals can be set as $b_i \pm z^*se$ where z is the table value of Standard Normal Deviate (1.96 and 2.56 for $\alpha = 0.05$ and 0.01, respectively). If the limits of confidence intervals does not include zero, it is generally considered statistically significant. Even the numerical value and the direction of the b_i's are important for assessing their practical significance. Only b_i's (in other words x_i's) which have statistical significance **and** practical bearing have to be considered in the final multiple regression equation.

5.1.1.6 Standardized (beta, β) regression coefficients

As discussed earlier, the regression coefficients indicate the relative importance of each of the x_i's in determining y. But, direct comparison of them is restricted by the fact that the x_i's have different metric units and consequently different variance on original scale as well. Therefore, all the x_i's are converted to standard normal deviate (*see* Chapter "**Continuous Probability distributions**") so that they are not only free from units and also have unit variance. Regression coefficients developed by employing such x_i's are called Standardized or β regression coefficients. Comparison of relative importance of x_i's is accurate with β coefficients provided that collinearity between x_i's is minimal. However, care has to be exercised in interpretation because they do not reflect absolute values and are unique to the equation in question; hence, they also do change either by adding or deleting one or many x_i's.

5.1.1.7 Tolerance and variance inflation factor (VIF)

If R^2_i and R^{2*} refer to coefficient of determination by the ith and by the rest of the independent variables, then tolerance value for $x_i = 1 - R^{2*}$ and VIF = reciprocal of tolerance; the former should be as high as possible and latter, obviously, as close to unity as possible. $\sqrt{VIF}$ indicates degree of inflation of standard error of the equation due to multicollinearity. In other words, inflation of standard error due to multi-collinearity = se* $\sqrt{VIF}$; hence, if VIF = 1 (that means tolerance = 1 or absence of multi-collinearity), then $\sqrt{VIF}$ = 1 or there will be no change in standard error. On the contrary, if tolerance = 0.11, VIF = 9.09 and $\sqrt{VIF}$ ≈ 3; that means standard error will be tripled due to multicollinearity. Inflated standard error definitely offsets the estimation accuracy of the multiple regression equation. In addition, high multi-collinearity affects the significance and in extreme cases, even the sign of the regression coefficients. Hence, proper care has to be exercised in identifying x_i's for MRA.

In view of the above, it is the researcher who sets limit for VIF. However, suggested values of VIF range between 3 and 5; preferably the lower limit. If tolerance = 0.1, VIF = 10 and hence $\sqrt{VIF}$ = 3.16. But, most of the statistical softwares do allow a very low tolerance value of even 0.0001; in other words VIF of 10000 or $\sqrt{VIF}$ of 100. Hence, they hardly exclude any of the independent variables and it is the researcher's prerogative to indicate exclusion and/or inclusion of x_i's in MRA.

5.1.1.8 Validation

After obtaining the equation, it can be validated by another (additional) set of data, if available. Otherwise, split data from the one that was used for MRA can be employed.

5.1.2 *Canonical Correlation (CCR, R_c)*

The word "Canonical" means "Latent" and CCR is the correlation between two latent variables; one being a set of independent variables and the other of dependent variables (both in linear combinations); correlation between the canonical variables (or variates) being maximized. Each set of variables are formed in such a way that variance of each of the variables accounted for by the other variables within the set is removed. Hence, the variable is called latent variable.

The aim is to find a linear combination of a set of variables (referred to as "Root") having the maximum correlation (hence the maximum R^2) with the other set of variables. CCR is also referred to as "Characteristic Root". The root is obtained by a series of iterative process under the condition that linear combinations considered successively do not possess correlation with the preceding one.

The two sets of variables may have > 1 orthogonally distinct roots and understandably, the number of roots can not exceed the number of variables in the smaller set. The 1st CCR is generally the one that is numerically the highest and its square gives the R^2, the coefficient of determination. Many other meaningful CCRs can be estimated with their corresponding R^2 values. If all such R^2s are pooled, the R^2_p, so obtained explains predictability of one set by the other set of canonical variable.

Given two column vectors $\begin{bmatrix} x_1 \\ x_2 \\ \cdot \\ \cdot \\ x_n \end{bmatrix}$ and $\begin{bmatrix} y_1 \\ y_2 \\ \cdot \\ \cdot \\ y_m \end{bmatrix}$ of random variables with finite variances,

covariance can be described by $x_i y_j$ elements of an $m \times n$ matrix. In practice, the covariance matrix is estimated on sampled data from X and Y (i.e. from a pair of data matrices).

Canonical correlation analysis seeks vectors a and b such that the random variables $A = a'X$ and $B = b'Y$ maximize the correlation ρ between them (and indicate transpose of the vector). The random variables A and B are the first pair of canonical variables. Further, vectors (uncorrelated with the first pair of canonical variables) maximizing the same correlation gives the second pair of canonical variables. This procedure may be continued up to $\min\{m, n\}$ times and are represented serially in rows. Obviously, the canonical variables will be orthogonal.

5.1.2.1 Eigen values

These are similar and approximately equal to R^2_c; since CCRs are progressively decreasing, so will be the Eigen values as well. It is up to the researcher to accept or reject variables producing low CCR. Eigen values refer to the set of variables and therefore, the R^2_c refers to the entire set but not any particular variable(s) in the set.

5.1.2.2 Canonical weight (canonical coefficient/function coefficient)

These are similar to β coefficients in the sense that the original variables within a canonical variable (set) are standardized into Standard Normal variables with mean zero and unit variance. These weights help compare relative contribution of each of the variables to the root. Hence, each of the original variable in each of the canonical variables will have a canonical coefficient for each of the CCRs; therefore, if one of the sets has x variables and totally y CCRs are derived, there will be $x*y$ canonical coefficients.

5.1.2.3 Canonical scores

CCRs or roots are derived for several cases (combination of original variables). Summation of product of canonical coefficients and standardized scores of the cases gives canonical scores for the case in question.

5.1.2.4 Canonical factor loadings (structure correlation coefficients)

This is the correlation between canonical variable with the original variable contained in it. Further, it is the correlation between score for a canonical variable with standardized score of the original variable. Squared value of this correlation, analogous to R^2 value, explains the contribution of the variable to the R^2 value of the canonical variable to which it belongs.

Structure correlation coefficient should be at least 0.3 ($R^2 \approx 10\%$) to be included as a part of canonical variable. Average of all the structure correlation coefficients within a canonical set indicates average variance explained by the raw variables in the set.

5.1.2.5 Canonical community coefficient

This is Σ(structure correlation coefficients)^2 and represents the reproducibility of the variance of the original variable from the canonical variable. If community coefficient is low, original variable had better be deleted from analysis.

5.1.2.6 Canonical variable adequacy coefficient

Adequacy coefficient for a given canonical variable (dependent or independent set) is

calculated as $\sum \dfrac{(\text{Structure correlation coefficients})^2}{\text{Number of original variables}}$ with respect to the variable. The

formula clearly indicates that adequacy coefficient reflects % of variability extracted by the canonical variable (efficacy) representing the variability in the original variables.

5.1.2.7 Redundancy coefficient (d or R_d)

This is the % variance of original variables in one set predicted from the canonical variable (usually the 1st) of the other set. R_d corresponding to independent canonical variable in predicting original variables in dependent set $\neq R_d$ corresponding to dependent canonical variable in predicting original variables in independent set; the former being of practical importance and hence the latter is not generally calculated.

It is calculated as $R_d = R_C^2 \sum \dfrac{(\text{Structure correlation coefficients})^2}{\text{Number of original variables}}$.

It is noteworthy that R^2_C gives the % variability in the **dependent set of variables** explained by the **independent set of variables** and does not specify any particular variable(s). On the other hand, R_d explains the % variability in the **dependent original variables** explained by the **independent set of variables**. Obviously, the former only gives extent of relationship between the canonical variables whereas the latter indicates the extent to which the dependent/independent original variables can be predicted by the independent and/or dependent canonical variable.

5.1.2.7.1 Pooled R_d

This is the summation of all R_d's of all the variables in a set. This indicates the efficiency of all canonical variables identified as solution in explaining the variance in original dependent/independent variables, as the case may be; researcher is always interested in the former.

5.1.2.8 Assumptions

Most assumptions are similar to MRA *viz.* linearity of relationship, low multi-collinearity, homoscedasticity, multivariate Normality and adequate sample size. In addition, minimum measurement error, proper sampling to ensure unrestricted variance, similar underlying distributions of the canonical variable and non-redundancy of the original variables (but high redundancy among canonical variables) are also assumed for computation of CCR.

5.1.2.9 Graphical representation

5.1.2.9.1 CCR plot

Usually 1st CCR is considered; X- and Y-axes consist of standardized values of the latent values of independent and dependent canonical variable, respectively. Hence, the origin will be (–4, –4), center point will be (0, 0). Generally, a linear regression line (of canonical variables) will be drawn and if CCR is high, two distinct clusters will be formed at different points on the regression line (*see* graph below).

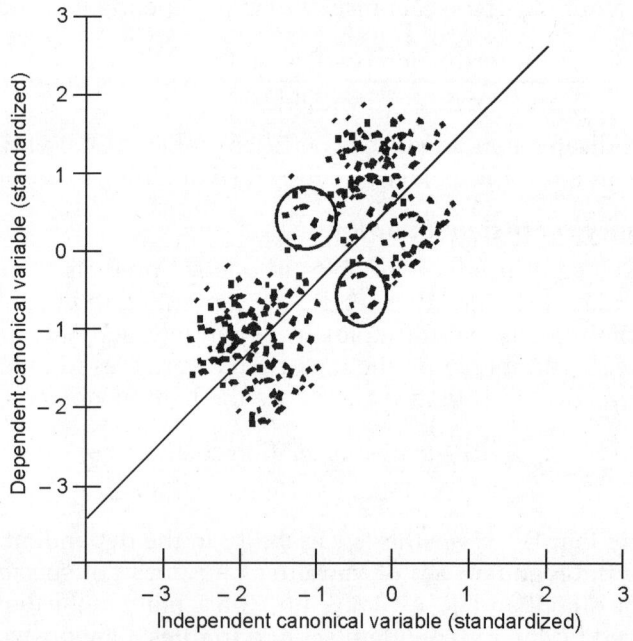

The graph above shows a case of high CCR and a few points encircled which are away from the clusters are referred to as "Outliers" which do not share the same pattern of association.

5.1.2.9.2 *Helio plot*

In a Helio plot canonical factor loadings (structural correlations) are shown. As in case of CCR plot, 1st CCR is considered. It consists of two concentric circles; both divided into semicircles. At the perimeter of the outer semicircle, original dependent and independent variables are marked; dependent on the left side and independent on the right. From the perimeter of the inner semicircles, structural correlations are represented by bars projecting inside (if negative) or outside (if positive); the length proportionate to the magnitude.

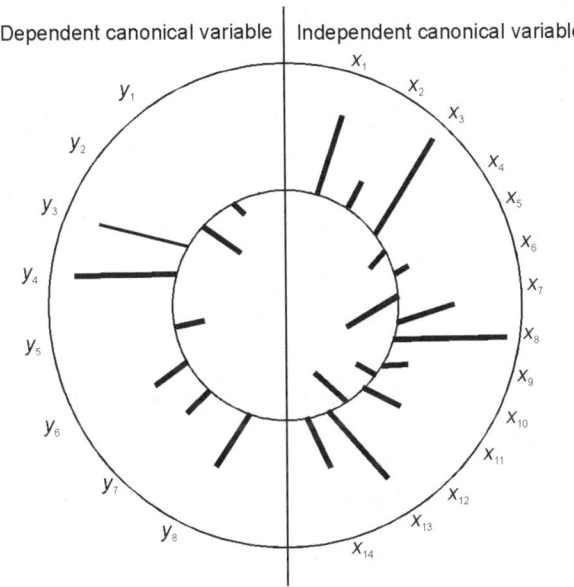

5.1.2.10 Testing of CCR

Generally 1st CCR is tested by employing Wilks' λ (lambda) test or U Statistic along with Bartlett's V test. However, to test all canonical variables (that means average linear relationship between canonical variables), Likelihood ratio test can be performed. However, likelihood ratio test is not suitable to test 1st CCR.

5.1.2.10.1 χ^2 *test*

Each row (CCR term) can be tested for $CCR_i = 0$; it further implies that all further correlations are also zero because they are smaller in magnitude than the preceding one. If we have p independent observations in a sample and is the estimated correlation

for $i = 1,2....\min\{m,n\}$. For the ith row, $\chi^2 = -\left[p-1-\frac{1}{2}(m+n+1) \right]\ln\prod_{j=1}^{p}\left(1-\rho_j^2\right)$ which

is asymptotically distributed as a χ^2 with $\upsilon = (m - i + 1)(n - i + 1)$ for large p.

5.1.2.10.2 *Wilks' λ or U statistic*

Wilks' λ is a distribution of two independent Wishart variables (*see* Section 3.1 above) $A \sim W_p(I,m)$ and $B \sim W_p(I,n)$; $m \geq p$ where p is the number of dimensions.

Then, $\lambda = \dfrac{\det|A|}{\det|A+B|} = \dfrac{1}{\det|I+A^{-1}B|} \sim \Lambda(p,m,n)$ where m and n are the υ for error and hypothesis, respectively (or $m + n$ is the total υ) and I is the identity matrix.

When m is large, Wilks' $\lambda \approx \chi^2$ on $\upsilon = np$ (Bartlett's approximation).

5.1.2.10.3 Likelihood ratio test

This test compares fit of two models when one of them is nested within the other. Nesting may occur due to imposition of linear constraints on parameters and simplify the model. Log likelihood of each of the models fit to the data is calculated. Hence, this test is not suitable to test 1st CCR.

Then, the statistic, D, is twice the difference in log likelihoods; i.e.,

$$D = 2\left[\ln(\text{Likelihood for null model}) - \ln(\text{Likelihood for alternate model})\right]$$

$$= 2\ln\left(\frac{\text{Likelihood for null model}}{\text{Likelihood for alternate model}}\right)$$

D approximately $\sim \chi^2$ on $\upsilon = (m - n)$ where m and n are the number of parameters in the alternative and the null model, respectively.

Notes:

CCR is calculated as a part of MANOVA in most statistical packages.

CCR or CCR^2 is not a measure of % variance in the original variables explained by the CCR; however, it is given by square of the structure correlation coefficient

CCR also does not accurately indicate as to which of the original variables is closely associated with it.

After computing CCR, one variable at a time can be eliminated to find out whether number of original variables can be reduced without affecting CCR or not. This procedure is called backward or stepwise canonical correlation.

5.1.3 Conjoint Analysis (CJA)

As the name suggests, CJA is study of joint effects. CJA is mainly applied for marketing research; for instance to know which characteristics of the products of the products (value-added products like sausages, nuggets, etc) determine in making a choice in favor of the product by consumers; i.e. preference criteria. Depending on the outcome, one can develop a product to create a market or increase the existing market. Hence, psychology of the consumers is also involved; hence, the independent variables involved generally non-metric and the dependent variable being metric or non-metric. It is because of the former, this analysis is also referred to as "Multi-attribute Compositional or Choice modeling or Stated Preference Research". Based on the findings, even newer products and/or advertisements for the products can be designed. CJA also helps develop model(s) for determining consumer preferences.

$y_i = x_1 + x_2 + x_3 + \dots x_n + \varepsilon_i$ where x_i are the attributes (non-metric), y_i is the dependent variable (metric or non-metric) and ε_i error associated with y_i.

For example, a value-added product may have attributes like acceptance, additives and different Brand names, each given scores by expert panels based on a scale developed for the purpose. These form the independent variables and actual sales (metric) or product preference (non-metric) can be the dependent variable. Hence, it is also called "Judgmental data". Since joint effects of several attributes are involved, it is referred to as "Conjoint analysis".

There are basically three conjoint methodologies *viz.*

Traditional: which assumes an additive model with a maximum of 9 attributes each evaluated one at a time for each individual

Hybrid: can accommodate up to 30 attributes in sets and subsets with additive effects; but requires computer assistance for data collection and analysis.

Choice-based: includes interaction effects with additive effects of a maximum of 6 attributes. If necessary, even aggregate effects can be analyzed. This method is most popular.

Note: Generally, only additive effects are considered.

A suitable profile(s) has(have) to be formulated for the respondents to evaluate; as a rule, if x factors each at y levels are involved, minimum number of profiles (combination of factors and levels) to be evaluated by the respondents will be $(xy - x + 1)$. It is the researcher who has to decide the number of factors depending on utility of each of them and also to minimize the number of factors as well to make the analysis simpler. Hence, he has to trade-off in selecting number and level of factors; hence, CJA is also referred to as "Trade-off" analysis.

Data for CJA is collected by market research/survey. The data can be subjected to any or many of the following statistical analysis to establish the combination of attributes that maximize the dependent variable:

1. ANOVA
2. Linear regression
3. MRA
4. LRA and
5. Maximum Likelihood Estimate (MLE) usually with LRA

Note: Dummy variables can be used to convert the attributes metric.

5.1.3.1 Estimating part-worth

For each of the attributes (independent variables, factors), range of scores (referred to as "Part-worth") given by each of the respondents (judges) is determined. The total of all the ranges is used to calculate relative importance of each of the factors as Factor

importance $= \dfrac{\text{Range for the Factor}}{\text{Total Range}} \times 100$ for each of the judges.

Utilizing values given by each of the judges for each combination of Factors, a predicted part-worth is estimated and they are allotted ranks depending on the magnitude. These are ranks are compared with the actual ranking given by each of the judges to obtain an idea about the consistency of judges with the preference structure (Pearson's or Kendall's Correlation Coefficient can be calculated depending on nature of variables; *see* **Chapter "Association between variables I")**. In the process, preferences of the individual judges are also determined.

The model is defined as $w_i = \sum_{j=1}^{k} p_j x_{ij}$ where w_i is the part-worth at level i, p_j is the part-worth of each of the levels, x_{ij} is the level of jth attribute for the ith judge and $k \leq 5$ (preferably) although it can range between 2 and 9.

Hence, CJA helps

1. Predict contribution of individual attributes and their levels in determining consumer preferences and
2. Establish a statistical model for consumer preferences. It is left to the prerogatives of the researcher to define the factors whose summation represents the total utility of the product. A sample size of 50 to 200 (generally 100) is advisable.

5.1.4 Multiple Discriminant Analysis (MDA)

As the name suggests "Discriminant Analysis" helps *discriminate* dependent (criterion or grouping) variable into ≥ 2 categories/groups. If a dependent categorical (nominal or non-metric) variable having only two categories (dichotomous, $\male$ Vs $\female$, Rich vs Poor, etc.) is classified using interval or dummy independent variables as predictors (discriminating variables, metric), it is called Discriminant Analysis (DA). An extension of DA with a categorical dependent variable having more than two categories (multichotomous) is referred to as MDA. MDA sometimes is also called as Discriminant Factor Analysis or Canonical Discriminant Analysis. DA has lesser type–II error and is an alternative to LRA; however, when the groups are uneven in numbers and normal distribution is not followed, LRA is preferred to DA (Note: MDA can not be substituted with LRA).

DA and/or MDA helps

1. Classify categorical data into groups based on an equation
2. Identify differences between and within groups
3. Identify independent variable(s) which can be used to accurately differentiate groups
4. R^2 Values
5. R^2 Values over above that by control variables (Sequential DA)
6. Relative importance of independent variables to classify dependent variables

The model can be represented as: $y = a + \sum_{i=1}^{n} b_i x_i$ where a is a constant, b_i's are the discriminating coefficients for the independent discriminating variables (x_i's), respectively. If the b_i's are standardized as in case of β coefficients in MRA, they are called *Standardized Discriminant Coefficients*.

It is easy to note that the model is similar to MRA; but, the b_i's in DA/MDA maximize the distance between the means of y. In case of DA, one discriminant function is possible because y is dichotomous and in case of MDA, $(k-1)$ discriminant functions are possible where k is the number of categories in y or n, the number of discriminating variables (x_i's), whichever is less; all functions being orthogonal (uncorrelated) to one another. Each discriminant function is also called *Dimension*.

Analogous to CCR, Eigen value is the characteristic root of the discriminant function. Obviously, in case of DA there will be only one Eigen value. In case of MDA, again analogous to CCR, the 1st function maximizes the distances between the values of y; the 2nd function maximizes those between values of y, controlling for the first factor; and so on. Therefore, as in case of CCR, importance of the functions will be in the descending order starting from the 1st one. In other words, ratio of Eigen values, indicates the relative discriminating power of the functions.

Ratio of Eigen value of a function to that of sum of all Eigen values is referred to as relative percentage of the function. CCR for each of the functions directly indicates the usefulness of the function to differentiate group differences; higher the better. This follows that in case of DA, CCR is simply the Pearson's r between discriminant scores and grouping variable.

5.1.4.1 Assumptions

DA/MDA is developed based on the following assumptions:
1. Multivariate normality of the independent (predictor) variables
2. Unknown but equal variance covariance matrices of the criterion (dependent) variable groups; in other words, linear and homoscedastic relationships. Thos can be tested by Box's M test
3. Data is interval type and untruncated
4. In case of DA, dependent variable is truly dichotomous

5.1.4.2 Graphical representation

Mean discriminant scores (centroids) for each of the categories of y, can be plotted (Discriminant function plots or canonical plots) with two x-axes; they have to be separated well apart to consider the function to be effective/useful. Each of the values are also plotted around the centroid. In effect, these plots represent the discriminant function space.

5.1.4.3 Tests of significance

5.1.4.3.1 Wilks' (Model) λ or U statistic

A significant Wilks' λ (*see* Section 5.1.2.10.1 above for details) indicates that H_0 (Two groups have the same discriminating function) can be rejected and hence, the discriminating function is effective in differentiating the categories of y.

5.1.4.3.2 Canonical correlation, R_C

A high R_C indicates the discriminating power of the function.

5.1.4.3.3 Mahalanobis D^2, Rao's V, Hotelling's trace, Pillai's trace and Roy's gcr

Mahalanobis D^2 is the distance of a case from the centroid of that group of y in Discriminant Function Space; smaller the Mahalanobis distance, more likely that it belongs to that group. Mahalanobis distance is measured in terms of standard deviations from the centroid. Mahalanobis $D^2 > 1.96$ and $D^2 > 2.58$ indicates that it has $< 5\%$ and $< 1\%$ chance of belonging to that group, respectively.

Mahalanobis D^2 and Rao's V are particularly appropriate when discriminant function is estimated stepwise; when simultaneous estimation is done, Wilks' λ (or U statistic), Hotelling's trace, Pillai's trace and Roy's gcr can be used. Hotelling's trace is outlined under Section 3.3.2.2 above and Section 5.1.6.2 below. Roy's gcr is outlined under Section 5.1.6.3 below.

5.1.4.4 Cutting score or critical Z value

This is the value based on which the object is discriminated into specific groups. In case of DA, the two groups are formed one whose discriminant score is less than cutting score and the other more than cutting score. In MDA, cutting score between the given two groups is utilized.

Cutting score is calculated based on the centroids and relative size of the groups; standardized discriminant function is utilized to calculate cutting scores as follows: $C_S = \dfrac{n_A C_A + n_B C_B}{n_A + n_B}$ where n_i and C_i ($i = A$ or B) are size and centroid of group i and C_S is the (weighted) cutting score. This follows that if group size is same, $C_S = \dfrac{C_A + C_B}{2}$.

5.1.4.4.1 Classification matrix

Utilizing the CS, the observations are classified into two groups and with number of objects correctly classified are formed into a matrix. With two groups (DA), a 2 × 2 matrix is formed thus:

Actual group	Prediction by discriminant function		Total (Actual)	Accuracy %
	A	**B**		
A	n_{AA}	n_{AB}	$n_{AA} + n_{AB}$	$\left(\dfrac{n_{AA}}{n_{AA} + n_{AB}}\right) \times 100$
B	n_{BA}	n_{BB}	$n_{BA} + n_{BB}$	$\left(\dfrac{n_{BB}}{n_{BA} + n_{BB}}\right) \times 100$
Total (Predicted)	$n_{AA} + n_{BA}$	$n_{AB} + n_{BB}$	$N = n_{AA} + n_{AB} + n_{BA} + n_{BB}$	$\left(\dfrac{n}{N}\right) \times 100$

$n = n_{AA} + n_{BB}$

After classification into two distinct groups, % of objects correctly classified can be calculated and is referred to as **Hit Ratio**. Proportion of correctly classified (i.e. p = Hit ratio ÷ 100) can be tested for significance as follows: $t = \dfrac{p - 0.5}{\sqrt{\dfrac{0.5(1.0 - 0.5)}{n}}} = 2(p - 0.5)\sqrt{n}$

where n is the group size; for unequal group sizes the formula will be modified as

$$t = \dfrac{2(p - 0.5)}{\sqrt{\dfrac{1}{n_A} + \dfrac{1}{n_B}}}.$$

5.1.4.4.2 Standards for hit ratio

When group sizes are equal, the probability that the correct classification can simply occur by chance is the reciprocal of number of groups.

When group sizes are unequal, proportional chance criterion can be calculated as $C_P = p_A^2 + (1 - p_A)^2$ where C_P is the proportionate chance criterion and P_A is the proportion of individuals in group A ($1 - P_A = P_B$).

To accept classification by the discriminant function as accurate, the classification accuracy achieved by the function should be $\geq 1.25 \times C_p$.

Discriminatory power of classification matrix *vis-à-vis* Chance matrix can be tested by Press's Q statistic (which follows χ^2 on $\upsilon = 1$) defined as $\text{Press's } Q = \dfrac{(N - nG)^2}{N(G-1)}$ where G is number of groups, N the total sample size and n total number correctly classified. Prediction is considered accurate if Press's Q value > table value of χ^2 on $\upsilon = 1$ at a defined α.

5.1.4.5 Interpretation in case of DA

5.1.4.5.1 Standardized discriminant weights

The magnitude of each of the standardized discriminant coefficients (ignoring sign) directly indicates relative importance of the predictor associated with it in determining the function. The sign is indicative of positive or negative contribution.

5.1.4.5.2 Discriminant loadings

These are the simple correlations between the predictor variable and the discriminant function; hence, indicate the root of the amount of variance of the discriminant function contributed by the predictor. A loading of at least 40% or $r = 0.63$ is desirable to consider an independent variable (predictor) being important in discriminating groups in criterion variable.

5.1.4.5.3 Partial F values

During stepwise DA/MDA, different F values are obtained. Based on the magnitude of F values, the functions (predictors) can be arranged in a descending order of importance because larger F values are suggestive of higher power of the discriminating function.

5.1.4.6 Interpretation in case of MDA

5.1.4.6.1 Rotation of functions

The discriminant functions developed can be rotated to redistribute variance and help interpretation.

5.1.4.6.2 Potency index

This index is developed to include contribution of each predictor to the discriminate function as well as relative importance of the function to overall solution.

Assuming that there are i predictors and j discriminating functions, relative eigen

$$\text{value}_j = \frac{\text{Eigen value}_j}{\sum\limits_{j} \text{Eigen value}} \text{ and potency value of } i \text{ on } j \text{ is given by:}$$

Potency value$_{i \to j}$ = Discriminant loading$_{ij}^2 \times$ Relative eigen value$_j$ and assuming that there are k significant discriminant functions, Potency index$_i$ = $\sum\limits_{j=1}^{k} \text{Potency value}_{i \to j}$.

It is clear from the derivation of the potency index that it is only a relative measure and its actual value has no meaning. Potency indices of each of the predictors can be arranged in a descending order for identifying their importance.

5.1.5 *Logistic Regression or* Logit *Analysis (LRA)*

That the dependent variable is not metric but binary categorical (nominal) is the major difference between LRA and other regression models. If dependent variable is multinomial, multinomial logistic regression or if dependent variable is ordinal, ordinal logistic regression analysis can be performed. In case of polytomous dependent variable with m alternatives ($m > 2$), $m - 1$ dichotomous *logit* equations can be developed and analyzed. Independent variables for logit regression can be continuous and/or categorical i.e. metric or non-metric.

As discussed under Section 5.1.4, DA/MDA/MRA requires that homoscedasticity and multivariate normality for application; however, multi-normality of distribution, linearity of relationship and homoscedasticity are not prerequisites for LRA. But, independent nature of observations and linearity of relationship of independent variables with the logit of the dependent variable are required conditions.

Further, LRA is similar to MRA and hence require application of familiar statistical tests. Thus, LRA is preferred to DA/MDA on most occasions.

The two groups (which are non-metric) of the dependent variable are assigned values "1" and "0". For instance, male *Vs* female, agree *Vs* disagree etc. The codes can be reversed as well. Unlike MRA, LRA predicts probability that an observation belongs to the group which is coded "1". Obviously, the probability will be ≤ unity.

Dependent variable so assigned is converted into logit variable by taking natural logarithm and hence the LRA estimates the odds that a particular event occurs. The model is represented as follows:

$$\hat{y}_i = a + \sum_{i=1}^{k} b_i x_i \text{ where } \hat{y} = \ln\left(\frac{\text{Probability of occurence of an event}}{\text{Probability of occurence of a non-event}}\right), a \text{ is the inter-}$$

cept, b_i's are the logistic coefficients referred to as **parameter estimates** and x_i's are the independent variables. In the above model, $\hat{y}$ is referred to as *Logit* variable.

On original scale i.e. $e^{\hat{y}}$ gives the probability that $\hat{y} = 1$ (dichotomous) or equals the assigned value and e^{b_i} indicates the **Odds Ratio (OR)**. Hence, the above model

can be written as $OR_i = e^{a + \sum_{i=1}^{k} b_i x_i}$. If OR = 1, the independent variable does not influence the dependent variable because ln (0) = 1 or $b_i = 0$. In case of continuous independent variables, $\hat{y}$ is the factor by which the odds that dependent variable = 1 increases/ decreases, as the case may be, per unit change in the independent variable. Again, if OR = 1, the independent variable does not influence the dependent variable. It is necessary to note that with dichotomous dependent variable, the reference is "0" and with polytomous dependent variable, the reference will be the highest value assigned.

Similar to DA/MDA/MRA, standardized (β) coefficients and coefficient of determination (pseudo R^2) can be calculated by employing Maximum Likelihood method involving iteration.

5.1.5.1 Tests of significance

5.1.5.1.1 Dichotomous dependent variable

5.1.5.1.1.1 Hosmer and lemeshow χ^2 goodness of fit

Applicable to test overall fit of the binary logistic regression. The subjects are divided into deciles (10 groups) and observed and expected values for the groups are tabulated in a 10 × 2 contingency table for each of the dichotomous categories. χ^2 value is calculated and compared with the table value at $\upsilon = 8$. If the value is not significant at a given α (at least 0.05), it indicates that the model is a good fit.

5.1.5.1.1.2 Omnibus test

This is a traditional χ^2 to test whether the model with parameter estimates is significantly different from that without; obviously, for a model to be a good fit, the difference should be significant.

Note: Both the tests above can be done by introducing independent variables stepwise also called block–entry LRA.

5.1.5.1.2 Polytomous dependent variable

5.1.5.1.2.1 Pearson goodness test

This is analogous to Hosmer and Lemeshow test outlined above.

5.1.5.1.2.2 Likelihood ratio test

This test is based log likelihood (LL) and also known as deviance χ^2, scaled deviance, deviation χ^2, D_M or L^2. Understandably, LL being a probability value lies between 0 and 1; hence, LL lies between $-\infty$ and 0. On multiplication by (-2), LL not only becomes positive but also approximately follows χ^2 distribution. Further, $-2LL$ can function similar error sum of squares in linear regression to test the difference between two– 2LLs; hence, the name "Deviance χ^2, Scaled deviance, Deviation χ^{2}".

This test can be used to test:

1. Model with only intercept *vs* that with all parameter estimates–this is test of the overall model or model χ^2 test. A significance test indicates that the independent variables help predict the dependent.
2. Models with and without interaction effects can be compared to test interaction effects.
3. With stepwise or sequential introduction of independent variables, individual model parameters; in other words, relative importance of independent variables can be tested. As another alternative, independent variables can be introduced in blocks (nested under a common criterion).

5.1.5.1.2.3 Wald statistic

This test is similar to test of partial regression coefficients and is used to test each of the parameter estimates against a null hypothesis that $b_i = 0$. Wald statistic =

$$\left(\frac{\text{Unstandardized parameter coefficient}}{\text{Standard error of the unstandardized parameter coefficient}}\right)^2 \text{ and it follows } \chi^2 \text{ dis-}$$

tribution on $\upsilon = 1$.

Note: A parameter estimate can be significant; but the corresponding correlation coefficient (in other words, R^2) should also be significant to make general statements about the relationship between the dependent and the independent variable.

5.1.5.2 Probabilities

As indicated above, $e^{\hat{y}}$ gives the probability of an event and therefore, $1 - e^{\hat{y}}$ gives the probability of a non-event. By rearrangement, Probability (event) = $\dfrac{e^{\hat{y}}}{1+e^{\hat{y}}}$. This can be employed to calculate relative risk ratio (RRR) which is the probability that the selected level of the independent variable decreases/increases the dependent variable in comparison to the base line level ("0" in binary model).

5.1.5.3 Pseudo R² values

Variance in case of dichotomous or even polytomous variables will be highly dependent on frequency distribution. Hence, unlike linear or MRA, classical R^2 values are not available in LRA. However, values indicating strength of association can be calculated and hence, they are referred to as "R^2 - like or Pseudo R^2" values.

5.1.5.3.1 Pseudo R²

This is generally calculated as $\dfrac{-2LL_{Intercept} - \left(-2LL_{Final\ model}\right)}{-2LL_{Intercept}}$. In a perfectly fit model, $-2LL_{Final\ model}$ decreases to 0 making pseudo R^2 = 1.0 or 100%.

5.1.5.3.2 Cox and Snell's R²

This is the ratio of LL of final model to that of baseline model; hence, it will be < 1.

5.1.5.3.3 Nagelkerke's R²

To help interpretation of Cox and Snell's R^2, Negelkerke's R^2 is the ratio of the Cox and Snell's R^2 to maximum Cox and Snell's R^2; therefore, analogous to probability, Negelkerke's R^2 lies between 0 and 1 making interpretation easy.

5.1.5.3.4 McFadden's R²

This is the ratio of LL of the final model to that of model with only intercept.

5.1.5.3.5 R²

This is the R^2 obtained by the linear regression of predicted values from the final model with the original values. Generally used with dichotomous dependent variables. Care should be exercised in interpretation of these values because they can be very high with many independent variables.

5.1.5.4 Classification tables

A 2 × 2 or 2 × k table indicating the actual (in rows) and predicted value (in columns) for intercept only and final model can be formed followed by calculation of % accuracy as the ratio of correct classifications to sample size. In perfectly matched case, all values lie in the diagonals and off-diagonals will be zero. If the prediction by the final model is at least 25% more than the intercept (null) model, the final model is considered good and acceptable.

5.1.6 *Multivariate Analysis of Variance (MANOVA)*

Conceptually, MANOVA has many similarities to ANOVA and hence, it is discussed in relation to the latter. MANOVA is employed when

1. there are > 1 dependent variables (metric) and they are correlated; but a single statistical test is desired for the entire set
2. it is necessary to test the influence of independent variables (non-metric) on pattern of response in dependent variables

Unlike ANOVA where equality of group (treatment) means is tested, in MANOVA equality of mean vectors is tested; in other words, they are from the same multivariate

Normal population. It is represented as follows:
$$\begin{bmatrix} \mu_{11} \\ \mu_{21} \\ \cdot \\ \cdot \\ \cdot \\ \mu_{p1} \end{bmatrix} = \begin{bmatrix} \mu_{12} \\ \mu_{22} \\ \cdot \\ \cdot \\ \cdot \\ \mu_{p2} \end{bmatrix} = \ldots\ldots = \begin{bmatrix} \mu_{1k} \\ \mu_{2k} \\ \cdot \\ \cdot \\ \cdot \\ \mu_{pk} \end{bmatrix} \quad \text{where is}$$

the mean of variable p in group k. It is easy to note that there will be k column vectors of size $(p \times 1)$.

On the same lines, variances and covariances are represented in a $(p \times p)$ matrix with variances forming diagonals and covariances, off-diagonals *viz.*

$$M = \begin{bmatrix} \sigma_1^2 & \text{cov}_{12} & \cdot & \cdot & \text{cov}_{1p} \\ \text{cov}_{12} & \sigma_2^2 & \cdot & \cdot & \text{cov}_{2p} \\ \cdot & \cdot & \cdot & \cdot & \cdot \\ \cdot & \cdot & \cdot & \cdot & \cdot \\ \text{cov}_{1p} & \text{cov}_{2p} & \cdot & \cdot & \sigma_p^2 \end{bmatrix}.$$

In ANOVA, total variance is partitioned into variance due to main effects, variance due to interaction(s) and variance due to error; considering two main effects a and b with additivity of effects assumed, total variance, $\sigma_t^2 = \sigma_a^2 + \sigma_b^2 + \sigma_{a \times b}^2 + \sigma_e^2$; σ_e^2 representing error component of variance. In case of MANOVA, each of the above will be a variance-covariance matrix. For instance, the error variance-covariance matrix in this

case will be $\begin{bmatrix} \sigma_{e_a}^2 & \text{cov}_{e_a e_b} \\ \text{cov}_{e_b e_a} & \sigma_{e_b}^2 \end{bmatrix}$. The diagonals are the error variances as in case of

ANOVA and the off-diagonals are the within group covariances indicating within a group to what extent higher values of a in an object is associated with higher values of b also.

It is ideal to have $k > p$ and each of the means on at least 20 observations.

5.1.6.1 Assumptions for MANOVA

The following are the main assumptions for MANOVA:

1. Observations are independent
2. Variance-covariance matrices are equal in all treatment groups; in other words homoscedasticity-tested by Box's M test

3. Set of dependent variables follows multivariate normal distribution which also implies that any of the linear combination of dependent variables follows normal distribution.

5.1.6.2 Hotelling's T² Statistic

In ANOVA, the group means are tested by t-test and an extension of the same test called Hotelling's T² is employed in MANOVA to make a collective comparisons of all the variables and groups. It helps test a variate made of a combination of dependent variables which produces maximum group differences. In other words, it provides for single test across all dependent variables at a known α thereby minimizing Type I error expected when separate t–tests are conducted for each case.

A composite variate is formed say y' which is defined as follows: $y' = \sum_{i=1}^{p} w_i y_i$ where are the weightages for each of the dependent variables. With composite dependent variate, ordinary t-test can be performed to test difference between k groups. But, w_i's which maximize the t-value will be the same as the discriminant function (most discriminant linear combination of dependent variables) between the k groups. Square of such a maximum t-value obtained from discriminant function is the Hotelling's T² value. If T² is significant, it implies that the groups differ across the mean vectors. T² follows F distribution with $\upsilon_1 = p$ and $\upsilon_2 = \sum_{i=1}^{p} n_i - k - 1$ and critical value of T² is given

by $F_{Crit, \upsilon_1, \upsilon_2, \alpha} \left[\dfrac{p \left(\sum_{i=1}^{k} n_i - k \right)}{\sum_{i=1}^{p} n_i - p - 1} \right]$. Hotelling's T² is applied when $k = 2$.

5.1.6.3 Roy's greatest characteristic root (Roy's gcr)

When $k > 2$, Hotelling's T² is extended to suit many combinations; the test is referred to as Roy's gcr. With > 2 dependent variables with 1 or > 1 independent variables, the MANOVA becomes similar to DA/MDA. As discussed under Section 5.1.4, the first function maximizes the differences between groups and hence the F value designated

F_{Max} which is necessary to calculate Roy's gcr value as $\dfrac{F_{Max}(k-1)}{(p-k)}$. Roy's gcr has a distribution on the hypothesis that the group mean vectors are equivalent or over a set of dependent variables, group means are same. If the calculated value is significant from the Roy's gcr$_{crit}$ (table value), the H_0 is liable to be rejected.

Subsequent discriminant functions are orthogonal and maximize the differences among the groups based on the remaining variance; they can also be tested as explained earlier in Section 5.1.4 by Wilks' λ (or U Statistic) or Pillai's criterion.

5.1.7 Structural Equation Modeling (SEM) and Confirmatory Factor Analysis (CFA)

As the name is suggestive, SEM helps study structure of relationships in a series of equations (similar to MRA). Both dependent and independent variables involved can be either observable or latent; the latter being represented by other variable(s) as in case of FA (*see* Section 5.2.1 below). Latent variables are those which can not be measured and which are not generally observable as well. For instance, job satisfaction of a farm attendant; this in itself a latent dependent variable and can depend on several latent variables like attitude of his superior in allotting work, considering his welfare as well as his promotion, etc.

Thus, SEM is a combination of analysis of both dependence (MRA) and inter-dependence (FA). Hence, it is also referred to as "Covariance structure analysis", "Covariance structure modeling", "Analysis of Covariance structures" and "Latent variable analysis".

In SEM, variables can be independent or dependent; for instance, a dependent variable can be an independent variable in determining another variable in the set. Hence, it is left to the prerogatives of the researcher to identify a set of independents to determine a dependent; the latter can be an independent variable in another relationship. In addition, a set of designated independent variables may have many dependent variables but it need not have to influence all the dependent variables equally.

It is clear from the above that SEM analyses several aspects viz. interactions, non-linearities, correlated/latent independents, latent dependents with multiple indicators. SEM can also include time series data as well as non–normal and incomplete data. Further, it can use CFA to reduce measurement error and analyze error terms of indicator variables. It is obviously more powerful than MRA, FA and ANACOVA.

Maximum likelihood estimation (MLE) technique is employed to derive the series of equations. Other methods of estimation include Bayesian estimation, weighted/generalized/ordinary/unweighted least squares, standardized structural (path) coefficients, unstandardized structural (path) coefficients, Asymptotically Distribution Free (ADF) estimation, Elliptical Distribution Theory (EDT) estimation, Bootstrapped estimates etc.

5.1.7.1 Reliability

In methods for analyzing dependence, there is no provision to estimate measurement error i.e. error associated with reliability of data; the subjects might as well provide false information or hide some information. Theoretically, $\beta_{yx} = \beta_x \times \rho_x$ where β_{yx} is the regression coefficient, β_x is the true structural coefficient and ρ_x is the reliability index

of the independent variable. It follows that $\beta_x = \dfrac{\beta_{yx}}{\rho_x}$. Hence, unless ρ_x is 100% (or unity),

prediction ability of β_{yx} underestimates the relationship. SEM estimates β_x instead of β_{yx} and hence, indicates the relationship when there is no measurement error.

5.1.7.2 Assumptions

The following are the assumptions for SEM:
1. Multivariate normal distribution of both indicators and latent (dependent) variables
2. Linearity of relationship between indicators and latent variables as well as between latent variables; suitable transformation can be made in variables violating this assumption
3. All variables in the SEM are latent variables

4. At least 3 or more variables indicators for each of the latent variables to minimize measurement error
5. Mean of the residuals (mean difference between observed and estimated covariances) is zero
6. Error terms are assumed uncorrelated; but if such a correlation is expected, it can be included in the model itself
7. Absence of multicollinearity; as in case of error terms, if expected to be present, can be estimated by the model
8. Observed covariances are non-zero

5.1.7.3 Sample size

It is generally necessary that there are at least 15 respondents for each measure variable (p) or indicator in the model i.e. 15p. If multivariate normality of the data is doubtful, sample size needs to be increased. In addition, sample size increases as number of latent variables and/or covariances (communalities) as well as number of measured variables increases. Number of missing observations also affects the sample size. With p variables, a minimum of $\dfrac{p(p+1)}{2}$ sample size is essential to compute covariance matrix. Some authors suggest $8p + 50$ and others $10p$ to $20p$ as sample size.

5.1.7.4 Path diagram

A **construct** is defined as a latent concept that can not be measured directly but measurable indirectly and approximately by several indicators. An exogenous construct is a latent multi-item independent variable represented as a variate; they are not determined by the factors within the model or no other construct within the model explains it; hence, the term independent construct. Conversely, an endogenous construct is also a latent multi-item variable which is determined by the factors within the model.

Each endogenous construct is usually represented by **Path diagram** which indicates relationships between exogenous constructs and endogenous construct (dependence relationships). However, relationships between several endogenous and exogenous constructs (covariance relationship) as well as those of exogenous constructs with several endogenous constructs are also indicated in the path diagram. In short, the path diagram depicts all the relationships visually.

Two types of relationships can be shown:
1. Free pathways, in which relationships between variables are tested, and therefore are left 'free' to vary, and
2. Fixed pathways for relationships between variables that already have an estimated relationship, usually based on previous studies.

The following format is generally adopted while representing in a path diagram:
1. Constructs as ovals/circles
2. Measured variable as squares/rectangles
3. Measured variables for exogenous construct as x
4. Measured variables for endogenous construct as y
5. Relationship between x and/or y with their respective constructs as a straight unidirectional arrow from construct(s) to x and/or y

6. Correlation (covariance relationship) between constructs bidirectional arrow usually as a curved line or arc.

If it is assumed that latent constructs cause measured variables and in the process error results due to their failure to fully explain the latter, they are referred to as **reflective measures/constructs** and arrows are drawn from latent constructs to measured variables. On the contrary, if measured variables cause the construct and error is due to their inability to fully explain the construct, they are referred to as **formative measures/constructs** arrows are drawn from the measured variables to latent constructs. Formative constructs are more popular.

An example of path diagram with only one exogenous and endogenous construct is shown below to highlight the efficiency of SEM in exploring all relationships.

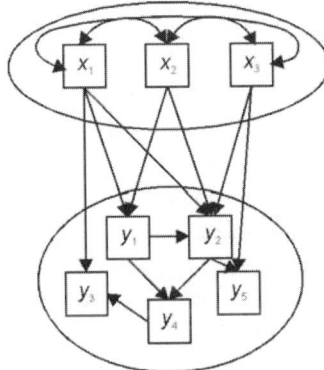

It is the responsibility of the researcher to first establish the cause-effect relationships as a prerequisite for deriving equations and testing them. In addition, correct sequence of relationships also needs to be established by carefully considering the nature of events; there could be events which are mutually exclusive. Similarly, only meaningful covariance(s) must be included in the model. It is evident from the above path diagram that such a complex relationship can not be studied either by DA/MDA or FA.

Number of parameters can be calculated as the total of number of:
a. exogenous variables
b. indicator variables
c. endogenous factors
d. correlations among latent variables (bidirectional arrows)
e. direct effects (straight arrows linking latent variables)
f. b number of latent variables

One parameter can be estimated for each unique variance and covariance in the variance-covariance matrix; hence the latter provides v. With p measure items,

$$\frac{1}{2} p (p + 1)$$ unique variance-covariance are possible.

5.1.7.4.1 *Measurement model*

Measurement model is all or part of SEM showing all possible straight unidirectional arrows between all possible latent variables with their indicators (but not between the latent variables) and there is unmeasured covariance between each possible pair latent variables or covariance matrix is assumed to be zero and hence, this model is usually considered as **Null model or Independence model**. In other words it is a Confirmatory Factor Analysis (CFA). CFA confirms the path diagram indicating the link between indicators and latent variables set by the researcher.

5.1.7.4.2 Structural model

This model includes both exogenous and endogenous variables with straight and curved unidirectional and bidirectional arrows. If all possible arrows are indicated it is referred to as **saturated model or Just Identified**; if covariances among all measured variables are zero (i.e. all paths in the structural model are 0), the structural model is called **independence model**. In a saturated model, number of parameters, p = number of elements in the covariance matrix. Hence, for saturated models and when $p >$ elements in the covariance matrix (**underidentified or unidentified model**), goodness of fit can not be calculated because υ becomes 0. For significance tests, number of knowns must be > number of unknowns.

For instance, a measurement model with two measured items can have two variances and one covariance; totally three unique values; but two each of factor and error loadings need to be estimated; hence, a unique solution is not possible and the model becomes underidentified. Similarly with three measured items, totally six unique values are available and three each of factor and error loadings need to be estimated resulting in a $\upsilon = 0$. Such a model becomes saturated model wherein testing is not possible. However, if other constructs have > 3 items, testing can be performed. On the same lines, with 4 measured items, $\upsilon = 2$ making it amenable for testing. Therefore, at least 3 – 4 items per construct are necessary; however, constructs with < 3 are permitted under special circumstances provided that overall $\upsilon \neq 0$.

5.1.7.4.3 Default model

This is structural model as decided by the researcher

5.1.7.4.4 Parsimony model or model parsimony

This is a model where no effect is constrained to be zero; a saturated model could be a parsimony model. As the number of variables considered increase and as more complex relationships are included in SEM, goodness of fit increases.

5.1.7.4.5 Recursive model

A model in which all arrows flow in one direction with no feedback looping (no covariances among endogenous variables) is referred to as recursive model. In this model number of parameters, p > number of observations and hence, has no solution.

5.1.7.5 Testing fitness of the model

Several measures to test the SEM have been developed and are being refined regularly.

5.1.7.5.1 Goodness of fit (model χ^2, discrepancy function, likelihood ratio χ^2, V fit index)

1. χ^2 goodness of fit (model χ^2, discrepancy function, likelihood ratio χ^2, χ^2 fit index):

calculated as $\chi^2 = (N-1)(M_{Obs} - M_{Est})$ on $\upsilon = \frac{1}{2}\left[p(p-1)\right] - k$ and set α level of significance where N is the overall sample size, M_{obs} and M_{Est} are the observed and estimated covariance matrix, respectively, p is the total number of observed variables and k is the number of parameters estimated in the SEM. With a model tested on H_0 that observed and estimated covariances are equal, χ^2 should be non-significant and should be close to 0. However, χ^2 increases even with sample size and is affected by deviations from multinormality. Hence, it is not a very reliable test.

Hoelter's critical N should be at least 75 to consider model χ^2 as a criterion for

goodness of fit. It is calculated as (for $\alpha = 0.05$): $\dfrac{\sqrt{[2.58+(2\upsilon-1)]^2}}{1+\left(2\chi^2 \big/ n-1\right)}$ where χ^2 is the

model χ^2 and n is the number of subjects.

Normed χ^2 is the ratio of χ^2 to the υ of the model. When the ratio is ≤ 3, the model is considered a good fit.

2. Goodness of fit index. GFI (Joreskog-Sorbom GFI, $\hat{\gamma}$): This is calculated as

$$1-\left(\frac{\chi^2_{\text{Default model}}}{\chi^2_{\text{Null model}}}\right);$$ GFI ≥ 0.95 is desirable to accept the model as a good fit. Even GFI

is affected by sample size or in other words υ. In spite of several variants are described like that proposed by Steiger and Adjusted GFI, it is now not popularly used. In

any case, Adjusted Goodness of Fit Index (AGFI): calculated as $1-(1-GFI)\left[\dfrac{p(p-1)}{2\upsilon}\right]$

where p is number of variables.

5.1.7.5.2 Based on information theory

1. Akaike Information Criterion (AIC) (*see* Section 3.6 **Chapter "Statistics in Specific**

Veterinary Fields") can be used by calculating $AIC = \dfrac{\chi^2}{n} + \dfrac{2k}{n-1}$ where k =

$\left[\frac{1}{2}p(p+1)\right]-\upsilon$, p being number of variables and υ, the degrees of freedom. AIC

values corrected for sample size like AICC (AIC$_C$) or Consistent AIC (CAIC), can also be employed. Similarly, AIC corrected for over-dispersion (QAIC) can also be used.

2. Bayesian information criterion (BIC) also called Akaike BIC (ABIC) which corrects for number of parameters is also available. In addition, rescaling of BIC to Akaike weights is also possible.

3. Browne-Cudeck criterion (BCC): This is a single sample cross validation index

calculated as $BCC = \dfrac{\chi^2}{n} + \dfrac{2k}{n-p-2}$ where $k = \left[\dfrac{1}{2}p(p+1)\right]-\upsilon$ and p is the number of

variables.

4. Others in this category include Expected Cross Validation Index (ECVI), Modified ECVI (MECVI) and Cross Validation Index (CVI).

5.1.7.5.3 Based on non-centrality

1. Non-centrality Parameter (NCP, McDonald NCP Index, DK): Corrects for complexities and is calculated as $\dfrac{\left(\chi^2 - \upsilon\right)_{Null} - \left(\chi^2 - \upsilon\right)_{SEM}}{\left(\chi^2 - \upsilon\right)_{Null}}$; this can be scaled to unity by $e^{-\left(\frac{NCP}{2}\right)}$.

2. Relative non-centrality index (RNI): This index accounts for both sample size and complexities in the model. This is computed as: $\dfrac{\left[\dfrac{\chi^2_{Null}}{n} - \dfrac{\upsilon}{n} - NCP\right]}{\left(\dfrac{\chi^2_{Null}}{n} - \dfrac{\upsilon}{n}\right)}$. McDonald's

NCI is given by $1 - \dfrac{\left(\chi^2 - \upsilon\right)_{SEM}}{\left(\chi^2 - \upsilon\right)_{Null}}$.

5.1.7.5.4 Given model vis-à-vis null/alternate model

In these tests, researcher's model is tested usually against independence model since the latter has the least fit.

1. Comparative Fit Index (CFI, Bentler's CFI): calculated as follows: $1 - \dfrac{\left(\chi^2 - \upsilon\right)_{SEM}}{\left(\chi^2 - \upsilon\right)_{Null}}$; a good fit is indicated by CFI ≥ 0.9

2. Incremental Fit Index (IFI, Bollen's IFI, BL89, Δ_2) which is computed as $\dfrac{\chi^2_{Null} - \chi^2_{Default}}{\chi^2_{Null} - \upsilon_{Default}}$; in a good fit, IFI ≥ 0.9

3. Normed Fit Index (NFI, Bentler-Bonett NFI, Δ_1) calculated as $\dfrac{\chi^2_{Null} - \chi^2_{Default}}{\chi^2_{Null}}$; it ranges between 0 and 1 and is influenced by complex relationships and hence not popular; an NFI > 0.95 is considered a good fit.

4. Bentler–Bonett Index (BBI) is given by $\dfrac{\chi^2_{Given\ Model} - \chi^2_{Null}}{\chi^2_{Null}}$; a value of > 0.9 is required for a good fit.

5. Tucker–Lewis Index (TLI, Non-normed Fit Index, NNFI, Tucker-Lewis ρ Index) given by $\dfrac{\left(\dfrac{\chi^2}{\upsilon}\right)_{Null} - \left(\dfrac{\chi^2}{\upsilon}\right)_{SEM}}{\left(\dfrac{\chi^2}{\upsilon}\right)_{Null} - 1}$; a value ≥ 0.95 is desirable. If the term "–1" is deleted

in the above formula, Bollen's 86 Fit Index is obtained which also should be > 0.9 for a good fit model.

6. Relative Fit Index (RFI, ρ_1) is given by $1 - \dfrac{\left(\dfrac{\chi^2}{\upsilon}\right)_{Default}}{\left(\dfrac{\chi^2_{Null}}{\upsilon_{Default}}\right)}$; a vlue as close to 1 as possible

is desirable.

5.1.7.5.5 *Based on lack of parsimony*

1. Parsimony ratio (PRATIO): is the ratio of υ of researcher's model to that of null model; for saturated model, the value will be 0 and conversely, for the independence model, it will be unity.
2. Indices from PRATIO: Product of PRATIO with other indices is also another index to test parsimony; they are tabulated below:

Multiplier	Index
NFI	Parsimony Normed Fit Index (PNFI$_1$)
IFI	PNFI$_2$
CFI	Parsimony Comparative Fit Index (PCFI)
GFI	PGFI
BBI	Parsimony Index, PI

In all the above indices, higher the value better is the fit of the model.
3. Root mean square error of approximation RMSEA, RMS, RMSE, and discrepancy

per degree of freedom): This is calculated as $\sqrt{\dfrac{\chi^2_{SEM} - \upsilon_{SEM}}{(n-1)}}$ where n is the number

of subjects.
4. Root mean square residuals (RMR, RMSR, RMS residuals): This is the mean absolute value of the covariance residuals i.e. $(M_{obs} - M_{Est})$ where M_{obs} and M_{Est} are the observed and estimated covariance matrix, respectively. In an ideal situation, it should be zero. Cut–off value to consider a model as a good fit has been highly varying from RMR < 0.04 to 0.10.
5. Standardized root mean square residual (SRMR): This is analogous to standard deviation (*see* **Chapter "Central tendency"**); each of the covariance residuals is squared and their mean is taken; the root of this mean value is the SRMR. Even for SRMR, cut–off value suggested is variable from 0.04 to 0.1.

5.1.7.5.6 *Pattern coefficients (factor loadings, factor pattern coefficients, validity coefficients)*

These are analogous to loadings described under Section 5.1.2.4 above. A loading of at least 0.7 is necessary on the latent variable because, communality which is the square of the loading indicates the proportion of variability in the given variable explained by the latent variable (similar to R^2 value in linear and multiple regression analysis). It is for this reason that factor loading can be used as an indicator of reliability.

If z_i's are standardized loadings and e_i is the error term or (1 – reliability) where

reliability $= z_i^2$, of the ith latent variable then **construct reliability** is given by $\dfrac{\sum\limits_{i=1}^{p} z_i^2}{\sum\limits_{i=1}^{p}\left(z_i^2 + e_i\right)}$

where p is the number of variables.

5.1.7.6 Confirmatory Factor Analysis (CFA)

From the path diagram, all straight arrows connecting latent variables are removed, curved arrows representing covariance between every pair of latent variables are added, and straight arrows from each latent variable to its indicator variables as well as leaving in the straight arrows from error and disturbance terms to their respective variables are retained. Using this as a measurement model, SEM is developed and tested as described above. CFA can be employed as a validation of relationships among latent variables before the main SEM. Hence, CFA is a part and parcel of SEM.

5.2 Multivariate Methods to Study Interdependence

5.2.1 Factor Analysis (FA), Principal Component Analysis (PCA), Exploratory Factor Analysis (EFA), and Principal Factor Analysis (PFA), Common Factor Analysis (CFA), Principal Axis Factoring (PAF)

Factor analysis (FA) is included in SEM itself. FA describes variability among observed variables in terms of fewer unobserved variables called **factors**. It helps identify tests that measure same factor thereby reduce the number of tests (attribute space) to derive the same result. It is also useful to identify items which load on > 1 factors so that the index can be improved by dropping such items. It follows that it can help identify subset of variables with highest correlation with principal components. In the process, it identifies variables with no correlations also so that multicollinearity can be handled. It is evident that factors are "extracted" from a set of variables to minimize attribute space.

In FA, none of the variable is considered dependent or independent but considered interdependent. Assumptions for FA are similar to those of MRA *viz.* multivariate normality, linear relationships, untruncated interval (or near interval) data and absence of high degree of multicollinearity.

5.2.1.1 Model

If $x_1, x_2 \ldots x_p$ are p random variables with means $\mu_1, \mu_2 \ldots \mu_p$, for k unknown random variables designated F_j and unknown constants (factor loadings) designated l_{ij}, given that $i \in 1, 2 \ldots p$ and $j \in 1, 2 \ldots k$ and $k < p$, then $\left(x_i - \mu_i\right) = \sum\limits_{i=1}^{p}\sum\limits_{j=1}^{k} l_{ij} F_j + e_i$ where e_i is

Normally and independently distributed with mean 0 and finite variance (ψ_i). This follows that $Cov_e = Diag\left(\psi_1, \psi_2, \ldots \psi_p\right) = \Psi$ and $E(e) = 0$. If L and F are matrices of factor loadings and random variables, respectively given that F and e are independent, E(F) = 0 and Cov (F) = unity, in terms of matrices we get $(x - \mu) = LF + e$ and any solution

for this model with constraints for F is defined as factors and L as loading matrix. If
Cov $(x) = M$, $M = Cov(LF + e) = LCov(F)L^T + Cov(e) = LL^T + \Psi$.

Variants of FA are PCA (for data reduction), EFA (study of structure of large set of variables and test a *a-priori* assumption that any indicator may be related to any factor), PFA (for causal analysis) and CFA (as a part of SEM to test *a-priori* assumption that number of factors and loadings of indicators or measured variables is as per the pre-established norms).

5.2.1.2 Assumptions

1. Interval data
2. No selection bias in inclusion/exclusion of variables
3. Valid imputation of factor labels
4. Linearity
5. Multivariate Normality
6. Homoscedasticity
7. In case of PFA, unique factors must be orthogonal to one another and also with other factors; not necessary for PCA
8. Absence of high multicollinearity
9. $p > k$; i.e., number of variables more than that of factors

5.2.1.3 PCA

PCA performs a variance-maximizing rotation of the variable space, whereas, FA estimates variability attributable due to common factors ("communality"). Basically PCA analyzes the variance into that explained by the components and that by the error, i.e. a correlation matrix (with diagonals as unity; not covariance matrix) through a series of linear equations. Analogous to CCR, PCA for first component accounts for maximum variance. PCA for second accounts for maximum variance after the variance explained by from first component is removed and so on till all the variance is explained. Generally, the linear equations are orthogonal to each other; otherwise, modification is required in the procedure. Addition of factors results in changes in factor loadings. Hence, PCA **explores** the causes and hence helps data reduction; for this reason, not used in SEM.

5.2.1.4 PFA

Unlike PCA but similar to SEM, PFA, analyzes correlation matrix with communalities as diagonals (equivalent of covariance matrix). It partitions covariance into that explained by the components and that by the error. PCA for first component accounts for maximum covariance. PCA for second accounts for maximum covariance after the covariance explained by from first component is removed and so on till all the covariance is explained. As with PCA, generally, the linear equations are orthogonal to each other; otherwise, modification is required in the procedure. Factors can be added without changing the factor loadings. Hence, PFA can be used to confirm *a-priori* assumed correlations and causal model by the researcher.

5.2.1.5 Other methods

Image factoring (using predicted variables), maximum likehood factoring (MLF, forming linear combination of variables as factors), α factoring (variables drawn random from universe of variables), unweighted/generalized least square factoring (minimizing differences between observed and estimated correlation matrix) and canonical factoring (Rao's canonical factoring, to identify factors having highest CCR with observed variables) are the other methods of extracting (minimizing) factors.

5.2.1.6 Interpretation

5.2.1.6.1 Factor loadings

These are correlation coefficients between variables (in rows) and factors (in columns) generally referred to as **component loadings**. Square of this correlation coefficient is analogous to R^2 in MRA indicating the proportion of variance in the concerned indicator variable explained by the factor. Hence, factor loading of at least 0.7 ($R^2 \approx 50\%$) is considered necessary to consider that an indicator is related to the factor.

This follows that proportion of variance in all variables explained by the given factor j can be computed as $\dfrac{\sum\limits_{i=1}^{p} l_{ij}^2}{p}$; if variances are standardized to unity, the denominator will be sum of the variances; in other words, ratio of Factor's Eigen value to p referred to as **percent of Trace.**

Factors can be rotated to maximize $\sum\limits_{i=1}^{p} l_{ij}^2$; several methods are available for this purpose.

5.2.1.6.2 Communality, h^2

Percent of variance in the variable jointly explained by all factors is given by the square of the multiple correlation coefficient; it is also called reliability of the indicator and designated h^2. Obviously, it indicates as to which of the measured variables is best explained by the factor analysis.

5.2.1.6.3 Uniqueness

Calculated as $1 - h^2$; it is converse of communality

5.2.1.6.4 Eigen values (characteristic roots)

This is the summation of variances of all variables accounted for by a given factor. It is expected to be as high as possible. If variables are standardized, Eigen value of any factor j is given by $\sum\limits_{i=1}^{p} l_{ij}^2$.

5.2.1.6.5 Trace

Trace is the sum of variances of all variables; since the variables are standardized, trace is simply p and percent of trace for a factor j is $\dfrac{\sum\limits_{i=1}^{p} l_{ij}^2}{p}$.

5.2.1.6.6 Factor scores (component scores in PCA)

These are scores on each variable (row) on each factor (column). If s_{ij} is the score for variable i and factor k, factor score $= \sum_{j=1}^{k} l_{ij} s_{ij}$.

5.2.2 Cluster Analysis (CSA, Segmentation Analysis, Q Analysis, Topology Construction, Taxonomy Analysis, Classification Analysis, Numerical Taxonomy)

CSA is used to identify homogenous groups in a population (even when number of such groups is not known in advance) based on distance by minimizing within group variation and maximizing between group variations. This is the only multivariate technique where variate is not estimated; instead used as specified by the researcher. It is a descriptive, non-theoretical and non-inferential analysis.

It is customary to standardize all variables to obviate those with higher magnitude to dominate the process. However, standardization is rather obligatory when the variables are not on the same scale. If the data represents ratings on a uniform scale say hedonic (10-point) scale, standardization is not required.

5.2.2.1 Assumptions

1. Randomization: especially for K-means and two-stage clustering.
2. Data: Interval or true dichotomous data for hierarchical and K-means clustering; two-stage clustering can include both categorical as well as continuous data.
3. Variables and observations are independent which can be tested by bivariate correlation matrix.
4. Absence of multicollinearity
5. Multinomial distribution for categorical data and normal distribution for continuous data.
6. Sample size: For K-means clustering > 200 and much larger for two-step clustering.

5.2.2.2 Hierarchical clustering

Distance is the criterion for grouping; distance is defined and number of groups is decided for the given data. Clusters so formed are represented as icicles and dendograms. At the beginning, each case is considered a cluster and then two clusters with distance ≤ the minimum distance are grouped together; likewise, all cases are assigned into the number of cases determined in advance. Clusters formed but close enough can be combined at the prerogatives of the researcher to achieve the desired number of clusters each being not only meaningful but also has sufficient cases. This method is suitable when sample size is < 250.

At the beginning wider cut-off can be used followed by relaxation to form more clusters (Forward clustering); alternatively, one can begin with narrow cut-off followed by merging of clusters closer enough (Backward clustering).

The "distance" can be interval, binary or count and for each of these separate methods are available.

5.2.2.2.1 Interval

Can be clustered based on euclidean or squared euclidean distance, cosine, Pearson's r, Chebychev distance, Block distance, etc. Pairs of variables are considered as x and y axes and cases are plotted. The distances are tabulated as a $(k \times k)$ similarity or proximity matrix with rows and columns representing the cases where k is the number of cases.

a. Euclidean and squared euclidean distance: Distance between each pair combination is calculated as per Pythagoras Theorem i.e. if a and b are distances on x and y axes,

Euclidean distance is given by $\sqrt{a^2 + b^2}$ and the squared euclidean distance is that without applying square root. The latter further magnifies the distances and hence facilitates the clustering procedure. The euclidean distance is most commonly used for formation of clusters.

b. Cosine: This is applicable for qualitative data (attributes). If θ is the angle between the two vectors of values, $\cos \theta$ is the cosine value between them. Hence, if values fall on the same line, $\theta = 0°$ and $\cos \theta = 1$ regardless of the "distance" between them. Similarly, if $\theta = 90°$, $\cos \theta = 0$.

c. Chebychev distance: This is the maximum of the absolute distances (coordinates of both x and y axes) between any pair cases on any one of the variables considered.

d. Block distance (city block distance, manhattan distance): Similar to chebychev distance; but coordinates of both x and y axes are added.

e. Mahalanobis D^2: This is similar to Euclidean distance utilizing standardized values and weightage given for correlations between variables

f. Pearson's r: Data with columns as variables and rows as cases are transposed to calculate Pearson's r between cases which can be used as similarity matrix. Since ± r can be significant, generally, absolute values are given in similarity matrix.

5.2.2.2.2 Counts

Can be classified by χ^2 or ψ^2 measure.

a. χ^2: Equality between two sets of frequencies as indicated by χ^2 is the criterion

b. ψ^2: By taking square root of combined frequency, ψ^2 normalizes χ^2 to yield distances with mean 0 and unit variance.

5.2.2.2.3 Binary

This is based on the value itself (0 or 1) between any pair of data; 1 indicating "Match" and 0 "No match". Several methods are available in this category viz. Size difference, Pattern difference, Goodman and Kruskal's λ, Variance, Dispersion, etc. Even Squared Euclidean Distance is employed.

5.2.2.2.4 Defining similarity between multiple–member clusters

It is necessary to study similarity between clusters for merging clusters (agglomeration) during the process of cluster formation. This is achieved by several methods as follows:

5.2.2.2.4.1 Single linkage (near neighborhood)

This is defined as the shortest distance between any object of one cluster and any object of another cluster.

5.2.2.2.4.2 Complete linkage (farthest neighborhood, greatest diameter method)

This is defined as the minimum distance (diameter) sphere that can enclose both clusters completely. In other words, this will be maximum distance between any object of one cluster and any object of another cluster.

5.2.2.2.4.3 Within groups linkage (average linkage within groups)

Average of all inter and intra pair distances is the within group linkage. This is made as low as possible to increase homogeneity within a cluster.

5.2.2.2.4.4 Between groups linkage (average linkage, ungrouped pair-group method, UGPMA)

The average linkage is the average of all inter-cluster pair distances (between all members of one cluster with those in another).

5.2.2.2.4.5 Centroid method

Centroid is the average of observations on the variables in the cluster; distance between centroids of the clusters is considered in this method. Centroid changes when as and when clusters merge.

5.2.2.2.4.6 Ward's method

Sum of squares over all variables within a cluster is the criterion in this method. Depending on which merger minimized the sum of squares within cluster, decision is taken for merging clusters.

Whenever clusters are merged, within cluster heterogeneity has to be checked either by estimating distance at which the clusters are formed or by observing change in within cluster sum of squares. Often, change in standard deviation between the original and merged clusters also help decision making.

5.2.2.2.4.7 Agglomeration coefficient

This measures increase in heterogeneity on merger of clusters and it is the distance between two closest observations among two clusters being merged. Agglomeration coefficient is useful in setting limits for merging process.

5.2.2.2.5 Dendograms (hierarchical tree, plot)

This is a graphical representation in which proximity matrix is represented with rows representing each case on y-axis. Variables with high similarity will be close together and *vice versa*; magnitude of similarity is indicated by the proportionate length of the line from left to right connecting the variables.

5.2.2.2.6 Icicle plots

These are usually horizontal plots depicting cases as rows and number of clusters as columns; when viewed from bottom upwards, the process of clustering can be visualized; initially there will be maximum number of clusters and as the process of cluster formation proceeds, number of clusters reduces and finally, all cases will be in one cluster. The icicle plot can be vertical as well; then, it is viewed right to left.

5.2.2.3 K-means clustering

Number of clusters (K) is decided and then assignment of cases into the clusters is through an algorithm developed for the purpose. Large sample size can be handled in this technique because developing proximity matrix is not a pre-requisite for cluster formation in this method. Since K number of cluster means are involved, it is called K-means clustering. The process is summarized below:

1. Researcher first decided the number of clusters
2. Cluster centers chosen at random after preliminary inspection of data
3. Based on euclidean distance to the mean of the cluster (centroid), through iteration, the observations (cases) are grouped in such a way that within cluster variance is minimized and between cluster variance is maximized.
4. Cluster means will continuously show changes as iteration progresses
5. Iteration process continued till cluster means stabilize and do not change beyond a pre-determined cut–off value.

5.2.2.4 Two-step clustering

Used for categorical data and is also suitable for continuous data. This method is also a method of choice when sample size is very large and/or when variables have ≥ 3 levels. Obviously, variable-wise and cluster-wise plots will be necessary for graphical representation. The steps involved are (a) Pre-clustering and (b) Hierarchical clustering for each of the pre–clusters.

5.2.2.5 Other methods of clustering

1. Expected Maximization (EM) Clustering: same as K-means clustering but MLE is employed for cluster determination. Suitable for both categorical and continuous data. Further, each case can be included in each of the clusters but with different probabilities.
2. Q–mode analysis: used when proximity matrix consists of correlation coefficients
3. MDS: MDS done by cases is a form of cluster analysis. MDS is outlined in a separate section below.
4. F–ratio methods: based on the ratio of variance between to that of within group variance; groups formed arbitrarily at the beginning whose means are the centroids of the clusters.

5.2.3 Multidimensional Scaling (MDS, Perceptual/Spatial Mapping)

MDS is a series of techniques that help detect the underlying dimensions for evaluation of objects by respondents and position the objects in the dimension defined by transforming them into distances. That means, MDS compares objects through following steps:

1. All measures of similarity or preferences are derived from all sets of objects
2. Estimation of relative position in the dimension through MDS
3. Identify and interpret multi-dimensional space in terms of attributes; objective or perceptual.

5.2.3.1 Object and Subject

Variables or stimuli are referred to as "Objects/Targets"; for instance, items, opinions, etc. which are to be compared. Individuals who are actually doing the comparison are referred to as "Subjects/Sources". Sometimes, subjects may rate themselves and become objects themselves.

An object can be characterized through measurable (metric or objective) attributes and/or through perceivable (subjective) attributes which can not be measured physically. Objective and perceived dimensions need not be independent of one another. Hence, they need to be related to the axes of the multidimensional space i.e. relative positioning.

MDS is unique in two ways:

1. Each respondent (individual) evaluates all objects and hence, solution for each individual is possible.

2. Variate is not formed. For instance, if one evaluates n egg preparations in all possible $\dfrac{n(n-1)}{2}$ pair combinations and ranks them depending on similarity of the pairs, researcher need not have to specify on what variables the respondent has to evaluate the preparations.

It can be visualized that as n increases, graphical representation of similarity of pairs becomes increasingly difficult on two dimensions (axes) and hence, multi-dimensional approach becomes necessary. It is clear from the above that MDS helps explore dimensions affecting behavior and compare objects without defining any basis for the same. Hence, the researcher has to make important decisions on selection of objects, attribute to be analyzed (similarity/preference) and type of analysis (individual/group level).

5.2.3.2 Selection of objects

Researcher should ensure that all relevant objects are included for MDS; inclusion of unnecessary objects as well as deletion of relevant ones makes considerable difference in the outcome of MDS

5.2.3.3 Attribute to be analyzed

If "similarity" is assessed by the respondents, good/bad aspects (preference) of the objects are not considered because bases for similarity may be completely independent of those for preference; *vice versa* is true if assessment is on "preference" of the respondents. Hence, researcher has to apply his mind depending on ultimate aim of his research.

5.2.3.4 Assumptions

Unlike most of the multivariate methods, MDS does not require linearity, metricity or multivariate normality; but, the primary assumption is that objects and subjects must be both representative and comparable.

5.2.3.5 Data collection

Most of the MDS data consists of objects being rated on an "Overall" basis by the subjects; in other words no specific criteria are defined by the researcher. Such data permit both aggregate and disaggregate analysis (*see* Section 5.2.3.6) through subject and object matrices. This is referred to as "Decompositional MDS". Alternatively, researcher may need subjects to evaluate objects through a series of defined attributes (color, taste, size, cost etc), it is necessary that data from all subjects is pooled and analyzed; i.e. aggregate analysis through only object matrices. This is referred to as "Compositional MDS"; however, data from compositional MDS is amenable for other statistical analysis like FA, DA, and CRA.

5.2.3.5.1 *Preference*

Subjects need to give whether a specified object is preferable over other object(s)

5.2.3.5.2 *Paired comparison*

If n objects are available, then all the $\dfrac{n(n-1)}{2}$ pair combinations are ranked depending on similarity of the pairs. Alternatively, subjects may be needed to evaluate each of the pairs for similarity on a hedonic (0 to 10) scale.

5.2.3.5.3 *Confusion data method*

Subjects are served with a card representing each of the objects and required to stack them into groups depending on similarities and space them in such a way that stacks closer to each other are similar than those farther away.

5.2.3.5.4 *Direct ranking*

Subjects rank n objects into ranks 1 to n in a descending order of preference.

5.2.3.5.5 *Objective data*

Frequencies, distances, proportions etc. are also possible to be subjected to MDS. A correlation matrix can be converted to dissimilarity matrix $(1 - r)$ and convert it into distance matrix suitable for MDS.

5.2.3.6 Distance

Similarity, dissimilarity, proximity, etc. between objects are depicted as "distance" between the object locations in the multidimensional space and hence, is the basic concept in MDS. Hence, distance means any of the following in MDS:

1. Similarity and dissimilarity matrices: generally, similarity matrix is converted to dissimilarity matrices indicating distance
2. Distance matrices: if the data collected itself is in the form of distance as in case of rankings, ratings, comparisons
3. Metric variables: are converted into distances by standardizing them into z variate.

Distance matrices may be subject matrices (one subject rating another) or object matrices (subjects rating objects) or objective matrices (distances between objects or a correlation matrix of objects)

5.2.3.7 Aggregate *vs* disaggregate analysis

As the name indicates, "Disaggregate analysis" analyses responses from each respondent separately and it follows that if analysis is performed aggregating responses of all the respondents, it is called "Aggregate analysis".

In disaggregate analysis perceptual maps are developed for each respondent to elucidate unique feature(s) in perception of each of the respondents, if any. But, it does not help develop a common perceptual map combining perceptions of all respondents.

There are three variants of aggregate analysis; *viz.*

1. Before scaling: Average evaluation of all the respondents can be utilized to develop a common perceptual map. However, average values may be clustered to identify

groups of respondents with similar perceptions and maps developed for average of each of the clusters. This is the most common method.

2. After individual MDS: In this method, perceptual maps of the individual respondents are clustered based on co-ordinates.
3. Combination approach: Available in some of the Statistical software. In this method, perceptual space shared by all respondents is derived (similar to aggregate analysis). A special group space map is also derived where respondent's position is determined depending on the respondent's weights for each dimension. Distance of the respondent's position from the origin is directly proportionate to the proportion of variance for that respondent accounted for by the solution.

Note: It is clear from the above that type of analysis is a function of research objectives set by the researcher.

5.2.3.8. Number of dimensions

Most MDS is either bi- or tri-dimensional. However, number of dimensions should be such that it minimizes stress or which is at the elbow of scree plot. If possible, PCA or FA can be employed to decide dimensions.

The MDS can be run for a sequence of dimensions and that which yields the most interpretable results can be picked up as the ideal dimension; this is the best method to define dimensions.

5.2.3.9 Goodness of fit

5.2.3.9.1 ψ (Phi) or stress

For MDS, goodness of fit is defined as ψ (*Phi*); as a difference between MDS-computed interpoint distances and corresponding actual input distances.

Therefore, smaller the ψ better the fit. When ψ is plotted against dimension, it is referred to as "Scree plot"; the number of dimensions corresponding to the elbow of the plot is the optimum dimension for the MDS.

There are two forms of stress measures: Young's stress (*S*-stress) based on squared distances and Kruskal's stress (Stress–1, Stress formula–1) based on distances. Average stress is the square root of mean of squared Kruskal's stress.

5.2.3.9.2 Squared correlation index, R^2

Squared correlation index is square of the correlation coefficient between input distance and scaled distance; analogous to coefficient determination it indicates proportion of variance in input data accounted for by the scaled data. R^2 is expected to be at least 0.6 to consider it significant.

5.2.3.9.3 Average R^2

This is average R^2 calculated from matrix obtained from values across respondents.

5.2.3.9.4 Individual R^2

R^2 calculated from matrix obtained from matrices of individual respondents. These values can be grouped into high and low or male and female or any such categories by the researcher, if needed by the objective of the experiment.

5.2.4. *Correspondence Analysis (CRA, Optimal Scaling or Scoring, Reciprocal Averaging, Homogeneity Analysis, Correspondence Mapping, Social Space Analysis, Correspondence Factor Analysis, PCA for Qualitative Data, Dual Scaling)*

Objectives of CRA are similar to those of MDS but differ in its approach because instead of similarities and preferences in MDA, CRA evaluates each object over a series of attributes (non-metric) and locates them in dimensional space for comparing objects and attributes simultaneously. CRA is used to study how one set of categorical entities are related to other sets and hence, CRA can also be viewed as a special case of CCR. For CRA, data should be discrete nominal or ordinal or continuous segmented into ranges. CRA is only an exploratory technique and is not a confirmatory analytical method.

In CRA also distance between any two points is the criterion and a distance matrix is the input to determine those categories which are closer to each other through a PCA and perceptual mapping based on CRA is developed in a two-dimensional correspondence map. CRA can help study association among only row or column categories or between both.

5.2.4.1 Assumptions

1. In CRA discrete data is involved and hence does not support usual methods of significance testing. Log-linear or LRA are used for testing.
2. χ^2 distance matrix is assumed to be equivalent of correlation matrix. Total variance in CRA is referred to as "Total Inertia" and closeness of any two points on correspondence map need not be associated with the proportion of inertia explained by the model.
3. Contingency tables consist of objects (categories) as rows and attributes (variables) as columns. Although $n \times n$ tables is possible, generally only 2 or 3 variables are optimum. Homogeneity of column variables across row variables is assumed. However, CRA is useful with many categories; otherwise, Log-linear regression will be more suitable.
4. Unlike other methods of FA, no underlying distribution is assumed. If continuous data has to be used, it must be segmented into ranges which may cause loss of information.
5. Cell values can not be negative.

Note: Total inertia is calculated as the ratio of total χ^2 to total sample size; χ^2 value for each of the cells is the inertia for the cell concerned.

5.2.4.2 Distance

Unlike MDA where euclidean distance is calculated, in CRA χ^2 distance is measured because discrete data is involved. χ^2 values are generally calculated as per usual χ^2 formula. Values of *Row profiles, Row/Column masses* and *Average Row/Column profiles* may be used instead of frequencies.

1. Cell values converted as % of row totals and are called *Row profiles*
2. Row totals converted as % of overall total (sample size) and are called *Row masses.*
3. Column totals converted as % of overall total (sample size) and are called *Average row profiles.*
4. Cell values converted as % of column totals and are called *Column profiles*

5. Column totals converted as % of overall total (sample size) and are called *Column masses*.

6. Row totals converted as % of overall total (sample size) and are called *Average column profiles*.

Note: Row masses = Average column profiles, and Column masses = Average row profiles. Row profiles are the ones which are to be explained and column profiles are explanatory in nature.

5.2.4.3. Number of dimensions

Eigen values (analogous to Stress values in MDS) are computed for each of the dimensions and plotted to obtain a Scree plot; the dimension referring to elbow of the Scree plot is the ideal number of dimensions. Ratio Eigen value of the dimension to total inertia estimates the proportion of variance explained by the dimension.

References

1. Amble, VN. Statistical methods in animal sciences. Indian Society of Agricultural Statistics, New Delhi, 1975.

2. Caughley, G and Sinclair, ARE. Wildlife ecology and management. Blackwell Scientific Publications, Boston 1994.

3. Chapman, AB. General and quantitative genetics. (Ed). World animal science series, A-4, Elsevier Pub. 1985.

4. Cornfield, J and Mantel, N. Some new aspects of the application of Maximum Likelihood for the calculation of the Disage–Response curve. J. Am. Stat. Assocn. 1950.

5. Falconer, DS. Introduction to quantitative genetics. III Ed. Longman Scientific & Technical, 1989.

6. Frankham, R, Ballou, JD and Briscoe, DA. Introduction to conservation genetics. Cambridge University press, 2002.

7. Gacula, Jr M. C and Singh, J., 1984 Statistical methods in food and consumer research. Academic Press, Orlando

8. Grossman, M and Koops, WJ. A model for individual egg production in chickens. Poultry Sci., 2001, **80**: 859–867.

9. Gupta, SC and Kapoor, VK. Fundamentals of applied statistics. Sultan Chand and Sons, New Delhi, 1994.

10. Gupta, SP and Gupta, A. Statistical methods. 2nd Revised Ed. Sultan Chand and Sons, New Delhi, 1996.

11. Hair, J.F.Jr., Black, W.C., Babin, B.J. and Anderson, R.E., 2010 Multivariate Data Analysis 10th Ed Prentice Hall

12. Johnson, R. A. and Dean, W.W. Applied multivariate statistical analysis 6th Ed. Pearson Education, Inc., NJ

13. Kaps, M and Lamberson, W. Biostatistics for animal science. CABI Publishing, 2004.

14. Katzung, BG. Basic and clinical pharmacology. 8th Ed. Lange Medical Books/McGraw-Hill, 2001.

15. Knapp, RG and Miller, MC III. Clinical epidemiology ad biostatistics. Harwal Publishing Co., Pennsylvania, 1992.

16. Male'cot, G. Cited from Pirchner, 1948, 1983.

17. Martin, SW, Mee, AH and Willeberg, P. Veterinary epidemiology. International Book Distributing Co., Lucknow, India, 1993.

18. McMillan, I, Earle, MF and Robson, DS. Quantitative genetics of fertility I and II. Genetics, 1970, **65**: 349–369.

19. McNally, DH. Mathematical model for egg production. Biometrics, 1971, **27**: 735–738.

20. Mead, R, Curnow, RN and Hasted, AM. Statistical methods in agriculture and biology. 2nd Ed. Chapman and Hall, London, 1993.
21. Morris, TR. Experimental Design and analysis in animal sciences. CABI Publishing, UK, 1999.
22. Noordhuizen, JPTM, Frankena, K, Thrusfield, MV and Graat, EAM. Application of quantitative methods in veterinary epidemioogy. International Book Distributing Co., Lucknow, India, 2003.
23. Nordskog, AW. Notes on poultry genetics and breeding. A.W Nordskog publication, 1976.
24. Pirchner, F. Population genetics in animal breeding. II Ed. Panima Publishing Corp. New Delhi, 1983.
25. Rosner, B. Fundamentals of biostatistics. 5th Ed. Duxbury Thomson Learning, USA, 2000.
26. Sharma, S., 1986 Applied multivariate techniques, John Wiley & Sons, New York
27. Short, J. Quoted from Caughley, G. and Sinclair, ARE, 1987, 1994.
28. Smith, RD. Veterinary clinical epidemiology: a problem–oriented approach. CRC press, 1994.
29. Snedecor, GW and Cochran, WG. Statistical methods. 8th Ed. East-West press, New Delhi, 1994.
30. Sreenivasaiah, PV. Studies on the growth rate, egg production, fertility and hatchability of Japanese quails (*Coturnix coturnix japonica*) hatched in different seasons. MVSc Thesis, Rohilkhand Univ., Uttar Pradesh, India, 1977,
31. Sreenivasaiah, PV. Studies on the use of sodium tri-polyphosphate (STPP) in chilling medium on selected quality characteristics of spent-hen meat during storage. PhD Thesis, Andhra Pradesh Agricultural Univ., Hyderabad, India, 1985.
32. Sreenivasaiah, PV. Scientific poultry production–a unique Encyclopedia. International Book Distributing Co., Lucknow, India, 2006.
33. Sreenivasaiah, PV and Krishnamurthy, KN. Japanese quails–mathematical model for egg production. Keral J. Vet. Sci., 1986, **17(1)**: 46–52.
34. Sreenivasaiah, PV, Krishnamurthy, KN, Prathapkumar, KS, Ramappa, BS and Chidananda, BL. Comparison of McMillan's and McNally's models for predicting egg production of Japanese quails. Indian Poultry Rev., 1985, **17(3)**: 19–23.
35. Strachan, T and Read, AP. Human molecular genetics. III Edition. Garland Science, London, New York, 2004.
36. Thapliyal, DC and Misra, DS. Fundamentals of animal hygiene and epidemiology. International Book Distributing Co., Lucknow, India, 1996.
37. Thomson, B., 1984 Canonical correlation analysis: uses and interpretations, Sage Publications
38. Thrusfield, M. Veterinary epidemiology. Blackwell Science Ltd., 1995.
39. Toma, B, Vaillancourt, JP, Dufour, B, Eliot, M, Moutou, F, Marsh, W, Benet, JJ, Sanna, M and Michel, P. Dictionary of veterinary epidemiology. Iowa State University Press, Ames, 1999.
40. Turner, DC and Bateson, P. The domestic cat–the biology of its behaviour. II Edition. Cambridge University Press, 2000.
41. van Vleck, D. Summary of methods for estimating genetic parameters using simple statistical models. Cornell Univ publication, 1979.
42. Wood, PDP. Algebraic model for the lactation curve in cattle. Nature (London), 1967, **216**: 164–165.
43. Wright, S. Systems of mating–I: Biometric relationship between parent and offspring. Genetics, 1921, **6**: 111 Cited from Pirchner, 1983
44. Yang, N, Wu, C and McMillan, I. New mathematical model of poultry egg production. Poultry Sci., 1989, **68**: 476–481.
45. Zar, JH. Biostatistical analysis. 4th Ed, Pearson Education, Singapore, New Delhi, 2003.

Appendices

APPENDIX 1

Area under the standard normal curve (Z)

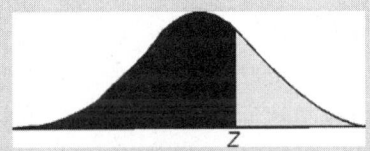

Cumulative area for Z < 0

Z	0	0.01	0.02	0.03	0.04	0.05	0.06	0.07	0.08	0.09
−3.40	0.0003	0.0003	0.0003	0.0003	0.0003	0.0003	0.0003	0.0003	0.0003	0.0002
−3.30	0.0005	0.0005	0.0005	0.0004	0.0004	0.0004	0.0004	0.0004	0.0004	0.0003
−3.20	0.0007	0.0007	0.0006	0.0006	0.0006	0.0006	0.0006	0.0005	0.0005	0.0005
−3.10	0.0010	0.0009	0.0009	0.0009	0.0008	0.0008	0.0008	0.0008	0.0007	0.0007
−3.00	0.0013	0.0013	0.0013	0.0012	0.0012	0.0011	0.0011	0.0011	0.0010	0.0010
−2.90	0.0019	0.0018	0.0018	0.0017	0.0016	0.0016	0.0015	0.0015	0.0014	0.0014
−2.80	0.0026	0.0025	0.0024	0.0023	0.0023	0.0022	0.0021	0.0021	0.0020	0.0019
−2.70	0.0035	0.0034	0.0033	0.0032	0.0031	0.0030	0.0029	0.0028	0.0027	0.0026
−2.60	0.0047	0.0045	0.0044	0.0043	0.0041	0.0040	0.0039	0.0038	0.0037	0.0036
−2.50	0.0062	0.0060	0.0059	0.0057	0.0055	0.0054	0.0052	0.0051	0.0049	0.0048
−2.40	0.0082	0.0080	0.0078	0.0075	0.0073	0.0071	0.0069	0.0068	0.0066	0.0064
−2.30	0.0107	0.0104	0.0102	0.0099	0.0096	0.0094	0.0091	0.0089	0.0087	0.0084
−2.20	0.0139	0.0136	0.0132	0.0129	0.0125	0.0122	0.0119	0.0116	0.0113	0.0110
−2.10	0.0179	0.0174	0.0170	0.0166	0.0162	0.0158	0.0154	0.0150	0.0146	0.0143
−2.00	0.0228	0.0222	0.0217	0.0212	0.0207	0.0202	0.0197	0.0192	0.0188	0.0183
−1.90	0.0287	0.0281	0.0274	0.0268	0.0262	0.0256	0.0250	0.0244	0.0239	0.0233
−1.80	0.0359	0.0351	0.0344	0.0336	0.0329	0.0322	0.0314	0.0307	0.0301	0.0294
−1.70	0.0446	0.0436	0.0427	0.0418	0.0409	0.0401	0.0392	0.0384	0.0375	0.0367

(Contd.)

Area under the standard normal curve (Z) (*Contd.*)

Cumulative area for Z < 0

Z	0	0.01	0.02	0.03	0.04	0.05	0.06	0.07	0.08	0.09
−1.60	0.0548	0.0537	0.0526	0.0516	0.0505	0.0495	0.0485	0.0475	0.0465	0.0455
−1.50	0.0668	0.0655	0.0643	0.0630	0.0618	0.0606	0.0594	0.0582	0.0571	0.0559
−1.40	0.0808	0.0793	0.0778	0.0764	0.0749	0.0735	0.0721	0.0708	0.0694	0.0681
−1.30	0.0968	0.0951	0.0934	0.0918	0.0901	0.0885	0.0869	0.0853	0.0838	0.0823
−1.20	0.1151	0.1131	0.1112	0.1093	0.1075	0.1056	0.1038	0.1020	0.1003	0.0985
−1.10	0.1357	0.1335	0.1314	0.1292	0.1271	0.1251	0.1230	0.1210	0.1190	0.1170
−1.00	0.1587	0.1562	0.1539	0.1515	0.1492	0.1469	0.1446	0.1423	0.1401	0.1379
−0.90	0.1841	0.1814	0.1788	0.1762	0.1736	0.1711	0.1685	0.1660	0.1635	0.1611
−0.80	0.2119	0.2090	0.2061	0.2033	0.2005	0.1977	0.1949	0.1922	0.1894	0.1867
−0.70	0.2420	0.2389	0.2358	0.2327	0.2296	0.2266	0.2236	0.2206	0.2177	0.2148
−0.60	0.2743	0.2709	0.2676	0.2643	0.2611	0.2578	0.2546	0.2514	0.2483	0.2451
−0.50	0.3085	0.3050	0.3015	0.2981	0.2946	0.2912	0.2877	0.2843	0.2810	0.2776
−0.40	0.3446	0.3409	0.3372	0.3336	0.3300	0.3264	0.3228	0.3192	0.3156	0.3121
−0.30	0.3821	0.3783	0.3745	0.3707	0.3669	0.3632	0.3594	0.3557	0.3520	0.3483
−0.20	0.4207	0.4168	0.4129	0.4090	0.4052	0.4013	0.3974	0.3936	0.3897	0.3859
−0.10	0.4602	0.4562	0.4522	0.4483	0.4443	0.4404	0.4364	0.4325	0.4286	0.4247
−0.00	0.5000	0.4960	0.4920	0.4880	0.4840	0.4801	0.4761	0.4721	0.4681	0.4641

Cumulative area for Z > 0

Z	0	0.01	0.02	0.03	0.04	0.05	0.06	0.07	0.08	0.09
0.00	0.5000	0.5040	0.5080	0.5120	0.5160	0.5199	0.5239	0.5279	0.5319	0.5359
0.10	0.5398	0.5438	0.5478	0.5517	0.5557	0.5596	0.5636	0.5675	0.5714	0.5753
0.20	0.5793	0.5832	0.5871	0.5910	0.5948	0.5987	0.6026	0.6064	0.6103	0.6141
0.30	0.6179	0.6217	0.6255	0.6293	0.6331	0.6368	0.6406	0.6443	0.6480	0.6517
0.40	0.6554	0.6591	0.6628	0.6664	0.6700	0.6736	0.6772	0.6808	0.6844	0.6879
0.50	0.6915	0.6950	0.6985	0.7019	0.7054	0.7088	0.7123	0.7157	0.7190	0.7224
0.60	0.7257	0.7291	0.7324	0.7357	0.7389	0.7422	0.7454	0.7486	0.7517	0.7549
0.70	0.7580	0.7611	0.7642	0.7673	0.7704	0.7734	0.7764	0.7794	0.7823	0.7852
0.80	0.7881	0.7910	0.7939	0.7967	0.7995	0.8023	0.8051	0.8078	0.8106	0.8133
0.90	0.8159	0.8186	0.8212	0.8238	0.8264	0.8289	0.8315	0.8340	0.8365	0.8389
1.00	0.8413	0.8438	0.8461	0.8485	0.8508	0.8531	0.8554	0.8577	0.8599	0.8621
1.10	0.8643	0.8665	0.8686	0.8708	0.8729	0.8749	0.8770	0.8790	0.8810	0.8830
1.20	0.8849	0.8869	0.8888	0.8907	0.8925	0.8944	0.8962	0.8980	0.8997	0.9015
1.30	0.9032	0.9049	0.9066	0.9082	0.9099	0.9115	0.9131	0.9147	0.9162	0.9177
1.40	0.9192	0.9207	0.9222	0.9236	0.9251	0.9265	0.9279	0.9292	0.9306	0.9319
1.50	0.9332	0.9345	0.9357	0.9370	0.9382	0.9394	0.9406	0.9418	0.9429	0.9441
1.60	0.9452	0.9463	0.9474	0.9484	0.9495	0.9505	0.9515	0.9525	0.9535	0.9545

(*Contd.*)

(Contd.)

Cumulative area for Z > 0

Z	0	0.01	0.02	0.03	0.04	0.05	0.06	0.07	0.08	0.09
1.70	0.9554	0.9564	0.9573	0.9582	0.9591	0.9599	0.9608	0.9616	0.9625	0.9633
1.80	0.9641	0.9649	0.9656	0.9664	0.9671	0.9678	0.9686	0.9693	0.9699	0.9706
1.90	0.9713	0.9719	0.9726	0.9732	0.9738	0.9744	0.9750	0.9756	0.9761	0.9767
2.00	0.9772	0.9778	0.9783	0.9788	0.9793	0.9798	0.9803	0.9808	0.9812	0.9817
2.10	0.9821	0.9826	0.9830	0.9834	0.9838	0.9842	0.9846	0.9850	0.9854	0.9857
2.20	0.9861	0.9864	0.9868	0.9871	0.9875	0.9878	0.9881	0.9884	0.9887	0.9890
2.30	0.9893	0.9896	0.9898	0.9901	0.9904	0.9906	0.9909	0.9911	0.9913	0.9916
2.40	0.9918	0.9920	0.9922	0.9925	0.9927	0.9929	0.9931	0.9932	0.9934	0.9936
2.50	0.9938	0.9940	0.9941	0.9943	0.9945	0.9946	0.9948	0.9949	0.9951	0.9952
2.60	0.9953	0.9955	0.9956	0.9957	0.9959	0.9960	0.9961	0.9962	0.9963	0.9964
2.70	0.9965	0.9966	0.9967	0.9968	0.9969	0.9970	0.9971	0.9972	0.9973	0.9974
2.80	0.9974	0.9975	0.9976	0.9977	0.9977	0.9978	0.9979	0.9979	0.9980	0.9981
2.90	0.9981	0.9982	0.9982	0.9983	0.9984	0.9984	0.9985	0.9985	0.9986	0.9986
3.00	0.9987	0.9987	0.9987	0.9988	0.9988	0.9989	0.9989	0.9989	0.9990	0.9990
3.10	0.9990	0.9991	0.9991	0.9991	0.9992	0.9992	0.9992	0.9992	0.9993	0.9993
3.20	0.9993	0.9993	0.9994	0.9994	0.9994	0.9994	0.9994	0.9995	0.9995	0.9995
3.30	0.9995	0.9995	0.9995	0.9996	0.9996	0.9996	0.9996	0.9996	0.9996	0.9997
3.40	0.9997	0.9997	0.9997	0.9997	0.9997	0.9997	0.9997	0.9997	0.9997	0.9998

Source: www.micquality.com

APPENDIX 2

Ordinates of standard normal curve (Z)

2nd decimal place in Z

Z	0.00	0.01	0.02	0.03	0.04	0.05	0.06	0.07	0.08	0.09
0.0	0.399	0.399	0.399	0.399	0.399	0.398	0.398	0.398	0.398	0.397
0.1	0.397	0.397	0.396	0.396	0.395	0.395	0.394	0.393	0.393	0.392
0.2	0.391	0.390	0.389	0.389	0.388	0.387	0.386	0.385	0.384	0.383
0.3	0.381	0.380	0.379	0.378	0.377	0.375	0.374	0.373	0.371	0.370
0.4	0.368	0.367	0.365	0.364	0.362	0.361	0.359	0.357	0.356	0.354
0.5	0.352	0.350	0.349	0.347	0.345	0.343	0.341	0.339	0.337	0.335
0.6	0.333	0.331	0.329	0.327	0.325	0.323	0.321	0.319	0.317	0.314
0.7	0.312	0.310	0.308	0.306	0.303	0.301	0.299	0.297	0.294	0.292
0.8	0.290	0.287	0.285	0.283	0.280	0.278	0.276	0.273	0.271	0.269
0.9	0.266	0.264	0.261	0.259	0.257	0.254	0.252	0.249	0.247	0.244
1.0	0.242	0.240	0.237	0.235	0.232	0.230	0.228	0.225	0.223	0.220
1.1	0.218	0.216	0.213	0.211	0.208	0.206	0.204	0.201	0.199	0.197
1.2	0.194	0.192	0.190	0.187	0.185	0.183	0.180	0.178	0.176	0.174
1.3	0.171	0.169	0.167	0.165	0.163	0.160	0.158	0.156	0.154	0.152
1.4	0.150	0.148	0.146	0.144	0.142	0.139	0.137	0.135	0.133	0.132
1.5	0.130	0.128	0.126	0.124	0.122	0.120	0.118	0.116	0.115	0.113
1.6	0.111	0.109	0.107	0.106	0.104	0.102	0.101	0.099	0.097	0.096
1.7	0.094	0.093	0.091	0.089	0.088	0.086	0.085	0.083	0.082	0.080
1.8	0.079	0.078	0.076	0.075	0.073	0.072	0.071	0.069	0.068	0.067
1.9	0.066	0.064	0.063	0.062	0.061	0.060	0.058	0.057	0.056	0.055
2.0	0.054	0.053	0.052	0.051	0.050	0.049	0.048	0.047	0.046	0.045
2.1	0.044	0.043	0.042	0.041	0.040	0.040	0.039	0.038	0.037	0.036
2.2	0.036	0.035	0.034	0.033	0.033	0.032	0.031	0.030	0.030	0.029
2.3	0.028	0.028	0.027	0.026	0.026	0.025	0.025	0.024	0.024	0.023
2.4	0.022	0.022	0.021	0.021	0.020	0.020	0.019	0.019	0.018	0.018
2.5	0.018	0.017	0.017	0.016	0.016	0.015	0.015	0.015	0.014	0.014
2.6	0.014	0.013	0.013	0.013	0.012	0.012	0.012	0.011	0.011	0.011
2.7	0.010	0.010	0.010	0.010	0.009	0.009	0.009	0.009	0.008	0.008
2.8	0.008	0.008	0.008	0.007	0.007	0.007	0.007	0.007	0.006	0.006
2.9	0.006	0.006	0.006	0.006	0.005	0.005	0.005	0.005	0.005	0.005

1st decimal place in Z

Z	0.0	0.1	0.2	0.3	0.4	0.5	0.6	0.7	0.8	0.9
3	0.0044	0.0033	0.0024	0.0017	0.0012	0.0009	0.0006	0.0004	0.0003	0.0002
4	0.0001	0.0001	0.0001	0.0000	0.0000	0.0000	0.0000	0.0000	0.0000	0.0000

Source: Snedecor and Cochran, 1994

APPENDIX 3

Area under student's t-distribution

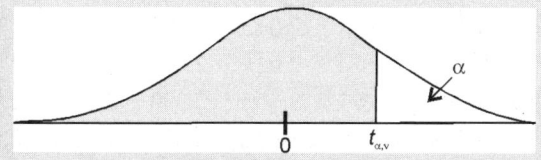

Level of significance α

υ	0.4	0.25	0.1	0.05	0.025	0.01	0.005	0.0025	0.001	0.0005
1	0.325	1.000	3.078	6.314	12.706	31.821	63.656	127.321	318.289	636.578
2	0.289	0.816	1.886	2.920	4.303	6.965	9.925	14.089	22.328	31.600
3	0.277	0.765	1.638	2.353	3.182	4.541	5.841	7.453	10.214	12.924
4	0.271	0.741	1.533	2.132	2.776	3.747	4.604	5.598	7.173	8.610
5	0.267	0.727	1.476	2.015	2.571	3.365	4.032	4.773	5.894	6.869
6	0.265	0.718	1.440	1.943	2.447	3.143	3.707	4.317	5.208	5.959
7	0.263	0.711	1.415	1.895	2.365	2.998	3.499	4.029	4.785	5.408
8	0.262	0.706	1.397	1.860	2.306	2.896	3.355	3.833	4.501	5.041
9	0.261	0.703	1.383	1.833	2.262	2.821	3.250	3.690	4.297	4.781
10	0.260	0.700	1.372	1.812	2.228	2.764	3.169	3.581	4.144	4.587
11	0.260	0.697	1.363	1.796	2.201	2.718	3.106	3.497	4.025	4.437
12	0.259	0.695	1.356	1.782	2.179	2.681	3.055	3.428	3.930	4.318
13	0.259	0.694	1.350	1.771	2.160	2.650	3.012	3.372	3.852	4.221
14	0.258	0.692	1.345	1.761	2.145	2.624	2.977	3.326	3.787	4.140
15	0.258	0.691	1.341	1.753	2.131	2.602	2.947	3.286	3.733	4.073
16	0.258	0.690	1.337	1.746	2.120	2.583	2.921	3.252	3.686	4.015
17	0.257	0.689	1.333	1.740	2.110	2.567	2.898	3.222	3.646	3.965
18	0.257	0.688	1.330	1.734	2.101	2.552	2.878	3.197	3.610	3.922
19	0.257	0.688	1.328	1.729	2.093	2.539	2.861	3.174	3.579	3.883
20	0.257	0.687	1.325	1.725	2.086	2.528	2.845	3.153	3.552	3.850
21	0.257	0.686	1.323	1.721	2.080	2.518	2.831	3.135	3.527	3.819
22	0.256	0.686	1.321	1.717	2.074	2.508	2.819	3.119	3.505	3.792
23	0.256	0.685	1.319	1.714	2.069	2.500	2.807	3.104	3.485	3.768
24	0.256	0.685	1.318	1.711	2.064	2.492	2.797	3.091	3.467	3.745
25	0.256	0.684	1.316	1.708	2.060	2.485	2.787	3.078	3.450	3.725
26	0.256	0.684	1.315	1.706	2.056	2.479	2.779	3.067	3.435	3.707
27	0.256	0.684	1.314	1.703	2.052	2.473	2.771	3.057	3.421	3.689
28	0.256	0.683	1.313	1.701	2.048	2.467	2.763	3.047	3.408	3.674
29	0.256	0.683	1.311	1.699	2.045	2.462	2.756	3.038	3.396	3.660

(Contd.)

Area under student's t-distribution *(Contd.)*

υ	\multicolumn{10}{c}{Level of significance α}
	0.4	0.25	0.1	0.05	0.025	0.01	0.005	0.0025	0.001	0.0005
30	0.256	0.683	1.310	1.697	2.042	2.457	2.750	3.030	3.385	3.646
40	0.255	0.681	1.303	1.684	2.021	2.423	2.704	2.971	3.307	3.551
60	0.254	0.679	1.296	1.671	2.000	2.390	2.660	2.915	3.232	3.460
120	0.254	0.677	1.289	1.658	1.980	2.358	2.617	2.860	3.160	3.373
∞	0.253	0.674	1.282	1.645	1.960	2.326	2.576	2.807	3.090	3.291

Source: www.micquality.com

APPENDIX 3.1

Computational Formula for Variance

As discussed already, $s^2 = \dfrac{\sum_{i=1}^{n}\left(x_i - \overline{x}\right)^2}{(n-1)}$; the numerator of this equation is difficult to compute especially when n is very large and / or mean value is not an integer. Hence, the numerator is rearranged as follows:

$$\sum_{i=1}^{n}\left(x_i - \overline{x}\right)^2 = \sum_{i=1}^{n}\left(x_i^2 - 2x_i\overline{x} + \overline{x}^2\right) = \sum_{i=1}^{n}x_i^2 - \sum_{i=1}^{n}2x_i\overline{x} + \sum_{i=1}^{n}\overline{x}^2 \; ; \quad \text{since 2 and } \overline{x} \text{ are}$$

constants, $\sum_{i=1}^{n}\left(x_i - \overline{x}\right)^2 = \sum_{i=1}^{n}x_i^2 - 2\overline{x}\sum_{i=1}^{n}x_i + n\overline{x}^2$; replacing $\overline{x} = \left(\dfrac{\sum_{i=1}^{n}x_i}{n}\right)$, we get

$$\sum_{i=1}^{n}\left(x_i - \overline{x}\right)^2 = \sum_{i=1}^{n}x_i^2 - \frac{2\left(\sum_{i=1}^{n}x_i\right)^2}{n} + n\left(\frac{\left(\sum_{i=1}^{n}x_i\right)^2}{n^2}\right).$$

Therefore, computation (machine) formula for $s^2 = \dfrac{\sum_{i=1}^{n}x_i^2 - \dfrac{\left(\sum_{i=1}^{n}x_i\right)^2}{n}}{(n-1)}$ where $\sum_{i=1}^{n}x_i^2$

refers to crude sum of squares or simply **sum of squares** and $\dfrac{\left(\sum_{i=1}^{n}x_i\right)^2}{n}$ is referred to as **correction factor**.

APPENDIX 3.2

Retransformation of Arcsin Values to the Original Scale

For retransformation of sd_{arc} values, no procedure appears to be available.

It is in the fitness of things to note that microbiological data are subjected to logarithmic transformation and as in *arcsin* transformation, the statistical analyses are performed utilizing the log values. The mean value on the logarithmic scale is retransformed to the original scale by taking the antilog of the log mean value. For retransformation of log *sd* value, the following procedure is shown: Let *s* be the standard deviation in the original scale; then, $s = \left[\dfrac{anti\log\left(\bar{X}+s\right) - anti\log\left(\bar{X}-s\right)}{2} \right]$. On the same lines, standard deviation in *arcsin* scale, s_{arc} can be retransformed to original scale by

$$s_{arc} = \left[\frac{\left\{100\sin^2\left(\bar{y} + s_{arc}\right)\right\} - 100\left\{\sin^2\left(\bar{y} + s_{arc}\right)\right\}}{2} \right] \qquad (1)$$

where $\bar{y} = arcsin$ mean. It is evident that retransformation of SD_{arc} values by the above formula is quite circuitous and hence time consuming. Therefore, it is necessary that by applying certain basic trigonometric rules, the equation (1) be simplified into a computational formula.; the same is enumerated below:

$$\text{Equation (1)} = 50\left[\sin^2\left(\bar{y} + s_{arc}\right)\right] - \left[\sin^2\left(\bar{y} - s_{arc}\right)\right] \qquad (2)$$

Let $A = y + s_{arc}$ and $B = y - s_{arc}$. Then, $s = 50(\sin^2 A) - (\sin^2 B)$ (3)

$\therefore sd = 50(\sin A + \sin B)(\sin A - \sin B)$ (4)

By applying trigonometric identity, we get

$$s = 50\left[2\sin\left(\frac{A+B}{2}\right)\cos\left(\frac{A-B}{2}\right)\right]\left[2\sin\left(\frac{A-B}{2}\right)\cos\left(\frac{A+B}{2}\right)\right] \qquad (5)$$

By rearranging the terms,

$$s = 50\left[2\sin\left(\frac{A+B}{2}\right)\cos\left(\frac{A-B}{2}\right)\right]\left[2\sin\left(\frac{A-B}{2}\right)\cos\left(\frac{A+B}{2}\right)\right] \qquad (6)$$

Since

$$\left[2\sin\left(\frac{A+B}{2}\right)\cos\left(\frac{A-B}{2}\right)\right] = \sin(A+B) \text{ and } \left[2\sin\left(\frac{A-B}{2}\right)\cos\left(\frac{A+B}{2}\right)\right] = \sin(A-B)$$

By substituting them in Equation (6), we get $s = 50[\sin(A+B)\sin(A-B)]$ (7)

Now, by substituting $A = \bar{y} + s_{arc}$ and $B = \bar{y} - s_{arc}$ and in Equation (7), the computational formula for retransforming the s values in *arcsin* scale to original % scale is obtained as

$$s = 50(\sin 2\bar{y})(\sin 2s_{arc}) \tag{8}$$

That means, standard deviation in percentage scale is equal to 50 times the product of the sine of twice the *arcsin* mean and sine of twice the *arcsin* standard deviation (Sreenivasaiah, 1985).

This short-cut method is accurate, simple and time-saving.

APPENDIX 4

Area under the χ^2 distribution

	α = Right hand tail area											
υ	0.999	0.995	0.99	0.975	0.95	0.9	0.1	0.05	0.025	0.01	0.005	0.001
1	0.00	0.00	0.00	0.00	0.00	0.02	2.71	3.84	5.02	6.63	7.88	10.83
2	0.00	0.01	0.02	0.05	0.10	0.21	4.61	5.99	7.38	9.21	10.60	13.82
3	0.02	0.07	0.11	0.22	0.35	0.58	6.25	7.81	9.35	11.34	12.84	16.27
4	0.09	0.21	0.30	0.48	0.71	1.06	7.78	9.49	11.14	13.28	14.86	18.47
5	0.21	0.41	0.55	0.83	1.15	1.61	9.24	11.07	12.83	15.09	16.75	20.51
6	0.38	0.68	0.87	1.24	1.64	2.20	10.64	12.59	14.45	16.81	18.55	22.46
7	0.60	0.99	1.24	1.69	2.17	2.83	12.02	14.07	16.01	18.48	20.28	24.32
8	0.86	1.34	1.65	2.18	2.73	3.49	13.36	15.51	17.53	20.09	21.95	26.12
9	1.15	1.73	2.09	2.70	3.33	4.17	14.68	16.92	19.02	21.67	23.59	27.88
10	1.48	2.16	2.56	3.25	3.94	4.87	15.99	18.31	20.48	23.21	25.19	29.59
11	1.83	2.60	3.05	3.82	4.57	5.58	17.28	19.68	21.92	24.73	26.76	31.26
12	2.21	3.07	3.57	4.40	5.23	6.30	18.55	21.03	23.34	26.22	28.30	32.91
13	2.62	3.57	4.11	5.01	5.89	7.04	19.81	22.36	24.74	27.69	29.82	34.53
14	3.04	4.07	4.66	5.63	6.57	7.79	21.06	23.68	26.12	29.14	31.32	36.12
15	3.48	4.60	5.23	6.26	7.26	8.55	22.31	25.00	27.49	30.58	32.80	37.70
16	3.94	5.14	5.81	6.91	7.96	9.31	23.54	26.30	28.85	32.00	34.27	39.25
17	4.42	5.70	6.41	7.56	8.67	10.09	24.77	27.59	30.19	33.41	35.72	40.79
18	4.90	6.26	7.01	8.23	9.39	10.86	25.99	28.87	31.53	34.81	37.16	42.31
19	5.41	6.84	7.63	8.91	10.12	11.65	27.20	30.14	32.85	36.19	38.58	43.82
20	5.92	7.43	8.26	9.59	10.85	12.44	28.41	31.41	34.17	37.57	40.00	45.31
21	6.45	8.03	8.90	10.28	11.59	13.24	29.62	32.67	35.48	38.93	41.40	46.80
22	6.98	8.64	9.54	10.98	12.34	14.04	30.81	33.92	36.78	40.29	42.80	48.27
23	7.53	9.26	10.20	11.69	13.09	14.85	32.01	35.17	38.08	41.64	44.18	49.73
24	8.08	9.89	10.86	12.40	13.85	15.66	33.20	36.42	39.36	42.98	45.56	51.18
25	8.65	10.52	11.52	13.12	14.61	16.47	34.38	37.65	40.65	44.31	46.93	52.62
26	9.22	11.16	12.20	13.84	15.38	17.29	35.56	38.89	41.92	45.64	48.29	54.05
27	9.80	11.81	12.88	14.57	16.15	18.11	36.74	40.11	43.19	46.96	49.65	55.48
28	10.39	12.46	13.56	15.31	16.93	18.94	37.92	41.34	44.46	48.28	50.99	56.89
29	10.99	13.12	14.26	16.05	17.71	19.77	39.09	42.56	45.72	49.59	52.34	58.30
30	11.59	13.79	14.95	16.79	18.49	20.60	40.26	43.77	46.98	50.89	53.67	59.70
32	12.81	15.13	16.36	18.29	20.07	22.27	42.58	46.19	49.48	53.49	56.33	62.49
34	14.06	16.50	17.79	19.81	21.66	23.95	44.90	48.60	51.97	56.06	58.96	65.25
36	15.32	17.89	19.23	21.34	23.27	25.64	47.21	51.00	54.44	58.62	61.58	67.98
38	16.61	19.29	20.69	22.88	24.88	27.34	49.51	53.38	56.90	61.16	64.18	70.70
40	17.92	20.71	22.16	24.43	26.51	29.05	51.81	55.76	59.34	63.69	66.77	73.40

(Contd.)

Area under the χ^2 distribution

	α = Right hand tail area											
υ	0.999	0.995	0.99	0.975	0.95	0.9	0.1	0.05	0.025	0.01	0.005	0.001
42	19.24	22.14	23.65	26.00	28.14	30.77	54.09	58.12	61.78	66.21	69.34	76.08
44	20.58	23.58	25.15	27.57	29.79	32.49	56.37	60.48	64.20	68.71	71.89	78.75
46	21.93	25.04	26.66	29.16	31.44	34.22	58.64	62.83	66.62	71.20	74.44	81.40
48	23.29	26.51	28.18	30.75	33.10	35.95	60.91	65.17	69.02	73.68	76.97	84.04
50	24.67	27.99	29.71	32.36	34.76	37.69	63.17	67.50	71.42	76.15	79.49	86.66
55	28.17	31.73	33.57	36.40	38.96	42.06	68.80	73.31	77.38	82.29	85.75	93.17
60	31.74	35.53	37.48	40.48	43.19	46.46	74.40	79.08	83.30	88.38	91.95	99.61
65	35.36	39.38	41.44	44.60	47.45	50.88	79.97	84.82	89.18	94.42	98.10	105.99
70	39.04	43.28	45.44	48.76	51.74	55.33	85.53	90.53	95.02	100.43	104.21	112.32
75	42.76	47.21	49.48	52.94	56.05	59.79	91.06	96.22	100.84	106.39	110.29	118.60
80	46.52	51.17	53.54	57.15	60.39	64.28	96.58	101.88	106.63	112.33	116.32	124.84
85	50.32	55.17	57.63	61.39	64.75	68.78	102.08	107.52	112.39	118.24	122.32	131.04
90	54.16	59.20	61.75	65.65	69.13	73.29	107.57	113.15	118.14	124.12	128.30	137.21
95	58.02	63.25	65.90	69.92	73.52	77.82	113.04	118.75	123.86	129.97	134.25	143.34
100	61.92	67.33	70.06	74.22	77.93	82.36	118.50	124.34	129.56	135.81	140.17	149.45

Source: www.micquality.com

APPENDIX 4.1

Permutation and Combination

Let us assume that for formulating a certain ration, 2 energy sources and 6 protein sources are available. If the ration has to contain one energy source and a protein source, we need to find out number of possible ways to make it; It is clear that there are 2 (k_1) and 6 (k_2) ways for choosing energy and protein source, respectively. When chosen together, each of the energy sources can be combined with 6 possible ways of protein source; that means, totally 2 × 6=12 ways or $k_1 k_2$ ways. This can be extended to any number of objects.

An important example is the triplet codes in DNA formed by 3 nitrogen bases; at each position of the triplet, any one of the 4 nitrogen bases (Adenine, Cytosine, Guanine and Thymine) can occupy; i.e. for each location in the triplet, there are 4 possible alternatives or $k_1 = 4$, $k_2 = 4$ and $k_3 = 4$. Therefore, the number of triplet codons = 4 × 4 × 4 or $4^3 = 64$.

1. PERMUTATION (Zar, 2003)

Arrangement of objects in a particular sequence (linear arrangement) is permutation.

Example 4.1.1: Suppose a cow (C), a horse (H) and a sheep (S) have to be arranged linearly; First position can be occupied by any one of the three animals (C or H or S). If 1st position is occupied by C, there only 2 ways to fill the 2nd position (H or S) and after the second position is occupied, there is only one way to fill the 3rd (if 2nd is H, third will be S else if the 2nd is S, the 3rd has to be H). In other words, $k_1 = 3, k_2 = 2$ and $k_3 = 1$; hence, total permutations possible is $k_1 \times k_2 \times k_3 = 3 \times 2 \times 1 = 6$.

To generalize, if there are n positions to be filled with n objects, total permutations, $^nP_n = n(n-1)(n-2) \ldots (3)(2)(1)$; the right-hand side of the equation is denoted mathematically with a **sign '!' called 'Factorial' meaning a product of all integers from 1 to n.** Hence, $^nP_n = n!$. It should be noted that $0! = 1$

Example 4.1.2: If there are fewer than n positions (say r positions) to permute n objects, then $^nP_r = \dfrac{n!}{(n-r)!}$. To illustrate this, let us consider that there are only two positions to be filled by a cow (C), a horse (H), a pig (P) and a sheep (S); for each of the animals in 1st position ($k_1 = 4$), there are only 3 alternatives ($k_2 = 3$). Therefore, total permutations possible is $4 \times 3 = 12$. Let us check this with the formula; $^4P_2 = \dfrac{4!}{(4-2)!}$

$$= \frac{4!}{2!} = \frac{(1)(2)(3)(4)}{(1)(2)} = 12.$$

Suppose in **Example 4.1.2**, there are 2 H's, one C and one S, it is easy to note that presence of 2 H's are indistinguishable as to whether the linear arrangement is 1st H, 2nd H or 2nd H and 1st H; hence, number of permutations of 4 animals will not be 4! = 24 but only 12. Mathematically, it can be represented thus: If n_i represents number of like individuals in category i, then $^nP_{n_1,n_2 \ldots n_i} = \dfrac{n!}{n_1!n_2! \ldots n_i!}$; in the above example,

$$^4P_{1,2,1} = \frac{4!}{1!\ 2!\ 1!} = 12.$$

2. COMBINATION

Let us consider **Example 4.1.2** and write down various permutations possible: CH, CP, CS, HC, HP, HS, PC, PS, PH, SC, SH and SP. It is clear that CH and HC, CP and PC, CS and SC, HP and PH, HS and SH and PS and SP are different only in order of arrangement; i.e. only 6 arrangements are possible. If order of arrangement is not important, the number of combinations can be calculated as follows:

$$^nC_r = \frac{n!}{r!(n-r)!}; \text{ in Example 4.1.2, it will be } \quad ^4C_2 = \frac{4!}{2!(4-2)!} = \frac{4!}{2!2!} = 6$$

3. SETS

Example 4.1.3: A collection of items is referred to as a **set**; say, for example, animals in a livestock farm. Each of the items (animals, in this case) is called an **element**. The animals may include buffaloes (B), cows (C), dogs (D), fowls (F), Goats (G), Horse (H) etc. If another set contains same elements (not necessarily same number or sequence of elements), the two sets are said to be **equal sets**.

Suppose, we classify the above set into ruminants and non-ruminants; we get two **subsets**; B, C and G under ruminants and D, F and H under non-ruminants. It is clear that a subset is also a set and its elements are elements of a larger set. If a set/subset is used for experiment, it is referred to as **outcome set**. For example, if one uses ruminant set, and draws two animals, the possible outcomes are: BB, BC, BG, CC, CB, CC, GG, GB and GC.

It can be noted that each of the outcomes itself is a set and hence, subset of the outcome set is called **event**; in the above example, occurrence of BB, BC, CB and CC is an event. Further characterization of an event is possible depending on the nature of the event and the experiment in question. For instance, in the above case, drawing one buffalo can be an event which includes BC, BG, CB and GB; in the same way, the event could be drawing both of same kind which will then include events BB, CC and GG.

Further, in the **Example 4.1.3**, subsets ruminants and non-ruminants **complementary to each other**; it means, when ruminants are defined, the rest of the animals in the set are, obviously, non-ruminants and *vice versa*.

Let us consider another situation; for example, in a livestock farm, one is interested to know the possibility (probability) of drawing at least two ruminants; it means that it includes the possibility of drawing B or C or G two at a time. Naturally, if possibility values are available for drawing B, C and G, they have to be added to get the desired possibility; hence, such situations are referred to as **union of events**.

APPENDIX 5

Area under the F distribution

Degrees of freedom for numerator (v_1)

(v_2)	1	2	3	4	5	6	7	8	9	10	12	15	20	24	30	40	60	120	∞
1	4052	4999	5404	5624	5764	5859	5928	5981	6022	6056	6107	6157	6209	6234	6260	6286	6313	6340	6366
2	98.5	99.0	99.2	99.3	99.3	99.3	99.4	99.4	99.4	99.4	99.4	99.4	99.4	99.5	99.5	99.5	99.5	99.5	99.5
3	34.1	30.8	29.5	28.7	28.2	27.9	27.7	27.5	27.3	27.2	27.1	26.9	26.7	26.6	26.5	26.4	26.3	26.2	26.1
4	21.2	18.0	16.7	16.0	15.5	15.2	15.0	14.8	14.7	14.5	14.4	14.2	14.0	13.9	13.8	13.7	13.7	13.6	13.5
5	16.3	13.3	12.1	11.4	11.0	10.7	10.5	10.3	10.2	10.1	9.89	9.72	9.55	9.47	9.38	9.29	9.20	9.11	9.02
6	13.7	10.9	9.78	9.15	8.75	8.47	8.26	8.10	7.98	7.87	7.72	7.56	7.40	7.31	7.23	7.14	7.06	6.97	6.88
7	12.2	9.55	8.45	7.85	7.46	7.19	6.99	6.84	6.72	6.62	6.47	6.31	6.16	6.07	5.99	5.91	5.82	5.74	5.65
8	11.3	8.65	7.59	7.01	6.63	6.37	6.18	6.03	5.91	5.81	5.67	5.52	5.36	5.28	5.20	5.12	5.03	4.95	4.86
9	10.6	8.02	6.99	6.42	6.06	5.80	5.61	5.47	5.35	5.26	5.11	4.96	4.81	4.73	4.65	4.57	4.48	4.40	4.31
10	10.0	7.56	6.55	5.99	5.64	5.39	5.20	5.06	4.94	4.85	4.71	4.56	4.41	4.33	4.25	4.17	4.08	4.00	3.91
11	9.65	7.21	6.22	5.67	5.32	5.07	4.89	4.74	4.63	4.54	4.40	4.25	4.10	4.02	3.94	3.86	3.78	3.69	3.60
12	9.33	6.93	5.95	5.41	5.06	4.82	4.64	4.50	4.39	4.30	4.16	4.01	3.86	3.78	3.70	3.62	3.54	3.45	3.36
13	9.07	6.70	5.74	5.21	4.86	4.62	4.44	4.30	4.19	4.10	3.96	3.82	3.66	3.59	3.51	3.43	3.34	3.25	3.17
14	8.86	6.51	5.56	5.04	4.69	4.46	4.28	4.14	4.03	3.94	3.80	3.66	3.51	3.43	3.35	3.27	3.18	3.09	3.00
15	8.68	6.36	5.42	4.89	4.56	4.32	4.14	4.00	3.89	3.80	3.67	3.52	3.37	3.29	3.21	3.13	3.05	2.96	2.87
16	8.53	6.23	5.29	4.77	4.44	4.20	4.03	3.89	3.78	3.69	3.55	3.41	3.26	3.18	3.10	3.02	2.93	2.84	2.75
17	8.40	6.11	5.19	4.67	4.34	4.10	3.93	3.79	3.68	3.59	3.46	3.31	3.16	3.08	3.00	2.92	2.83	2.75	2.65
18	8.29	6.01	5.09	4.58	4.25	4.01	3.84	3.71	3.60	3.51	3.37	3.23	3.08	3.00	2.92	2.84	2.75	2.66	2.57
19	8.18	5.93	5.01	4.50	4.17	3.94	3.77	3.63	3.52	3.43	3.30	3.15	3.00	2.92	2.84	2.76	2.67	2.58	2.49
20	8.10	5.85	4.94	4.43	4.10	3.87	3.70	3.56	3.46	3.37	3.23	3.09	2.94	2.86	2.78	2.69	2.61	2.52	2.42
21	8.02	5.78	4.87	4.37	4.04	3.81	3.64	3.51	3.40	3.31	3.17	3.03	2.88	2.80	2.72	2.64	2.55	2.46	2.36
22	7.95	5.72	4.82	4.31	3.99	3.76	3.59	3.45	3.35	3.26	3.12	2.98	2.83	2.75	2.67	2.58	2.50	2.40	2.31
23	7.88	5.66	4.76	4.26	3.94	3.71	3.54	3.41	3.30	3.21	3.07	2.93	2.78	2.70	2.62	2.54	2.45	2.35	2.26
24	7.82	5.61	4.72	4.22	3.90	3.67	3.50	3.36	3.26	3.17	3.03	2.89	2.74	2.66	2.58	2.49	2.40	2.31	2.21
25	7.77	5.57	4.68	4.18	3.85	3.63	3.46	3.32	3.22	3.13	2.99	2.85	2.70	2.62	2.54	2.45	2.36	2.27	2.17
26	7.72	5.53	4.64	4.14	3.82	3.59	3.42	3.29	3.18	3.09	2.96	2.81	2.66	2.58	2.50	2.42	2.33	2.23	2.13
27	7.68	5.49	4.60	4.11	3.78	3.56	3.39	3.26	3.15	3.06	2.93	2.78	2.63	2.55	2.47	2.38	2.29	2.20	2.10
28	7.64	5.45	4.57	4.07	3.75	3.53	3.36	3.23	3.12	3.03	2.90	2.75	2.60	2.52	2.44	2.35	2.26	2.17	2.06
29	7.60	5.42	4.54	4.04	3.73	3.50	3.33	3.20	3.09	3.00	2.87	2.73	2.57	2.49	2.41	2.33	2.23	2.14	2.03
30	7.56	5.39	4.51	4.02	3.70	3.47	3.30	3.17	3.07	2.98	2.84	2.70	2.55	2.47	2.39	2.30	2.21	2.11	2.01
40	7.31	5.18	4.31	3.83	3.51	3.29	3.12	2.99	2.89	2.80	2.66	2.52	2.37	2.29	2.20	2.11	2.02	1.92	1.80
60	7.08	4.98	4.13	3.65	3.34	3.12	2.95	2.82	2.72	2.63	2.50	2.35	2.20	2.12	2.03	1.94	1.84	1.73	1.60
120	6.85	4.79	3.95	3.48	3.17	2.96	2.79	2.66	2.56	2.47	2.34	2.19	2.03	1.95	1.86	1.76	1.66	1.53	1.38
∞	6.64	4.61	3.78	3.32	3.02	2.80	2.64	2.51	2.41	2.32	2.18	2.04	1.88	1.79	1.70	1.59	1.47	1.32	1.00

v_2 is v for denominator

Source: www.micquality.com

Degrees of freedom for numerator (v_1)

(v_2)	1	2	3	4	5	6	7	8	9	10	12	15	20	24	30	40	60	120	∞
1	161	199	216	225	230	234	237	239	241	242	244	246	248	249	250	251	252	253	254
2	18.5	19.0	19.2	19.2	19.3	19.3	19.4	19.4	19.4	19.4	19.4	19.4	19.4	19.5	19.5	19.5	19.5	19.5	19.5
3	10.1	9.55	9.28	9.12	9.01	8.94	8.89	8.85	8.81	8.79	8.74	8.70	8.66	8.64	8.62	8.59	8.57	8.55	8.53
4	7.71	6.94	6.59	6.39	6.26	6.16	6.09	6.04	6.00	5.96	5.91	5.86	5.80	5.77	5.75	5.72	5.69	5.66	5.63
5	6.61	5.79	5.41	5.19	5.05	4.95	4.88	4.82	4.77	4.74	4.68	4.62	4.56	4.53	4.50	4.46	4.43	4.40	4.37
6	5.99	5.14	4.76	4.53	4.39	4.28	4.21	4.15	4.10	4.06	4.00	3.94	3.87	3.84	3.81	3.77	3.74	3.70	3.67
7	5.59	4.74	4.35	4.12	3.97	3.87	3.79	3.73	3.68	3.64	3.57	3.51	3.44	3.41	3.38	3.34	3.30	3.27	3.23
8	5.32	4.46	4.07	3.84	3.69	3.58	3.50	3.44	3.39	3.35	3.28	3.22	3.15	3.12	3.08	3.04	3.01	2.97	2.93
9	5.12	4.26	3.86	3.63	3.48	3.37	3.29	3.23	3.18	3.14	3.07	3.01	2.94	2.90	2.86	2.83	2.79	2.75	2.71
10	4.96	4.10	3.71	3.48	3.33	3.22	3.14	3.07	3.02	2.98	2.91	2.85	2.77	2.74	2.70	2.66	2.62	2.58	2.54
11	4.84	3.98	3.59	3.36	3.20	3.09	3.01	2.95	2.90	2.85	2.79	2.72	2.65	2.61	2.57	2.53	2.49	2.45	2.40
12	4.75	3.89	3.49	3.26	3.11	3.00	2.91	2.85	2.80	2.75	2.69	2.62	2.54	2.51	2.47	2.43	2.38	2.34	2.30
13	4.67	3.81	3.41	3.18	3.03	2.92	2.83	2.77	2.71	2.67	2.60	2.53	2.46	2.42	2.38	2.34	2.30	2.25	2.21
14	4.60	3.74	3.34	3.11	2.96	2.85	2.76	2.70	2.65	2.60	2.53	2.46	2.39	2.35	2.31	2.27	2.22	2.18	2.13
15	4.54	3.68	3.29	3.06	2.90	2.79	2.71	2.64	2.59	2.54	2.48	2.40	2.33	2.29	2.25	2.20	2.16	2.11	2.07
16	4.49	3.63	3.24	3.01	2.85	2.74	2.66	2.59	2.54	2.49	2.42	2.35	2.28	2.24	2.19	2.15	2.11	2.06	2.01
17	4.45	3.59	3.20	2.96	2.81	2.70	2.61	2.55	2.49	2.45	2.38	2.31	2.23	2.19	2.15	2.10	2.06	2.01	1.96
18	4.41	3.55	3.16	2.93	2.77	2.66	2.58	2.51	2.46	2.41	2.34	2.27	2.19	2.15	2.11	2.06	2.02	1.97	1.92
19	4.38	3.52	3.13	2.90	2.74	2.63	2.54	2.48	2.42	2.38	2.31	2.23	2.16	2.11	2.07	2.03	1.98	1.93	1.88
20	4.35	3.49	3.10	2.87	2.71	2.60	2.51	2.45	2.39	2.35	2.28	2.20	2.12	2.08	2.04	1.99	1.95	1.90	1.84
21	4.32	3.47	3.07	2.84	2.68	2.57	2.49	2.42	2.37	2.32	2.25	2.18	2.10	2.05	2.01	1.96	1.92	1.87	1.81
22	4.30	3.44	3.05	2.82	2.66	2.55	2.46	2.40	2.34	2.30	2.23	2.15	2.07	2.03	1.98	1.94	1.89	1.84	1.78
23	4.28	3.42	3.03	2.80	2.64	2.53	2.44	2.37	2.32	2.27	2.20	2.13	2.05	2.01	1.96	1.91	1.86	1.81	1.76
24	4.26	3.40	3.01	2.78	2.62	2.51	2.42	2.36	2.30	2.25	2.18	2.11	2.03	1.98	1.94	1.89	1.84	1.79	1.73
25	4.24	3.39	2.99	2.76	2.60	2.49	2.40	2.34	2.28	2.24	2.16	2.09	2.01	1.96	1.92	1.87	1.82	1.77	1.71
26	4.23	3.37	2.98	2.74	2.59	2.47	2.39	2.32	2.27	2.22	2.15	2.07	1.99	1.95	1.90	1.85	1.80	1.75	1.69
27	4.21	3.35	2.96	2.73	2.57	2.46	2.37	2.31	2.25	2.20	2.13	2.06	1.97	1.93	1.88	1.84	1.79	1.73	1.67
28	4.20	3.34	2.95	2.71	2.56	2.45	2.36	2.29	2.24	2.19	2.12	2.04	1.96	1.91	1.87	1.82	1.77	1.71	1.65
29	4.18	3.33	2.93	2.70	2.55	2.43	2.35	2.28	2.22	2.18	2.10	2.03	1.94	1.90	1.85	1.81	1.75	1.70	1.64
30	4.17	3.32	2.92	2.69	2.53	2.42	2.33	2.27	2.21	2.16	2.09	2.01	1.93	1.89	1.84	1.79	1.74	1.68	1.62
40	4.08	3.23	2.84	2.61	2.45	2.34	2.25	2.18	2.12	2.08	2.00	1.92	1.84	1.79	1.74	1.69	1.64	1.58	1.51
60	4.00	3.15	2.76	2.53	2.37	2.25	2.17	2.10	2.04	1.99	1.92	1.84	1.75	1.70	1.65	1.59	1.53	1.47	1.39
120	3.92	3.07	2.68	2.45	2.29	2.18	2.09	2.02	1.96	1.91	1.83	1.75	1.66	1.61	1.55	1.50	1.43	1.35	1.25
∞	3.84	3.00	2.60	2.37	2.21	2.10	2.01	1.94	1.88	1.83	1.75	1.67	1.57	1.52	1.46	1.39	1.32	1.22	1.00

v_2 is v for denominator

Source: www.micquality.com

APPENDIX 6

Critical values of the Spearman's rank correlation coefficients (r_s)

n	Level of significance (α), one-tail					
	0.10	0.05	0.025	0.01	0.005	0.001
4	1.000	1.000	–	–	–	–
5	0.800	0.900	1.000	1.000	–	–
6	0.657	0.829	0.886	0.943	1.000	–
7	0.571	0.714	0.786	0.893	0.929	1.000
8	0.524	0.643	0.738	0.833	0.881	0.952
9	0.483	0.600	0.700	0.783	0.833	0.917
10	0.455	0.564	0.648	0.745	0.794	0.879
11	0.427	0.536	0.618	0.709	0.755	0.845
12	0.406	0.503	0.587	0.678	0.727	0.818
13	0.385	0.484	0.560	0.648	0.703	0.791
14	0.367	0.464	0.538	0.626	0.679	0.771
15	0.354	0.446	0.521	0.604	0.654	0.750
16	0.341	0.429	0.503	0.582	0.635	0.729
17	0.328	0.414	0.488	0.566	0.618	0.711
18	0.317	0.401	0.472	0.550	0.600	0.692
19	0.309	0.391	0.460	0.535	0.584	0.675
20	0.299	0.380	0.447	0.522	0.570	0.662
21	0.292	0.370	0.436	0.509	0.556	0.647
22	0.284	0.361	0.425	0.497	0.544	0.633
23	0.278	0.353	0.416	0.486	0.532	0.621
24	0.271	0.344	0.407	0.476	0.521	0.609
25	0.265	0.337	0.398	0.466	0.511	0.597
26	0.259	0.331	0.390	0.457	0.501	0.586
27	0.255	0.324	0.383	0.449	0.492	0.576
28	0.250	0.318	0.375	0.441	0.483	0.567
29	0.245	0.312	0.368	0.433	0.475	0.558
30	0.240	0.306	0.362	0.425	0.467	0.549
31	0.236	0.301	0.356	0.419	0.459	0.540
32	0.232	0.296	0.350	0.412	0.452	0.532
33	0.229	0.291	0.345	0.405	0.446	0.525
34	0.225	0.287	0.340	0.400	0.439	0.517
35	0.222	0.283	0.335	0.394	0.433	0.510
36	0.219	0.279	0.330	0.388	0.427	0.503
37	0.215	0.275	0.325	0.383	0.421	0.497
38	0.212	0.271	0.321	0.378	0.415	0.491

(Contd.)

Critical values of the Spearman's rank correlation coefficients (r_s) *(Contd.)*

n	Level of significance (α), one-tail					
	0.10	0.05	0.025	0.01	0.005	0.001
39	0.210	0.267	0.317	0.373	0.410	0.485
40	0.207	0.264	0.313	0.368	0.405	0.479
41	0.204	0.261	0.309	0.364	0.400	0.473
42	0.202	0.257	0.305	0.359	0.396	0.468
43	0.199	0.254	0.301	0.355	0.391	0.462
44	0.197	0.251	0.298	0.351	0.386	0.457
45	0.194	0.248	0.294	0.347	0.382	0.452
46	0.192	0.246	0.291	0.343	0.378	0.448
47	0.190	0.243	0.288	0.340	0.374	0.443
48	0.188	0.240	0.285	0.336	0.370	0.439
49	0.186	0.238	0.282	0.333	0.366	0.434
50	0.184	0.235	0.279	0.329	0.363	0.430
51	0.182	0.233	0.276	0.326	0.359	0.426
52	0.180	0.231	0.274	0.323	0.356	0.422
53	0.179	0.228	0.271	0.320	0.352	0.418
54	0.177	0.226	0.268	0.317	0.349	0.414
55	0.175	0.224	0.266	0.314	0.346	0.411
56	0.174	0.222	0.264	0.311	0.343	0.407
57	0.172	0.220	0.261	0.308	0.340	0.404
58	0.171	0.218	0.259	0.306	0.337	0.400
59	0.169	0.216	0.257	0.303	0.334	0.397
60	0.168	0.214	0.255	0.301	0.331	0.394

Source: Zar, 2003

APPENDIX 7

Critical values of top-down correlation coefficients (r_T)

n	$\alpha = 0.05$	$\alpha = 0.01$
3	1.000	1.000
4	0.942	1.000
5	0.959	1.000
6	0.810	0.943
7	0.738	0.906
8	0.692	0.865
9	0.654	0.826
10	0.620	0.793
11	0.589	0.762
12	0.560	0.735
13	0.535	0.711
14	0.513	0.689
15	0.486	0.680
16	0.470	0.656
17	0.454	0.635
18	0.440	0.615
19	0.428	0.598
20	0.416	0.581
21	0.405	0.566
22	0.395	0.552
23	0.386	0.538
24	0.377	0.526
25	0.368	0.515
26	0.361	0.504
27	0.354	0.494
28	0.347	0.484
29	0.340	0.475
30	0.334	0.466

Source: Zar, 2003

APPENDIX 8

Critical values of Friedman's χ^2_r distribution

$a\ (n)$	$b\ (M)$	$\alpha = 0.05$	$\alpha = 0.01$
3	3	6.000	–
3	4	6.500	8.000
3	5	6.400	8.400
3	6	7.000	9.000
3	7	7.143	8.857
3	8	6.250	9.000
3	9	6.222	9.556
3	10	6.200	9.600
3	11	6.545	9.455
3	12	6.167	9.500
3	13	6.000	9.385
3	14	6.143	9.000
3	15	6.400	8.933
4	2	6.000	—
4	3	7.400	9.000
4	4	7.800	9.600
4	5	7.800	9.960
4	6	7.600	10.200
4	7	7.800	10.371
4	8	7.650	10.350
4	9	7.800	10.867
4	10	7.800	10.800
4	11	7.909	11.073
4	12	7.900	11.100
4	13	7.985	11.123
4	14	7.886	11.143
4	15	8.040	11.240
5	2	7.600	8.000
5	3	8.533	10.133
5	4	8.800	11.200
5	5	8.960	11.60
5	6	9.067	11.867
5	7	9.143	12.114
5	8	9.300	12.300
5	9	9.244	12.444
5	10	9.280	12.480

(Contd.)

Critical values of Friedman's χ^2_r distribution

$a\ (n)$	$b\ (M)$	$\alpha = 0.05$	$\alpha = 0.01$
6	2	9.143	9.714
6	3	9.857	11.762
6	4	10.286	12.714
6	5	10.486	13.229
6	6	10.571	13.619
6	7	10.674	13.857
6	8	10.714	14.000
6	9	10.778	14.143
6	10	10.800	14.299

Adapted from: Zar, 2003

APPENDIX 9

Orthogonal polynomials

Levels of x (n)	Degree	Orthogonal coefficients, ξ_i										SS, ξ_i^2	λ_i
3	Linear	−1	0	1								2	1
	Quadratic	1	−2	1								6	3
4	Linear	−3	−1	1	3							20	2
	Quadratic	1	−1	−1	1							4	1
	Cubic	−1	3	−3	1							20	10 ÷ 3
5	Linear	−2	−1	0	1	2						10	1
	Quadratic	2	−1	−2	−1	2						14	1
	Cubic	−1	2	0	−2	1						10	5 ÷ 6
	Quartic	1	−4	6	−4	1						70	35 ÷ 12
6	Linear	−5	−3	−1	1	3	5					70	2
	Quadratic	5	−1	−4	−4	−1	5					84	3 ÷ 2
	Cubic	−5	7	4	−4	−7	5					180	5 ÷ 3
	Quartic	1	−3	2	2	−3	1					28	7 ÷ 12
	Quintic	−1	5	−10	10	−5	1					252	21 ÷ 10
7	Linear	−3	−2	−1	0	1	2	3				28	1
	Quadratic	5	0	−3	−4	−3	0	5				84	1
	Cubic	−1	1	1	0	−1	−1	1				6	1 ÷ 6
	Quartic	3	−7	1	6	1	−7	3				154	7 ÷ 12
	Quintic	0	−5	4	−1	0	5	−4	1			84	7 ÷ 20
8	Linear	−7	−5	−3	−1	1	3	5	7			168	2
	Quadratic	7	1	−3	−5	−5	−3	1	7			168	1
	Cubic	−7	5	7	3	−3	−7	−5	7			264	2 ÷ 3
	Quartic	7	−13	−3	9	9	−3	−13	7			616	7 ÷ 12
	Quintic	−7	23	−17	−15	15	17	−23	7			2184	7 ÷ 10
9	Linear	−4	−3	−2	−1	0	1	2	3	4		20	1
	Quadratic	28	7	−8	−17	−20	−17	−8	7	28		2772	3
	Cubic	−14	7	13	9	0	−9	−13	−7	14		990	5 ÷ 6
	Quartic	14	−21	−11	9	18	9	−11	−21	14		2002	7 ÷ 12
	Quintic	−4	11	−4	−9	0	9	4	−11	4		468	3 ÷ 20
10	Linear	−9	−7	−5	−3	−1	1	3	5	7	9	330	2
	Quadratic	6	2	−1	−3	−4	−4	−3	−1	2	6	132	½
	Cubic	−42	14	35	31	12	−12	−31	−35	−14	42	8580	5 ÷ 3
	Quartic	18	−22	−17	3	18	18	3	−17	−22	18	2860	5 ÷ 12
	Quintic	−6	14	−1	−11	−6	6	11	1	−1	6	780	1 ÷ 10

(Contd.)

Orthogonal polynomials

Levels of x (n)	Degree	Orthogonal coefficients, ξ_i												SS, ξ_i^2	λ_i
11	Linear	−1	−2	−3	−4	−5	0	1	2	3	4	5		110	1
	Quadratic	15	6	−1	−6	−9	−10	−9	−6	−1	6	15		858	1
	Cubic	−30	6	22	23	14	0	−14	−23	−22	−6	30		4290	5 ÷ 6
	Quartic	6	−6	−6	−1	4	6	4	−1	−6	−6	6		286	1 ÷ 12
	Quintic	−3	6	1	−4	−4	0	4	4	−1	−6	3		156	1 ÷ 40
12	Linear	−11	−9	−7	−5	−3	−1	1	3	5	7	9	11	572	2
	Quadratic	55	25	1	−17	−29	−35	−35	−29	−17	1	25	55	12012	3
	Cubic	−33	3	21	25	19	7	−7	−19	−25	−21	−3	33	5148	2 ÷ 3
	Quartic	33	−27	−33	−13	12	28	28	12	−13	−33	−27	33	8008	7 ÷ 24
	Quintic	−33	57	21	−29	−44	−20	20	44	29	−21	−57	33	15912	3 ÷ 20

Note: Linear, cubic and quintic are odd–power equations

Adapted from: Snedecor and Cochran, 1994

APPENDIX 10

Duncan's significant studentized range values

v									Number of means in the range ($\alpha = 0.05$)										
	2	3	4	5	6	7	8	9	10	11	12	13	14	15	16	17	18	19	20
3	4.501	4.516	4.516	4.516	4.516	4.516	4.516	4.516	4.516	4.516	4.516	4.516	4.516	4.516	4.516	4.516	4.516	4.516	4.516
4	3.926	4.013	4.033	4.033	4.033	4.033	4.033	4.033	4.033	4.033	4.033	4.033	4.033	4.033	4.033	4.033	4.033	4.033	4.033
5	3.635	3.749	3.796	3.814	3.814	3.814	3.814	3.814	3.814	3.814	3.814	3.814	3.814	3.814	3.814	3.814	3.814	3.814	3.814
6	3.460	3.586	3.649	3.680	3.694	3.697	3.697	3.697	3.697	3.697	3.697	3.697	3.697	3.697	3.697	3.697	3.697	3.697	3.697
7	3.344	3.477	3.548	3.588	3.611	3.622	3.625	3.625	3.625	3.625	3.625	3.625	3.625	3.625	3.625	3.625	3.625	3.625	3.625
8	3.261	3.398	3.475	3.521	3.549	3.566	3.575	3.579	3.579	3.579	3.579	3.579	3.579	3.579	3.579	3.579	3.579	3.579	3.579
9	3.199	3.339	3.420	3.470	3.502	3.523	3.536	3.544	3.547	3.547	3.547	3.547	3.547	3.547	3.547	3.547	3.547	3.547	3.547
10	3.151	3.293	3.376	3.430	3.465	3.489	3.505	3.516	3.522	3.525	3.525	3.525	3.525	3.525	3.525	3.525	3.525	3.525	3.525
11	3.113	3.256	3.341	3.397	3.435	3.462	3.480	3.493	3.501	3.506	3.509	3.510	3.510	3.510	3.510	3.510	3.510	3.510	3.510
12	3.081	3.225	3.312	3.370	3.410	3.439	3.459	3.474	3.484	3.491	3.495	3.498	3.498	3.498	3.498	3.498	3.498	3.498	3.498
13	3.055	3.200	3.288	3.348	3.389	3.419	3.441	3.458	3.470	3.478	3.484	3.488	3.490	3.490	3.490	3.490	3.490	3.490	3.490
14	3.033	3.178	3.268	3.328	3.371	3.403	3.426	3.444	3.457	3.467	3.474	3.479	3.482	3.484	3.484	3.484	3.484	3.484	3.484
15	3.014	3.160	3.250	3.312	3.356	3.389	3.413	3.432	3.446	3.457	3.465	3.471	3.476	3.478	3.480	3.480	3.480	3.480	3.480
16	2.998	3.144	3.235	3.297	3.343	3.376	3.402	3.422	3.437	3.449	3.457	3.465	3.470	3.473	3.476	3.477	3.477	3.477	3.477
17	2.984	3.130	3.222	3.285	3.331	3.365	3.392	3.412	3.429	3.441	3.449	3.458	3.465	3.470	3.473	3.474	3.475	3.475	3.475
18	2.971	3.117	3.210	3.274	3.320	3.356	3.383	3.404	3.421	3.435	3.445	3.454	3.459	3.465	3.469	3.472	3.473	3.473	3.474
19	2.960	3.106	3.199	3.264	3.311	3.347	3.375	3.397	3.415	3.429	3.440	3.449	3.456	3.462	3.466	3.469	3.472	3.473	3.474
20	2.950	3.097	3.190	3.255	3.303	3.339	3.368	3.390	3.409	3.423	3.435	3.445	3.452	3.459	3.463	3.467	3.470	3.472	3.473
21	2.941	3.088	3.181	3.247	3.295	3.332	3.361	3.385	3.403	3.418	3.431	3.441	3.449	3.456	3.461	3.465	3.469	3.471	3.473
22	2.933	3.080	3.173	3.239	3.288	3.326	3.355	3.379	3.398	3.414	3.427	3.437	3.446	3.453	3.459	3.464	3.467	3.470	3.472
23	2.926	3.072	3.166	3.233	3.282	3.320	3.350	3.374	3.394	3.410	3.423	3.434	3.443	3.451	3.457	3.462	3.466	3.469	3.472

(Contd.)

Duncan's significant studentized range values (*Contd.*)

v	2	3	4	5	6	7	8	9	10	11	12	13	14	15	16	17	18	19	20
24	2.919	3.066	3.160	3.226	3.276	3.315	3.345	3.370	3.390	3.406	3.420	3.431	3.441	3.449	3.455	3.461	3.465	3.469	3.472
25	2.913	3.059	3.154	3.221	3.271	3.310	3.341	3.366	3.386	3.403	3.417	3.429	3.439	3.447	3.454	3.459	3.464	3.468	3.471
26	2.907	3.054	3.149	3.216	3.266	3.305	3.336	3.362	3.382	3.400	3.414	3.426	3.436	3.445	3.452	3.458	3.463	3.468	3.471
27	2.902	3.049	3.144	3.211	3.262	3.301	3.332	3.358	3.379	3.397	3.412	3.424	3.434	3.443	3.451	3.457	3.463	3.467	3.471
28	2.897	3.044	3.139	3.206	3.257	3.297	3.329	3.355	3.376	3.394	3.409	3.422	3.433	3.442	3.450	3.456	3.462	3.467	3.470
29	2.892	3.039	3.135	3.202	3.253	3.293	3.326	3.352	3.373	3.392	3.407	3.420	3.431	3.440	3.448	3.455	3.461	3.466	3.470
30	2.888	3.035	3.131	3.199	3.250	3.290	3.322	3.349	3.371	3.389	3.405	3.418	3.429	3.439	3.447	3.454	3.460	3.466	3.470
31	2.884	3.031	3.127	3.195	3.246	3.287	3.319	3.346	3.368	3.387	3.403	3.416	3.428	3.438	3.446	3.453	3.460	3.465	3.470
32	2.881	3.028	3.123	3.192	3.243	3.284	3.317	3.344	3.366	3.385	3.401	3.415	3.426	3.436	3.445	3.452	3.459	3.465	3.470
33	2.877	3.024	3.120	3.188	3.240	3.281	3.314	3.341	3.364	3.383	3.399	3.413	3.425	3.435	3.444	3.452	3.459	3.465	3.470
34	2.874	3.021	3.117	3.185	3.238	3.279	3.312	3.339	3.362	3.381	3.398	3.412	3.424	3.434	3.443	3.451	3.458	3.464	3.469
35	2.871	3.018	3.114	3.183	3.235	3.276	3.309	3.337	3.360	3.379	3.396	3.410	3.423	3.433	3.443	3.451	3.458	3.464	3.469
36	2.868	3.015	3.111	3.180	3.232	3.274	3.307	3.335	3.358	3.378	3.395	3.409	3.421	3.432	3.442	3.450	3.457	3.464	3.469
37	2.865	3.013	3.109	3.178	3.230	3.272	3.305	3.333	3.356	3.376	3.393	3.408	3.420	3.431	3.441	3.449	3.457	3.463	3.469
38	2.863	3.010	3.106	3.175	3.228	3.270	3.303	3.331	3.355	3.375	3.392	3.407	3.419	3.431	3.440	3.449	3.456	3.463	3.469
39	2.861	3.008	3.104	3.173	3.226	3.268	3.301	3.330	3.353	3.373	3.391	3.406	3.418	3.430	3.440	3.448	3.456	3.463	3.469
40	2.858	3.005	3.102	3.171	3.224	3.266	3.300	3.328	3.352	3.372	3.389	3.404	3.418	3.429	3.439	3.448	3.456	3.463	3.469
48	2.843	2.991	3.087	3.157	3.211	3.253	3.288	3.318	3.342	3.363	3.382	3.398	3.412	3.424	3.435	3.445	3.453	3.461	3.468
60	2.829	2.976	3.073	3.143	3.198	3.241	3.277	3.307	3.333	3.355	3.374	3.391	3.406	3.419	3.431	3.441	3.451	3.460	3.468
80	2.814	2.961	3.059	3.130	3.185	3.229	3.266	3.297	3.323	3.346	3.366	3.384	3.400	3.414	3.427	3.438	3.449	3.458	3.467
120	2.800	2.947	3.045	3.116	3.172	3.217	3.254	3.286	3.313	3.337	3.358	3.377	3.394	3.409	3.423	3.435	3.446	3.457	3.466
240	2.786	2.933	3.031	3.103	3.159	3.205	3.243	3.276	3.304	3.329	3.350	3.370	3.388	3.404	3.418	3.432	3.444	3.455	3.466
∞	2.772	2.918	3.017	3.089	3.146	3.193	3.232	3.265	3.294	3.320	3.343	3.363	3.382	3.399	3.414	3.428	3.442	3.454	3.466

Number of means in the range (α = 0.05)

Note: For degrees of freedom for MS_E (v) = 1 and 2, for all ranges, table value is 17.969 and 6.085, respectively.

Source: http://cse.niaes.affrc.go.jp/miwa/probcalc/index.html

Duncan's significant studentized range values (*Contd.*)

Number of means in the range ($\alpha = 0.01$)

v	2	3	4	5	6	7	8	9	10	11	12	13	14	15	16	17	18	19	20
4	6.511	6.677	6.740	6.755	6.755	6.755	6.755	6.755	6.755	6.755	6.755	6.755	6.755	6.755	6.755	6.755	6.755	6.755	6.755
5	5.702	5.893	5.989	6.040	6.065	6.074	6.074	6.074	6.074	6.074	6.074	6.074	6.074	6.074	6.074	6.074	6.074	6.074	6.074
6	5.243	5.439	5.549	5.614	5.655	5.680	5.694	5.701	5.703	5.703	5.703	5.703	5.703	5.703	5.703	5.703	5.703	5.703	5.703
7	4.949	5.145	5.260	5.333	5.383	5.416	5.439	5.454	5.464	5.470	5.472	5.472	5.472	5.472	5.472	5.472	5.472	5.472	5.472
8	4.745	4.939	5.056	5.134	5.189	5.227	5.256	5.276	5.291	5.302	5.309	5.313	5.316	5.317	5.317	5.317	5.317	5.317	5.317
9	4.596	4.787	4.906	4.986	5.043	5.086	5.117	5.142	5.160	5.174	5.185	5.193	5.199	5.202	5.205	5.206	5.206	5.206	5.206
10	4.482	4.671	4.789	4.871	4.931	4.975	5.010	5.036	5.058	5.074	5.087	5.098	5.106	5.112	5.117	5.120	5.122	5.123	5.124
11	4.392	4.579	4.697	4.780	4.841	4.887	4.923	4.952	4.975	4.994	5.009	5.021	5.031	5.039	5.045	5.050	5.054	5.057	5.059
12	4.320	4.504	4.622	4.705	4.767	4.815	4.852	4.882	4.907	4.927	4.944	4.957	4.969	4.978	4.986	4.993	4.998	5.002	5.005
13	4.260	4.442	4.560	4.643	4.706	4.754	4.793	4.824	4.850	4.871	4.889	4.904	4.917	4.927	4.936	4.944	4.950	4.955	4.960
14	4.210	4.391	4.508	4.591	4.654	4.703	4.743	4.775	4.802	4.824	4.843	4.859	4.872	4.884	4.894	4.902	4.909	4.916	4.921
15	4.167	4.346	4.463	4.547	4.610	4.660	4.700	4.733	4.760	4.783	4.803	4.820	4.834	4.846	4.857	4.866	4.874	4.881	4.887
16	4.131	4.308	4.425	4.508	4.572	4.622	4.662	4.696	4.724	4.748	4.768	4.785	4.800	4.813	4.825	4.835	4.843	4.851	4.858
17	4.099	4.275	4.391	4.474	4.538	4.589	4.630	4.664	4.692	4.717	4.737	4.755	4.771	4.785	4.797	4.807	4.816	4.824	4.832
18	4.071	4.246	4.361	4.445	4.509	4.559	4.601	4.635	4.664	4.689	4.710	4.729	4.745	4.759	4.771	4.782	4.792	4.801	4.808
19	4.046	4.220	4.335	4.418	4.483	4.533	4.575	4.610	4.639	4.664	4.686	4.705	4.722	4.736	4.749	4.760	4.771	4.780	4.788
20	4.024	4.197	4.312	4.395	4.459	4.510	4.552	4.587	4.617	4.642	4.664	4.684	4.701	4.716	4.729	4.741	4.751	4.761	4.769
21	4.004	4.177	4.291	4.374	4.438	4.489	4.531	4.567	4.597	4.622	4.645	4.664	4.682	4.697	4.711	4.723	4.734	4.743	4.752
22	3.986	4.158	4.272	4.355	4.419	4.470	4.513	4.548	4.578	4.604	4.627	4.647	4.664	4.680	4.694	4.706	4.718	4.728	4.737
23	3.970	4.141	4.254	4.337	4.402	4.453	4.496	4.531	4.562	4.588	4.611	4.631	4.649	4.665	4.679	4.692	4.703	4.713	4.723
24	3.955	4.126	4.239	4.322	4.386	4.437	4.480	4.516	4.546	4.573	4.596	4.616	4.634	4.651	4.665	4.678	4.690	4.700	4.710
25	3.942	4.112	4.224	4.307	4.371	4.423	4.466	4.502	4.532	4.559	4.582	4.603	4.621	4.638	4.652	4.665	4.677	4.688	4.698
26	3.930	4.099	4.211	4.294	4.358	4.410	4.452	4.489	4.520	4.546	4.570	4.591	4.609	4.626	4.640	4.654	4.666	4.677	4.687
27	3.918	4.087	4.199	4.282	4.346	4.397	4.440	4.477	4.508	4.535	4.558	4.579	4.598	4.615	4.630	4.643	4.655	4.667	4.677

(*Contd.*)

Duncan's significant studentized range values (*Contd.*)

v										Number of means in the range (α = 0.01)									
	2	3	4	5	6	7	8	9	10	11	12	13	14	15	16	17	18	19	20
28	3.908	4.076	4.188	4.270	4.334	4.386	4.429	4.465	4.497	4.524	4.548	4.569	4.587	4.604	4.619	4.633	4.646	4.657	4.667
29	3.898	4.065	4.177	4.260	4.324	4.376	4.419	4.455	4.486	4.514	4.538	4.559	4.578	4.595	4.610	4.624	4.637	4.648	4.659
30	3.889	4.056	4.168	4.250	4.314	4.366	4.409	4.445	4.477	4.504	4.528	4.550	4.569	4.586	4.601	4.615	4.628	4.640	4.650
31	3.881	4.047	4.159	4.241	4.305	4.357	4.400	4.436	4.468	4.495	4.519	4.541	4.560	4.577	4.593	4.607	4.620	4.632	4.643
32	3.873	4.039	4.150	4.232	4.296	4.348	4.391	4.428	4.459	4.487	4.511	4.533	4.552	4.570	4.585	4.600	4.613	4.625	4.635
33	3.865	4.031	4.142	4.224	4.288	4.340	4.383	4.420	4.452	4.479	4.504	4.525	4.545	4.562	4.578	4.592	4.606	4.618	4.629
34	3.859	4.024	4.135	4.217	4.281	4.333	4.376	4.413	4.444	4.472	4.496	4.518	4.538	4.555	4.571	4.586	4.599	4.611	4.622
35	3.852	4.017	4.128	4.210	4.273	4.325	4.369	4.405	4.437	4.465	4.490	4.511	4.531	4.549	4.565	4.579	4.593	4.605	4.616
36	3.846	4.011	4.121	4.203	4.267	4.319	4.362	4.399	4.431	4.459	4.483	4.505	4.525	4.543	4.559	4.573	4.587	4.599	4.611
37	3.840	4.005	4.115	4.197	4.260	4.312	4.356	4.393	4.425	4.452	4.477	4.499	4.519	4.537	4.553	4.568	4.581	4.594	4.605
38	3.835	3.999	4.109	4.191	4.254	4.306	4.350	4.387	4.419	4.447	4.471	4.493	4.513	4.531	4.548	4.562	4.576	4.589	4.600
39	3.830	3.993	4.103	4.185	4.249	4.301	4.344	4.381	4.413	4.441	4.466	4.488	4.508	4.526	4.542	4.557	4.571	4.584	4.595
40	3.825	3.988	4.098	4.180	4.243	4.295	4.339	4.376	4.408	4.436	4.461	4.483	4.503	4.521	4.537	4.552	4.566	4.579	4.591
48	3.793	3.955	4.064	4.145	4.209	4.261	4.304	4.341	4.374	4.402	4.427	4.450	4.470	4.489	4.506	4.521	4.535	4.548	4.561
60	3.762	3.922	4.030	4.111	4.174	4.226	4.270	4.307	4.340	4.368	4.394	4.417	4.437	4.456	4.474	4.489	4.504	4.518	4.530
80	3.732	3.890	3.997	4.077	4.140	4.192	4.236	4.273	4.306	4.335	4.360	4.384	4.405	4.424	4.442	4.458	4.473	4.487	4.500
120	3.702	3.858	3.964	4.044	4.107	4.158	4.202	4.239	4.272	4.301	4.327	4.351	4.372	4.392	4.410	4.426	4.442	4.456	4.469
240	3.672	3.827	3.932	4.011	4.073	4.125	4.168	4.206	4.239	4.268	4.294	4.318	4.339	4.359	4.378	4.394	4.410	4.425	4.439
∞	3.643	3.796	3.900	3.978	4.040	4.091	4.135	4.172	4.205	4.235	4.261	4.285	4.307	4.327	4.345	4.363	4.379	4.394	4.408

Note: For degrees of freedom for MS_E (v) = 1, 2 and 3, for all ranges, table value is 90.024, 14.036 and 8.321, respectively.

Source: http://cse.niaes.affrc.go.jp/miwa/probcalc/index.html

APPENDIX 11

Kruskal-Wallis *H* distribution

n_1	n_2	n_3	$\alpha = 0.05$	$\alpha = 0.01$
3	2	2	4.714	–
3	3	1	5.142	–
3	3	2	5.361	–
3	3	3	5.6	7.2
4	2	2	5.333	–
4	3	1	5.208	–
4	3	2	5.444	6.444
4	3	3	5.727	6.746
4	4	1	4.967	6.667
4	4	2	5.455	7.036
4	4	3	5.599	7.144
4	4	4	5.692	7.654
5	2	1	5	–
5	2	2	5.16	6.533
5	3	1	4.96	–
5	3	2	5.251	6.909
5	3	3	5.649	7.079
5	4	1	4.986	6.955
5	4	2	5.273	7.118
5	4	3	5.631	7.445
5	4	4	5.618	7.76
5	5	1	5.127	7.309
5	5	2	5.339	7.269
5	5	3	5.706	7.543
5	5	4	5.643	7.791
5	5	5	5.78	7.98
6	2	1	4.822	–
6	2	2	5.345	6.982
6	3	1	4.855	–
6	3	2	5.348	6.970
6	3	3	5.615	7.410
6	4	1	4.947	7.106
6	4	2	5.340	7.340
6	4	3	5.610	7.500
6	4	4	5.681	7.795
6	5	1	4.990	7.182

(Contd.)

Kruskal-Wallis *H* distribution (*Contd.*)

n_1	n_2	n_3	$\alpha = 0.05$	$\alpha = 0.01$
6	5	2	5.338	7.376
6	5	3	5.602	7.590
6	5	4	5.661	7.936
6	5	5	5.729	8.028
6	6	1	4.945	7.121
6	6	2	5.410	7.467
6	6	3	5.625	7.725
6	6	4	5.724	8.000
6	6	5	5.765	8.124
6	6	6	5.801	8.222
7	7	7	5.819	8.387
8	8	8	5.805	8.465

Adapted from Zar, 2003

APPENDIX 12

SPC–Factors for control charts

n	A	A_2	D_1	D_2	D_3	D_4	A_3	B_3	B_4	d_2	c_4
2	2.121	1.880	0	3.686	0	3.267	2.659	0	3.267	1.128	0.7979
3	1.732	1.023	0	4.358	0	2.574	1.954	0	2.568	1.693	0.8862
4	1.500	0.729	0	4.698	0	2.282	1.628	0	2.266	2.059	0.9213
5	1.342	0.577	0	4.918	0	2.114	1.427	0	2.089	2.326	0.9400
6	1.225	0.483	0	5.078	0	2.004	1.287	0.030	1.970	2.534	0.9515
7	1.134	0.419	0.204	5.204	0.076	1.924	1.182	0.118	1.882	2.704	0.9594
8	1.061	0.373	0.388	5.306	0.136	1.864	1.099	0.185	1.815	2.847	0.9650
9	1.000	0.337	0.547	5.393	0.184	1.816	1.032	0.239	1.761	2.970	0.9693
10	0.949	0.308	0.687	5.469	0.223	1.777	0.975	0.284	1.716	3.078	0.9727
11	0.905	0.285	0.811	5.535	0.256	1.744	0.927	0.321	1.679	3.173	0.9754
12	0.866	0.266	0.922	5.594	0.283	1.717	0.886	0.354	1.646	3.258	0.9776
13	0.832	0.249	1.025	5.647	0.307	1.693	0.850	0.382	1.618	3.336	0.9794
14	0.802	0.235	1.118	5.696	0.328	1.672	0.817	0.406	1.594	3.407	0.9810
15	0.775	0.223	1.203	5.741	0.347	1.653	0.789	0.428	1.572	3.472	0.9823
16	0.750	0.212	1.282	5.782	0.363	1.637	0.763	0.448	1.552	3.532	0.9835
17	0.728	0.203	1.356	5.820	0.378	1.622	0.739	0.466	1.534	3.588	0.9845
18	0.0707	0.194	1.424	5.856	0.391	1.608	0.718	0.482	1.518	3.640	0.9854
19	0.688	0.187	1.487	5.891	0.403	1.597	0.698	0.497	1.503	3.689	0.9862
20	0.671	0.180	1.549	5.921	0.415	1.585	0.680	0.510	1.490	3.735	0.9869
21	0.655	0.173	1.605	5.951	0.425	1.575	0.663	0.523	1.477	3.778	0.9876
22	0.640	0.167	1.659	5.979	0.434	1.566	0.647	0.534	1.466	3.819	0.9882
23	0.626	0.162	1.710	6.006	0.443	1.557	0.633	0.545	1.455	3.858	0.9887
24	0.612	0.157	1.759	6.031	0.451	1.548	0.619	0.555	1.445	3.895	0.9892
25	0.600	0.153	1.806	6.056	0.459	1.541	0.606	0.565	1.435	3.931	0.9896

Factors for computing center line and three sigma limits

Source: Try Free eLearning module "Introduction to Statistics"

APPENDIX 13

Method of Three Selected Points

Let us consider fitting modified Exponential curve $y_t = a + bc^t$: In this method we must select the values of t, say t_1, t_2 and t_3 which are equally spaced; that means, $t_2 - t_1 = t_3 - t_2$. Now, by substituting t_1, t_2 and t_3 into the equation we get:

$$y_1 = a + bc^{t_1}$$

$$y_2 = a + bc^{t_2} \text{ and}$$

$$y_3 = a + bc^{t_2} \text{ ; hence } y_2 - y_1 = b\left(c^{t_2} - c^{t_1}\right) = bc^{t_1}\left(c^{t_2 - t_1} - 1\right); \text{similarly,}$$

$$y_3 - y_2 = b\left(c^{t_3} - c^{t_1}\right) = bc^{t_2}\left(c^{t_3 - t_1} - 1\right).$$

Since $t_2 - t_1 = t_3 - t_2$, $\dfrac{y_3 - y_2}{y_2 - y_1} = c^{(t_2 - t_1)}$; therefore, $c = \left[\dfrac{y_3 - y_2}{y_2 - y_1}\right]^{\left(\frac{1}{t_2 - t_1}\right)}$.

Substituting the value of c in $y_2 - y_1 = bc^{t_1}\left(c^{t_2 - t_1} - 1\right)$ we get

$$y_2 - y_1 = b\left[\dfrac{y_3 - y_2}{y_2 - y_1}\right]^{\frac{1}{(t_2 - t_1)}t_1}\left[\left(\dfrac{y_3 - y_2}{y_2 - y_1}\right)^{\frac{1}{(t_2 - t_1)}t_1} - 1\right].$$

This gets simplified to $y_2 - y_1 = b\left[\dfrac{y_3 - y_2}{y_2 - y_1}\right]^{\frac{t_1}{(t_2 - t_1)}}\left(\dfrac{y_3 - 2y_2 + y_1}{y_2 - y_1}\right)$. Rearranging the

terms we get $b = \dfrac{y_2 - y_1}{\left[\dfrac{y_3 - y_2}{y_2 - y_1}\right]^{\frac{t_1}{(t_2 - t_1)}}\left(\dfrac{y_3 - 2y_2 + y_1}{y_2 - y_1}\right)}$ which upon further rearrangement

condenses to $b = \dfrac{\left(y_2 - y_1\right)^2}{y_3 - 2y_2 + y_1}\left[\dfrac{y_2 - y_1}{y_3 - y_2}\right]^{\frac{t_1}{(t_2 - t_1)}}$. Finally, by rearranging $y_1 = a + bc^{t_1}$,

we get $a = y_1 - bc^{t_1}$ and substituting b and c in this equation, we get

$$a = y_1 - \left[\dfrac{\left(y_2 - y_1\right)^2}{y_3 - 2y_2 + y_1}\left[\dfrac{y_2 - y_1}{y_3 - y_2}\right]^{\frac{t_1}{(t_2 - t_1)}}\right]\left[\left[\dfrac{y_3 - y_2}{y_2 - y_1}\right]^{\frac{1}{(t_2 - t_1)}}\right];$$

then ; $a = y_1 - \left[\dfrac{(y_2 - y_1)^2}{y_3 - 2y_2 + y_1} \left[\dfrac{y_2 - y_1}{y_3 - y_2} \right]^{\frac{t_1}{(t_2 - t_1)}} \right] \left[\dfrac{1}{\left[\dfrac{y_2 - y_1}{y_3 - y_2} \right]^{\frac{1}{(t_2 - t_1)}}} \right]$; therefore, the equa-

tion simplifies to $a = y_1 - \left[\dfrac{(y_2 - y_1)^2}{y_3 - 2y_2 + y_1} \right]$ and on further simplification

$a = \dfrac{y_1 y_3 - y_2^2}{y_3 - 2y_2 + y_1}$ which is the computational formula for a.

APPENDIX 14

Method of Partial Sums

Let us consider fitting modified Exponential curve $y_t = a + bc^t$: In this method we must divide the number of observations into three equal parts containing (equal number of) n consecutive values of t and y; then the partial sums are $S_1 = \sum_{t=1}^{n} y_t, S_2 = \sum_{t=n+1}^{2n} y_t$

and $S_3 = \sum_{t=2n+1}^{3n} y_t$. Now, substituting $y_t = a + bc^t$ in S_1.

$$S_1 = \sum_{t=1}^{n} a + bc' = na + b\left(c + c^2 ... + c^n\right); \text{ or } S_1 = na + bc\left(\frac{c^n - 1}{c - 1}\right);$$

similarly, $S_2 = na + bc^{n+1}\left(\frac{c^n - 1}{c - 1}\right)$ and $S_3 = na + bc^{2n+1}\left(\frac{c^n - 1}{c - 1}\right)$.

Then, $S_2 - S_1 = bc^{n+1}\left(\frac{c^n - 1}{c - 1}\right) - bc\left(\frac{c^n - 1}{c - 1}\right)$; this cab $= n$ be simplified as

$$S_2 - S_1 = b\left(\frac{c^n - 1}{c - 1}\right)\left(c^{n+1} - c\right) \text{ and further to } S_2 - S_1 = bc\left(\frac{c^n - 1}{c - 1}\right).(c^n - 1)$$

or $S_2 - S_1 = bc\frac{\left(c^n - 1\right)^2}{c - 1}$; on the same lines it can be shown that $S_3 - S_2 = bc^{n+1}\frac{\left(c^n - 1\right)^2}{c - 1}$;

it is therefore obvious that $\frac{S_3 - S_2}{S_2 - S_1} = c^n$ or $c = \left(\frac{S_3 - S_2}{S_2 - S_1}\right)^{\frac{1}{n}}$; substituting this value in

$S_2 - S_1 = bc\frac{\left(c^n - 1\right)^2}{c - 1}$ and rearranging we get $b = \frac{(c - 1)(S_2 - S_1)^2}{c(S_3 - 2S_2 + S_1)}$ and finally

substituting for b and c in $S_1 = na + bc\left(\frac{c^n - 1}{c - 1}\right)$ and rearranging the terms we get

$a = \frac{1}{n}\left(\frac{S_1 S_3 - S_2^2}{S_3 - 2S_2 + S_1}\right)$. Similarities in the formulae with those of Method of three selected points can be noticed.

APPENDIX 15

Fitting Logistic Curve by Three Selected Points

Principle of Method of three selected points is essentially the same to the one used for modified Exponential curve (Appendix 13); but, the formula to which it is applied is different. Following are the derivations with respect to Logistic curve: $y_t = \dfrac{k}{1 + e^{a+bt}}$.

Three values of values of t, say t_1, t_2 and t_3 which are equally spaced are selected; that means, $t_2 - t_1 = t_3 - t_2$. Now, by substituting t_1, t_2 and t_3 into the equation we get:

$$y_t = \frac{k}{1 + e^{a+bt_1}}, \; y_t = \frac{k}{1 + e^{a+bt_2}} \text{ and } y_t = \frac{k}{1 + e^{a+bt_3}}. \text{ Taking Natural logarithm, we get}$$

$a + bt_1 = \ln\left(\dfrac{k}{y_1} - 1\right)$, $a + bt_2 = \ln\left(\dfrac{k}{y_2} - 1\right)$ and $a + bt_3 = \ln\left(\dfrac{k}{y_3} - 1\right)$, respectively; sub-

tracting the first from the second equation and second from the third equation, we get

$$b(t_2 - t_1) = \ln\left[\frac{\frac{k}{y_2} - 1}{\frac{k}{y_1} - 1}\right] \quad \text{and} \quad b(t_3 - t_2) = \ln\left[\frac{\frac{k}{y_3} - 1}{\frac{k}{y_2} - 1}\right]; \quad \text{since } t_2 - t_1 = t_3 - t_2,$$

$$\ln\left[\frac{\frac{k}{y_2} - 1}{\frac{k}{y_1} - 1}\right] = \ln\left[\frac{\frac{k}{y_3} - 1}{\frac{k}{y_2} - 1}\right]. \text{ Now, raising both sides to the power of } e \text{ (base of natural}$$

logarithm), and cross multiplying, we get $\left(\dfrac{k}{y_3} - 1\right)\left(\dfrac{k}{y_1} - 1\right) = \left(\dfrac{k}{y_2} - 1\right)$; on simpli-

fication, $\dfrac{(k - y_1)(k - y_3)}{y_1 y_3} = \left(\dfrac{k - y_2}{y_2}\right)^2$ or $y_2^2(k - y_1)(k - y_3) = y_1 y_3 (k - y_2)^2$. Segregating

terms containing k and that $k \neq 0$, and finally solving for k gives

$$k = \frac{y_2^2(y_1 + y_3) - 2y_1 y_2 y_3}{y_2^2 - y_1 y_3}.$$

Substitution of k in suitable equations gives $b = \dfrac{1}{t_2 - t_1} \ln\left[\dfrac{y_1(k - y_2)}{y_2(k - y_1)}\right]$ and

$a = \ln\left(\dfrac{k}{y_t} - 1\right) - bt_1.$

Index